Wohlbefinden und Gesundheit im Jugendalter

Andreas Heinen · Robin Samuel ·
Claus Vögele · Helmut Willems
(Hrsg.)

Wohlbefinden und Gesundheit im Jugendalter

Theoretische Perspektiven,
empirische Befunde
und Praxisansätze

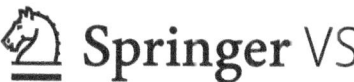 Springer VS

Hrsg.

Andreas Heinen
Fachbereich Sozialwissenschaften
Universität Luxemburg
Esch-sur-Alzette, Luxemburg

Robin Samuel
Fachbereich Sozialwissenschaften
Universität Luxemburg
Esch-sur-Alzette, Luxemburg

Claus Vögele
Fachbereich Verhaltens- und
Kognitionswissenschaften
Universität Luxemburg
Esch-sur-Alzette, Luxemburg

Helmut Willems
Fachbereich Verhaltens- und
Kognitionswissenschaften
Universität Luxemburg
Esch-sur-Alzette, Luxemburg

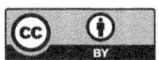

ISBN 978-3-658-35743-6   ISBN 978-3-658-35744-3   (eBook)
https://doi.org/10.1007/978-3-658-35744-3

Die Deutsche Nationalbibliothek verzeichnet diese Publikation in der Deutschen Nationalbibliografie; detaillierte bibliografische Daten sind im Internet über http://dnb.d-nb.de abrufbar.

Planung/Lektorat: Katrin Emmerich
Springer VS ist ein Imprint der eingetragenen Gesellschaft Springer Fachmedien Wiesbaden GmbH und ist ein Teil von Springer Nature.
Die Anschrift der Gesellschaft ist: Abraham-Lincoln-Str. 46, 65189 Wiesbaden, Germany

Inhaltsverzeichnis

Autorinnen- und Autorenverzeichnis

Aixa Aleman-Diaz, PhD fellow, Copenhagen Business School, Denmark. Research focus: Child and adolescent health, Policy, Governance, Innovation. E-Mail: aixa.aleman@gmail.com

Conchita D'Ambrosio, PhD, Professor of Economics at the Department of Behavioural and Cognitive Sciences, University of Luxembourg, Luxembourg. Main research interests: Income and Wealth Distributions, Individual Well-being, Social Exclusion and Economic Insecurity. E-Mail: conchita.dambrosio@uni.lu

Joël Billieux, Prof. Dr., Professor of Clinical Psychology, University of Lausanne, Switzerland. Research focus: Psychological factors (cognitive, affective, motivational, interpersonal) involved in the etiology of addictive behaviors. E-Mail: Joel.Billieux@unil.ch

Liyousew Borga, PhD, Research Associate at the Department of Behavioural and Cognitive Sciences, University of Luxembourg, Luxembourg. Main research interests: Child development, Intrahousehold allocation, Program evaluation, Poverty analysis. E-Mail: liyousew.borga@uni.lu

Matthias Böhmer, Dr., Diplompsychologe, Psychologischer Psychotherapeut, Research Scientist am Department of Behavioural and Cognitive Sciences der Universität Luxemburg. Forschung im Bereich der empirischen Bildungsforschung sowie zur REVT. E-Mail: matthias.boehmer@uni.lu

Damien Brevers, PhD, Professor at the Faculty of Psychology and Educational Sciences at UCLouvain, Belgium. Main research interests: the study of self-regulation processes involved in physical activity habits, addictions, and pro-ecological behaviours. E-Mail: damien.brevers@uclouvain.be

Andreas Bund, Prof. Dr., Associate Professor am Department of Education and Social Work der Universität Luxemburg, Luxemburg. Forschungsschwerpunkte: Körperliche Aktivität im Kindes- und Jugendalter, Sportunterricht, Motorische Entwicklung, Motorische Diagnostik. E-Mail: andreas.bund@uni.lu

Susanne Carai, MA, Consultant, Child and Adolescent Health. Area of work: WHO Regional office for Europe Child and adolescent health. E-Mail: carais@who.int

Jeanne Chomé, Psychologue diplomée, Psychothérapeute, im Ruhestand, ehemals Mitarbeiterin im Service Consultation Omega 90, Luxemburg.

Lisa Clees, Diplompsychologin, Psychotherapeutin für Kinder und Jugendliche in eigener Praxis, Mamer, Luxemburg. Arbeitsschwerpunkte: systemische Familientherapie, Psychotraumatherapie mit Kindern und Jugendlichen. E-Mail: lisa.clees@pt.lu

Alessandro Decarli, PhD, Clinical Psychologist at the Divison of Youth Psychiatry at the Centre Hospitalier Neuro-Psychiatrique (CHNP), Luxembourg and the Department of Clinical Psychology and Psychotherapy at the University of Trier, Germany; Former Research Associate at the Department of Cognitive and Behavioural Sciences at the University of Luxembourg, Luxembourg. Research focus: Developmental Psychopathology, Attachment, Mentalization. E-Mail: s1aldeca@uni-trier.de

Marco Deepen, Dipl.-Päd., M.A. Management und Coaching. Direktor, Luxemburgisches Rotes Kreuz, Bereich non-formale Bildung, Luxemburg. Arbeitsbereich: Mitglied des Direktionskomitees und Verantwortlicher für die Aktivitäten der non-formalen Bildung im Kinder- und Jugendbereich, u. a. Jugendhäuser, Kinderkrippen, Maisons Relais und weitere Jugendstrukturen. E-Mail: marco.deepen@croix-rouge.lu

Dina Dias, Dipl.-Psych., Psychotherapeutin bei Service Psy-Jeunes Croix-Rouge luxembourgeoise, Luxemburg. Arbeitsbereich: Psychotherapie von Jugendlichen und jungen Erwachsenen. E-Mail: Dina.dias@croix-rouge.lu

Elitsa Dimitrova, PhD, Associate Professor at the Institute for Population and Human Studies at the Bulgarian Academy of Sciences & Plovdiv University Paisii Hilendarski, Plovdiv, Bulgaria. Research focus: fertility and family studies, adolescent health behaviors, family policy, qualitative and quantitative research methods. E-Mail: e.dimitrova@iphs.eu

Melanie Eckelt, M.Sc., Doktorandin am Department of Education and Social Work an der Universität Luxemburg. Forschungsschwerpunkte: Körperliche Aktivität, Akzelerometrie, Sportunterricht. E-Mail: melanie.eckelt@uni.lu

Pascale Esch, Dr., Research Scientist at the LUCET, University of Luxembourg. Research focus: Coordination of the Luxembourg school monitoring programme „Épreuves Standardisées", educational pathways, neuro-cognitive abilities and educational performance. E-Mail: pascale.esch@uni.lu

Heike Eschenbeck, Prof. Dr., Professorin in der Abteilung Pädagogische Psychologie und Gesundheitspsychologie der Pädagogischen Hochschule Schwäbisch Gmünd, Deutschland. Forschungsschwerpunkte: Emotionen, Stress und Stressbewältigung, Prävention und Gesundheitsförderung bei Kindern und Jugendlichen. E-Mail: heike.eschenbeck@ph-gmuend.de

Antoine Fischbach, Prof. Dr., Head of LUCET & Associate Professor in Educational and Psychological Measurement at the University of Luxembourg. Research focus: Educational measurement, large-scale assessment, psychometrics, computer-based/assisted testing & learning. E-Mail: antoine.fischbach@uni.lu

Uwe C. Fischer, Dr. phil., Akademischer Oberrat am Institut für Psychologie der Otto-Friedrich-Universität Bamberg, Deutschland. Forschungsschwerpunkte: Gesundheitsförderung und Prävention, Gemeindepsychologie, Evaluation, Ästhetik, Lehre in Statistik und Forschungsmethoden. E-Mail: uwe.fischer@uni-bamberg.de

Barbara Gorges-Wagner, Dipl.-Päd., Direktionsbeauftragte des KJT (Kanner-Jugendtelefon), Luxemburg. E-Mail: bgorgeswagner@kjt.lu

Henri Grün, Psychologue diplomé. Arbeitsbereiche: Psychotherapeut in eigener Praxis, bis 2017 Direktor von Omega 90, Luxemburg. E-Mail: henri.gruen@pt.lu

Simone Grün, Diplom-Pädagogin mit Zusatzausbildungen als systemische Beraterin, Mediatorin, Suchtpräventionsbeauftragte, Sozialmanagerin, Personal Coach. Leiterin des „Centre Biergop" (Wohnstruktur für junge Erwachsene) und ehemalige Leiterin des DLJ (Daachverband vun de Lëtzebuerger Jugendstrukturen). Arbeitsbereiche: Sozialmanagement, Jugendarbeit, psychopädagogische Therapie. E-Mail: simone.gruen@biergop.lu

Anne-Catherine Guio, PhD, Senior Reseracher at LISER, Luxembourg. Research focus: material deprivation, poverty, social exclusion and well-being, social policies – applied to both the overall population and the specific situation of children, at the national and European levels. E-Mail: anne-catherine.guio@liser.lu

Andreas Hadjar, Prof. Dr. phil. habil., Ordentlicher Professor für Soziologie, Sozialpolitik und Sozialforschung an der Université de Fribourg, Schweiz & Professor für Bildungssoziologie an der Universität Luxemburg, Luxemburg. Forschungsschwerpunkte: Ungleichheiten nach sozialer Herkunft, Geschlecht und Migrationshintergrund; Bildungs- und Sozialsysteme; Werthaltungen/ Einstellungen; politische Partizipation; subjektives Wohlbefinden. E-Mail: andreas.hadjar@unifr.ch

Miriam-Linnea Hale, M.Sc., Doktorandin im Department of Behavioural and Cognitive Sciences der Universität Luxemburg. Forschungsschwerpunkte: Geschlechterstereotype, benevolenter und hostiler Sexismus in online Kontexten, Genderunterschiede und -stereotype bei der Nutzung sozialer Medien. E-Mail: miriam-linnea.hale@uni.lu

Viviane Hansen, B.A. Sozialpädagogik. Arbeitsbereiche: Direktionsbeauftragte des Centre Formida, Esch-sur-Alzette, Luxemburg. Leitung von stationären und teilstationären Einrichtungen des AEF Bereiches bei arcus. E-Mail: viviane.hansen@arcus.lu

Aline Hartz, Dipl.-Psych., Mitarbeiterin am Kanner-Jugendtelefon (KJT), Luxemburg. E-Mail: ahartz@kjt.lu

Andreas Heinen, Dipl.-Soz., Research and development specialist am Zentrum für Kindheits- und Jugendforschung an der Universität Luxemburg. Forschungsschwerpunkte: Jugendforschung, Jugendpolitikforschung, Jugendberichterstattung sowie Qualitative Forschungsmethoden. E-Mail: andreas.heinen@uni.lu

Martine Hentges, Psychologue diplomée, Psychothérapeute. Arbeitsbereich: Mitarbeiterin im Service Consultation, verantwortlich für den Kannerservice Omega 90, Luxemburg. E-Mail: MartineHentges@omega90.lu

Laura Hoffmann, Dr. phil., wissenschaftliche Mitarbeiterin an der Martin-Luther-Universität Halle-Wittenberg, Deutschland. Forschungsschwerpunkte: Medizin- und Gesundheitssoziologie, Suchtforschung, Kinder- und Jugendgesundheitsforschung, Qualitative Methoden der empirischen Sozialforschung, Versorgungsforschung. E-Mail: laura.hoffmann@medizin.uni-halle.de

Elisabeth Holl, M.Sc., Doktorandin im Department of Behavioural and Cognitive Sciences der Universität Luxemburg. Forschungsschwerpunkte: Moralisches Entscheidungsverhalten in Videospielen, Gaming-Motivation, Grundmechanismen und Effekte von Virtual Reality. E-Mail: elisabeth.holl@uni.lu

Djenna Hutmacher, Dr., Externe wissenschaftliche Mitarbeiterin des Fachbereichs Verhaltens- und Kognitionswissenschaften an der Universität Luxemburg. Forschungsschwerpunkte: Motivation, Gesundheitsförderung, Psychosomatik. E-Mail: djenna.hutmacher.001@student.uni.lu

Andreas Hück, Psychologue diplomé, Psychothérapeute. Arbeitsbereich: Responsable Service Consultation Omega 90, Luxemburg. E-Mail: AndreasHueck@omega90.lu

Ulrich Keller, Dipl.-Psych., Research and Development Specialist at the University of Luxembourg. Research focus: Educational assessment, Psychometrics, Determinants of educational success. E-Mail: ulrich.keller@uni.lu

Yvonne Kelly, FhD, Professor of Lifecourse Epidemiology at the University College London, United Kingdom. Research focus: Causes and consequences of socioeconomic and ethnic inequalities in health, influence of digital technologies for healthy development including physical and mental health in children and young people. E-Mail: y.kelly@ucl.ac.uk

Claude Kohll, Dipl. Heilpädagogin. Arbeitsbereich: Direktionsbeauftragte Centre Movida, Fouhren/Luxemburg. E-Mail: claude.kohll@arcus.lu

Tatyana Kotzeva, PhD, Professor at the Institute for Population and Human Studies at the Bulgarian Academy of Sciences & Burgas Free University, Burgas, Bulgaria. Research focus: family studies, family policy, adolescent risk behaviors, gender studies, women's health. E-Mail: t.kotzeva@iphs.eu

Andreas König, Dr. phil., Chargé de Direction, Zenter fir exzessiivt Verhalen an Verhalenssucht, Luxemburg. Arbeitsschwerpunkte: Prävention, Beratung und Therapie bei exzessiven und süchtigem Verhalten (Schwerpunkt digitale Medien und Glücksspiel). E-Mail: akoenig@zev.lu

Caroll Kremer, MA Pädagogik, Direktionsbeauftragte DLJ asbl, Luxemburg. Arbeitsbereich: Direktion, Koordination, Personalmanagement, Organisationsberatung, Projektmanagement, Netzwerkarbeit, Öffentlichkeitsarbeit, Offene Jugendarbeit, Weiterbildungsangebote. E-Mail: caroll.kremer@dlj.lu

Anthony Lepinteur, PhD, Scientific Researcher at the Department of Behavioural and Cognitive Sciences, University of Luxembourg, Luxembourg. Main research interests: Economic Insecurity, Individual Well-being, Program Evaluation, Working Time. E-Mail: anthony.lepinteur@uni.lu

Arnold Lohaus, Prof. Dr., Professor für Entwicklungspsychologie und Entwicklungspsychopathologie an der Universität Bielefeld, Deutschland. Forschungsschwerpunkte: Gesundheitsförderung im Kindes- und Jugendalter; Emotionsregulation und Stressbewältigung bei Kindern und Jugendlichen. E-Mail: arnold.lohaus@uni-bielefeld.de

Annika P. C. Lutz, Dr., Research Scientist at the University of Luxembourg. Research focus: Eating disorders, Body image, Interoception, Self-regulation, Electroencephalography/Event-Related Potentials. E-Mail: annika.lutz@uni.lu

Jérôme Mailliet, MA Pädagogik, Direktionsassistent DLJ asbl, Luxemburg. Arbeitsbereich: Offene Jugendarbeit, Projektmanagement, Organisationsberatung, Netzwerkarbeit, Öffentlichkeitsarbeit, Weiterbildungsangebote. E-Mail: jerome.mailliet@dlj.lu

André Melzer, Prof. Dr. rer. nat., Assistant Professor in Psychology; Studiendirektor Bachelor of Science in Psychology an der Universität Luxemburg. Forschungsschwerpunkte: Die Nutzung und Auswirkungen interaktiver Medien (z. B. Videospiele), die Beziehung zwischen Geschlechterstereotypen und Mediennutzung, sowie die Nutzung des Internets durch Kinder und Jugendliche. E-Mail: andre.melzer@uni.lu

Thérèse Michaelis, Dipl.-Psych., ehemalige Direktorin des CePT (Centre de Prévention des Toxicomanies), Luxemburg. Arbeitsbereiche: Schulpsychologie, Suchtprävention, Psychotherapie, Ethik im Bereich Psychologie, Kinder- und Jugendbereich.

Irene Moor, Dr. PH, wissenschaftliche Mitarbeiterin an der Martin-Luther-Universität Halle-Wittenberg, Deutschland. Forschungsschwerpunkte: Soziale Determinanten von Gesundheit und Krankheit, soziale Ungleichheit und Gesundheit, Kinder- und Jugendgesundheitsforschung, Prävention & Gesundheitsförderung in der Schule. E-Mail: irene.moor@medizin.uni-halle.de

Frederick de Moll, Dr. phil., Assistant Postdoktorant am Institute of Education and Society des Department of Social Sciences der Universität Luxemburg. Forschungsschwerpunkte: Bildungsungleichheit, Familie, Kindheit, Gesellschafts- und Ungleichheitstheorie, subjektives Wohlbefinden. E-Mail: frederick.demoll@uni.lu

Solveig Nicolas, Psychologue diplomée, Psychothérapeute. Arbeitsbereiche: Mitarbeiterin im Service Consultation und im Kannerservice Omega 90, Luxemburg. E-Mail: SolveigNicolas@omega90.lu

Jean-Paul Nilles, Dr. phil., ehemals selbständiger Kommunikationspädagoge, Lehrbeauftragter an den Universitäten Wien, Graz und Luxemburg sowie Direktor im CePT (Centre de Prévention des Toxicomanies). Arbeitsbereiche: Beratung, Supervision, Seminar- und Lehrtätigkeit in den Settings Schule, Universität, Sozialorganisationen, Wirtschaft zu den Schwerpunktthemen Kommunikation, betriebliche Gesundheitsförderung und Suchtprävention.

Meinolf Noeker, Prof. Dr., Psychologischer Psychotherapeut für Kinder und Jugendliche sowie Erwachsene; Dezernent für Krankenhäuser und Gesundheitswesen (Landesrat) für den LWL-PsychiatrieVerbund des Landschaftsverbandes Westfalen-Lippe, Deutschland. Forschungsschwerpunkte: Psychiatrische Versorgungsforschung und Versorgungspolitik; Funktionelle und somatoforme Störungen; Adaptation und klinisch-psychologische Intervention bei chronisch-somatischer Erkrankung; Konversionsstörungen; Gesundheitspsychologie und Verhaltensmedizin. E-Mail: meinolf.noeker@googlemail.com

Alain Origer, PhD, National Drug Coordinator at the Ministry of Health, Luxembourg. Research focus: Substance use, Addiction, Drug demand and harm reduction, Drug markets, New psychoactive substances, Social medicine, Epidemiology, Drug related infections diseases, Social determinants and inequalities. E-Mail: alain.origer@ms.etat.lu

Nabila Özen, M.A. Klinische Sozialarbeit. Arbeitsbereich: Mitarbeiterin des Dienstes „assistance en famille" bei arcus, Luxemburg. E-Mail: nabila.oezen@arcus.lu

Gudrun Paulsen, Psychologue diplomée, Psychothérapeute. Arbeitsbereiche: Mitarbeiterin im Service Consultation und im Kannerservice Omega 90, Luxemburg. E-Mail: GudrunPaulsen@omega90.lu

Blaise Pierrehumbert, PhD, Former Head of the Research Unit of the Service Universitaire de Psychiatrie de l'Enfant et de l'Adolescent (SUPA) at the University of Lausanne, Switzerland Research focus: Developmental Psychopathology, Attachment, Emotion Regulation, Stress Reactions, Trauma, Hyperactivity, Substance Abuse, Perinatal Problems, Parenting, Prematurity. E-Mail: blapier@gmail.com

Ineke M. Pit-ten Cate, Dr., Research Scientist in the Luxembourg Centre for Educational Testing (LUCET) at the University of Luxembourg. Research focus: Child development, inclusive education, special education, teacher decision making, family adjustment to chronic illness and physical disability, social cognition, psychodiagnostic assessment, test construction. E-Mail: ineke.pit@uni.lu

Cathy Reuter, Dipl.-Psych., Mitarbeiterin am Kanner-Jugendtelefon (KJT), Luxemburg. E-Mail: creuter@kjt.lu

Matthias Richter, Prof. Dr., Universitätsprofessor an der Martin-Luther-Universität Halle-Wittenberg, Deutschland. Forschungsschwerpunkte: Soziale Determinanten von Gesundheit und Krankheit, soziale Ungleichheit und Gesundheit über den Lebenslauf, vergleichende Kinder- und Jugendgesundheitsforschung, Prävention und Versorgungsforschung. E-Mail: m.richter@medizin.uni-halle.de

Katariina Salmela-Aro, PhD, Academy Professor at the University of Helsinki, Finland. Research focus: academic wellbeing, longitudinal studies, socioemotional skills, motivation, burnout, engagement, digital skills, young people. E-Mail: katariin.salmela-ari@helsinki.fi

Robin Samuel, Prof. Dr., Soziologe, Professor für Jugendforschung und Leiter des Zentrums für Kindheits- und Jugendforschung an der Universität Luxemburg. Forschungsschwerpunkte: Wohlbefinden, Gesundheit, Soziale Ungleichheit, Nachhaltigkeit und Forschungsmethoden. E-Mail: robin.samuel@uni.lu

René Schmit, Dipl.-Psych., Psychotherapeut, von 2003 bis 2017 Leiter der Staatlichen Kinderheime (heute: Institut étatique d'aide à l'enfance et à la famille / AITIA), Luxemburg. E-Mail: rene.schmit@education.lu

André Schulz, Dr., Assistant Professor in Psychology at the Department of Behavioural and Cognitive Sciences and Head of the Clinical Psychophysiology Laboratory (CLIPSLAB) at the University of Luxembourg, Luxembourg. Research focus: Interception, Psychobiology of Stress, Mental Disorders associated with Physical Symptoms, Mental Health in Chronic Conditions, Psychophysiological Research Methods. E-Mail: andre.schulz@uni.lu

Eileen Scott, Dr., Principal Public Health Intelligence Adviser, Public Health Scotland. Research focus: Child and Adolescent Health, Public health. E- Mail: eileen.scott1@phs.scot

Philipp E. Sischka, Dr., Research Scientist am Fachbereich für Verhaltens- und Kognitionswissenschaften an der Universität Luxemburg. Forschungsschwerpunkte: Qualität des Arbeitslebens und psychosoziale Arbeitsbedingungen, Ursachen und Konsequenzen von Arbeitsplatzaggression, Fragebogenentwicklung und -testung, Modellierung von latenten Variablen (z. B. Strukturgleichungsmodelle, Item Response Theorie, Mischverteilungsmodelle), Online-Survey-Forschung. E-Mail: philipp.sischka@uni.lu

Georges Steffgen, Prof. Dr., Professor für Psychologie am Fachbereich Verhaltens- und Kognitionswissenschaften an der Universität Luxemburg. Forschungsschwerpunkte: Aggression, Ärger, Emotionsregulation, (cyber) bullying, Gesundheitsförderung. E-Mail: georges.steffgen@uni.lu

Sally Stephany, Dipl.-Psych., Mitarbeiterin am Kanner-Jugendtelefon (KJT), Luxemburg. E-Mail: sstephany@kjt.lu

Zoé van Dyck, Dr., Research Scientist at the University of Luxembourg. Research focus: Interoceptive processes in eating disorders, Attentional processing of food cues, Food decision-making and overeating, Psychophysiological research methods. E-Mail: zoe.vandyck@uni.lu

Claus Vögele, Prof. Dr., Professor of Clinical and Health Psychology, Head of Department, Department of Behavioural and Cognitive Sciences, University of Luxembourg. Reserch interests: interoception, eating disorders, chronic pain, nudging and boosting, and eHealth. E-Mail: claus.voegele@uni.lu

Martin W. Weber, Dr., Programme Manager, Child and Adolescent Health. Area of work: WHO Regional office for Europe. Child and adolescent health. E-Mail: weberm@who.int

Christiane Weintzen, Dipl.-Psych., Kinder- und Jugendpsychotherapeutin und Chargée de Direction vom Service Psy-Jeunes Croix-Rouge luxembourgeoise, Luxemburg. Arbeitsbereich: Psychotherapie von Säuglingen, Kleinkindern, Kindern, Jugendlichen und jungen Erwachsenen. E-Mail: Christiane weintzen@croix-rouge.lu

Ross Whitehead, Dr., Public Health Intelligence Adviser, Public Health Scotland. Research focus: Public Mental Health, Child and Adolescent Health. E-Mail: ross.whitehead1@phs.scot

Helmut Willems, Prof. Dr. phil. habil., Soziologe, Professor für Soziologie an der Universität Luxemburg. Forschungsschwerpunkte: Jugendforschung, Migrationsforschung, Gewalt- und Konfliktforschung. E-Mail: helmut.willems@uni.lu

Manuela Woll, Dipl.-Psych., Psychologische Psychotherapeutin bei Service Psy-Jeunes Croix-Rouge luxembourgeoise, Luxemburg. Arbeitsbereich: Psychotherapie von Jugendlichen und jungen Erwachsenen. E-Mail: Manuela.woll@croix-rouge.lu

Rachel Wollschläger, Dr., Postdoctoral Researcher at LUCET, University of Luxembourg. Research focus: Coordination of the Test Development and Large Scale Statistics Laboratories in the frame of the Luxembourg school monitoring programme „Épreuves Standardisées", Academic achievement (assessment, development, and stability), Psychological and educational assessment, Specific learning disorders. E-Mail: rachel.wollschlaeger@uni.lu

Malou Zeyen, Dipl.-Psych., Psychotherapeutin bei Service Psy-Jeunes Croix-Rouge luxembourgeoise, Luxemburg. Arbeitsbereich: Psychotherapie von Kindern, Jugendlichen und jungen Erwachsenen. E-Mail: Malou.zeyen@croix-rouge.lu

Einleitung

Andreas Heinen, Robin Samuel, Claus Vögele
und Helmut Willems

Wohlbefinden und Gesundheit im Kindheits- und Jugendalter haben in den vergangenen Jahren in der sozialwissenschaftlichen Forschung an Bedeutung
gewonnen. Im Vordergrund steht dabei vor allem die Erforschung der
Bedingungsfaktoren für die Entwicklung eines „guten" Wohlbefindens und einer
„guten" Gesundheit bei Kindern und Jugendlichen. Die verschiedenen Fach-
disziplinen beschäftigen sich mit Fragen zu Wohlbefinden und Gesundheit von
Jugendlichen aus ihrer jeweiligen Perspektive. Psychologische Ansätze richten
den Fokus insbesondere auf persönliche Faktoren und individuelle Prozesse
(Abraham et al. 2016). Soziologische Ansätze konzentrieren sich stärker auf
die sozialen Faktoren und die Mechanismen der Entstehung ungleicher Ausprägungen von Wohlbefinden und Gesundheit (Hurrelmann und Richter 2013).
Bei den ökonomischen Ansätzen wiederum stehen wirtschaftliche Erklärungs-
faktoren für Gesundheit und Wohlbefinden im Mittelpunkt, wobei zunehmend
auch nicht-monetäre Faktoren an Bedeutung gewinnen (D'Ambrosio 2018).

A. Heinen (✉) · R. Samuel
Fachbereich Sozialwissenschaften, Universität Luxemburg, Esch-sur-Alzette,
Luxemburg
E-Mail: andreas.heinen@uni.lu

R. Samuel
E-Mail: robin.samuel@uni.lu

C. Vögele · H. Willems
Fachbereich Verhaltens- und Kognitionswissenschaften, Universität Luxemburg,
Esch-sur-Alzette, Luxemburg
E-Mail: claus.voegele@uni.lu

H. Willems
E-Mail: helmut.willems@uni.lu

Die Bedeutung der Thematik zeigt sich im mittlerweile beachtlichen Umfang der vorliegenden Forschung. Hervorzuheben ist unter anderem die internationale Kinder- und Jugendgesundheitsstudie „Health Behaviour in School-aged Children" (HBSC) (Inchley et al. 2020). Sie liefert mit ihrer langfristig und international ausgerichteten Datenerhebung eine umfassende Grundlage zum Gesundheitszustand und gesundheitsrelevanten Verhalten von Kindern und Jugendlichen in weit über 40 Ländern. In der Literatur gibt es eine Reihe von Überblicksarbeiten zu Wohlbefinden und Gesundheit von Kindern und Jugendlichen; zum Beispiel das „Handbook of Child Well-Being" (Ben-Arieh et al. 2014), die Schriftenreihe „Children's Well-Being: Indicators and Research" (Ben-Arieh 2010–2021) und „The Mental Health and Well-being of Children and Adolescents" (Hornby 2019–2021). Diese Beiträge beschäftigen sich vor allem mit dem Kindesalter. Es liegen aber auch einige Beiträge vor, die den Fokus stärker auf das Jugend- und junge Erwachsenenalter legen; so etwa das „International Handbook on Adolescent Health and Development" (Cherry et al. 2017), das „Handbook of Adolescent Health Psychology" (O'Donohue et al. 2013), der Band „Psychological, Educational, and Sociological Perspectives on Success and Well-Being in Career Development" (Keller et al. 2014) und der Band „Adolescent Health and Wellbeing" (Pingitore et al. 2019).

In der Forschung zu Wohlbefinden und Gesundheit von Jugendlichen lassen sich drei große Entwicklungslinien identifizieren. Erstens: Die Konzepte Wohlbefinden und Gesundheit werden umfassend verstanden und beschränken sich nicht auf die körperliche Dimension. Sie beschreiben nicht nur die Abwesenheit einer (diagnostizierten) körperlichen Krankheit, sondern berücksichtigen auch die psychologische und soziale Dimension von Wohlbefinden und Gesundheit. Zweitens: Bei der Erforschung von Wohlbefinden und Gesundheit steht die subjektive Sicht der Betroffenen verstärkt im Vordergrund. Jugendliche werden zu ihrem Wohlbefinden und ihrem Gesundheitsempfinden befragt. „Objektive", medizinisch diagnostizierte Krankheiten geben zwar Aufschluss über den Gesundheitszustand von Jugendlichen, werden aber um die subjektive Perspektive erweitert. Dahinter steht die Überlegung, dass die eigene Wahrnehmung und die individuelle Einschätzung der eigenen Befindlichkeit von zentraler Bedeutung ist und ein gutes Maß für die Lebensqualität und die weitere Entwicklung von Wohlbefinden und Gesundheit darstellen. Drittens: Die Forschung zu Wohlbefinden und Gesundheit richtet den Blick nicht nur auf Probleme oder Defizite, sondern zunehmend auch auf die Gesundheitsressourcen und -kompetenzen von Jugendlichen. In diesem Zusammenhang geht es etwa um die Frage, welche Handlungsmöglichkeiten Jugendlichen zur Verfügung stehen („Capabilities") um Wohlbefinden oder Gesundheit zu erhalten bzw. zu verbessern, beispielsweise Sport und Bewegung (Vögele 2019) und die Nutzung digitaler Medien (Domin et al. 2021). Der vorliegende Herausgeberband greift diese Entwicklungslinien auf.

Die Idee zu dem Band ist bei den Vorbereitungen zur Erstellung des Nationalen Berichtes zur Situation der Jugend in Luxemburg 2020 (Samuel und Willems 2021) entstanden. Dieser Bericht präsentiert vor allem luxemburgische Befunde zu Wohlbefinden und Gesundheit von Jugendlichen. Ergänzend zu diesem Jugendbericht bietet der vorliegende Band Fachbeiträge mit einer internationalen Perspektive auf Wohlbefinden und Gesundheit.

Die Beiträge bilden ein breites thematisches Spektrum ab. Neben theoretischen Beiträgen finden sich auch empirische Überblicks- und Originalarbeiten sowie Beiträge aus gesundheitsrelevanten Praxisfeldern in Luxemburg. Der Band spiegelt den vielfältigen Forschungsstand und den mitunter kontroversen Diskurs zu Wohlbefinden und Gesundheit von Jugendlichen wider. Er stellt kein systematisches Überblickswerk dar und erhebt nicht den Anspruch auf Repräsentativität oder Vollständigkeit. Die Beiträge sollen vielmehr Anregung geben für die Diskussion über die vielschichtigen Aspekte sowie die aktuellen und zukünftigen Herausforderungen im Zusammenhang mit Wohlbefinden und Gesundheit von Jugendlichen.

Der Band untergliedert sich in insgesamt fünf Teile.

Die Beiträge im ersten Teil *Wohlbefinden und Gesundheit: Theoretische Perspektiven* präsentieren zentrale theoretische Konzepte und disziplinäre Perspektiven aus Psychologie, Soziologie und Ökonomie. Die Beiträge im zweiten Teil *Wohlbefinden und Gesundheit in jugendlichen Lebenswelten* diskutieren Forschungsbefunde zu Wohlbefinden und Gesundheit von Jugendlichen in verschiedenen jugendrelevanten Lebensbereichen wie der Familie, der Schule, der Arbeitswelt sowie den Strukturen der Fremdunterbringung. Im dritten Teil *Jugendliches Handeln als Ressource oder Risiko für Wohlbefinden und Gesundheit* liegt der Schwerpunkt der Beiträge auf den gesundheitsrelevanten Handlungen der Jugendlichen. Dabei werden unterschiedliche thematische Schwerpunkte gesetzt. Diese betreffen Themen wie Ernährung, Bewegungsverhalten und Substanzkonsum, Mediennutzung, Spielsucht und Mobbing. Die Beiträge beschreiben die damit verbundenen Probleme und Risiken, diskutieren aber auch die Frage, inwieweit jugendliches Handeln eine Ressource für Wohlbefinden und Gesundheit darstellen kann. Die Beiträge im vierten Teil *Praxisansätze zur Förderung von Wohlbefinden und Gesundheit in Luxemburg* widmen sich verschiedenen gesundheitsrelevanten Praxisfeldern in Luxemburg. Auf der Grundlage von Praxisberichten und Erfahrungswissen von Fachexperten zeigen die Beiträge auf, mit welchen Angeboten, Konzepten und Methoden in den verschiedenen Praxisfelder das Wohlbefinden und die Gesundheit der Jugendlichen gefördert werden. Darüber hinaus reflektieren die Beiträge die gegenwärtigen Problemlagen und Herausforderungen von Jugendlichen im Zusammenhang mit ihrem Wohlbefinden und ihrer Gesundheit. Die Beiträge im fünften Teil *Internationale Befunde und Policy-Ansätze* richten den Blick auf empirische Befunde zu Wohlbefinden und Gesundheit von Jugendlichen mit dem Fokus auf ausgewählten europäischen Ländern und Policy-Ansätzen.

Wir bedanken uns bei den Autorinnen und Autoren dieses Bandes für die konstruktive Zusammenarbeit. Ohne deren Arbeit und Geduld hätte dieser Band nicht realisiert werden können. Unser Dank gilt auch Frau Simone Charles für ihre gewohnt zuverlässige und engagierte Unterstützung bei der Vorbereitung des Bandes. Danken möchten wir außerdem der studentischen Mitarbeiterin Marielle Baumgarten für ihre wertvolle Mithilfe.

Wir hoffen, dass der Band Fachleuten aus Forschung, Lehre und Praxis eine Anregung gibt, sich mit dem Thema Wohlbefinden und Gesundheit von Jugendlichen kritisch und konstruktiv auseinanderzusetzen. Die Beiträge sollen Ausgangspunkt für Diskussionen und Reflexionen sein, aber auch Anknüpfungspunkt für weiterführende Forschung.

Introduction

The topics of well-being and health in childhood and adolescence have gained importance in social science research in recent years. The main focus is on the investigation of the factors that contribute to the development of well-being and "good" health in children and adolescents. Disciplines focusing on questions of the well-being and health of adolescents do so from their respective perspectives. Psychological studies tend to focus on personal factors and individual processes (Abraham et al. 2016), while sociological approaches concentrate more on social factors and the mechanisms of the emergence of unequal outcomes of well-being and health (Hurrelmann und Richter 2013). In contrast to Psychology and Sociology, research carried out within the discipline of Economics explores economic factors important for health and well-being, with non-monetary factors gaining in importance (D'Ambrosio 2018).

The increasing importance of the topic of health and well-being in adolescence is reflected in the considerable volume of available research. The international child and youth health study "Health Behaviour in School-aged Children" (HBSC) (Inchley et al. 2020) is an exemplar. With its long-term and cross-country data collection, this international project provides a comprehensive data set of the health status and health-relevant behaviours of children and adolescents in more than 40 countries. There are a number of overviews of child and adolescent well-being and health in the literature; for example, the "Handbook of Child Well-Being" (Ben-Arieh et al. 2014), the "Children's Well-Being: Indicators and Research series" (Ben-Arieh 2010–2021) and "The Mental Health and Well-being of Children and Adolescents" (Hornby 2019–2021). These contributions mainly concern childhood. There are also some volumes that focus more on adolescence and young adulthood; for example, the "International Handbook on Adolescent Health and Development" (Cherry et al. 2017), the "Handbook of Adolescent Health Psychology" (O'Donohue et al. 2013), "Psychological, Educational, and Sociological Perspectives on Success and Well-Being in Career Development" (Keller et al. 2014) and "Adolescent Health and Wellbeing" (Pingitore et al. 2019).

Three major trends can be identified in research on well-being and health in adolescence. Firstly, the concepts of well-being and health are used comprehensively, and are not limited to the physical dimension. They not only describe the absence of a (diagnosed) physical illness, but also take into account the psychological and social dimensions of well-being and health. Secondly, research into well-being and health increasingly focuses on the view of those affected. Young people are asked about their well-being and their perception of health. Medical assessments may provide objectifiable information on the health status of young people, but these are increasingly expanded to include people's perceptions. The reason for this is that one's own perceptions and self-rated health have been shown to be related to mortality, and that self-assessments of health are the best predictors of quality of life and future well-being and health. Thirdly, research on well-being and health does not only focus on problems or deficits, but also takes health resources and competences of young people into account. For example, this concerns the possibilities for action that are available to young people ("capabilities") to maintain or improve their well-being and health, for example sport and exercise (Vögele 2019) and the use of digital media (Domin et al. 2021). This edited volume takes up these developments.

The idea for the present volume arose during the preparations for the National Report on the Situation of Youth in Luxembourg 2020 (Samuel und Willems 2021). This report presents mainly Luxembourgish findings on the well-being and health of young people. Complementary to this youth report, the present volume offers expert contributions with an international perspective on well-being and health.

The contributions cover a broad thematic spectrum. In addition to theoretical contributions, there are also empirical overviews and original works as well as contributions from health-relevant fields of practice in Luxembourg. The volume reflects the diverse state of research and the sometimes-controversial discourse on the well-being and health of young people. It is not a systematic overview and does not claim to be representative or complete. Rather, the contributions are intended to stimulate discussion on the multi-layered aspects as well as the current and future challenges related to the well-being and health of adolescents. The volume is divided into five parts.

The contributions in the first part, *Well-being and Health: Theoretical Perspectives,* present central theoretical concepts and disciplinary perspectives from Psychology, Sociology and Economics. The contributions in the second part, *Well-being and health in youth life environments,* discuss research findings on the well-being and health of adolescents in various life areas relevant to adolescents, such as the family, school, the world of work and the structures of foster care. In the third part, *Youth action as a resource or risk for well-being and health,* the focus of the contributions is on the health-relevant actions of young people. Different thematic focuses are set. These concern topics such as nutrition, physical activity and substance use, media use, gambling addiction and bullying. The contributions describe the associated problems and risks, but also discuss the question of the extent to which youth actions can be a resource for well-being and health. The contributions in the fourth part, *Practical approaches to promoting well-being and health in Luxembourg,* are dedicated to various health-relevant fields of practice in Luxembourg. On the basis of practical reports and the experience of experts, the contributions show which offers, concepts and methods are used to promote the well-being and health of young people in the various fields of practice. In addition, the contributions reflect on the current problems and challenges of young people in connection with their well-being and health. The contributions in the fifth part, *International findings and policy approaches,* focus on empirical findings on the well-being and health of young people with a focus on selected European countries and policy approaches.

We would like to thank the authors of this volume for their constructive collaboration. Without their work and patience, this volume could not have been realised. We would also like to thank Ms Simone Charles for her usual reliable and committed support in the preparation of the volume. We are also grateful for the valuable assistance provided by the student assistant Marielle Baumgarten.

We hope that the volume will provide professionals from research, teaching and practice with ideas to engage critically and constructively with the topic of young people's well-being and health. We would hope for the contributions in the present volume to stimulate discussion and reflection, but to also serve as a starting point for further research.

Literature

Abraham, C., Conner, M., Jones, F. & O'Connor, D. (2016). Health Psychology (2nd ed.). Topics in Applied Psychology: Routledge.

Ben-Arieh, A. (Ed.) (2010–2021). Children's Well-Being: Indicators and Research Series (Children's Well-Being: Indicators and Research Series).

Ben-Arieh, A., Casas, F., Frønes, I. & Korbin, J. E. (Eds.) (2014). Handbook of child well-being. Theories, methods and policies in global perspective. Dordrecht: Springer Netherlands.

Cherry, A. L., Baltag, V. & Dillon, M. E. (Eds.) (2017). International Handbook on Adolescent Health and Development. The Public Health Response. Cham, s.l.: Springer International Publishing

D'Ambrosio, C. (Ed.) (2018). Handbook of research on economic and social well-being. Cheltenham, UK, Northampton, MA, USA: Edward Elgar Publishing.

Domin, A., Spruijt-Metz, D., Theisen, D., Ouzzahra, Y. & Vögele, C. (2021). Smartphone-based interventions for physical activity promotion: scoping review of the evidence over the last 10-years. Journal of Medical Internet Research mHealth and uHealth, 9(7), e24308. doi: https://doi.org/10.2196/24308.

Hurrelmann, K., & Richter, M. (Hrsg.) (2013). Grundlagentexte Soziologie. Gesundheits- und Medizinsoziologie: Eine Einführung in sozialwissenschaftliche Gesundheitsforschung (8., überarb. Aufl.). Weinheim: Beltz Juventa.

Hornby, G. (Ed.) (2019–2021). The Mental Health and Well-being of Children and Adolescents: Routledge.

Inchley, J., Currie, D, Budisavljevic, S., Torsheim, T., Jåstad, A. & Cosma, A. (2020). Spotlight on adolescent health and well-being. Findings from the 2017/2018 Health Behaviour in School-aged Children (HBSC) survey in Europe and Canada. International report. Volume 1. Key findings. Copenhagen. WHO Regional Office for Europe.

Keller, A. C., Samuel, R., Bergman, M. M. & Semmer, N. K. (Eds.) (2014). Psychological, Educational, and Sociological Perspectives on Success and Well-Being in Career Development. Dordrecht, s.l.: Springer Netherlands.

O'Donohue, W. T., Benuto, L. T. & Woodward Tolle, L. (2013). Handbook of Adolescent Health Psychology. New York, NY: Springer

Pingitore, A., Mastorci, F. & Vassalle, C. (2019). Adolescent Health and Wellbeing. Current Strategies and Future Trends. 1st ed. 2019. Cham: Springer International Publishing; Imprint: Springer.

Samuel, R. & Willems, H. (Hrsg.) (2021). Wohlbefinden und Gesundheit von Jugendlichen in Luxemburg. Ministère de l'Éducation nationale, de l'Enfance et de la Jeunesse & Université du Luxembourg. Esch-sur-Alzette (Nationaler Bericht zur Situation der Jugend in Luxemburg).

Vögele, C. (2019). Die Rolle von Sport und Bewegung für die körperliche und psychische Gesundheit. In: S. Schneider & J. Margraf (Hrsg.), Lehrbuch der Verhaltenstherapie, Band 3: Psychologische Therapie bei Indikationen im Kindes- und Jugendalter (2. rev. Auflage, S. 967–977). Berlin, Heidelberg, New York: Springer

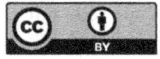

Wohlbefinden und Gesundheit: Theoretische Perspektiven

Health and Well-being from a Psychological Perspective

Claus Vögele

1   Introduction

Health and well-being are concepts of high contemporary interest, locally, nationally and globally (Anderson et al. 2012). Yet, at the same time, their conceptualizations, and related to this, their operationalisation and assessment as well as their relationship to each other remain highly contested in the literature (McAllister 2005). Historically, the Romans equated concepts of health and well-being, while the ancient Greeks distinguished between them, understanding good health to be a necessary, but not in itself sufficient, component of *eudaemonic* well-being. Eudaemonic in this context refers to human flourishing and realisation of potential, in contrast to *hedonic* well-being, which refers to pleasure, avoidance of pain and happiness (Ryan and Deci 2001; Carlisle et al. 2009). In 19th century utilitarianism, and in 20th century liberalism and socialism the debate focused on well-being alongside and arguably beyond the economic and material needs of individuals (Bacon et al. 2010).

These considerations are not only of theoretical interest for these concepts, but have practical implications for their operationalisations in terms of assessment methods. It follows from this range of concepts for both health and well-being, that there is a similarly wide range of different assessments. In this chapter we provide a description, clarification and integration of these concepts from a Psychology perspective, highlighting areas that need further development and

C. Vögele (✉)
Department of Behavioural and Cognitive Sciences, University of Luxembourg, Esch-sur-Alzette, Luxembourg
E-Mail: Claus.voegele@uni.lu

© Der/die Autor(en) 2022
A. Heinen et al. (Hrsg.), *Wohlbefinden und Gesundheit im Jugendalter,*
https://doi.org/10.1007/978-3-658-35744-3_2

outlining complementary assessment approaches. Though overlapping in very many aspects we argue that health and well-being are related but nevertheless distinct concepts, which are operationalised and assessed accordingly.

2   Conceptual Issues

2.1   Health

In 1946 the World Health Organisation defined health as a "complete state of physical, social and mental well-being, and not just the absence of disease or infirmity" (WHO 2009; p. 1), thus establishing a close relationship between the two concepts. This definition has remained almost unchanged over the last 7 decades, but has attracted criticism since, especially in view of the fact that an ever-larger proportion of the world's population reach an age at which multi-morbidity is the rule rather than the exception (Barnett et al. 2012). As a consequence of our aging societies, therefore, fewer and fewer people would be considered "healthy" according to this definition, thereby rendering it diagnostically obsolete and stigmatizing.

In contrast to the WHO definition of 1946 the focus has shifted from health as a state of complete physical, mental and social well-being to one of health as the capacity to adapt and to self-manage when facing physical, mental and social challenges (Huber et al. 2011). This applies to us both as individuals and as members of a community. Health in general is increasingly understood as the ability of an individual or community to adapt and to self-manage, even in the face of adversity, e.g. chronic disease or disability (Huber et al. 2011).

This new conceptualization of health has some important implications. Firstly, it illustrates the limitations of the "diagnose-and-fix" approach that still dominates most health care systems throughout the world, and helps to recognize that such an approach is of value only to a small fraction of people who face acute, curable conditions. Secondly, if health is understood as the ability to adapt and to self-manage, many new interesting possibilities emerge. A key one is that it is possible for health and disease to co-exist. In other words, it is possible to be ill and healthy at the same time.

Support for this view comes from a number of studies suggesting that most people, including seniors living with multiple chronic diseases, consider themselves to be healthy. For example, a Canadian survey of over 3000 people aged 65 years or older (Terner et al. 2011) illustrates this point clearly, as it showed that 86% of those with one chronic disease, 77% of those with two diseases and 51% of those with three or more regarded their health to be good, very good or excellent. These findings have been replicated several times in quality-of-life studies that include self-assessments of health. In addition, self-rated health seems to be related to mortality: a meta-analysis of 22 cohort studies revealed that individuals who rated their health as "poor" had a two-fold higher mortality risk compared with those who considered their health as "excellent" (DeSalvo et al. 2006). An Australian study goes ever further, by showing not only that most people (62%) living with advanced incurable cancer consider their health to be good or better, but also that their self-assessments are the best predictors of their survival (Shadbolt et al. 2002).

A third consequence of this paradigm shift concerns the (re-)organization and (new) focus of health care systems. As a result of the dramatic increase in life expectancy in the 20th century, there is a shift towards chronic, incurable diseases, which now account for most of the morbidity and mortality worldwide. With the rising prevalence of multiple chronic diseases, challenges for health care systems rise that are much more than the sum of the consequences of each of the individual conditions. The needs of those with multiple conditions cannot be met through diagnostic tests, curative interventions, or health care services that are focused on individual organs (e.g., cardiology), systems (e.g., gastroenterology) or diseases (e.g., cancer). Instead, services are required that enable a holistic view of people, that are responsive to the culture context, and that are sensitive to unique individual needs and, therefore, deliver personalized care at the individual level (Phillips and Vögele 2015). Responsible and integrated services are needed that take into account not only physical, but also mental, spiritual and social needs. There is an urgent need for sustainable support systems that enable a full life. The increasing number of people worldwide who live with multimorbid conditions emphasizes the realization that it is not enough to put more years into lives, but that it is essential, and perhaps even more important, to put more life into years.

2.2 Well-being

While individual well-being seems to be included in these conceptualisations of health, it is widely acknowledged that the two constructs are related but distinct. Even if health is conceptualised as the ability to self-manage and adapt, it can be assessed at the physiological, emotional, cognitive and behavioural level. In contrast, well-being emphasises the experiential aspect, which describes a feeling that is often referred to as "subjective well-being" (SWB). SWB is, therefore, primarily a psychological construct as it is concerned with people's evaluation of their lives; however, it includes a wide range of notions, from momentary moods to global life satisfaction judgments.

Well-being is also of increasing importance as a concept in public health (Dooris et al. 2018; La Plaza and Knight 2014). This perspective not only considers well-being as a matter of individual lifestyle and its subjective experience, but also its wider contextual determinants (Aked and Thompson 2011; Huppert, 2009). McNaught (2011), for example, considers health as only one component of well-being, and proposes a definitional framework comprising individual, family, community and society levels. He defines well-being as a "macro concept concerned with the objective and subjective assessment of how human beings survive, thrive and function" (p. 11).

There is a growing debate on the relationship between individual, collective and ecological well-being (Dooris et al. 2018). One aspect of this debate concerns the question to what degree the pursuit of personal well-being (particularly when defined in hedonic terms) threatens well-being of communities, societies and the ecosystems on which we depend (Carlisle 2009). Jones-Devitt (2011) takes this argument further by raising the question whether a valid commitment to well-being can be entered in a globalised neo-liberal ideology, which prioritises individual self-interest.

The increasing use of well-being as a core concept in public health is related to a number of factors, including the growing acknowledgment of mental health as a key element of health in general (Prince et al. 2007), the shift of public health to local authorities, and the establishment of health and well-being boards (HM Government 2010).

2.3   Health and Well-being: A Proposed Synthesis

Based on the definition proposed by Huber et al. (2011), health could be considered fundamentally as a mental phenomenon that can only be assessed in the presence of a challenge. Because of its reactive nature, the reformulation of health as "the ability to adapt and to self-manage" opens the door for the concept of wellness as its proactive complement, which reflects our ability to fulfil our personal and collective human potential, and to pursue a joyful life.

From this perspective, health and wellness, as complementary entities, would constitute the conceptual building blocks of well-being, which is conceived of as a state, not an ability. Its building blocks, which are already built into the word, contain its meaning: being well.

3   Operationalisation and Assessment

3.1   Health

3.1.1 Mental Health

Self-report health assessments and diagnoses (i.e. excluding medical examinations) are carried out using interviews and questionnaires that determine the presence, severity, frequency, and duration of a broad range of mental and physical symptoms, and health-related behaviours. From a psychological perspective this concerns mainly mental symptoms and conditions, as reflected in a classification system such as the Diagnostic and Statistical Manual of Mental Disorders (DSM-5) (American Psychiatric Association 2013), which pre-defines mental health symptoms, and groups them into nosological entities. In contrast to the DSM-5 the International Statistical Classification of Diseases and Related Health Problems (ICD-11) (World Health Organization, 2018) also includes physical symptoms and disorders. Nevertheless, in terms of mental disorders both classification systems have converged ever since their respective inceptions (DSM: 1952; ICD: 1900), so that they are now almost identical concerning diagnostic categories, with very few exceptions.

Assessment tools to explore and quantify mental symptoms range from structured clinician-led interviews typically used to make a formal clinical diagnosis (e.g., SCID) (First et al. 2016), to more quantitatively designed questionnaires (e.g., PHQ-9) (Spitzer et al. 1999) that provide multidimensional assessments of symptom experience and severity to support diagnosis and treatment evaluation in clinical practice and research. Both approaches are, therefore, used in clinical practice and also in the investigation of underlying aetiologies and treatment efficacy and effectiveness in clinical trials and other studies.

A closer inspection of this array of mental health assessment reveals a large range of interviews and questionnaires available for use This diversity of choice means that there is no shortage of options when searching for assessment tools for clinical use or research. This diversity, however, can also make it difficult to decide which questionnaire(s) or interview(s) to select for clinical diagnosis or evaluation. For example, there have been more than 280 different questionnaires developed over the last century to assess symptoms of depression (Santor et al. 2006), which differ in terms of which version of the DSM they align to, the degree to which they consider co-morbid symptoms, whether they are computer- or paper-based, and whether they are self-rated, parent-rated or clinician-led. Knowing which questionnaire to choose to obtain a suitable assessment of an individual's mental and physical health is, therefore, not always a straightforward exercise for even the most experienced researcher or clinician. As a consequence, diagnoses may differ dependent on the assessment method used thus introducing variability and inconsistency between clinicians (Wisco et al. 2016). This heterogeneity of assessment options also hampers progress in research, as different assessment methods render study results potentially incomparable.

A recent analysis of the most commonly used assessment tools to diagnose and screen for the most prevalent mental health conditions illustrates this issue (Newson et al. 2020). Altogether 126 different questionnaires and interviews were included in the analysis, which demonstrates substantial inconsistency in the inclusion and emphasis of symptoms assessed within disorders as well as considerable symptom overlap across disorder-specific tools. Furthermore, there were large differences in assessments in terms of emphasising emotional, cognitive, physical or behavioural symptoms, adding to the heterogeneity across assessments. Analysis of other characteristics such as the time period over which symptoms were assessed, as well as whether there was a focus on frequency, severity or duration of symptoms also varied substantially across assessment tools. In summary, this analysis underscores the need for standardized assessment tools that are more disorder agnostic and span the full spectrum of mental health symptoms to aid the understanding of underlying aetiologies and the improvement of treatments for mental disorders.

3.1.2 General Health

Over and beyond self-report measures of mental health, self-report measures of general health play an important role in social, behavioural, and health studies. Results over decades of research suggest that self-rated health is strongly associated with both physical, and mental and cognitive health (Latham and Peek 2013; Mavaddat et al. 2014; Singh-Manoux et al. 2006; Schnittker 2005), and shows a graded relationship with many clinically-relevant biomarkers, even at "subclinical" levels not directly associated with increased health risk (Goldman et al. 2004; Jylhä et al. 2006).

While the precise nature of the processes underlying self-reports of individuals' overall health remains unknown (Jylhä 2009), many researchers justify their use of these measures with the strong predictive validity of self-report health measures for poor health and early mortality across many surveys, populations, and sociodemographic groups, often over and above the potential influences of more "objective" health conditions or diagnoses (Dowd and Zajacova 2007; Franks et al. 2003; Singh-Manoux et al. 2007). In addition, self-report measures of health are easily implemented in large-scale studies and in clinical practice. Nevertheless, the widespread use of measures of self-reported health is not commensurate with our knowledge of its measurement properties (Grol-Prokopczyk et al. 2011; Hardy et al. 2014; Idler and Cartwright 2018), in particular their validity and reliability. For example, self-report measures of health are subject to self-report bias (e.g. social desirability, self-concept etc.). It could be argued, for example, that answers to questions concerning health behaviours and anthropometric characteristics, for example alcohol consumption and body weight, respectively, reflect the respondent's beliefs about number of drinks per week or weight, rather than their "actual" alcohol intake or body weight (sensu "meta-cognitive beliefs": Lenzo et al. 2020; Wells and Purdon 1999), thus questioning the validity of self-report measures of health. In addition, the reliability of self-reported health measures has received relatively limited attention (Boardman 2006; Zajacova and Dowd 2011), as the majority of studies use such items without considering measurement error. In a recent analysis of data from the *National Longitudinal Study of Adolescent to Adult Health Study* (Add Health) (Bollen et al. 2021) the authors report estimates for the measurement reliability of self-reported health relative to proxy assessments and respondents' recollections of past health. The best indicators—contemporaneous self-reports—had a modest reliability of only 0.6, with retrospective and proxy assessments being even lower, with reliability less than 0.2. Not correcting for measurement error led to a 20–40% reduction in the correlation of self-reported health with other measures of health. Considering the substantial measurement error of self-reported health assessments is, therefore, crucial for the correct interpretation of results obtained with such measures.

3.1.3 Complementary Assessment Approaches

If there is justified interest, the necessary resources are available, and feasibility is provided, self-report measures of health can be complemented by assessments at other levels such as behavioural observations and psychophysiological assessments, both in experimental and clinical settings. Such direct observations of behaviour and/or physiological responses, mostly to selected and standardized challenging situations and paradigms, can provide data un-affected by social desirability and self-concepts and contribute to a better understanding of underlying mechanisms (Vögele 1998). Based on the definition of health as described previously in this chapter, i.e. as "the ability to adapt and to self-manage", the operationalisation and assessment of health as a response to a defined challenge gains more importance, in contrast to the assessment of health as a more general and stable trait. Nevertheless, non-self-report measures are not more "objective" than self-report ones, in that there are no true or false responses, but only different observation levels, which ideally complement each other in providing a comprehensive assessment of health.

3.2   Well-being

Subjective well-being (SWB) refers to the various ways in which people experience and evaluate their lives positively (Diener et al. 1999). It includes feelings of pleasant or positive affect (PA), and feelings of unpleasant or negative affect (NA). Together, PA and NA constitute the *affective components* of SWB. In addition to affect, evaluations of life (e.g., life satisfaction) are also important. In contrast to affective experiences evaluations often require reflection on circumstances and standards. Assessment of life satisfaction or life evaluation are, therefore, called the *cognitive component* of SWB. Though the affective and cognitive components are often correlated with each other, they are also associated with different outcomes (Tay and Diener 2011). Thus, the assessment of SWB, ideally involves the measurement of these components separately (Pavot 2008).

SWB is sometimes referred to as hedonic well-being because of its emphasis on a pleasant and satisfying quality of life (Tov 2018). This contrasts with eudaemonic well-being, which includes a variety of constructs like meaning, personal growth, and authenticity (Huta and Waterman 2014; Vittersø 2016). Concepts of eudaemonic well-being focus less on the pleasantness of experience, but more on the needs that people must fulfil to reach their full potential. In contrast, the SWB approach does not specify the "ingredients" required for well-being. The assessment of SWB is subjective in the sense that people report their own happiness and satisfaction without reference to any particular template of life conditions or experiences. Instead, they assess their well-being using whichever standards are personally relevant and important to them. As discussed in the previous section on measures of self-reported health, the distinction between subjective and objective does not imply that one is more true than the other, but simply refers to the level of observation.

As is the case for self-report measures of health, SWB measures are associated with important outcomes, despite a lack of knowledge of the mediating mechanisms or factors. For example, higher levels of life satisfaction and PA predict lower susceptibility to health problems and increased longevity, whereas higher levels of NA tend to predict poorer health outcomes (Diener et al. 2017). Self-reports of well-being provide valuable information beyond objective economic indicators in the evaluation of social and economic policies (Diener and Tov 2012).

There is a range of measures that have been used in the assessment of SWB. Tov et al. (in press) provide a review and meta-analysis of the reliability and validity of the four most commonly used measures of SWB (two cognitive and two affective), based on studies published between 1999 to 2019, and, therefore, with a strong empirical foundation: the Satisfaction with Life Scale (SWLS; Diener et al. 1985), which is a widely used measure of global cognitive well-being; Cantril's ladder or The Self-Anchoring Striving Scale (Cantril 1965; Kilpatrick and Cantril 1960), which requests respondents to evaluate their life according to their own goals, values, and standards; the Positive and Negative Affect Schedule (PANAS; Watson et al. 1988) consisting of two 10-item scales, focusing on positive and negative states; and the Scale of Positive and Negative Experiences (SPANE; Diener et al. 2010), consisting of 12 items with six items each measuring PA (SPANE-P scale) and NA (SPANE-N scale).).

The SWLS, PANAS, and SPANE generally exhibited acceptable levels of reliability (alphas > .80) across most samples, time frame instructions, and age groups. All measures were substantially correlated with each other. However, SWLS was more strongly correlated with SPANE-P than with PANAS-PA.

3.2.1 Complementary Assessment Approaches

Although this analysis (Tov et al., in press) provides a good foundation for the further use of these scales to assess SWB, SWB measures share the same shortcomings with self-report measures of health in that they are open to reporting biases, e.g. recall bias etc. To reduce recall biases, for example, methods for assessing online affect are increasingly popular. For example, the experience sampling method (ESM) makes use of handheld devices (e.g., smartphones) to survey people on how they are feeling at randomly selected or predefined moments during the day (Trull and Ebner-Priemer 2014). Another approach concerns the Day Reconstruction Method (DRM; Kahneman et al. 2004), in which respondents recall the events they experienced the previous day and rate how they felt during these events. These developments have good potential to overcome some of the limitations of traditional questionnaire-based assessments, but they come with their own challenges and complex problems, that require significant advance planning and numerous decisions on the part of the researcher. On the one hand, and as in other studies, power and sample-size calculations are required (although rarely reported; Trull and Ebner-Priemer 2020; van Roekel et al. 2019), but these are made more complex in ESM research because of the multilevel nature of the data (Bolger et al. 2012). In addition, the use of ESM methods raises considerations regarding item selection, psychometrics, and analytic strategy (Wright and Zimmermann 2019).

Furthermore, ESM methods put considerable burden on the respondents as they are prompted several times per day to respond to questions, thus increasing risk of attrition and affecting the very phenomenon under investigation by the method of investigation (sensu Heisenberg's uncertainty principle; Stamm 1985), which can be experienced as intrusive. The DRM, on the other hand, might be less burdensome on respondents than ESM, and might reduce memory biases that are inherent in global recall of feelings. Nevertheless, evidence for the validity and reliability of the DRM is limited and is not entirely supportive (Diener and Tay 2013). For one of the first direct comparisons between ESM and DRM, see Lucas et al. (2021).

4   Summary and Outlook

Concepts of health and well-being have evolved ever since ancient Greek and Roman history. Based on new approaches, which define health as the ability to adapt and manage even in the face of adversity (Huber et al. 2011), the concept of wellness can be understood as its proactive complement, which reflects our ability to fulfil our personal and collective human potential, and to pursue a joyful life. From this perspective, health and wellness, as complementary entities, would constitute the conceptual building blocks of well-being, which is conceived of as a state, not an ability.

These considerations not only have theoretical but also practical implications in terms of the operationalisation and assessment of these concepts. Non-medical assessments of health include interviews and questionnaires that determine the presence, severity, frequency, and duration of a broad range of mental and physical symptoms, and health-related behaviours. Self-reported (also called "subjective") health has been shown over decades of research to be strongly associated with both physical, and mental and cognitive health, although the mechanisms underlying these associations remain elusive. Despite their strong predictive validity for poor health and early mortality, the validity and reliability of measures of self-reported health is only modest, even for the best indicators. The same seems to hold for self-assessments of well-being (also called "subjective well-being", SWB). Similar to self-reported measures of health, SWB measures are associated with important outcomes, despite a lack of knowledge of the mediating mechanisms or factors. In a similar vein, SWB measures share the same shortcomings with self-report measures of health in that they are open to reporting biases, e.g. recall bias etc. Complementary approaches that reflect the reactive nature of the new definition of health include observations at behavioural and physiological levels to standardized challenges; in terms of well-being these concern methods for assessing online affect such as the experience sampling method (ESM) and the Day Reconstruction Method (DRM), with the advantage that they reduce recollection bias and the risk of assessing meta-cognitive beliefs rather than well-being itself.

It should be noted that both measures of health and well-being are denoted "subjective" in the literature in the sense that assessments are made without reference to any particular template of life conditions or experiences. Instead, respondents are asked to assess their own health and well-being in terms of whichever standards are personally relevant and important to them. As the term "subjective" is not supposed to imply that these measures are less true than "objective" measures, it stands to reason that this distinction is somewhat misleading. Alternatives to "subjective health" or "subjective well-being" that avoid such misinterpretations, could be terms such as "personal health and well-being" or "individual health and well-being", thus emphasising the personal assessment context without implying false notions of "true" (sensu "objective") versus "imagined" (sensu "subjective"). After all, health and well-being should be understood as private experiences, and not as objectifiable states, as purported by a medicalised health system for the last centuries.

References

Aked, J. & Thompson, S. (2011). *Five Ways to Wellbeing: New applications, new ways of thinking*. London: New Economics Foundation.

Anderson, P., Cooper, C., Layard, R., Litchfield, P. & Jane-Llopis, E. (2012). *Well-being and global success: a report prepared by the World Economic Forum Global Agenda Council on Health & Well-being*. World Economic Forum, Geneva, Switzerland.

APA. (2013). *Diagnostic and statistical manual of mental disorders, 5th ed.* (Arlington, VA: American Psychiatric Association).

Bacon, N., Brophy, M., Mguni, N., Mulgan, G. & Shandro, A. (2010). *The State of Happiness: Can public policy shape people's wellbeing and resilience?* London: The Young Foundation.

Barnett, K., Mercer, S.W., Norbury, M., Watt, G., Wyke, S., & Guthrie, B. (2012). Epidemiology of multimorbidity and implications for health care, research, and medical education: a cross-sectional study. *Lancet, 380*, 37–43.

Boardman, J.D. (2006). Self-rated health among US adolescents. *The Journal of Adolescent Health, 38 (4)*, 401–408.

Bolger, N., Stadler, G., & Laurenceau, J.-P. (2012). Power analysis for intensive longitudinal studies. In M. R. Mehl & T. S. Conner (Eds.), *Handbook of research methods for studying daily life* (pp. 285–301). Guilford Press.

Bollen, K.A., Gutin, I., Halpern, C.T., & Harris, K.M. (2021). Subjective health in adolescence: Comparing the reliability of contemporaneous, retrospective, and proxy reports of overall health. *Social Science Research, May 2021, 96,* 102538. doi: https://doi.org/10.1016/j.ssresearch.2021.102538. Epub 2021 Feb 16.

Cantril, H. (1965). *The pattern of human concerns.* New Brunswick, NJ: Rutgers University Press.

Carlisle, S., Henderson, G., & Hanlon, P.W. (2009). "Wellbeing": A collateral casualty of modernity? *Social Science and Medicine, 69(10),* 1556–1560.

DeSalvo, K.B., Bloser, N., Reynolds, K., He, J., & Muntner, P. (2006). Mortality prediction with a single general self-rated health question: A meta-analysis. *Journal of General Internal Medicine, 21,* 267–75.

Diener, E., Emmons, R. A., Larsen, R. J., & Griffin, S. (1985). The Satisfaction With Life Scale. *Journal of Personality Assessment, 49,* 71–75. doi: https://doi.org/10.1207/s15327752jpa4901_13.

Diener, E., Pressman, S. D., Hunter, J., & Delgadillo-Chase, D. (2017). If, why, and when subjective well-being influences health, and future needed research. *Applied Psychology: Health and Well-Being, 9,* 133–167. doi: https://doi.org/10.1111/aphw.12090.

Diener, E. & Tay, L. (2013). Review of the Day Reconstruction Method (DRM). *Social Indicators Research, 116,* 255–267.

Diener, E., Suh, E. M., Lucas, R. E., & Smith, H. L. (1999). Subjective well-being: three decades of progress. *Psychological Bulletin, 125,* 276–302. doi: https://doi.org/10.1037/0033-2909.125.2.276.

Diener, E., Wirtz, D., Tov, W., Kim-Prieto, C., Choi, D., Oishi, S., & Biswas-Diener, R. (2010). New well-being measures: short scales to assess flourishing and positive and negative feelings. *Social Indicators Research, 97,* 143–156.

Diener, E., & Tov, W. (2012). National accounts of wellbeing. In K. C. Land, A. C. Michalos, & M. J. Sirgy (Eds.), *Handbook of social indicators and quality of life research* (pp. 137–156). New York, NY: Springer.

Dooris, M., Farrier, A., & Froggett, L. (2018). Wellbeing: the challenge of 'operationalising' a holistic concept within a reductionist public health programme. *Perspectives in Public Health, 138(2),* 93–99.

Dowd, J.B., & Zajacova, A. (2007). Does the predictive power of self-rated health for subsequent mortality risk vary by socioeconomic status in the US? *International Journal of Epidemiology, 36 (6),* 1214–1221.

First, M., Williams, J., Karg, R., & Spitzer R. (2016). *Structured Clinical Interview for DSM-5 Disorders, Clinician Version (SCID-5-CV).* Arlington, VA: American Psychiatric Association.

Franks, P., Gold, M.R., & Fiscella, K. (2003). Sociodemographics, self-rated health, and mortality in the US. *Social Science and Medicine, 56 (12),* 2505–2514.

Goldman, N., Glei, D.A., & Chang, M.C. (2004). The role of clinical risk factors in understanding self-rated health. *Annals of Epidemiology, 14(1),* 49–57. doi: https://doi.org/10.1016/s1047-2797(03)00077-2.

Grol-Prokopczyk, H., Freese, J., & Hauser, R.M. (2011). Using anchoring vignettes to assess group differences in general self-rated health. *Journal of Health and Social Behavior, 52 (2),* 246–261.

Hardy, M.A., Acciai, F., & Reyes, A.M. (2014). How health conditions translate into self-ratings: a comparative study of older adults across Europe. *Journal of Health and Social Behavior, 55 (3),* 320–341.

HM Government (2010). *Healthy Lives, Healthy People: Our strategy for public health in England.* London: Department of Health (Mental Health D vision).

Huber, M., Knottnerus, J.A., Green, L., Horst, H., Jadad, A.R., Kromhout, D., Leonard, B., Lorig, K., Loureiro, M.I., Meer, J.W., Schnabel, P., Sm th, R., Weel, C., & Smid, H. (2011). How should we define health? *British Medical Journal, 343,* d4163.

Huppert F. (2009). *Psychological Well-Being: Evidence Regarding its Causes and its Consequences.* London: Foresight.

Huta, V., & Waterman, A. S. (2014). Eudaimonia and its distinction from hedonia: Developing a classification and terminology for understanding conceptual and operational definitions. *Journal of Happiness Studies, 15,* 1425–1456. doi: https://doi.org/10.1007/s10902-013-9485-0.

Idler, E., & Cartwright, K. (2018). What do we rate when we rate our health? Decomposing age-related contributions to self-rated health. *Journal of Health and Social Behavior, 59 (1),* 74–93.

Jylhä, M. (2009). What is self-rated health and why does it predict mortality? Towards a unified conceptual model. *Social Science and Medicine, 69 (3),* 307–316.

Jylhä, M., Volpato. S., & Guralnik, J.M. (2006). Self-rated health showed a graded association with frequently used biomarkers in a large population sample. *Journal of Clinical Epidemiology, 59 (5),* 465–471.

Jones-Devitt, S. (2011). Wellbeing and health. In A. Knight & A. McNaught (Eds.), *Understanding Wellbeing: An Introduction for Students and Practitioners of Health and Social Care* (pp. 23–36). Banbury: Lantern.

Kahneman, D., Krueger, A. B., Schkade, D. A., Schwarz, N., & Stone, A. A. (2004). A survey method for characterizing daily life experience: The Day Reconstruction Method. *Science, 306,* 1776–1780.

Kilpatrick, F. P., & Cantril, H. (1960). Self-anchoring scaling: a measure of individuals' unique reality worlds. *Journal of Individual Psychology, 16,* 158–173.

La Placa, V. & Knight, A. (2014). Well-being: Its influence and local impact on public health. *Public Health, 128(1),* 38–42.

Latham, K. & Peek, C.W. (2013). Self-rated health and morbidity onset among late midlife US adults. *The Journals of Gerontology. Series B, Psychological Sciences and Social Sciences, 68 (1),* 107–116.

Lenzo, V., Sardella, A., Martino, G., & Quattropani, M.C. (2020). A systematic review of metacognitive beliefs in chronic medical conditions. *Frontiers in Psychology, Jan 10, 10,* 2875. doi: https://doi.org/10.3389/fpsyg.2019.02875. eCollection 2019.

Lucas, R. E., Wallsworth, C., Anusic, I., & Donnellan, M. B. (2021). A direct comparison of the day reconstruction method (DRM) and the experience sampling method (ESM). *Journal of Personality and Social Psychology, 120(3),* 816–835. https://doi.org/10.1037/pspp0000289.

Mavaddat, N., Valderas, J.M., van Der Linde, R., Khaw, K.T., & Kinmonth, A.L. (2014). Association of self-rated health with multimorbidity, chronic disease and psychosocial factors in a large middle-aged and older cohort from general practice: a cross-sectional study. *BMC Family Practice, 15 (1),* 185.

McAllister F. (2005). Wellbeing Concepts and Challenges. *SDRN Briefing, 3,* 1–8.

McNaught, A. (2011). Defining wellbeing. In A. Knight & A. McNaught (Eds.), Understanding Wellbeing: An Introduction for Students and Practitioners of Health and Social Care (pp. 7–22). Banbury: Lantern.

Newson, J.J., Hunter, D., & Thiagarajan, T.C. (2020). The Heterogeneity of mental health assessment. *Front. Psychiatry, 11,* 76. https://doi.org/10.3389/fpsyt.2020.00076.

Pavot, W. (2008). The assessment of subjective well-being: Successes and shortfalls. In M. Eid & R. J. Larsen (Eds.), *The science of subjective well-being* (pp. 124–140). New York, NY: Guilford Press. (2008-00541-007).

Phillips, R., & Vögele, C. (2015). Personalized Medicine. In J. D. Wright (Ed.), *International Encyclopedia of the Social and Behavioral Sciences* (2nd revised edition, pp. 925–931). Amsterdam: Elsevier.

Stamm, J.S. (1985). The uncertainty principle in psychology. *Behavioral and Brain Sciences 8 (4),* 553–554.

Tay, L., & Diener, E. (2011). Needs and subjective well-being around the world. *Journal of Personality and Social Psychology, 101,* 354–365. doi: https://doi.org/10.1037/a0023779.

Terner, M., Reason, B., McKeag, A.M., Tipper, B., & Webster, G. (2011). Chronic conditions more than age drive health system use in Canadian seniors. *Healthcare Quarterly, 14,* 19–22.

Trull, T.J. & Ebner-Priemer, U.W. (2020). Ambulatory assessment in psychopathology research: A review of recommended reporting guidelines and current practices. *Journal of Abnormal Psychology, 129(1),* 56–63. https://doi.org/10.1037/abn0000473.

Prince, M., Patel, V., Saxena, S., Maj, M., Maselko, J., Phillips, M.R. & Rahman, A. (2007). No health without mental health. *Lancet, 370,* 859–877.

Ryan, R.M. & Deci, E.L. (2001). On happiness and human potentials: a review of research on hedonic and eudaemonic well-being. *Annual Review of Psychology, 52,* 141–166.

Santor, D.A., Gregus, M., & Welch, A. (2006). Eight decades of measurement in depression. *Measurement: Interdisciplinary Research and Perspectives, 4(3),* 135–155. doi: https://doi.org/10.1207/s15366359mea0403_1.

Schnittker, J. (2005). Cognitive abilities and self-rated health: is there a relationship? Is it growing? Does it explain disparities? *Social Science Research, 34 (4),* 821–842.

Shadbolt, B., Barresi, J., & Craft, P. (2002). Self-rated health as a predictor of survival among patients with advanced cancer. *Journal of Clinical Oncology, 20,* 2514–2519.

Singh-Manoux, A., Dugravot, A., Shipley, M.J., Ferrie, J.E., Martikainen, P., Goldberg, M., & Zins, M. (2007). The association between self-rated health and mortality in different socioeconomic groups in the GAZEL cohort study. *International Journal of Epidemiology, 36 (6),* 1222–1228.

Singh-Manoux, A., Martikainen, P., Ferrie, J., Zins, M., Marmot, M., & Goldberg, M. (2006). What does self-rated health measure? Results from the British Whitehall II and French Gazel cohort studies. *Journal of Epidemiology and Community Health, 60(4),* 364–372.

Spitzer, R.L., Kroenke, K., Williams, J.B.W. and the Patient Health Questionnaire Primary Care Study Group (1999). Validation and utility of a self-report version of PRIME-MD: the PHQ primary care study. *Journal of the American Medical Association, 282(18),* 1737–1744. doi: https://doi.org/10.1001/jama.282.18.1737

Tov, W. (2018). Well-being concepts and components. In E. Diener, S. Oishi, & L. Tay (Eds.), *Handbook of subjective well-being* (pp. –15). Salt Lake City, UT: DEF. nobascholar.com.

Tov, W., Keh, J. S., Tan, Y. Q., Tan, Q. Y., & Indra Alam Syah, A. (in press). The assessment of subjective well-being: A review of common measures. In W. Ruch, A. B. Bakker, L. Tay, & F. Gander (Eds.), *Handbook of positive psychology assessment*. European Association of Psychological Assessment. https://www.researchgate.net/publication/348078354_The_Assessment_of_Subjective_Well-Being_A_Review_of_Common_Measures [Accessed Mar 16 2022].

Trull, T. J., & Ebner-Priemer, U. (2014). The role of ambulatory assessment in psychological science. *Current Directions in Psychological Science, 23(6),* 466–470. https://doi.org/10.1177/0963721414550706.

van Roekel, E., Keijsers, L., & Chung, J. M. (2019). A review of current ambulatory assessment studies in adolescent samples and practical recommendations. *Journal of Research on Adolescence, 29(3),* 560–577. https://doi.org/10.1111/jora.12471.

Vitterø, J. (Ed.). (2016). *Handbook of eudaemonic well-being.* doi: https://doi.org/10.1007/978-3-319-42445-3.

Vögele, C. (1998). Klinische Psychophysiologie: Psychophysiologische Methoden in der Diagnostik und Therapie psychischer und psychophysiologischer Störungen. In F. Rösler (Hrsg.) *Enzyklopädie der Psychologie, Band 5: Ergebnisse und Anwendungen der Psychophysiologie* (S. 573–618). Göttingen: Hogrefe.

Watson, D., Clark, L. A., & Tellegen, A. (1988). Development and validation of brief measures of positive and negative affect: The PANAS scales. *Journal of Personality and Social Psychology, 54,* 1063–1070.

Wells, A., & Purdon, C. L. (1999). Metacognition and cognitive-behaviour therapy: a special issue. *Clinical Psychology & Psychotherapy, 6,* 71–72.

Wisco, B.E., Miller, M.W., Wolf, E.J., Kilpatrick, D., Resnick, H.S., Badour, C.L., Marx, B.P., Keane, T.M., Rosen, R.C., & Friedman, M.J. (2016). The impact of proposed changes to ICD-11 on estimates of PTSD prevalence and comorbidity. *Psychiatry Research, 24,* 226–233. doi: https://doi.org/10.1016/j.psychres.2016.04.043.

World Health Organization (2009). *Basic Documents. 47th Edition.* Geneva: WHO.

World Health Organization (2018). *International statistical classification of diseases and related health problems (11th Revision).* Geneva: WHO.

Wright, A. G. C., & Zimmermann, J. (2019). Applied ambulatory assessment: Integrating idiographic and nomothetic principles of measurement. *Psychological Assessment, 31(12),* 1467–1480. https://doi.org/10.1037/pas0000685.

Zajacova, A., & Dowd, J.B. (2011). Reliability of self-rated health in US adults. *American journal of epidemiology, 174(8),* 977–983.

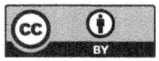

Gesundheit und Wohlbefinden aus soziologischer Perspektive

Laura Hoffmann, Irene Moor und Matthias Richter

1 Einleitung

Aus Sichtweise der immer noch stark *naturwissenschaftlich orientierten Medizin* werden Krankheiten und Krankheitssymptome als Abweichungen mit physiologischen und biologischen Ursachen verstanden und Gesundheit entsprechend als das Fehlen dieser Normabweichungen. Ein Blick in unsere Alltagskultur verdeutlicht, dass Gesundheit jedoch viel mehr beinhaltet als alleine die Abwesenheit von Krankheit. So dreht sich die heutige „gesundheitsbesessene Welt" (Richter und Hurrelmann 2016) um komplexe Themen von gesunder Ernährung und Körperoptimierung bis hin zu Fitnessuhren und Apps, die permanent die Bewegung und den Puls ihrer Nutzer messen und dokumentieren (Nettleton 2013; Richter und Hurrelmann 2016). Es scheint nahezu als wären Gesundheit und Wohlbefinden zu allgegenwärtigen Motiven der heutigen Gesellschaft geworden (Nettleton 2013). Dies spiegelt sich unter anderem auch darin wieder, dass Gesundheit und Wohlbefinden durch unterschiedlichste Kanäle transportiert und kommuniziert werden, sei es über Fernseh- oder Radiosendungen, Zeitungen und Magazine (Nettleton 2013; Richter und Hurrelmann 2016) oder die immer bedeutsamer werdenden sozialen Medien, wie z. B. Instagram und Facebook.

L. Hoffmann (✉) · I. Moor · M. Richter
Institut für Medizinische Soziologie, Martin-Luther-Universität Halle-Wittenberg,
Halle (Saale), Deutschland
E-Mail: laura.hoffmann@medizin.uni-halle.de

I. Moor
E-Mail: irene.moor@medizin.uni-halle.de

M. Richter
E-Mail: m.richter@medizin.uni-halle.de

© Der/die Autor(en) 2022
A. Heinen et al. (Hrsg.), *Wohlbefinden und Gesundheit im Jugendalter,*
https://doi.org/10.1007/978-3-658-35744-3_3

Gesundheit, Wohlbefinden und Krankheit sind also längst keine Themen mehr, die allein unter „Experten" diskutiert werden, sondern nehmen einen immer größeren Stellenwert in gesellschaftlichen Debatten und Laiendiskursen ein (Nettleton 2013).

Die Weltgesundheitsorganisation (WHO) definierte Gesundheit 1946 als „einen Zustand des vollständigen körperlichen, psychischen und sozialen Wohlbefindens und nicht nur [als] die Abwesenheit von Krankheit und Gebrechen" (WHO 1946 zitiert nach Hornberg 2016, S. 63). Damit sind eben nicht nur physische Faktoren von Gesundheit angesprochen, die in der naturwissenschaftlich orientieren Medizin im Vordergrund stehen, sondern es werden auch die sozialen und psychischen Komponenten sowie das Wohlbefinden ausdrücklich eingeschlossen. Es besteht jedoch bis heute kein Konsens darüber, was Wohlbefinden überhaupt ist und eine einheitliche Definition sucht man vergeblich (Weltgesundheitsorganisation 2013; Diener und Ryan 2009).

Welche Rolle spielt nun in diesem Kontext eine soziologische Perspektive auf Gesundheit und Wohlbefinden? Die meisten Menschen nehmen die Welt, in der wir leben, hauptsächlich aus ihrer eigenen Perspektive wahr, wohingegen die Soziologie über diese individuelle Sichtweise hinausgeht und die Gesellschaft aus einem größeren Blickwinkel zu beschreiben versucht (Richter und Hurrelmann 2016; Giddens und Griffiths 2006). Diese Perspektive hat C. Wright Mills (1959) auch als „sociological imagination" beschrieben (Mills 1959; Richter und Hurrelmann 2016). Anders als die naturwissenschaftliche Medizin, geht die Soziologie davon aus, dass Gesundheit und Krankheit weniger individuell sind und versucht deshalb überindividuelle Strukturen zu identifizieren, die wiederum das jeweilige individuelle Handeln maßgeblich beeinflussen (Bittlingmayer 2016).

Anthony Giddens (2006), einer der bedeutsamsten Vertreter der Soziologie, definiert diese als „[...] the scientific study of human social life, groups and societies. It is a dazzling and compelling enterprise, as its subject matter is our own behaviour as social beings. The scope of sociological study is extremely wide, ranging from the analysis of passing encounters between individuals on the street to the investigation of global social processes [...]." (Giddens und Griffiths 2006). Die Soziologie untersucht also „die Strukturen des sozialen Handelns und die Formen der Vergemeinschaftung und Vergesellschaftung, unter Berücksichtigung der jeweils vorherrschenden Normen und Werte. Sie untersucht die sozialen Prozesse und Institutionen, die die Integration der Gesellschaft bewirken. Sozialer Wandel und soziale Ungleichheit gehören zu den grundlegenden Phänomenen der soziologischen Theorie und Empirie." (Schäfers 2016). Sie ist zudem eine empirische Wissenschaft, denn ihr Wissen basiert auf einem

Ansatz, dem empirische Forschung zugrunde liegt (Schäfers 2016; Richter und Hurrelmann 2016). Aufgabe einer soziologischen Perspektive auf Gesundheit und Wohlbefinden ist es unter anderem, soziale Strukturen und Verhaltensmuster in Bezug auf Gesundheit und Krankheit zu untersuchen. Antworten und Erklärungen auf die ihr zugrunde gelegten Fragen sucht die soziologische Sichtweise dabei nicht in der Untersuchung biologischer oder psychologischer Faktoren, sondern mithilfe der Erforschung sozialer Determinanten, wie zum Beispiel den Lebens- oder Arbeitsbedingungen von Menschen, die maßgeblich ihre Gesundheit beein- flussen (Germov 2009; White 2009). Auch unsere Einstellungen gegenüber Gesundheit und Wohlbefinden sind beeinflusst durch gesellschaftliche Diskurse und eng mit dem jeweiligen soziokulturellen Kontext verbunden (Nettleton 2013).

Diese Beispiele zeigen eindrucksvoll, dass es nicht ausreicht, allein der bio- medizinischen Perspektive, die den Menschen als biologischen Organismus versteht, zu folgen. Ebenso wichtig ist ein sozialer Blick auf Gesundheit und Wohlbefinden, ein Blick auf die soziale Konstruktion von Gesundheit und Krankheit, die soziale Organisation der gesundheitlichen Versorgung sowie die systematische wissenschaftliche Analyse der sozialen Ursachen von Gesund- heit und Krankheit, um zu einem besseren und umfassenden Verständnis dieser komplexen Thematik zu gelangen. Die soziologische Perspektive auf Gesund- heit und Wohlbefinden stellt somit eine „second opinion" (Germov 2009), eine zweite Perspektive gegenüber dem konventionellen medizinischen Blickwinkel zur Erforschung von Gesundheit und Wohlbefinden zur Verfügung und betont die Wichtigkeit des Verstehens des Sozialen – den Menschen also als soziales Wesen und eben nicht „nur" als biologischen Organismus zu verstehen (Germov 2009; Richter und Hurrelmann 2016).

Die allgemeine Soziologie stellt dabei verschiedene, miteinander konkurrierende Theorien und Ansätze zur Verfügung, mithilfe einiger auch Gesundheit und Wohlbefinden untersucht werden können (Richter und Hurrelmann 2016). So existieren zum Beispiel neben strukturtheoretischen Ansätzen, die den Einfluss der Gesellschaft auf das individuelle Handeln in den Mittelpunkt rücken, hand- lungstheoretische Ansätze, die den Einfluss des Einzelnen auf die Gesellschaft fokussieren (Richter und Hurrelmann 2016; Germov 2009; Bittlingmayer 2016; Sperlich 2016). Aufgrund der Komplexität und Vielfalt soziologischer Theorien ist es jedoch nicht möglich, all diese in einem Beitrag ausführlich zu betrachten. Deshalb beschränkt sich die folgende Darstellung soziologischer Theorien und Perspektiven zunächst einmal auf solche, die auf Gesundheit und Wohlbefinden anwendbar sind. Zum anderen handelt es sich bei den im Folgenden vorgestellten Theorien wohl um einige der Bekanntesten aus diesem Bereich. Im Mittelpunkt stehen dabei Klassiker wie materialistische Theorien bzw. der Marxismus, die

Strukturtheorie und der Strukturfunktionalismus, der symbolische Interaktionismus sowie als Beispiel für eine moderne Theorie, die feministische Theorie. Im Anschluss wird auf das Verhältnis zur naturwissenschaftlich dominierten Medizin eingegangen und das soziale Modell von Gesundheit ausführlich erläutert sowie dem biomedizinischen Modell gegenübergestellt. Der Beitrag schließt mit einem Fazit zur Soziologie von Gesundheit und Krankheit sowie Wohlbefinden.

2 Soziologische Theorien im Kontext von Gesundheit und Krankheit

Aufgabe einer soziologischen Theorie ist es, möglichst allgemeingültige Aussagen zum Zustand und zur Entwicklung von Gesellschaften zu treffen. Soziologische Theorien sind also grundlagenorientiert und können auf unterschiedliche Untersuchungsbereiche angewendet werden (Treibel 2006). Sie unterscheiden sich dabei deutlich von Alltagstheorien, denn sie sind in der Regel systematisch und empirisch überprüfbar (Barry und Yuill 2012; Germov 2009). Alltagstheorien beruhen hingegen überwiegend auf eigenen Erfahrungen und weniger auf überprüfbaren Fakten (Germov 2009). Auf diese Art und Weise ermöglichen es soziologische Theorien, Phänomene zu untersuchen und zu verstehen, die der Forschende selbst nicht konkret erlebt hat (Barry und Yuill 2012) und liefern damit das Grundgerüst, um über die individuelle Sichtweise hinauszugehen und die Gesellschaft aus einem weiteren Blickwinkel zu betrachten – mithin die „sociological imagination" (Mills 1959) anzuwenden. Germov (2009) fasst Theorien zusammen als „an explanation of how things work and why things happen. Theories allow us to make sense of our world – they provide answers to the ‚how' and ‚why' questions of life – by showing the way certain facts are connected to one another." (Germov 2009).

Wie bereits angedeutet, existiert nicht *die* soziologische Theorie, sondern es konkurrieren ganz unterschiedliche Paradigmen und Ansätze miteinander, welche die Gesellschaft jeweils auf unterschiedliche Art und Weise und aus unterschiedlichen Blickwinkeln zu erklären versuchen. Grob lässt sich zwischen „Strukturorientierten Theorien" und „Handlungsorientierten Theorien" unterscheiden (Bittlingmayer 2016; Sperlich 2016; Germov 2009). Bei den strukturtheoretischen Ansätzen steht der Einfluss gesellschaftlicher Strukturen auf das individuelle Verhalten im Vordergrund (Sperlich 2016). Sie gehen davon aus, dass individuelle Entscheidungen vor allem aufgrund von gesellschaftlichen Strukturen getroffen werden (Bittlingmayer 2016; Germov 2009). Der sozialwissenschaftliche Strukturbegriff beruhte bis in die 1970er Jahre auf der

Vorstellung, dass die Gesellschaft durch eine vertikale Klassen- und Schicht-
struktur geprägt sei und eben jene Zugehörigkeit zu einer bestimmten Klasse
auch gleichzeitig das individuelle Verhalten maßgeblich beeinflusst (Sperlich
2016; Bittlingmayer 2016). Germov (2009) definiert soziale Strukturen als „the
recurring patterns of social interaction through which people are related to each
other, such as social institutions and social groups." (Germov 2009). So wird
zum Beispiel auch die Geschlechtszugehörigkeit wie „Mann" oder „Frau" als
Struktur definiert (Bittlingmayer 2016). Aktuelle Forschungsergebnisse zeigen
deutlich, dass Strukturen, wie die soziale Herkunft, das Geschlecht, die ethnische
Zugehörigkeit sowie das Einkommen, maßgeblich Einfluss auf das individuelle
Gesundheitsverhalten, psychische Erkrankungen sowie das subjektive Wohlbefinden nehmen (Bittlingmayer 2016; Lampert et al. 2019, 2018). Bittlingmayer
(2016) verweist dabei auf zwei Merkmale eines modernen sozialwissenschaftlichen Strukturbegriffes:

- Erstens ist zu beachten, dass die Zugehörigkeit zu einer Struktur nicht
  determinierend wirkt, d. h. die Eigenschaft zur Ober- oder Unterschicht zu
  gehören, lässt verschiedene Erkrankungen oder Verhaltensweisen unterschiedlich wahrscheinlich werden, legt diese jedoch nicht automatisch fest.
- Zweitens werden soziale Strukturen vom Menschen selbst erzeugt und sind
  somit grundsätzlich wandel- und gestaltbar. Obwohl sie einerseits über lange
  Zeiträume Kontinuität und Beständigkeit aufweisen, können sie sich dennoch
  im historischen Verlauf verändern (Bittlingmayer 2016).

Handlungsorientierte Theorien oder auch Agency-Ansätze stellen hingegen das
individuelle Handeln von Menschen in den Mittelpunkt und gehören zu den
mikrosoziologischen Theorieansätzen (Sperlich 2016; Cockerham 2013; Germov
2009). Dem Agency-Ansatz „liegt die Annahme zugrunde, dass soziale Sach-
verhalte über das individuelle Verhalten erklärt werden können und demzufolge
soziale Wirklichkeit primär durch menschliches Handeln hervorgebracht wird."
(Sperlich 2016). Agency bezeichnet dabei die Fähigkeit von Menschen sowohl
individuell als auch kollektiv ihr eigenes Leben sowie die Gesellschaft, in der
sie leben, zu beeinflussen (Germov 2009). Aus handlungsorientierter Sichtweise werden im Kontext von Gesundheit und Krankheit z. B. individuelles
Gesundheits- und Krankheitsverhalten sowie soziale Interaktionsprozesse (u. a.
Arzt-Patient-Kommunikation) und Krankenrollenverhalten untersucht (Sperlich
2016). Die Agency-Perspektive geht zudem davon aus, „dass Handeln ein
absichtsvolles Tun der Akteure darstellt, was sowohl ein bewusst rationales als

auch ein gewohnheitsmäßiges oder an Wertvorstellungen orientiertes Handeln einschließt." (Sperlich 2016).

Die Trennung von Struktur und Agency wurde in der Vergangenheit stark kritisiert. Gefordert wurde, dass der Bezug auf das Individuum gemeinsam mit der Untersuchung der strukturellen Gegebenheiten erforscht werden muss, um Gesundheit und Krankheit ganzheitlich zu verstehen (Sperlich 2016). So kann beispielsweise das Konzept des Habitus von Pierre Bourdieu (Bourdieu 1982) genutzt werden, um Struktur und Agency miteinander zu verbinden (Sperlich 2016). Stefanie Sperlich (2016) beschreibt dies wie folgt: „Nach Bourdieu kann der Habitus als ein sozial erworbenes psychisches Dispositionssystem verstanden werden, welches das Wahrnehmen, Denken und Empfinden strukturiert (Bourdieu 1982). [...]. Mit dem Habituskonzept wird einerseits betont, dass Handlungen jenseits eines ‚blinden' Ausübens von Regeln oder Normen von den Subjekten ausgeführt werden, weil sie sinnvoll und situationsangemessen und in diesem Sinne auch rational sind. Gleichzeitig werden Handlungen jedoch nicht als Ausdruck autonomer Subjektivität betrachtet, vielmehr ist der handlungsleitende ‚Praxis-Sinn' das Ergebnis der Auseinandersetzung mit der gesellschaftlichen Realität." (Sperlich 2016, S. 46 ff.).

Nachdem nun die zwei grundlegenden Theorieausrichtungen Struktur und Agency erläutert wurden, soll im Folgenden auf einige ausgewählte soziologische Theorien und ihren Bezug zu Gesundheit und Krankheit eingegangen werden. Es sei an dieser Stelle darauf verwiesen, dass der Fokus der hier vorgestellten Theorien in erster Linie auf „Krankheit" liegt und diese vor allem in der medizinsoziologischen Forschung und weniger in der Gesundheitssoziologie Anwendung finden, welche ein noch verhältnismäßig junges Feld darstellt.

2.1 Marxismus/Materialistische Theorie

Der Marxismus (oder auch materialistische Theorie) gehört zu den strukturtheoretischen Theorien und geht zurück auf die Arbeiten von Karl Marx (1818 bis 1883) und Friedrich Engels (1820 bis 1895) (Germov 2009). Die zentrale These dieser Theorie besagt, dass soziale Phänomene in erster Linie durch die ökonomischen Strukturen einer Gesellschaft bestimmt werden (Barry und Yuill 2012). Entscheidend dabei ist die ungleiche Verteilung bzw. der Besitz von Produktionsgütern, wodurch unterschiedliche gesellschaftliche Machtverhältnisse entstehen (Barry und Yuill 2012). Marx hat dabei moderne, westliche Gesellschaften als Kapitalistische beschrieben, in denen die Machtverhältnisse ungleich verteilt sind; d. h. eine Minderheit besitzt die Produktionsmittel, die sie nutzt, um Profit zu generieren, wohingegen die Mehrheit – die nicht Besitzenden – ihre Arbeitskraft einsetzen müssen, um ihren Lebensunterhalt zu verdienen (Barry und Yuill 2012). Auf diese Art und Weise entstehen zwei soziale Klassen: die Bourgeoisie (Besitzer der Produktionsmittel) und das Proletariat (Arbeiter) (Barry und Yuill 2012). Aus Besitz und nicht-Besitz von Produktionsmitteln resultieren wiederum soziale Ungleichheiten, wie zum Beispiel ungleiche Lebens- und Wohnbedingungen, die als Ausgangspunkt für die Analyse gesundheitlicher Ungleichheiten zwischen der herrschenden und der arbeitenden Klasse gesehen werden können (Barry und Yuill 2012). Die marxistische Theorie wurde dabei vielfach zur Untersuchung des Einflusses von Arbeits- und Lebensbedingungen in kapitalistischen Gesellschaften auf die Gesundheit genutzt (Germov 2009; Engels 1845/1958). Es konnte gezeigt werden, wie das Streben nach immer mehr Profit durch die Bourgeoisie zur Ausbeutung der Arbeiter, gefährlichen Arbeitsbedingungen und ärmlichen Lebensbedingungen des Proletariats führt und dies wiederum in höheren Morbiditäts- sowie Mortalitätsraten der arbeitenden Klasse resultiert (Germov 2009; Engels 1845/1958). Auch heute hat dieser theoretische Strang überraschend wenig an Aktualität eingebüßt. Trotz ihrer bestehenden Aktualität und Anwendbarkeit auf derzeitige gesellschaftliche Entwicklungen (z. B bei der fortschreitenden Ökonomisierung des Gesundheitswesens, insbesondere bei den ökonomischen und strukturellen Veränderungen im Krankenhaussektor, die zu immer schlechter werdenden Arbeitsbedingungen der Beschäftigten in den Kliniken führen (Simon 2016)), wurde die Marxistische Theorie auch vielfach kritisiert. Insbesondere der ausschließliche Fokus auf die ökonomischen Einflussfaktoren sozialer Ungleichheiten und somit das außer Acht lassen anderer möglicher Determinanten stehen dabei im Mittelpunkt (Barry und Yuill 2012).

2.2 Strukturfunktionalismus

Der Strukturfunktionalismus gehört ebenfalls zu den strukturtheoretischen Ansätzen und beschäftigt sich in erster Linie mit der Frage, wie es Gesellschaften gelingt dauerhaft stabil zu bleiben und die soziale Ordnung beständig und auch unter sich wandelnden Bedingungen aufrecht zu erhalten (Germov 2009). Berühmte Vertreter sind z. B. Émile Durkheim (1858 bis 1917), Talcott Parsons (1902 bis 1972) und Robert Merton (1910 bis 2003) (Germov 2009). Der Strukturfunktionalismus geht davon aus, dass die Gesellschaft in unterschiedliche Subsysteme (z. B. soziales System, kulturelles System) unterteilt ist, die sich gegenseitig beeinflussen (Barry und Yuill 2012). Barry und

Yuill (2012) beschreiben in diesem Zusammenhang eine Analogie der struktur-funktionalistischen Sicht vom Aufbau einer Gesellschaft und eines biologischen Organismus: „Just as the body is made up of different but interrelated and inter-dependent parts, so society is made up of a number of different systems and subsystems." (Barry und Yuill 2012). Jedes einzelne Subsystem muss demnach seine Aufgaben erfüllen, um die Gesellschaft und soziale Ordnung aufrecht zu erhalten (Germov 2009; Cockerham 2013). Der Fokus des Strukturfunktionalis-mus liegt also in der Untersuchung der einzelnen gesellschaftlichen Subsysteme, um zu verstehen wie diese sich gegenseitig beeinflussen und zusammenwirken, um somit wiederum die Gesellschaft dauerhaft und stabil aufrecht zu erhalten (Germov 2009). Dabei geht es weniger um die Erforschung von Einstellungen oder Verhaltensweisen auf individueller Ebene, sondern vielmehr darum, wie diese die Subsysteme als Ganzes beeinflussen. So hat jedes Individuum ver-schiedene Funktionen oder Rollen zu erfüllen (z. B. die Elternrolle, die Rolle des Erwerbstätigen) und sozialen Erwartungen zu entsprechen (d. h. wie man sich in bestimmten Situationen rollenkonform verhält), um die gesellschaftliche Ordnung aufrecht zu erhalten (Barry und Yuill 2012).

Im Kontext von Gesundheit und Krankheit stellte Parsons heraus, dass soziale Rollen und Erwartungen nur erfüllt werden können, wenn das Individuum gesund ist. Er definierte damit Krankheit als eine Form der Abweichung von der Norm, die die Menschen davon abhält ihren alltäglichen Rollenerwartungen nachzu-kommen (Germov 2009). In diesem Zusammenhang hat Parsons das Konzept der „sick role" (Barry und Yuill 2012; Germov 2009) eingeführt, welches es dem „abweichenden" Individuum ermöglicht, aus seinen gewohnten Rollen zeitweilig „auszusteigen", um wieder gesund zu werden: „When a person takes on the ‚sick role', they are excused from their normal roles and responsibilities. The medical professions determines who is legitimately ‚sick'. This regulatory role ensures that not too many people are unable to fulfil their normal roles – otherwise illness would have a detrimental effect on the society as a whole." (Barry und Yuill 2012). Vor allem bei der Analyse von Arzt-Patienten-Beziehungen kommt dieses Konzept häufiger zum Einsatz, z. B. in Form von einer Krankschreibung und damit der Legitimation von der Rolle des Erwerbstätigen in diesem Zeitraum auszusetzen. Ein wichtiger Kritikpunkt an der „Rolle des Kranken" ist allerdings, dass bisher unklar ist in welcher Weise sie auf chronisch Erkrankte, dauerhaft Beeinträchtigte oder moribunde Patienten Anwendung finden kann (Germov 2009).

2.3   Symbolischer Interaktionismus

Der symbolische Interaktionismus gehört zu den handlungstheoretischen Ansätzen und fokussiert das individuelle Verhalten von Menschen und ihre Fähigkeit das eigene Leben sowie die Gesellschaft zu gestalten (Germov 2009). Berühmte Vertreter des symbolischen Interaktionismus sind zum Beispiel George Herbert Mead (1863 bis 1931), Anselm Strauss (1916 bis 1996) sowie Howard Becker (*1928) (Germov 2009). Die Grundannahme des symbolischen Interaktionismus ist, dass Menschen die soziale Wirklichkeit über Kommunikation, Sprache, Symbole und die jeweiligen Bedeutungszuschreibungen erzeugen (Germov 2009; Charmaz und Belgrave 2013). Die Theorie des symbolischen Interaktionismus beschäftigt sich also damit, wie Menschen ihre soziale Welt sehen, wahrnehmen und selbst gestalten, sie fokussiert damit weniger auf die Analyse größerer sozialer Systeme oder Strukturen (Barry und Yuill 2012). Im Kontext von Gesundheit und Krankheit macht der symbolische Interaktionismus deutlich, dass das was als „krank" oder das was als „gesund" gilt, subjektiv wahrgenommen und somit gesellschaftlich durch die handelnden Individuen konstruiert wird (Germov 2009). Solche Zuschreibungen können sich im Laufe der historischen Entwicklung maßgeblich ändern und unterscheiden sich zudem zwischen verschiedenen Kulturen. Wurde z. B. Homosexualität im vergangenen Jahrhundert noch als Krankheit verstanden, so ist dies heute in den westlichen Gesellschaften längst nicht mehr der Fall. Was sozial konstruiert als „krank" oder „gesund" wahrgenommen wird, ist zudem weniger abhängig von biologischen Faktoren (Germov 2009). Hier können die Analysen zu abweichendem Verhalten von Howard Becker herangezogen werden, um die Perspektive des symbolischen Interaktionismus deutlicher zu machen (Barry und Yuill 2012). Becker (2008) zeigt in seiner Definition von abweichendem Verhalten auf, dass das, was als abweichend bezeichnet wird, gesellschaftlich konstruiert ist und sich von Gruppe zu Gruppe oder auch Gesellschaft zu Gesellschaft unterscheiden kann. Folgt man also der Perspektive des symbolischen Interaktionismus, sind auch Gesundheit und Krankheit stets gesellschaftlich konstruiert und wandelbar. Bekannte Untersuchungsbereiche sind beispielsweise das subjektive Krankheitsempfinden oder aber auch die Arzt-Patient-Kommunikation (Germov 2009).

2.4   Feministische Theorie

Die feministische Theorie ist eine verhältnismäßig neue Theorie, die erst in den 1960er Jahren entstanden ist. Dabei existiert jedoch nicht *die* feministische Theorie, sondern sehr heterogene Strömungen, wie z. B. der liberale Feminismus, der radikale Feminismus oder der postmoderne Feminismus (Germov 2009). All diesen Theoriesträngen ist gemein, dass das Geschlecht – vor allem das weibliche – im Mittelpunkt der Untersuchung steht. Dem feministischen Ansatz liegt die Kritik zu Grunde, dass vorherige soziologische Theorien vor allem auf die Erforschung männlicher Akteure fokussierten und die Frau als Forschungsgegenstand tendenziell unterrepräsentiert war bzw. ist (Germov 2009). Germov (2009) weist zudem darauf hin, dass frühere theoretische Ansätze ein sexistisches Frauenbild vermitteln und führt dabei z. B. Parsons Rollenverständnis der Frau an, welche die gesellschaftlichen Aufgaben der Fürsorge für den Mann und die Familie zu erfüllen habe. Auch patriarchalische Gesellschaftsstrukturen und die Unterdrückung der Frauen werden stark kritisiert. Feministische Theorien beziehen sich also vor allem auf die Frage „What about the woman?" (Germov 2009) und stellen soziale Ungleichheiten zwischen Männern und Frauen in den Untersuchungsfokus. Im Kontext von Gesundheit und Krankheit finden feministische Theorien Anwendung in der Untersuchung gesundheitlicher Ungleichheiten zwischen Männern und Frauen, die nicht auf biologische, sondern eben auf soziale Unterschiede, z. B. ungleiche Arbeitsbedingungen oder die Doppelbelastung in Beruf und Familie, zurückzuführen sind (Germov 2009). Im Kontext unserer immer noch eher patriarchalisch ausgerichteten Gesellschaft verweisen Barry und Yuill (2012) zudem auf ein weiteres Untersuchungsfeld, in dem feministische Theorien Anwendung finden: „Particular examples can be seen in relation to pregnancy and childbirth, where what was previously seen as a ‚natural' event attended by women rapidly became the focus of medical intervention, and now principally takes place in hospital, with the profession of obstetrics being dominated by men." (Barry und Yuill 2012).

3   Das soziologische Modell von Gesundheit

Nachdem verschiedene soziologische Theorien, die zur Erforschung von Gesundheit und Krankheit genutzt werden können, erläutert wurden, soll im Folgenden spezifischer auf das soziologische Modell von Gesundheit im Vergleich zum biomedizinischen Modell eingegangen werden. Es sollen dabei die unterschiedlichen Perspektiven und Denkrichtungen gegenübergestellt werden. Tab. 1 stellt das biomedizinische und das soziale Modell zusammenfassend gegenüber. Hier wird beschrieben, welche unterschiedlichen Annahmen, Schwerpunkte oder auch Ursachen von Krankheiten jeweils angelegt werden als auch welche Kritik hierzu geäußert wurde. Einige Beispiele dieser differenzierten Betrachtungsweisen werden im Folgenden genauer erläutert.

In der Medizin herrscht als zentraler Erklärungs- und Therapieansatz von Gesundheit und Krankheit nach wie vor das biomedizinische Krankheitsmodell vor. Dieses widmet sich einer naturwissenschaftlichen Herangehensweise bei der Erklärung von Gesundheit und Krankheit und fand seinen Ursprung Ende des 19. Jahrhunderts (Roch und Hampel 2019). Dem biomedizinischen Modell – auch biologisches oder medizinisches Modell genannt – liegen Annahmen und Erkenntnisse der Bakteriologie der letzten Hälfte des 19. Jahrhunderts zu Grunde. Hierbei werden Krankheiten auf bestimmte Erreger, wie Keime und Bakterien, zurückgeführt und können damit einem kausalen Grund zugesprochen werden (Franke 2012). Menschen werden – dem biomedizinischen Modell folgend – vor allem als biologische Organismen verstanden. Krankheiten können nach diesem Verständnis durch die Untersuchung der Symptome erkannt und entsprechend therapiert werden.

Dieser Ansatz ist natürlich nicht falsch, er berücksichtigt pathophysiologische, biochemische und auch molekulargenetische Prozesse, die für die Entstehung und Entwicklung von Krankheiten essentiell sind (Franke 2012). Dennoch stößt das Modell auch an Grenzen, die im Folgenden aufgezeigt und zudem um weitere Perspektiven ergänzt werden sollen. Folgende Herausforderungen und Kritikpunkte an dem biomedizinischen Modell können angeführt werden (Richter und Hurrelmann 2016; Nettleton 2013; Germov 2009): Zum einen gibt es zwar Erkrankungen (z. B. Infektionskrankheiten), die auf *eine* Ursache zurückzuführen sind, der Großteil gegenwärtig vorherrschender Krankheiten in Industrienationen ist jedoch das Ergebnis *multifaktorieller* Ursachen, welche neben biomedizinischen Hintergründen auch soziale Faktoren einschließen. Zum anderen entspricht die Sichtweise auf Patienten nicht mehr dem aktuellen gesellschaftlichen Bild. Vorherrschend war die auf die Erkrankung (oder den Körper) reduzierte Sichtweise der Patienten als passive Objekte, anstatt den Patienten als ganzheitliche Person zu sehen. Darüber hinaus setzt sich auch zunehmend die Ansicht durch, dass Gesundheit nicht nur von den vermeintlichen Experten beurteilt werden kann, sondern dass auch „Laien" also die Menschen selbst ihre Erfahrungen und subjektive Interpretation über ihren Körper und ihre Gesundheit hegen und dies auch einen wichtigen Teilbereich darstellt. Eng verbunden ist damit auch ein weiterer Punkt, der steigenden Kosten des Gesundheitssystems.

Tab. 1 Das biomedizinische und soziale Modell von Gesundheit im Vergleich. (Quelle: Germov 2009: 17 zitiert nach Richter und Hurrelmann 2016: 12 f)

	Biomedizinische Modell	Soziales Modell
Fokus	• Individueller Fokus, akute Behandlung kranker Individuen	• Gesellschaftlicher Fokus, Lebens- und Arbeitsbedingungen, die Gesundheit beeinflussen
Annahmen	• Gesundheit und Krankheit sind objektive biologische Zustände • Individuelle Verantwortung für Gesundheit	• Gesundheit und Krankheit sind soziale Konstruktionen • Soziale Verantwortung für Gesundheit
Schlüsselindikatoren	• Individuelle Pathologie • Vererbung, Geschlecht (Sex), Alter • Risikofaktoren	• Soziale Ungleichheit • Soziale Gruppen: Klasse, Geschlecht, Migration, Alter, Beruf, Arbeitslosigkeit • Risikoinduzierende Faktoren
Ursachen von Erkrankungen	• Gendefekte und Mikroorganismen (Viren/Bakterien) • Trauma (Unfälle) • Verhalten/Lebensstil	• Politische/ökonomische Faktoren: Verteilung von Wohlstand, Einkommen, Macht, Armut • Beschäftigungsfaktoren: arbeits- und bildungsbezogene Möglichkeiten, stressreiche und gefährliche Arbeit • Kulturelle und strukturelle Faktoren
Intervention	• Individuelle Behandlung durch Chirurgie und Pharmazie • Verhaltensmodifikation • Gesundheitserziehung und Immunisierung	• Öffentliche Politik • Interventionen des Staates zur Stärkung von Gesundheit und Abbau von sozialen Ungleichheiten • Community, Partizipation, Anwaltschaft und Lobbyismus

(Fortsetzung)

Tab. 1 (Fortsetzung)

	Biomedizinische Modell	Soziales Modell
Kritik	• Ein Fokus auf Krankheiten führt zu einem Mangel an präventiven Maßnahmen • Reduktionistisch; ignoriert die Komplexität von Gesundheit und Krankheit • Scheitert an der Berücksichtigung der sozialen Ursachen von Gesundheit und Krankheit • Expertenmeinung kann das „victim blaming" verstärken	• Utopisches Ziel von Gleichheit führt zu nicht umsetzbaren Forderungen sozialen Wandels • Überbetonung der schädigenden Nebeneffekte der Biomedizin • Die vorgeschlagenen Lösungen können sehr komplex und schwierig in der kurzfristigen Implementation sein • Soziologische Vorstellungen können die individuelle Verantwortung und psychologische Faktoren unterschätzen

So wird argumentiert, dass die Wirksamkeit der biomedizinischen Herangehensweise zur Behandlung und Reduzierung von Krankheiten überschätzt wird. Hier ist die evidenzbasierte Medizin gefragt, die an Bedeutung gewinnt.

Aus dieser Kritik heraus wird deutlich, dass es die soziologische Sichtweise ebenso braucht, um die Entstehung und Vermeidung von Krankheiten besser verstehen zu können und um gleichzeitig zu untersuchen, wie Gesundheit gefördert werden kann (siehe soziales Modell in Tab. 1). Das soziale Modell von Gesundheit und Krankheit betrachtet die gesellschaftlichen Bedingungen, in denen Menschen leben und arbeiten, statt die alleinige Verantwortung beim Individuum zu sehen. Während im biomedizinischen Modell vor allem die pathologischen und biologischen Prozesse als auch Risikofaktoren (z. B. Tabakkonsum) im Mittelpunkt stehen, so fokussiert das soziale Modell vor allem den sozialen Kontext und soziale Ungleichheiten, die zu einer Ungleichverteilung von Gesundheit und Krankheit führen (Richter und Hurrelmann 2016). Damit ist gemeint, dass jene mit einem hohen sozialen Status (hohe Bildung, hohes Einkommen, hohe berufliche Position) insgesamt eine bessere Gesundheit aufweisen, als jene mit niedrigem Sozialstatus. Damit ist beispielsweise gemeint, dass jene mit einem hohen sozialen Status (hohe Bildung, hohes Einkommen, hohe berufliche Position) weniger gesundheitsschädlichen Wohn- und Arbeitsbedingungen ausgesetzt sind, mehr psychosoziale Ressourcen (u. a. soziale Unterstützung, personale Kompetenzen) und weniger Risikoverhaltensweisen aufweisen, die letztlich zu einer besseren gesundheitlichen Lage führen (Granström et al. 2015; Lampert et al. 2019; Lampert et al. 2016; Marmot und Wilkinson 2001; Moor et al. 2017; Pförtner und Moor 2017) (Tab. 1).

Der soziologische Blick berücksichtigt also die sozialen Verhältnisse, ebenso wie die risiko-induzierenden Faktoren, d. h. jene Faktoren, die zu Risikofaktoren führen. Selbstverständlich gibt es auch beim sozialen Modell Kritikpunkte, wie beispielsweise, dass die WHO Gesundheit als „vollständigen körperlichen, psychischen und sozialen Wohlbefindens" definiert, welcher nicht erreicht werden kann. Daher sollte es eher als Idealvorstellung angesehen werden.

4 Fazit

In den letzten 150 Jahren hat die Medizin- und Gesundheitssoziologie herausragende Erkenntnisse über die sozialen Dimensionen von Gesundheit und Krankheit hervorgebracht. Der vorliegende Beitrag hat gezeigt, dass die Soziologie dabei wichtige Theorien zur Erforschung von Gesundheit und Krankheit zur Verfügung stellt. Neben strukturtheoretischen Ansätzen, welche den Einfluss der Gesellschaft auf das individuelle Handeln untersuchen, wurden auch handlungstheoretische Ansätze vorgestellt, die den Zusammenhang des Individuums auf die Gesellschaft fokussieren. Im Mittelpunkt standen dabei einige der bekanntesten soziologischen Theorien und Perspektiven, welche bei der Erforschung von Gesundheit und Krankheit Anwendung finden. Beispielhaft wurde zusammenfassend auf Klassiker, wie materialistische Theorien bzw. den Marxismus, die Strukturtheorie und den Strukturfunktionalismus, den symbolischen Interaktionismus sowie die moderne feministische Theorie eingegangen. Zudem wurden wichtige Untersuchungsschwerpunkte der Medizin- und Gesundheitssoziologie angerissen. Das gesamte Themenspektrum ist jedoch noch um ein Vielfaches größer und differenzierter, weswegen hier nur erste Einblicke in die soziologische Perspektive von Gesundheit und Krankheit gegeben werden können. Weitere Forschungsthemen, die im vorliegenden Beitrag nicht zur Sprache gekommen sind, sind zum Beispiel medizinische Technologien und ihre gesellschaftlichen Konsequenzen, die Bioethik sowie die Prävention und Gesundheitsförderung. Der Beitrag konnte zudem zeigen, dass die Untersuchungsschwerpunkte der Soziologie – speziell der Medizin- und Gesundheitssoziologie – nicht auf der biomedizinischen Sichtweise der medizinischen Behandlung oder Heilung einer Krankheit oder „beeinträchtigten" Gesundheit liegen, sondern vielmehr auf den sozialen Faktoren, Ursachen und Kontexten von Gesundheit und Krankheit (Richter 2014). Dazu wurde auch auf das Verständnis der naturwissenschaftlich dominierten Medizin eingegangen und dem biomedizinischen Modell das soziale Modell von Gesundheit gegenübergestellt. Auch das Wohlbefinden spielt im Kontext von Gesundheit und Krankheit eine immer bedeutsamere Rolle. Es zeigt sich jedoch, dass die zur Verfügung stehenden soziologischen Theorien sich eher auf „Gesundheit und Krankheit" als auf das Wohlbefinden fokussieren. Obwohl Wohlbefinden oftmals in Bezug zu Gesundheit gesetzt wird, wird dieses Konstrukt jedoch noch zu selten genutzt und definiert und es bleibt vage, was Wohlbefinden aus soziologischer Perspektive genau ist.

Das Konstrukt des Wohlbefindens muss also zukünftig stärker in den Vordergrund gerückt werden, denn bei der Beurteilung von Gesundheit spielen aus soziologischer Sicht weniger objektive Befunde von Krankheiten eine Rolle, sondern vielmehr steht die subjektive Wahrnehmung im Mittelpunkt. Auch bezüglich des Wohlbefindens steht dies im Vordergrund „denn wer diagnostiziert krank ist, kann sich nichtsdestotrotz gesund *fühlen* (vice versa)." (Ohlbrecht und Winkler 2018, S. 3). Während eine Erkrankung oftmals durch Symptome objektivier- und messbar ist, verhält es sich mit der Gesundheit und ebenso mit dem Wohlbefinden anders, da es sich hier um die individuelle Wahrnehmung des Individuums handelt (Ohlbrecht und Winkler 2018). Insgesamt herrscht in der Wissenschaft noch kein Konsens darüber, wie Wohlbefinden und (subjektive) Gesundheit definiert werden (Hornberg 2016; Erhart et al. 2009), vielmehr existieren eine Bandbreite an verschiedenen Konzepten und Konstrukten, die, je nach Fachdisziplin und theoretischen Annahmen, ähnliche Komponenten umfassen. Mittlerweile ist die Literatur so stark angewachsen und die Dimensionen so divers, dass Pollard und Lee (2003) bereits von einer „confusing and contradicotry research base" sprechen. Dodge et al. (2012) betiteln ihre Übersichtsarbeit zu den Definitionen und der Beschreibung von Wohlbefinden nicht ohne Grund als „The challenge of defining wellbeing". In der Soziologie scheint die Forschung zu Wohlbefinden im Vergleich zu anderen Wissenschaften jedoch noch verhältnismäßig rückständig (Veenhoven 2008), auch wenn hier das Forschungsinteresse in den vergangenen Jahren angestiegen ist und z. B. in Bereichen wie der Erwerbstätigkeit (Arbeits- und Einkommenszufriedenheit) eingesetzt wird. Hier spielt vor allem die Zufriedenheit mit unterschiedlichen Lebensbereichen eine wichtige Rolle.

Zusammenfassend öffnet die Medizin- und Gesundheitssoziologie jedoch den Diskurs und zeigt, dass Gesundheit mehr als nur die Abwesenheit von Krankheit bedeutet und der Fokus vermehrt zu einer Berücksichtigung der subjektiven

Bewertung von Gesundheit und Wohlbefinden gelenkt wird. Es gibt mittlerweile eine Bandbreite an Beschreibungen und Dimensionen von Wohlbefinden, weniger gelungen ist es bislang eine eindeutige Definition von Wohlbefinden zu finden. Zukünftige Aufgabe der Medizin- und Gesundheitssoziologie, welche eine unverzichtbare Ergänzung des biowissenschaftlichen Forschungsprogramms der Medizin darstellt (Richter 2014; Richter und Hurrelmann 2016), ist es also das Konzept des Wohlbefindens stärker in den Kontext von Gesundheit und Krankheit zu integrieren sowie auch zu definieren.

Literatur

Barry, Anne-Marie; Yuill, Chris (2012). Understanding the sociology of health. An introduction. 3. ed. Los Angeles, Calif.: SAGE.
Becker, H. S. (2008). Outsiders. Studies in the sociology of deviance. New York: Free Press.
Bittlingmayer, Uwe H. (2016). Strukturorientierte Perspektiven auf Gesundheit und Krankheit. In: Matthias Richter und Klaus Hurrelmann (Hg.). Soziologie von Gesundheit und Krankheit. 1. Auflage. Wiesbaden: Springer VS (Lehrbuch), S. 23–40.
Bourdieu, Pierre (1982). Die feinen Unterschiede. Kritik der gesellschaftlichen Urteilskraft. Frankfurt/Main: Suhrkamp.
Charmaz, Kathy; Belgrave, Linda Liska (2013). Modern Symbolic Interaction Theory and Health. In: William C. Cockerham (Hg.). Medical Sociology on the Move. New Directions in Theory. Dordrecht: Springer, S. 11–39.
Cockerham, William C. (2013). Social causes of health and disease. Second edition. Cambridge, Malden: Polity.
Diener, Ed; Ryan, Katherine (2009). Subjective Well-Being. A General Overview. In: *South African Journal of Psychology* 39 (4), S. 391–406. DOI: https://doi.org/10.1177/008124630903900402.
Dodge, Rachel; Daly, Annette; Huyton, Jan; Sanders, Lalage (2012). The challenge of defining wellbeing. In. *Intnl. J. Wellbeing* 2 (3), S. 222–235. DOI: https://doi.org/10.5502/ijw.v2i3.4.
Engels, F. (1845/1958). The condition of the working class in England. Trans. W. O. Henderson & W.H. Chaloner. Oxford: Basil Blackwell.
Erhart, Michael; Wille, Nora; Ravens-Sieberer, Ulrike (2009). Die Messung der subjektiven Gesundheit. Stand der Forschung und Herausforderungen. In: Matthias Richter und Klaus Hurrelmann (Hg.). Gesundheitliche Ungleichheit: Grundlagen, Probleme, Perspektiven. Wiesbaden: VS Verlag für Sozialwissenschaften, S. 335–352. Online verfügbar unter https://doi.org/10.1007/978-3-531-91643-9_19.
Franke, Alexa (2012). Modelle von Gesundheit und Krankheit. 3., überarb. Aufl. Bern: Huber (Programmbereich Gesundheit). Online verfügbar unter http://sub-hh.ciando.com/book/?bok_id=471889.
Germov, John (2009). Second opinion: an introduction to health sociology. 4. Aufl. Victoria: Oxford University Press.

Giddens, A.; Griffiths, S. (2005). Sociology. Cambridge: Polity Press.

Granström, Fredrik; Molarius, Anu; Garvin, Peter; Elo, Sirkka; Feldman, Inna; Kristenson, Margareta (2015). Exploring trends in and determinants of educational inequalities in self-rated health. In: *Scandinavian journal of public health* 43 (7), S. 677–686. DOI: https://doi.org/10.1177/1403494815592271.

Hornberg, Claudia (2016). Gesundheit und Wohlbefinden. In: Ulrich Gebhard und Thomas Kistemann (Hg.) Landschaft, Identität und Gesundheit. Zum Konzept der therapeutischen Landschaften. Wiesbaden: Springer VS, S. 63–69.

Lampert, Thomas; Hoebel, Jens; Kuntz, Benjamin; Waldhauer, Julia (2019). Soziale Ungleichheit und Gesundheit. In. Robin Haring (Hg.). Gesundheitswissenschaften. Berlin, Heidelberg: Springer Berlin Heidelberg, S. 155–164. Online verfügbar unter https://doi.org/10.1007/978-3-662-58314-2_14.

Lampert, Thomas; Kroll, Lars Eric; Kuntz, Benjamin; Hoebel, Jens (2018). Gesundheitliche Ungleichheit in Deutschland und im internationalen Vergleich. Zeitliche Entwicklungen und Trends. In. Journal of Health Monitoring, Bd. 3: Robert Koch-Institut, Epidemiologie und Gesundheitsberichterstattung.

Lampert, Thomas; Richter, Matthias; Schneider, Sven; Spalek, Jacob; Dragano, Nico (2016). Soziale Ungleichheit und Gesundheit. Stand und Perspektiven der sozial-epidemiologischen Forschung in Deutschland. In. *Bundesgesundheitsblatt, Gesundheitsforschung, Gesundheitsschutz* 59 (2), S. 153–165. DOI: https://doi.org/10.1007/s00103-015-2275-6.

Marmot, M.; Wilkinson, R. G. (2001). Psychosocial and material pathways in the relation between income and health: a response to Lynch et al. In. *BMJ (Clinical research ed.)* 322 (7296), S. 1233–1236. DOI: https://doi.org/10.1136/bmj.322.7296.1233

Mills, C. Wright (1959). The sociological imagination. New York: Oxford University Press.

Moor, Irene; Spallek, Jacob; Richter, Matthias (2017). Explaining socioeconomic inequalities in self-rated health. A systematic review of the relative contribution of material, psychosocial and behavioural factors. In. *Journal of epidemiology and community health* 71 (6), S. 565–575. DOI: https://doi.org/10.1136/jech-2016-207589.

Nettleton, Sarah (2013). The sociology of health and illness. Third edition. Cambridge, Malden: Polity Press.

Ohlbrecht, Heike; Winkler, Torsten (2018). Gesundheit und Wohlbefinden im Kindes- und Jugendalter. In. Andreas Lange, Herwig Reiter, Sabina Schutter und Christine Steiner (Hg.). Handbuch Kindheits- und Jugendsoziologie. Wiesbaden: Springer Fachmedien Wiesbaden, S. 607–618. Online verfügbar unter https://doi.org/10.1007/978-3-658-04207-3_67.

Pförtner, Timo-Kolja; Moor, Irene (2017). Wie kommt die Gesellschaft unter die Haut? Eine Mediatoranalyse gesundheitlicher Ungleichheit mit den Daten des Sozioökonomischen Panels 2011. In. *Psychotherapie, Psychosomatik, medizinische Psychologie* 67 (1), S. 9–18. DOI: https://doi.org/10.1055/s-0042-116153.

Pollard, Elizabeth L.; Lee, Patrice D. (2003). Child Well-being: A Systematic Review of the Literature. In. *Social Indicators Research* 61 (1), S. 59–78. DOI: https://doi.org/10.1023/A:1021284215801.

Richter, Matthias (2014). Medizin- und Gesundheitssoziologie. In. Günter Endruweit, Gisela Trommsdorff und Nicole Burzan (Hg.). Wörterbuch der Soziologie. 3., völlig überarb. Aufl. Konstanz, Stuttgart: UVK-Verl.-Ges; UTB (UTB, 8566), S. 287–293.

Richter, Matthias; Hurrelmann, Klaus (2016). Die soziologische Perspektive auf Gesundheit und Krankheit. In. Matthias Richter und Klaus Hurrelmann (Hg.). Soziologie von Gesundheit und Krankheit. 1. Auflage. Wiesbaden: Springer VS (Lehrbuch), S. 1–19.

Roch, Svenja; Hampel, Petra (2019). Modelle von Gesundheit und Krankheit. In. Robin Haring (Hg.): Gesundheitswissenschaften. Berlin, Heidelberg: Springer Berlin Heidelberg, S. 247–255. Online verfügbar unter https://doi.org/10.1007/978-3-662-58314-2_23.

Schäfers, Bernhard (2016). Einführung in die Soziologie. 2. Auflage. Wiesbaden: Springer VS (Lehrbuch). Online verfügbar unter https://doi.org/10.1007/978-3-658-13699-4.

Simon, Michael (2016). Die ökonomischen und strukturellen Veränderungen des Krankenhausbereichs seit den 1970er Jahren. In: Ingo Bode und Werner Vogd (Hg.). Mutationen des Krankenhauses. Soziologische Diagnosen in organisations- und gesellschaftstheoretischer Perspektive. Wiesbaden: Springer VS (Gesundheit und Gesellschaft), S. 29–45.

Sperlich, Stefanie (2016). Handlungsorientierte Perspektiven auf Gesundheit und Krankheit. In. Matthias Richter und Klaus Hurrelmann (Hg.). Soziologie von Gesundheit und Krankheit. 1. Auflage. Wiesbaden: Springer VS (Lehrbuch), S. 41–54.

Treibel, Annette (2006). Einführung in soziologische Theorien der Gegenwart. 7., aktualisierte Aufl. Wiesbaden: VS Verl. für Sozialwiss (Einführungskurs Soziologie, / hrsg. von Hermann Korte …; Bd. 3).

Veenhoven, Ruut (2008). Sociological Theories of subjective well-being. In. Michael Eid und Randy J. Larsen (Hg.). The science of subjective well-being. New York: Guilford Press, S. 44–61.

Weltgesundheitsorganisation (2013). Zusammenfassung. Der Europäische Gesundheitsbericht 2020. Ein Wegweiser zu mehr Wohlbefinden. Hg. v. Regionalbüro für Europa.

White, Kevin (2009). An introduction to the sociology of health and illness. 2.ed. Los Angeles: SAGE.

WHO (World Health Organization) (1946). Preamble to the Constitution of the World Health Organization. http://www.who.int/about/definition/en/print.html (Zugegriffen: 07. Februar 2015).

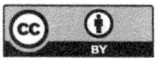

Economic Perspectives on Individual Well-being

Liyousew Borga, Conchita D'Ambrosio
und Anthony Lepinteur

1 Introduction

Individual well-being is a central concept of Economics, and there are several approaches for its measurement and inclusion in studies investigating its determinants and consequences on behaviour. In this chapter we will focus on the analysis of the contributions in the so-called income distribution literature and economics of happiness. The two are related since they examine what are there known as "objective" and "subjective" aspects of well-being, that are respectively what the analyst thinks individual well-being is, based on command over economic resources, and what the individual herself says it is, when asked to report on it. The distinction between objective and subjective well-being is by no means a distinction between reality and imagination, as well-being is always an experience made by the individual. Economists use these two terms to simply distinguish between measures of well-being computed by the analyst from the command the individual has over economic resources, and measures of well-being that are stated by the individual directly when asked to report on it. In this chapter devoted to Economics we will analyse both in details and refer to it as custom in the literature.

L. Borga (✉) · C. D'Ambrosio · A. Lepinteur
Department of Behavioural and Cognitive Sciences, University of Luxembourg,
Esch-sur-Alzette, Luxembourg
E-Mail: Liyousew.Borga@uni.lu

C. D'Ambrosio
E-Mail: Conchita.Dambrosio@uni.lu

A. Lepinteur
E-Mail: Anthony.Lepinteur@uni.lu

© Der/die Autor(en) 2022
A. Heinen et al. (Hrsg.), *Wohlbefinden und Gesundheit im Jugendalter,*
https://doi.org/10.1007/978-3-658-35744-3_4

45

Traditionally, economists have dealt with the question of well-being through the lens of the concept of utility. Assuming that individuals are rational and fully informed, and seek to maximise utility, economists inferred the well-being of individuals from the decisions that they make (the revealed preferences) and from their behaviour. However, a burgeoning strand of the literature in Economics utilizes self-reported well-being as an indicator of economic and social progress. In this chapter, we provide a detailed review of this literature. We first outline the different measures of subjective well-being used by the literature and we assess the nature and cross-cultural validity of these measures. Second, a theoretical framework that serves as a basis for empirical analysis of subjective well-being is set. We then review the most influential articles exploring the determinants of subjective well-being. The last part of our chapter presents a summary of the evidence regarding the behaviour of happy people. We conclude with measures of objective well-being from the income distribution literature, such as uni-dimensional and multidimensional poverty.

2 "Subjective" Well-being in Economics: Measurement, Objectives and Limits

2.1 Measurement of Subjective Well-being in Economics

There are two main types of measures of subjective well-being in Economics. The first type of subjective well-being measures is cognitive (or evaluative).[1] Individuals are directly asked to make statements about how well their life is going. The objective of the cognitive measures of well-being is to capture the reflective process of an individual judging herself, her satisfaction with respect to her life, or a particular aspect of it. The most popular cognitive measures of well-being in Economics are the Cantril Ladder and the life-satisfaction question. The first one is usually stated as follows: *Please imagine a ladder with steps numbered from 0 at the bottom to 10 at the top. The top of the ladder represents the best possible life for you and the bottom of the ladder represents the worst possible life for you. On which step of the ladder would you say you personally*

---

[1] Note that the terminology differs from Psychology as the term cognitive by itself usually refers to basic cognitive processes such as attention or memory. What economists call "cognitive" is what psychologists would call "meta-cognitive".

feel you stand at this time?" The life-satisfaction question is generally stated as follows: *"How satisfied are you with your life, all things considered?"* The scale the respondents use to answer this question varies across surveys. For instance, in the British Household Panel Survey, the life-satisfaction question's scale goes from one to seven while it goes from zero to ten in the German Socio Economic Panel. Similar questions are also used to measure the satisfaction of individuals regarding different domains of life such as work, finance or family life.

The second type of self-reported well-being measures is referred to as affective (or hedonic) well-being and refers to a specific point in time. There are two types of affective measures of well-being: positive affect and negative affect. The former includes elements such as the frequency of experiencing positive feelings or smiling; the latter encompasses negative emotions (stress, anxiety etc.). Contrary to evaluative measures, affective well-being are not supposed to capture a reflective process but a personal emotional state at a precise moment. Questions measuring affect usually are of the following kind: *"From 0–6, where a 0 means you were not stressed at all and a 6 means you were very stressed, how stressed did you feel during this time?"* The U-index is one of the most-used measures of affect in the literature. This index, going from 0 to 1, represents the proportion of time spent in activities where negative feelings were more intense than positive feelings during a given day. As they usually concern a particular moment or activity, affective well-being is more sensitive to variations in the short-run than evaluative measures.

2.2 Measurement Issues and Reliability

The conditions of the collection of subjective well-being data has been shown to be important. In Conti and Pudney (2011), the level of satisfaction reported by survey respondents is on average higher during oral interviews as compared to computer-assisted self-interviews and when children are present during the interview. It confirms that self-reported scores of well-being are likely to be inflated because of a social desirability bias. In the same study, Conti and Pudney (2011) demonstrate that the presence of the interviewee's partner during the interview lowers the level of reported satisfaction. This is seen by the authors as a way for the respondent to maintain a strong bargaining power in the household. The date of the interview as well as the question ordering (Deaton 2012) are also crucial and potential sources of biases. One may also raise conceptual questions such as the issues of cardinality or inter-personal comparisons.

Economists, however, have extensively discussed these various issues and the validity of the well-being measures.

There are two important elements to note regarding the reliability of measures of subjective well-being. First, both cognitive and hedonic measures of subjective well-being are highly correlated (Clark 2016). Albeit they are measured using different questions, different scales and they refer to different time horizons, the relatively high levels of correlation between these two families of measures mean that they are arguably capturing the same concept, i.e. well-being. Note also that the different measures of subjective well-being also share a large set of determinants. Nevertheless, cognitive and hedonic measures of well-being are never perfectly correlated; this is expected as they are meant to measure aspects of well-being that are arguably different.

Second, experimental studies confirm that measures like life satisfaction capture the concept of well-being. Using a series of hypothetical pairwise-choice scenarios, Benjamin et al. (2012) show that options that are perceived by individuals as the better choice in terms of life satisfaction score are also those they would choose in real life in roughly 80% of the cases.

Convergent validity tests have been performed too. One of the most famous examples is the cross-rating exercise: in Pavot and Diener (1993), the level of correlation between the interviewer ratings and self-ratings goes from 0.43 to 0.66. In the same study, one can find that family members and friends are also able to predict accurately the happiness of the main respondent.

The question of the interpersonal comparability of subjective well-being has been addressed in various ways. First, most of the researchers in Economics make use of longitudinal dataset to run within-regressions. This estimation method focuses on individual changes (within-variation) and neutralises differences between individuals (between-variance). It is also possible to neutralise a variety of reporting biases using longitudinal data (e.g. questionnaire changes, bias due to the day of the interview). Last, it is worth mentioning that individuals tend to use the scales of subjective well-being measures in a comparable since observed behaviours can be predicted by levels of happiness in cross-section (Clark 2001; O'Connor, 2020).

3   The Use of Subjective Well-being Data in Economics: Theoretical Considerations

Theoretical models in Economics are based on the concept of utility. Utility can be interpreted as a measure of satisfaction an individual derives from the consumption of commodities. It usually takes the following form: U = U(X) where U is the utility that depends on the vector of determinants X. While the use of utility as a theoretical tool is widespread, its empirical measurement is problematic. According to Marshall (1920) and Samuelson (1938), utility cannot be directly measured but it can be indirectly observed from individual choices. This is what economists call the *revealed preferences* approach.

The use of subjective well-being in Economics in the past forty years can be seen as an alternative way of measuring utility. According to Hirschauer et al. (2015), considering subjective well-being as a proxy for utility brings utility back to its utilitarian definition. Bentham (1789) stated that *"Nature has placed mankind under the governance of two sovereign masters, pain and pleasure. It is for them alone to point out what we ought to do, [...]. By the principle of utility is meant that principle which approves or disapproves of every action whatsoever according to the tendency it appears to have to augment or diminish the happiness of the party whose interest is in question: [...]. I say of every action whatsoever, and therefore not only of every action of a private individual, but of every measure of government."* According to Bentham, the empirical measure of utility, or *"felicific utility"*, should incorporate different elements such as the intensity of pain and pleasures as well as their duration. Subjective well-being data arguably appear as a proxy for the measurement of the utility a la Bentham.

The standard approach in applied Economics is to use large databases and econometrics methods to estimate the following model:

$$SWB_{it} = \beta' X_{it} + \varepsilon_{it}$$

where SWB_{it}, the subjective well-being of an individual (or a country) i at time t. The objective of this type of model is to estimate to what extent a given vector of characteristics, X_{it}, influences significantly the utility function. It might also be used to estimate empirically marginal rates of substitution and to test for the existence of concepts such as the interdependence of utilities.

4   The Easterlin Paradox and the Concept
         of Relative Utility

Richard Easterlin is one of the first researchers who brought measures of
subjective well-being to academic research in the field of Economics. The so-
called 'Easterlin Paradox' (1974, 1995) suggested that, despite substantial real
income growth in Japan and Western countries over time, average happiness
levels remained roughly constant. This paradox seems to contradict causal
evidence and a parallel body of work that has shown three main facts: 1) within
each country at a single point in time, richer individuals are more satisfied with
their life (Blanchflower and Oswald 2004; Graham and Pettinato 2002). This
correlation holds both for developed and developing countries. 2) Using panel
data to control for individual fixed effects, Winkelmann and Winkelmann (1998),
Ferrer-i-Carbonell (2005) and others concluded that not only the level of income
matters, but also changes in income are positively correlated with changes in
life satisfaction. Within this framework, Frijters et al. (2004) established the
causal impact of income changes exploiting quasi-natural experiments. 3) Life
satisfaction is also positively correlated with macroeconomic variables such as
GDP in very large cross-time cross-country samples (Di Tella et al. 2003; Alesina
et al. 2004). One way to reconcile the above evidence on the positive relation
between income and life satisfaction with the Easterlin Paradox is to consider the
existence of a relative component in the utility function (Clark et al. 2008). This
means that income is evaluated relative to others or to oneself in the past.

The standard *comparison effect* states that individuals report on average lower
levels of well-being when the income of their peers increases. Defining who
the peers (or the reference group) are is crucial here. The standard approach in
Economics is to consider that individuals with the same age, the same sex, the
same education or living in the same region can be seen as peers. Using wage
regressions to estimate the comparison income, Clark and Oswald (1996) show
that a similar increase in own income and comparison income has no effect on
well-being: the positive effect of the former is totally reduced by the negative
effect of the latter. With a similar method but different datasets, Sloane and
Williams (2000) and Levy-Garboua and Montmarquette (2004) confirmed that
comparison income is negatively correlated with job satisfaction. The literature
in Economics also extensively used cell averages to estimate the comparison
income (McBride 2001; Blanchflower and Oswald 2004; Ferrer-i-Carbonell
2005; Luttmer 2005; Graham and Felton 2006). While these articles use data
from different countries, different periods, and define the reference group in

various ways, they all confirm that the lower the comparison income, the higher the own well-being. Card et al. (2012) address causality issues by exploiting a quasi-natural experiment setting. The state of California made the salary of any state employee public knowledge and a local newspaper set up a website to ease the access to this information. Card et al. (2012) informed a random subset of employees of three different campuses at the University of California about the existence of the website. Some days later, Card et al. (2012) surveyed all the employees from the three campuses and found that the informed employees whose wage was lower than their colleagues (defined as co-workers in the same occupation group and administrative unit) reported lower level of job satisfaction and a higher probability to quit. Note that they found no effect for employees at the top of the wage distribution.

A second bulk of the literature documents a positive relationship between one's own well-being and the comparison income (Senik 2004; Clark et al. 2009). This phenomenon is referred as the *information effect.* Here researchers follow Hirshman's (1973) interpretation and appeal to the information content that economic advances of others have: the presence of richer individuals signals that there is a possibility for oneself to get richer in the future, which increases own happiness even before any actual enrichment takes place. On this point see also D'Ambrosio and Frick (2012). These authors incorporate in the analysis the effects of time, that is of passing and being passed by others and, relying on panel data from Germany, they show that comparison and signal effects can coexist: the first is found with respect to those whose relative position did not change over time, while those who moved play an information role.

We also know that comparisons are not only interpersonal but also intra-personal. Using panel data, Clark (1999) and Grund and Sliwka (2007) show that past level of income has a negative effect on current well-being. Using German data, Di Tella et al. (2010) find that most of the effect on an increase in income vanishes after a year. *Habituation* refers to the evidence that people adapt to having more income, a phenomenon known as hedonic adaptation, or hedonic treadmill (see Lyubomirsky 2011, for an excellent survey).

5 The Main Individual Determinants of Well-being

5.1 Unemployment

Unemployment is probably the most widely studied of all personal characteristics, after income. The standard microeconomic model assumes that utility only depends on consumption and leisure, and labour affects utility only indirectly, i.e. it increases consumption but reduces leisure. In this model, unemployment is seen as voluntary. Consequently, we shall expect no effect of unemployment on well-being once controlling for income. The empirical literature, however, unanimously confirms that, keeping income constant, unemployment does reduce well-being. This is true both in cross-sections and panels (Clark and Oswald 1994; Winkelmann and Winkelmann 1998; Dolan et al. 2008; Frey and Stutzer 2010). Kassenboehmer and Haisken-DeNew (2009) used plant-closure as natural experiments and found similar results. Those findings are important because they suggest that unemployment is mostly involuntary.

Past unemployment also affects well-being today. This *scarring effect* has been extensively discussed (see Clark et al. 2001; Bell and Blanchflower 2011). In a recent work, Clark and Lepinteur (2019) find that the overall unemployment experience between the end of full-time education and age 30 significantly reduces life satisfaction at age 30.

The unemployment of other people matters too. Clark (2003) showed that the effect of unemployment on well-being is smaller for those with an unemployed partner or who live in higher-unemployment regions. He also showed that those whose well-being fell the most on entering unemployment leave unemployment faster, consistent with hysteresis in unemployment.

Having a job significantly increases well-being but job characteristics are of importance too. Job security is one of the most important job characteristics (Clark 2001). The more protected the better but, as income, relative job security matters (Clark and Postel-Vinay 2009; Georgieff and Lepinteur 2018). The effect of working time has been widely discussed as well. Correlational studies yield contradictory evidence but Loog and Collewet (2014) used an instrumental variable approach to estimate the causal impact of work-week length on life satisfaction. They conclude that working time has an inversed-U shaped effect and the optimal work-week length is just below 30 h. Lepinteur (2019a) confirms this finding by showing that mandatory reductions in working time in France (from 39 h per week to 35) and in Portugal (from 44 h per week to 40) increased the well-being of workers. Once again, relative working time also influences well-being (Booth and Van Ours 2008; Collewet et al. 2017, Lepinteur 2019b).

5.2   Health

Layard et al. (2014) and Clark et al. (2019) developed a life-course model of well-being and demonstrate that the most important determinant of well-being is health. Dolan et al. (2008) show that both physical and mental health matters. Shields and Price (2005) find that the levels of well-being reported after a heart attack or a stroke are on average lower. Well-being is positively correlated with life expectancy (Danner et al. 2001) and negatively correlated with cardiovascular diseases (Steptoe et al. 2015).

Using longitudinal data, Oswald and Powdthavee (2008) show that individuals adapt only partially to negative health shocks, e.g. disability. While severe disability reduces well-being immediately, there is no full recovery in terms of well-being during the three subsequent years. Moreover, Clark et al. (2019) find that living with an ill partner reduces well-being.

5.3   Marital Status

Married individuals are found to be happier than the rest of the population in a variety of studies (see Stutzer and Frey 2006, for an excellent review). Their higher level of happiness, however, does not come from marriage per se. In Clark and Georgellis (2013), it appears that the positive effect of getting married fades away after the first 3 years. The observed premium in happiness among married individuals comes from the absence of adaptation to partnership.

In the same study, Clark and Georgellis (2013) show that divorce brings back individuals to the average level of happiness of the rest of the population. Widowhood has a negative impact on well-being that does not last.

5.4   Education

There is no consensus in the Economics literature about the effect of education on well-being (Blanchflower and Oswald 2004; Stutzer 2004). Using mandatory increases in school-leaving age as natural experiments to address endogeneity concerns, Oreopoulos and Salvanes (2011) report that education has a positive effect on well-being in the US while Clark and Jung (2017) found no effect in the UK. One way to explain such results is to consider that not only education increases earnings, but it also raises expectations (Clark et al. 2015). Using

Australian data, Nikolaev (2018) showed that the reference group education is negatively correlated with well-being. This result is robust to a variety of definitions of the reference group and goes beyond the effect of relative income: this suggests that a higher education-level has the role of a desirable social status. Note that individuals with high levels of education are less prone to comparisons. Clark et al. (2019) replicated this analysis with British, German and American data and confirmed these results.

5.5   Age and Sex

One of the most stable findings in the literature is the U-shape curve between well-being and age (Gerdtham and Johannesson 2001; Hayo and Seifert 2003; Blanchflower and Oswald 2004) but convincing explanations are still missing today.

Women often report higher levels of cognitive well-being (Helliwell et al. 2016) but also more negative affect and stress (Nolen-Hoeksema and Rusting 1999; Kahneman and Deaton 2010). In a similar vein, Clark (1997) found that women are happier than men on the labour market and showed that the gender gap cannot be fully explained by factors such as observable characteristics and selection. He suggests that the gender gap might be explained by the fact that women have on average lower expectations on the labour market and evaluate the quality of their job more positively. Note that recent studies found that the gender gap in well-being decreases (Stevenson and Wolfers 2009) or has disappeared (Green et al. 2018).

6   Predicting the Behaviour of Happy People

Another strand of the literature in Economics considers subjective well-being as a factor that is likely to influence individual's behaviour instead of treating it as an outcome. The standard model here is the following:

$$Y_{it+1} = \gamma_1 SWB_{it} + \gamma_2' X_{it} + \epsilon_{it}$$

In this framework, Y_{it} is a future objective behaviour or decision that is plausibly influenced by current subjective well-being. It is important to mention here that γ_1 is estimated keeping the vector of objective characteristics X_{it} constant as it allows isolating the contribution of subjective well-being and shows to what extent it incorporates a meaningful and independent information about individual behaviour. We here present a non-exhaustive list of papers that applied this approach.

There are different behaviours and outcomes that are influenced by the current level of subjective well-being. Individuals with higher levels of well-being have better health outcomes. One famous contribution here is the "Nun Study," in which nuns who wrote more positive short descriptions of their life in their late teens and early twenties were significantly more likely to still be alive 60 years later (Danner et al. 2001). Using larger samples and more sophisticated statistical methods, Diener and Chan (2011) and Banks et al. (2012) find that life satisfaction is significantly associated with better future health outcomes.

Subjective well-being predicts a variety of outcomes and behaviours on the labour market. Conditional on current employment, higher levels of life satisfaction today reduce the probability of being unemployed in the future (O'Connor 2020). Similarly, keeping the objective job characteristics constant, Clark (2001) showed that a low level of job satisfaction predicts a higher probability of job quit.

Finally, Liberini et al. (2017) showed that measures of subjective well-being can be used to predict individual voting behaviours. Using British data and an instrumental variable approach, they demonstrate that the higher the well-being scores, the higher the probability to support the incumbent. Using worldwide data, Ward (2020) finds similar results. At the macroeconomic level, national happiness was a better predictor of the incumbent government vote share than the GDP growth rate, unemployment rate and inflation rate.

---

7 "Objective" Well-being in Economics: Unidimensional and Multidimensional Poverty

Poor individuals have an objectively low level of well-being since they are not able to satisfy their basic needs, that may, or may not, depend on the society they live in. When this is the case, poverty is said to be relative, when this is not the case, poverty is absolute. These considerations are captured by the choice of the level of income (or consumption) that determines who is poor, the so-called, poverty line. An absolute poverty line is a number that is fixed according to some criterion and does not change constantly over time, such as, for example, the international poverty line set by the World Bank of $1.90 a day. A relative poverty line is a number that depends on the distribution of resources of the country of residence of the individual under analysis, such as the poverty lines set by the EU member states equal to 50% of the median of the distribution of equivalent household disposable income of the year under analysis. Any change in the median income will be automatically reflected in an update of the poverty line.

The fundamental contribution to the measurement of unidimensional poverty, that is of poverty that looks only at one dimension of well-being such as income or consumption, is based on Sen (1976). Sen (1976) viewed poverty measurement as involving two exercises: (i) the identification problem: the identification of the poor, and (ii) the aggregation problem: the aggregation of the characteristics of the poor into an overall indicator of poverty. The identification problem was discussed above and requires the specification of a poverty line—a demarcation line separating poor individuals from non-poor persons in the population. Once the poor persons are identified, the next step is to aggregate the information on the poor into an indexthat will quantify the extent of poverty.

Many indices of poverty have been proposed in the literature. The most popular include headcount, poverty gap and squared poverty gap indices. Headcount measures the proportion of the population that is poor, that is, it consists of a simple count of the poor as a fraction of the total number of individuals in society. This index, of the incidence of poverty, is very simple and easy to understand but it lacks any consideration of the depth of poverty, that is, of how poor the individual is. The poverty gap index was proposed to overcome this shortcoming and to capture the intensity of poverty, that is the amount of money the poor needs to cross the poverty line. This difference is known as the individual poverty gap. The poverty gap index is equal to the average, over the population, of the individual's poverty gaps as a proportion of the poverty line. The third index of poverty, the squared poverty gap, averages the poverty gap squared relative to the poverty line. It is a measure that considers inequality among the poor since it gives much more weight to people with larger poverty gaps. These three indices look at the three I's of poverty: incidence, intensity and inequality.

Researchers are in agreement that well-being is multidimensional; to assess all aspects of poverty, more than one dimension needs to be considered, such as, for example, income, health and education of the individual. The measurement of multidimensional poverty is much more complicated that what we summarized above for the unidimensional case. Multiple poverty lines should be set, one for each dimension of poverty, and the aggregation stage is more complex given the possible associations existing between the dimensions that need to be included (going back to the example above, a positive correlation exists between income, health and education). An additional difficulty is given by the type of variables relevant for the measurement of poverty that are very often ordinal or categorical, adding an additional layer of difficulty to the measurement of association between dimensions and the aggregation step. We refer the reader interested to know more to the handbook edited by D'Ambrosio (2018).

References

Alesina, A., Di Tella, R. & MacCulloch, R. (2004). "Inequality and happiness: are Europeans and Americans different?" *Journal of Public Economics, 88,* 2009–2042.

Banks, J., Nazroo, J. & Steptoe, A. (2012). *The dynamics of ageing: Evidence from the English Longitudinal Study of Ageing 2002–10 (Wave 5).* Institute for Fiscal Studies.

Bell, D. N. & Blanchflower, D. G. (2011). "Young people and the Great Recession." *Oxford Review of Economic Policy. 27,* 241–267.

Benjamin, D. J., Heffetz, O., Kimball, M. S. & Rees-Jones, A. (2012). "What do you think would make you happier? What do you think you would choose?" *American Economic Review, 102,* 2083–2110.

Bentham, J. (1789). *An Introduction to the Principles of Morals and Legislation,* Reprinted by The Athlone Press, 1970.

Blanchflower, D.G. & Oswald, A.J. (2004). "Well-being over time in Britain and the USA." *Journal of Public Economics, 88,* 1359–1386.

Booth, A. L. & Van Ours, J. C. (2008). "Job satisfaction and family happiness: the part-time work puzzle." *Economic Journal, 118,* F77–F99.

Card, D., Mas, A., Moretti, E. & Saez, E. (2012). "Inequality at work: The effect of peer salaries on job satisfaction." *American Economic Review, 102,* 2981–3003.

Clark, A. E. (1997). "Job satisfaction and gender: why are women so happy at work?" *Labour Economics, 4,* 341–372.

Clark, A. E. (1999). "Are wages habit-forming? Evidence from micro data." *Journal of Economic Behavior and Organization, 39,* 179–200.

Clark, A. E. (2001). "What really matters in a job? Hedonic measurement using quit data." *Labour Economics, 8,* 223–242.

Clark, A. E. (2003). "Unemployment as a social norm: Psychological evidence from panel data." *Journal of Labor Economics, 21,* 323–351.

Clark, A. E. (2016). "SWB as a measure of individual well-being." In *Oxford Handbook of Well-Being and Public Policy,* M. Adler & M. Fleurbaey (Eds.), Oxford University Press, 518–52.

Clark, A. E. & Oswald, A. J. (1994). Unhappiness and unemployment. *Economic Journal, 104,* 648–659.

Clark, A. E. & Oswald, A. J. (1996). "Satisfaction and comparison income." *Journal of Public Economics, 61,* 359–381.

Clark, A., Georgellis, Y. & Sanfey, P. (2001). "Scarring: The psychological impact of past unemployment." *Economica, 68,* 221–241.

Clark, A.E., Frijters, P. & Shields, M.A. (2008). "Relative income, happiness, and utility: an explanation for the Easterlin paradox and other puzzles." *Journal of Economic Literature, 46,* 95–144.

Clark, A. & Postel-Vinay, F. (2009). "Job security and job protection." *Oxford Economic Papers, 61,* 207–239.

Clark, A. E., Westergård-Nielsen, N. & Kristensen, N. (2009). "Economic satisfaction and income rank in small neighbourhoods." *Journal of the European Economic Association, 7*, 519–527.

Clark, A. E. & Georgellis, Y. (2013). "Back to baseline in Britain: adaptation in the British household panel survey." *Economica, 80*, 496–512.

Clark, A. E., Kamesaka, A. & Tamura, T. (2015). "Rising aspirations dampen satisfaction." *Education Economics, 23*, 515–531.

Clark, A. E. & Jung, S. (2017). *"Does Compulsory Education Really Increase Life Satisfaction?"* Inha University IBER Working Paper Series, 2017–6.

Clark, A. E., Flèche, S., Layard, R., Powdthavee, N. & Ward, G. (2019). *The origins of happiness: the science of well-being over the life course.* Princeton University Press.

Clark, A. E. & Lepinteur, A. (2019). "The causes and consequences of early-adult unemployment: Evidence from cohort data." *Journal of Economic Behavior and Organization, 166*, 107–124.

Collewet, M. & Loog, B. (2014). *"The effect of weekly working hours on life satisfaction."* Working Paper—Maastricht University.

Collewet, M., de Grip, A. & de Koning, J. (2017). "Conspicuous work: Peer working time, labour supply, and happiness." *Journal of Behavioral and Experimental Economics, 68*, 79–90.

Conti, G. & Pudney, S. (2011). "Survey design and the analysis of satisfaction." *Review of Economics and Statistics, 93*, 1087–1093.

D'Ambrosio, C. & Frick, J.R. (2012). "Individual well-being in a dynamic perspective". *Economica, 79*, 284–302.

D'Ambrosio, C. (2018). *Handbook of Research on Economic and Social Well-being.* Edward Elgar.

Danner, D. D., Snowdon, D. A. & Friesen, W. V. (2001). "Positive emotions in early life and longevity: findings from the nun study." *Journal of Personality and Social Psychology, 80*, 804.

Deaton, A. (2012). "The financial crisis and the well-being of Americans—2011 OEP Hicks Lecture." *Oxford Economic Papers, 64*, 1–26.

Di Tella, R., MacCulloch, R.J. & Oswald, A.J. (2003). "The macroeconomics of happiness." *Review of Economics and Statistics, 85*, 809–827.

Di Tella, R., Haisken-De New, J. & MacCulloch, R. (2010). "Happiness adaptation to income and to status in an individual panel." *Journal of Economic Behavior and Organization, 76*, 834–852.

Diener, E. & Chan, M. Y. (2011). "Happy people live longer: Subjective well-being contributes to health and longevity." *Applied Psychology: Health and Well-Being, 3*, 1–43.

Dolan, P., Peasgood, T. & White, M. (2008). "Do we really know what makes us happy? A review of the economic literature on the factors associated with subjective well-being." *Journal of Economic Psychology, 29*, 94–122.

Easterlin, R.A., 1974. Does economic growth improve the human lot? Some empirical evidence. In *Nations and households in economic growth: Essays in Honor of Moses Abramowitz.,* P.A. David and M.W. Reder (Eds.). New York: Academic Press, 89–125.

Easterlin, R.A. (1995). "Will raising the incomes of all increase the happiness of all?" *Journal of Economic Behavior and Organization, 27*, 35–47.

Ferrer-i-Carbonell, A. (2005). "Income and well-being: an empirical analysis of the comparison income effect." *Journal of Public Economics, 89*, 997–1019.

Frey, B. S. & Stutzer, A. (2010). *Happiness and economics: How the economy and institutions affect human well-being*. Princeton University Press.

Frijters, P., Haisken-DeNew, J.P. & Shields, M.A. (2004). "Money does matter! Evidence from increasing real income and life satisfaction in East Germany following reunification." *American Economic Review, 94*, 730–740.

Georgieff, A. & Lepinteur, A. (2018). "Partial employment protection and perceived job security: evidence from France." *Oxford Economic Papers, 70*, 846–867.

Gerdtham, U. G. & Johannesson, M. (2001). "The relationship between happiness, health, and socio-economic factors: results based on Swedish microdata." *Journal of Socio-Economics, 30*, 553–557.

Graham, C. & Pettinato, S. (2002). "Frustrated achievers: winners, losers and subjective well-being in new market economies." *Journal of Development Studies, 38*, 100–140.

Graham, C. & Felton, A. (2006). "Inequality and happiness: insights from Latin America." *Journal of Economic Inequality, 4*, 107–122.

Green, C. P., Heywood, J. S., Kler, P. & Leeves, G. (2018). "Paradox lost: the disappearing female job satisfaction premium." *British Journal of Industrial Relations, 56*, 484–502.

Grund, C. & Sliwka, D. (2007). "Reference-dependent preferences and the impact of wage increases on job satisfaction: Theory and evidence." *Journal of Institutional and Theoretical Economics, 313*–335.

Hayo, B. & Seifert, W. (2003). "Subjective economic well-being in Eastern Europe." *Journal of Economic Psychology, 24*, 329–348.

Hirschauer, N., Lehberger, M. & Musshoff, O. (2015). "Happiness and utility in economic thought or: What can we learn from happiness research for public policy analysis and public policy making?" *Social Indicators Research, 121*, 647–674.

Helliwell, J. F., Huang, H. & Wang, S. (2016). "The distribution of world happiness." *World Happiness Report*.

Hirschman, A.O. (1973). "The changing tolerance for income inequality in the course of economic development." *Quarterly Journal of Economics, 87*, 544–566.

Kahneman, D. & Deaton, A. (2010). "High income improves evaluation of life but not emotional well-being." *Proceedings of the National Academy of Sciences, 107*, 16489–16493.

Kassenboehmer, S. C. & Haisken-DeNew, J. P. (2009). "You're fired! The causal negative effect of entry unemployment on life satisfaction." *Economic Journal, 119*, 448–462.

Layard, R., Clark, A. E., Cornaglia, F., Powdthavee, N. & Vernoit, J. (2014). "What predicts a successful life? A life-course model of well-being." *The Economic Journal, 124*, F720–F738.

Lepinteur, A. (2019a). "The shorter workweek and worker wellbeing: Evidence from Portugal and France." *Labour Economics, 58*, 204–220.

Lepinteur, A. (2019b). Working time mismatches and self-assessed health of married couples: Evidence from Germany. *Social Science & Medicine, 235*, 112410.

Lévy-Garboua, L. & Montmarquette, C. (2004). "Reported job satisfaction: what does it mean?" *Journal of Socio-Economics, 33*, 135–151.

Luttmer, E. F. (2005). "Neighbors as negatives: Relative earnings and well-being." *Quarterly Journal of Economics, 120*, 963–1002.

Liberini, F., Redoano, M. & Proto, E. (2017). "Happy voters." *Journal of Public Economics, 146*, 41–57.

Lyubomirsky, S. (2011). "Hedonic adaptation to positive and negative experiences." In *The Oxford Handbook on Stress, Health and Coping*, S. Folkman (Ed.), Oxford Unversity Press, 200–224.

Marshall, A. (1920). *Principles of Economics (Revised ed.).* Reprinted by Prometheus Books, 1997.

McBride, M. (2001). "Relative-income effects on subjective well-being in the cross-section." *Journal of Economic Behavior and Organization, 45*, 251–278.

Nolen-Hoeksema, S., Rusting, C. L., Kahneman, D., Diener, E. & Schwarz, N. (1999). *Well-being: The foundations of hedonic psychology.* Russell Sage Foundation.

Nikolaev, B. (2018). "Does higher education increase hedonic and eudaimonic happiness?" *Journal of Happiness Studies, 19*, 483–504.

O'Connor, K. J. (2020). Life satisfaction and noncognitive skills: Effects on the likelihood of unemployment. *Kyklos, 73*, 568-604.

Oreopoulos, P. & Salvanes, K. G. (2011). "Priceless: The nonpecuniary benefits of schooling." *Journal of Economic Perspectives, 25*, 159–84.

Oswald, A. J. & Powdthavee, N. (2008). "Does happiness adapt? A longitudinal study of disability with implications for economists and judges." *Journal of Public Economics, 92*, 1061–1077.

Pavot, W. & Diener, E. (1993). "The affective and cognitive context of self-reported measures of subjective well-being." *Social Indicators Research, 28*, 1–20.

Samuelson, P. A. (1938). "A note on the pure theory of consumer's behaviour." *Economica, 5*, 61–71.

Sen, A. (1976). "Poverty: an ordinal approach to measurement." *Econometrica, 44*, 219–231.

Senik, C. (2004). "When information dominates comparison: Learning from Russian subjective panel data." *Journal of Public Economics, 88*, 2099–2123.

Shields, M. A. & Price, S. W. (2005). "Exploring the economic and social determinants of psychological well-being and perceived social support in England." *Journal of the Royal Statistical Society: Series A (Statistics in Society), 168*, 513–537.

Sloane, P. J. & Williams, H. (2000). "Job satisfaction, comparison earnings, and gender." *Labour, 14*, 473–502.

Steptoe, A., Deaton, A. & Stone, A. A. (2015). "Subjective wellbeing, health, and ageing." *Lancet, 385*, 640–648.

Stevenson, B. & Wolfers, J. (2009). "The paradox of declining female happiness." *American Economic Journal: Economic Policy, 1*, 190–225.

Stutzer, A. (2004). "The role of income aspirations in individual happiness." *Journal of Economic Behavior and Organization, 54*, 89–109.

Stutzer, A. & Frey, B. S. (2006). "Does marriage make people happy, or do happy people get married?" *Journal of Socio-Economics, 35*, 326–347.

Urry, H. L., Nitschke, J. B., Dolski, I., Jackson, D. C., Dalton, K. M., Mueller, C. J., Rosen-kranz, M. A., Ryff, C. D., Singer, B. H. & Davidson, R. J. (2004). "Making a life worth living: Neural correlates of well-being." *Psychological science, 15*, 367–372.

Ward, G. (2020). Happiness and voting: Evidence from four decades of elections in Europe. *American Journal of Political Science, 64*, 504-518.

Winkelmann, L. & Winkelmann, R. (1998). "Why are the unemployed so unhappy? Evidence from panel data." *Economica, 65*, 1–15.

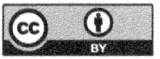

Wohlbefinden und Gesundheit in jugendlichen Lebenswelten

Psychische Gesundheit und Anpassung bei chronisch-körperlicher Erkrankung

Meinolf Noeker

1 Chronische Erkrankung als Modellfall zur Klärung des Verhältnisses von körperlichem und psychischem Wohlbefinden

Die Beziehung zwischen körperlicher Gesundheit einerseits und psychischem Wohlbefinden und Gesundheit andererseits ist komplex und unterliegt vielen Einflussfaktoren und Wechselwirkungen. Ein wichtiger methodischer Zugang liegt in der Untersuchung von gesundheitsbezogenen Daten einerseits und psychometrischen Daten andererseits in möglichst repräsentativen Kollektiven aus der Normalbevölkerung mit einem entsprechend hohen Anteil an gesunden Personen. Ein Beispiel für einen solchen methodischen Zugang mit einem hohen Stichprobenumfang, und einem längsschnittlich angelegten Design stellt die HBSC-Studie dar (vgl. aktuell: Heinz et al. 2020; Kern et al. 2020). Solche epidemiologisch ausgerichteten Studien können basierend auf einer hohen statistischen Power subtile Unterschiede im Gesundheitszustand, dem gesundheitsrelevanten Verhalten sowie dem Wohlbefinden bei Kindern und Jugendlichen und deren Prädiktoren identifizieren.

Ein methodisch komplementärer Zugang sind Studien bei spezifischen Risikogruppen, bei denen von einer besonderen Relevanz des körperlichen Gesundheitszustandes für die psychische Gesundheit auszugehen ist. Psychische Gesundheit soll hier nicht verkürzt in einem kategorialen Sinne verstanden werden als Abwesenheit von psychischer Störung entsprechend der Störungskriterien zum Beispiel nach ICD oder DSM. Analog zur Begriffsbestimmung von körperlichen

M. Noeker (✉)
LWL-PsychiatrieVerbund, Landschaftsverband Westfalen-Lippe, Münster, Deutschland

© Der/die Autor(en) 2022 65
A. Heinen et al. (Hrsg.), *Wohlbefinden und Gesundheit im Jugendalter*,
https://doi.org/10.1007/978-3-658-35744-3_5

Gesundheit und Krankheit soll auch psychische Gesundheit und Krankheit vielmehr als Kontinuum eines Anpassungsergebnisses und als multidimensionales Konstrukt eines biopsychosozialen Anpassungsprozesses verstanden werden (vgl. Hurrelmann et al. 2018; Hurrelmann und Richter 2013; Richter und Hurrelmann 2016). Die Übersicht 1 führt solche vielschichtigen biopsychosozialen und damit auch interdisziplinär relevanten Entwicklungsbedingungen und Entwicklungsergebnisse von Krankheit und Gesundheit auf.

Übersicht 1:
Acht interdisziplinär tragfähige Maximen von Gesundheit und Krankheit nach Hurrelmann (vgl. Hurrelmann und Richter 2013, 139–146)

1. Gesundheit und Krankheit ergeben sich aus einem Wechselspiel von sozialen und personalen Bedingungen, welches das Gesundheitsverhalten prägt.
2. Die sozialen Bedingungen (Gesundheitsverhältnisse) bilden den Möglichkeitsraum für die Entfaltung der personalen Bedingungen für Gesundheit und Krankheit.
3. Gesundheit ist das Stadium des Gleichgewichts, Krankheit das Stadium des Ungleichgewichts von Risiko- und Schutzfaktoren auf körperlicher, psychischer und sozialer Ebene.
4. Gesundheit und Krankheit als jeweilige Endpunkte von Gleichgewichts- und Ungleichgewichtsstadien haben eine körperliche, psychische und soziale Dimension.
5. Gesundheit ist das Ergebnis einer gelungenen, Krankheit einer nicht gelungenen Bewältigung von inneren und äußeren Anforderungen.
6. Persönliche Voraussetzung für Gesundheit ist eine körperbewusste, psychisch sensible und umweltorientierte Lebensführung.
7. Die Bestimmung der Ausprägungen und Stadien von Gesundheit und Krankheit unterliegt einer subjektiven Bewertung.
8. Fremd- und Selbsteinschätzung von Gesundheits- und Krankheitsstadien können sich auf allen drei Dimensionen – der körperlichen, der psychischen und der sozialen – voneinander unterscheiden.

Das Leben mit einer chronisch-somatischen Erkrankung ist eine solche Konstellation, bei der die Wirkmächtigkeit des körperlichen Krankheits/Gesundheitszustandes auf die psychische Gesundheit sehr eindrücklich hervortritt. Wenn die körperliche Gesundheit dauerhaft gefährdet und beeinträchtigt ist, resultiert ein Leidensdruck, der Anpassungsprozesse herausfordert. Die statistische Power der großen Zahl in epidemiologischen Studien wird hier komplementär gespiegelt durch die klinische „Power" bzw. Effektstärke der intensiven Betroffenheit im Einzelfall („impact").

Ein viel zitiertes Sprichwort besagt: „Gesundheit ist nicht alles. Aber ohne Gesundheit ist alles nichts." Das Sprichwort soll anzeigen, dass die Wirkung des körperlichen Wohlbefindens im Zustand der Gesundheit in der Wahrnehmung nicht sonderlich hervorsticht, dies sich aber bei ernsthaften gesundheitlichen Beschwerden schlagartig ändern kann. Dies gilt umso eindrücklicher, wenn es sich um eine chronische Erkrankung handelt, die mit besonders aversiven Schmerzen oder Beschwerden einhergeht und viele Sorgen nicht nur um den Erkrankungszustand im engeren Sinne, sondern auch um dessen Vereinbarkeit mit vielen Rollen und Bedürfnissen des Alltagslebens einhergeht. Beschwerden, Befürchtungen und Sorgen binden wiederkehrend und selektiv die Aufmerksamkeit des Bewusstseins an den körperlichen Krankheitszustand. Bei Jugendlichen kreisen die Sorgen nicht nur um die Einschränkungen in der Gegenwart, sondern auch um Zukunftsentwürfe in allen relevanten Domänen wie Partnerschaft und Intimität, Ausbildung und Beruf, Freizeit und Hobbys sowie Loslösung von der Herkunftsfamilie und Autonomiemotive. Die Salienz, also der emotionale und motivationale Stellenwert der körperlichen Befindlichkeit innerhalb der persönlichen Motivations- und Wertehierarchie steigt bei Krankheit zusätzlich an, insbesondere wenn eine chronische Erkrankung absehbar nicht heilbar ist und Anpassungserfordernisse geradezu erzwingt. Ein chinesisches Sprichwort bringt dies für die Situation des gesunden Menschen schön zum Ausdruck: „Der Schuh, der passt, den spürt man nicht!". Man mag komplementär für den chronisch kranken Menschen vervollständigen: „Der Schuh, der drückt, den spürt man stetig."

Chronisch-somatische Erkrankungen mit ihrer zentralen Wertigkeit des körperlichen Wohlbefindens für das psychische Wohlbefinden stellen damit neben epidemiologischen Populationsstudien ein ausgezeichnetes Modellbeispiel zur Klärung der Beziehung zwischen körperlicher und psychischer Gesundheit dar. Im Mittelpunkt des vorliegenden Beitrags soll daher ein Entwicklungsmodell zur psychischen Adaptation an chronisch-somatische Erkrankung stehen, das die vielschichtigen biopsychosozialen Bedingungsfaktoren für einen positiven wie negativen psychischen Status ausdifferenziert. Die Einflussfaktoren sind sehr vielschichtig, können aber in einem Modell so geordnet werden können, dass die Entwicklung eines bestimmten, individuellen psychischen Anpassungsergebnisses nachvollziehbar wird. Der Bewältigungsprozess kann erfolgreich verlaufen und in eine Wiederherstellung des psychischen Gleichgewichts münden. Er kann aber auch scheitern, so dass das psychische Wohlbefinden und in Folge auch der körperliche Gesundheitszustand nachhaltig in Mitleidenschaft gezogen werden.

2   Prävalenz chronischer Erkrankungen

Zu den chronischen Erkrankungen können Krankheitsbilder gezählt werden (Noeker und Petermann 2008a, 2013; Shapiro et al. 2017),

- deren Dauer mindestens ein Jahr überschreitet,
- die mit Einschränkungen der Funktionsfähigkeit und sozialen Rollen einhergehen und
- bei denen die betroffenen Kinder und Jugendlichen wiederkehrend auf kompensatorische Hilfen (Medikation, Diät, Hilfsmittel, persönliche Anleitung) sowie auf wiederholte medizinisch-pflegerische und/oder psychologisch-pädagogische Unterstützung angewiesen sind.

Die Häufigkeitsangaben variieren in der Literatur je nach Einschluss oder Ausschluss spezifischer Krankheitsbilder und der Berücksichtigung von überdauernden Behinderungen (Barker et al. 2019). Chronisch-somatische Erkrankungen nehmen international kontinuierlich zu. Auf der Basis der deutschen KiGGS-Studie betragen die Lebenszeitprävalenzen bei Kindern und Jugendliche im Alter von null bis 17 Jahren bei atopischer Dermatitis 13,2 %, bei Asthma 4,7 %, bei Diabetes mellitus 0,14 % und bei Krampfanfällen/epileptischen Anfällen 3,6 %. Noch stärker als die Inzidenzraten (Neuerkrankungen pro Jahr) steigen die Prävalenzraten, also der Anteil chronisch kranker Kinder an der Gesamtbevölkerung (Klauber et al. 2016; Noeker 2019b; Noeker und Petermann 2013). Medizinischer Fortschritt senkt weniger den Versorgungsbedarf durch Heilung einer chronischen Krankheit, sondern erhöht ihn vielmehr vor allem durch die Verlängerung der Lebenserwartung von Kindern, die früher an ihrer Krankheit verstorben wären und heute zu Dauerpatienten werden. Viele Erkrankungen wie Diabetes, Asthma, Epilepsie, Hämophilie können zwar medizinisch noch nicht geheilt, aber effektiv symptomatisch behandelt werden. Viele Patienten gewinnen eine fast normale Lebenserwartung, benötigen dazu aber dauerhaft medizinische Therapie und Pflege sowie zunehmend komplementäre klinisch-psychologische Beratung, Anleitung, Edukation, Schulung und Therapie (Bal et al. 2016; Bennet et al. 2015; Eccleston et al. 2015; Härter Baumeister und Bengel 2007; Kirk et al. 2012; Kompetenznetz Patientenschulung im Kindes und Jugendalter 2016; Lindsay et al. 2014; Noeker 2008a, 2013, 2019, 2020; Shapiro et al. 2017). In gesundheitsökonomischer Hinsicht geht dies mit dem nur vordergründigen Paradox einher, dass medizinischer Fortschritt weniger die Behandlungskosten durch Heilung senkt, sondern vielmehr durch eine verlängerte Lebenserwartung chronisch kranker Patienten und damit Leistungsempfängern insgesamt erhöht (Noeker 2019b; Suryavanshi und Yang 2016).

3 Typologie eines gemeinsamen Auftretens körperlicher und psychischer Symptomatik

Nicht in jedem Fall liegt bei einem Zusammentreffen von körperlichen und psychischen Symptomen eine chronische Erkrankung zugrunde. Vielmehr können körperliche Symptome in sehr unterschiedlicher Weise mit psychischen Ursachen, Begleiterscheinungen und Folgestörungen in Verbindung stehen. Das Kapitel F des Klassifikationssystems ICD-10 führt hierzu unterschiedliche Konstellationen bzw. Diagnosegruppen auf. Diese gilt es differenzialdiagnostisch klar zu unterscheiden. Die Übersicht 2 gruppiert diese Störungsbilder entsprechend ihrer Strukturierung und Klassifikation im ICD-10.

Übersicht 2:
Typologie einer Koinzidenz von körperlichen Symptomen mit psychischen Ursachen, Begleiterscheinungen und Folgestörungen im Sinne der Störungskategorien des ICD-10

1. Komorbidität von somatischer Erkrankung (also Erkrankungsbilder, die außerhalb des F-Kapitels im ICD 10 kategorisiert werden, z. B. Morbus Crohn) und psychischer Störung (Störungsbilder kategorisiert innerhalb des F-Kapitels im ICD 10, z. B. depressive Episode während eines erneuten Schubs der chronisch-entzündlichen Darmerkrankung).
2. Psychologische Faktoren und Verhaltensfaktoren bei andernorts klassifizierten somatischen Krankheiten (ICD-10 F54). Diese Kategorie wird verwendet, wenn eine körperliche Erkrankung (z. B. Diabetes mellitus) durch Verhaltensfaktoren (wie zum Beispiel eine unzureichende Therapiemitarbeit) in ihrem Verlauf nachhaltig beeinträchtigt wird. Die

dysfunktionalen Verhaltensfaktoren sind für den Verlauf der körperlichen Erkrankung abträglich, erreichen aber selbst keine psychopathologische Störungswertigkeit.

3. Verhaltensauffälligkeiten mit körperlichen Störungen und Faktoren
   (ICD-10 F5). Die Verhaltensauffälligkeiten manifestieren sich hier vor-
   rangig in Form von körperlichen Symptommanifestationen wie zum
   Beispiel bei nicht-organischen Schlafstörungen oder Essstörungen wie
   Anorexie oder Bulimie (vgl. z. B. Legenbauer et al. 2018).

4. Spezifische Verhaltens- und emotionale Störungen mit Beginn in Kindheit & Jugend (ICD-10 F98.0). Hierzu zählt zum Beispiel die nicht-
   organische Enuresis, die sich zwar körperlich in Form des Einnässens
   manifestiert, die aber abgesehen von einer möglichen körperlichen
   Reifungsverzögerung nicht wesentlich durch eine strukturelle biologische Schädigung verursacht ist (vgl. z. B. Gontard 2018).

5. Entwicklung körperlicher Symptome aus psychischen Gründen (synonym:
   artifizielle Störung/Münchhausen by proxy Syndrom; Simulation;
   ICD-10 F68.0; Noeker et al. 2010). Hier erfolgt eine manipulierte und
   aktiv fabrizierte, aber gegenüber den Ärzten nicht offen kommunizierte
   Schädigung des eigenen Körpers bzw. des Körpers des Kindes durch
   eine Bezugsperson aus der Motivation heraus, so stellvertretend über
   das geschädigte Kind eine Krankenrolle einnehmen und daraus einen
   psychischen Gewinn ziehen zu können.

6. Motorische bzw. sensorische Konversionsstörungen sowie nichtepi-
   leptische Anfälle (ICD-10 F44; Noeker 2020). In der Regel gehen
   unbewusste bzw. nicht lösbare Konflikte und Belastungssituationen
   der Manifestation von solchen Konversionssymptomen voraus. Die
   Störungen zählen zur übergeordneten Gruppe der dissoziativen
   Störungen.

7. Somatoforme Störungen (Noeker 2008) bzw. Somatische Belastungs-
   störungen (ICD F45). Funktionelle körperliche Symptome erzeugen
   einen überproportionalen Leidensdruck, Einschränkungen der psychosozialen Funktionsfähigkeit bzw. eine übersteigerte Angst, an einer
   bedrohlichen Erkrankung zu leiden und in Folge ein übertriebenes Inan-
   spruchnahmeverhalten von Praxen und Kliniken.

4 Besondere Bewältigungsanforderungen in Abhängigkeit vom medizinischen Verlaufsmuster der Erkrankung

Chronische Erkrankungen zeichnen sich je nach individuellem Krankheitsbild durch ein spezifisches Verlaufsmuster aus. Dieses Verlaufsmuster umfasst verschiedene Dimensionen, deren jeweilige Ausprägung die psychischen Belastungseffekte wiederum intensivieren oder abschwächen können (Noeker und Petermann 2003; Mitchell et al. 2015). Zu diesen Dimensionen zählen:

- Erkrankungsbeginn: angeboren versus erworben
- Dauer: zeitlich limitiert versus lebenslang
- Prognose: stabil versus progredient versus remittierend
- Akute Lebensbedrohlichkeit: Hohes oder niedriges Risiko von Krisenzuständen mit potenziell letalem Ausgang
- Mehr oder weniger auftretende, beängstigende, akute Exazerbationen: häufig versus selten
- Verfügbarkeit von Therapieoptionen
  - Grad der langfristigen Beeinflussung des Krankheitsverlaufs: heilbar versus unheilbar
  - Grad der eigenständigen Kontrollierbarkeit von plötzlichen Notfallsituationen versus Angewiesenheit auf professionelle Notfallmedizin.

Je nach Ausprägung dieser medizinischen Verlaufsdimensionen und deren Kombination im Rahmen der individuellen Grunderkrankung ergibt sich eine gewisse Übergangswahrscheinlichkeit für bestimmte psychische Folgebelastungen. Im Extremfall ist von einer besonders intensiven Belastung bei einer Erkrankung auszugehen, die lebenslang bzw. progredient mit einer verkürzten Lebenserwartung, einem hohen Risiko an plötzlichen, schwer vorhersehbaren und kontrollierbaren Symptomverschlechterungen sowie geringen Behandlungsoptionen der Grunderkrankung, ihrer Krisenzustände sowie der Beschwerden oder Schmerzen einhergeht.

5 Äquifinalität und Multifinalität des Anpassungsprozesses

Chronizität bedeutet Dauer, damit Veränderung über dem Entwicklungsverlauf, damit das Erfordernis einer längsschnittlichen und damit nicht nur
klinisch-psychologischen, sondern auch entwicklungspsychologischen bzw. ent-
wicklungspsychopathologischen Perspektive. Literatur wie klinische Erfahrung
dokumentieren gleichermaßen eine ausgeprägte Varianz der psychischen
Gesundheit innerhalb von Patientengruppen mit einer chronischen Erkrankung
(vgl. Barker et al. 2019; Petermann et al. 1987; Silva et al. 2019). Die Abb. 1
illustriert in exemplarischer Weise die interindividuelle Heterogenität über den
Entwicklungs- und Anpassungsverlauf bis hin zu einem Anpassungsergebnis
(Outcome). Aus entwicklungspsychopathologischer Sicht kann diese Varianz
sinnvoll mit den beiden komplementären Prinzipien der Äquifinalität und Multifinalität abgebildet werden:

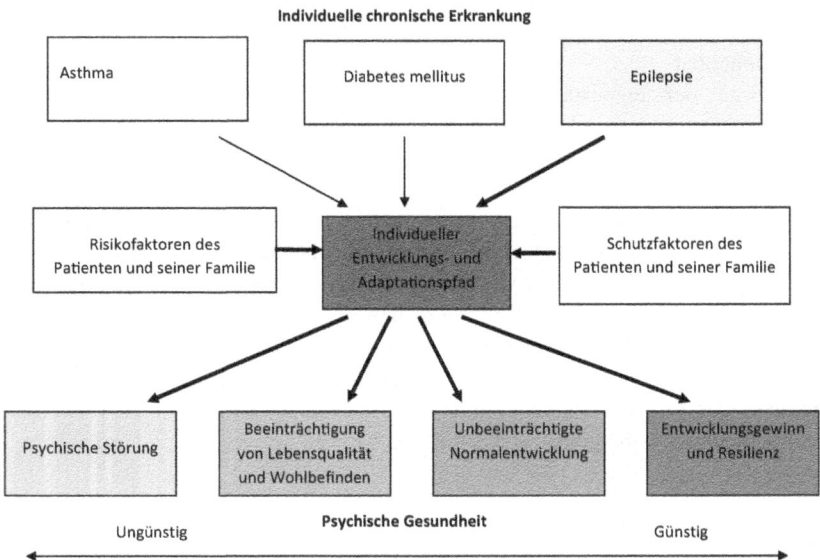

Abb. 1 Aquifinalität und Multifinalität des Adaptationsprozesses und der resultierenden
psychischen Gesundheit bei unterschiedlichen chronisch-somatischen Grunderkrankungen.
(Quelle: Eigene Abbildung)

- Das Entwicklungsprinzip der Äquifinalität kann an drei Personen illustriert werden, die trotz individuell unterschiedlicher Krankheitsbilder über einen ähnlich verlaufenden Adaptationspfad im Ergebnis einen vergleichbaren psychischen Status herausbilden. In dem Beispiel der Abb. 1 bedeutet dies, dass drei Jugendliche, von denen einer an einem Asthma bronchiale, ein zweiter an einem Diabetes mellitus und ein dritter an einer Epilepsie leiden, im Verlauf ihres Bewältigungs- und Anpassungsprozesses an ihre jeweils individuelle Erkrankung alle ein sehr vergleichbares psychisches Anpassungsergebnis entwickeln können. Dies könnte zum Beispiel eine psychopathologisch identische depressive Störung im Sinne einer Dysthymie sein. Äquifinalität bezeichnet hier ein gleiches psychisches Entwicklungsergebnis trotz unterschiedlichem körperlichem Ausgangsbefund.
- Das komplementäre Prinzip zur Äquifinalität ist das Prinzip der Multifinalität. Multifinalität bezeichnet das Phänomen, dass verschiedene Personen mit der gleichen chronischen Erkrankung, hier also zum Beispiel vier Jugendliche, die alle an einer Epilepsie leiden, gleichwohl sehr unterschiedliche Entwicklungs- und Adaptationsverläufe nehmen und einen sehr unterschiedlichen psychischen Status herausbilden können. So kann ein Jugendlicher eine psychische Störung, ein anderer Beeinträchtigungen seiner Lebensqualität und seines Wohlbefindens, ein weiterer eine unbeeinträchtigte Normalentwicklung vergleichbar zu gesunden Kontrollen und ein vierter Jugendlicher eine akzelerierte Reifungsentwicklung nehmen.

Beide Prinzipien der Äqui- und der Multifinalität verdeutlichen, dass der resultierende psychische Entwicklungsoutcome nicht verkürzt als Funktion der biomedizinischen Merkmale der jeweiligen Grunderkrankung verstanden werden darf. Vielmehr modulieren interindividuell variierende psychosoziale Risiko- und Schutzfaktoren als Mediatoren und Moderatoren den jeweiligen Entwicklungsverlauf und -ausgang (Petermann et al. 2020). Methodisch formuliert bedeutet dies, dass der Varianzanteil zu Lasten sozialmedizinischer, psychosozialer und kompetenzbezogener Variablen in der Regel höher ist als der Varianzanteil zu Lasten von Merkmalen der jeweiligen Grunderkrankung (Compas et al. 2012; Didsbury et al. 2016; Jaser et al. 2017; Noeker und Petermann 2003, 2008). Solche vielschichtigen Risiko- und Schutzfaktoren beim Patienten wie seiner Familie gilt es wissenschaftlich wie klinisch im Rahmen von Anamnese und Befunderhebung zu identifizieren (Noeker 2002b, 2006; 2011). Sie bieten neben der medizinischen Therapie der Grunderkrankung entscheidende Ansatzpunkte zur Einflussnahme auf den Adaptationsverlauf und damit den langfristigen Outcome im Sinne des Risikos einer psychopathologischen Störungsentwicklung bzw. von Beeinträchtigungen der Lebensqualität und des Wohlbefindens (Nolte und Osborne 2013; Trivedi 2013). Diese Variabilität der Entwicklungsverläufe wird besonders erkennbar bei einer Subgruppe, die trotz des Lebens mit einer schwerwiegenden und bedrohlichen Grunderkrankung unter Anwendung kompensatorischer Bewältigungsstrategien mit effektiver Problemlösung, Krankheitsmanagement, Emotions- und Selbstregulation einen befriedigenden, ja mitunter sogar besonders gereiften psychischen Gesundheitszustand herausbilden kann. Diese kann in Einzelfällen sogar besser als bei gesunden Kontrollen sein. Diese Subgruppe kann als Beleg dienen, dass die Adaptation an eine starke gesundheitliche Beeinträchtigung solche intensiven Herausforderungen und Lernerfahrungen vermitteln kann, dass sich letztlich sogar die Chance auf einen psychisch gestärkten, resilienten Verlauf ergibt. Die Konfrontation mit den Stressoren aus Krankheit und Behandlung birgt daher in Einzelfällen auch die Möglichkeit zu einer Stimulierung und Ausdifferenzierung von spezifisch-gesundheitsbezogenen wie allgemein-psychosozialen Bewältigungskompetenzen, die ohne die unausweichliche Konfrontation mit den körperlichen Beeinträchtigungen sich nicht herausgebildet hätten (Noeker und Petermann 2008b).

6 Operationalisierung der psychischen Gesundheit bei chronischer Erkrankung

Psychische Gesundheit bei chronisch-körperlicher Krankheit kann unterschiedlich operationalisiert werden (Janssens et al. 2015; Morris et al. 2015). Abb. 1 führt ein Spektrum von vier in der Literatur verwendeten Parametern ein. Diese vier Parameter folgen einer dimensionalen Abstufung von einem besonders ungünstigen bis zu einem besonders günstigen Outcome. Sie spiegeln gleichzeitig bestimmte Paradigmen der empirischen Untersuchung der Beziehung von chronisch-somatischer Erkrankung und psychischer Gesundheit. Personen mit chronischer Erkrankung können sich von gesunden Kontrollen unterscheiden hinsichtlich einer psychopathologischen Komorbidität bzw. hinsichtlich subklinischer Beeinträchtigungen der gesundheitsbezogenen Lebensqualität und des Wohlbefindens bzw. hinsichtlich weitgehend fehlender psychologischer Unterschiede bis hin zu erhöhten Chancen auf Entwicklungsgewinne und Resilienzentwicklungen im Zuge einer gelingenden Auseinandersetzung mit den gesundheitlichen Herausforderungen.

Psychopathologische Komorbidität

Eine Reihe von Studien hat die psychische Gesundheit im Sinne eines Auftretens einer Komorbidität von psychischer Störung bei vorliegender chronisch-somatischer Erkrankung operationalisiert. Demnach wird der psychische Status als beeinträchtigt bewertet, wenn sich im Zuge eines fehlschlagenden Anpassungsprozesses eine zusätzliche psychische Störung im Sinne psychiatrischer Klassifikationssysteme wie DSM bzw. ICD herausbildet. Dieser Parameter setzt einen vergleichsweise hohen Schwellenwert, um eine Beeinträchtigung der psychischen Gesundheit zu bestätigen. In methodischer Hinsicht liegt eine niedrige Sensitivität vor. Psychische Beeinträchtigungen, die keine psychopathologische Störungswertigkeit im Sinne einer Diagnose nach den Klassifikationskriterien nach ICD bzw. DSM erreichen, werden im Zuge dieser Operationalisierung (noch) als Abwesenheit einer Beeinträchtigung bzw. als Normalbefund erfasst.

Nach Studienlage wird die Prävalenz psychischer Störungen bei Kindern mit einer chronisch-somatischen Erkrankung im Vergleich zu gesunden Gleichaltrigen als zwei- bis dreifach erhöht angegeben (vgl. Barlow und Ellard 2006; Noeker und Petermann 2013). Dieser Befund weist eine chronische Erkrankung damit zwar als statistischer Risikofaktor für die Entwicklung einer psychischen Störung aus, verweist aber umgekehrt ebenso darauf, dass die Mehrzahl der Betroffenen eben keine psychopathologische Störungswertigkeit herausbildet. Insbesondere im Rahmen der klinischen Diagnostik ist es für die Therapieplanung besonders relevant zu verstehen, aus welchen Gründen sich im jeweiligen Einzelfall eine psychische Komorbidität herausbildet oder eben nicht (Noeker 2016). Drei Entwicklungspfade auf dem Weg zu einer psychopathologischen Komorbidität sind zu unterscheiden:

- **Ätiopathogenetisch unabhängige Komorbidität von somatischer Krankheit und psychischer Störung.** Diese Konstellation ist sehr wahrscheinlich, wenn in der Anamnese die Herausbildung der psychischen Störung (z. B. eines ADHS im Vorschulalter) der Manifestation der somatischen Erkrankung (z. B. der Manifestation eines Diabetes mellitus im Jugendalter) zeitlich schon vorausgeht. Eine unabhängige Komorbidität ist weiterhin wahrscheinlich, wenn die somatische und die psychische Störung keine gemeinsamen Ursachen aufweisen wie z. B. beim gemeinsamen Auftreten von ADHS und Diabetes mellitus, deren Entstehung vollkommen unabhängig ist.
- **Ätiopathogenetisch einheitliche Komorbidität.** Die zugrunde liegende biologische Ätiologie der somatischen Erkrankung manifestiert sich hier zusätzlich zu den körperlichen Symptomen auch in Form einer Entwicklungsretardierung und/oder Verhaltensstörung. Diese Konstellation ergibt sich

vor allem bei chronischen neuropädiatrischen Krankheitsbildern mit ZNS-Beteiligung (Holtmann 2007; Noeker 2005; Sarimski 2019). Viele genetische Syndrome und angeborene bzw. früh erworbene Stoffwechselerkrankungen erzeugen nicht nur körperliche Fehlbildungen und organische Funktionsbeeinträchtigungen, sondern auch einen charakteristischen kognitiven, affektiven oder behavioralen Phänotyp im Sinne erkrankungstypischer (pathognomischer) Verhaltensstörungen. Beispiele sind das Fragile X-Syndrom (u. a. Aufmerksamkeitsstörungen), das Prader-Willi-Syndrom (u. a. eines unstillbaren Appetits), die Phenylketonurie (u. a. Lernbeeinträchtigungen bei unzureichender Diätadhärenz) oder das Fetofetale Alkoholsyndrom (u. a. Aufmerksamkeits- und Verhaltensstörungen). Es ergeben sich fließende Übergänge von einer chronischen Erkrankung über eine Retardierung bzw. Störung der ZNS-Entwicklung bis hin zu einer geistigen, lernbezogenen, sensorischen oder motorischen Behinderung. Körperliche Erkrankung, funktionelle Behinderung zum Beispiel in der Fein- und Grobmotorik, neuropsychologische Defizite in den Bereichen Aufmerksamkeit, Gedächtnis, Lernen und Intelligenz sowie Verhaltensstörungen gehen hier vielfach auf eine gemeinsame angeborene oder früh erworbene Ursache zurück. In manchen Fällen besteht die Option, über eine optimierte medizinische Behandlung der Grunderkrankung auch den Schweregrad der psychischen Störung positiv zu beeinflussen. Dies ist z. B. der Fall, wenn die Gabe eines Antikonvulsivums (Medikament zur Kontrolle epileptischer Anfälle) bei einem Kind mit Epilepsie und ADHS die Symptomatik des assoziierten ADHS besser kontrolliert als die Gabe von Psychostimulanzien (Noeker et al. 2005).

• **Konsekutive Komorbidität.** Die größte Subgruppe bezieht sich auf diejenigen Kinder, bei denen eine kumulative Fehlanpassung an die Herausforderungen der chronischen Grunderkrankung im Zusammenwirken mit weiteren krankheitsunabhängigen Risikofaktoren bzw. dem Fehlen von Ressourcen sekundär zur Entwicklung einer psychischen Störung führt (vgl. Übersicht 3 mit dem Beispiel einer Komorbidität von Diabetes mellitus und Depression). Bei diesem Entwicklungspfad geht in der Anamnese charakteristischerweise die somatische Erkrankung der psychischen Störung voraus. Zum Zeitpunkt der Manifestation der psychischen Störung finden sich in der Anamnese oft kritische Wendepunkte im Verlauf der chronischen Erkrankung (z. B. Diagnose- oder Rezidivmitteilung, Operation, wiederkehrende Stoffwechselentgleisungen mit der Folge intensiver familiärer Auseinandersetzungen) oder hinzutretende krankheitsunabhängige kritische Lebensereignisse (z. B. Trennung der Eltern, Klassenwiederholung).

Übersicht 3:
Erhöhte Komorbidität einer Depression bei vorliegendem Diabetes mellitus
  Verschiedene Studien identifizierten erhöhte Depressionswerte bei jugendlichen Diabetikern (Buchberger et al. 2016). In einer groß angelegten Untersuchung an 2672 Jugendlichen zeigten 14 % der jugendlichen Diabetiker leicht erhöhte Depressionswerte sowie 3,6 % eine mittel- bis schwergradige Depression (Hood et al. 2006). Eine begleitende depressive Störung bildet wiederum einen Prädiktor für eine schlechtere metabolische Kontrolle und diabetesassoziierte Komplikationen und Folgeerkrankungen. Beeinträchtigte somatische und eine beeinträchtigte psychische Gesundheit können sich also wechselseitig im Sinne eines Teufelskreises verstärken. Das Risiko für eine Depression sowie Beeinträchtigungen der Lebensqualität ist besonders stark bei Kindern und Jugendlichen mit weiteren krankheitsunabhängigen Risikofaktoren wie zum Beispiel einem niedrigeren sozioökonomischen Status verknüpft. Das Leben mit einem Diabetes mellitus kann mit Verstärkerverlusten, sozialem Rückzug und wiederholten Erfahrungen von gelernter Hilflosigkeit einhergehen, die allesamt Risikofaktoren für die Entwicklung einer depressiven Störung sind (Gonzalez et al. 2016; Noeker 2011a).

Bidirektional wirksame Komorbidität mit wechselseitiger Verlaufsbeeinträchtigung
Auch wenn in der Phase der Krankheitsmanifestation die Wirkungsrichtung von der somatischen zur psychischen Seite vielfach zunächst im Vordergrund steht, so ergibt sich über den weiteren langzeitigen Verlauf eine Dynamik wechselseitiger Beeinflussung zwischen somatischer und psychischer Gesundheit (Mitchell 2018). Dabei können wiederum unterschiedliche Wirkmechanismen beteiligt sein.
  Die Übersicht 4 zeigt am Beispiel des Asthma bronchiale, dass sich bidirektionale Mechanismen wechselseitig aufschaukeln und Teufelskreise herausbilden können. Aus dieser Erkenntnis ergibt sich für eine biopsychosozial und interdisziplinär ausgerichtete Behandlungsplanung die Schlussfolgerung, dass eine erfolgreiche medizinische Behandlung nicht nur direkt den biomedizinischen, sondern über eine Reduzierung der psychosozialen Folgebelastungen mittelbar auch den psychischen Statusverlauf positiv beeinflussen kann. Umgekehrt gilt, dass psychologische Interventionen zur Krankheitsbewältigung und zum Krankheitsmanagement nicht nur unmittelbar den psychischen, sondern auch mittelbar zum Beispiel über eine Verbesserung der

Selbstbehandlungskompetenz auch den biomedizinischen Verlauf verbessern
kann (Noeker 2002a).

Übersicht 4:
**Wechselseitige Effekte zwischen chronischer Erkrankung und
Psyche: Unterschiedliche Wirkungsmechanismen am Beispiel Asthma
bronchiale**

- Panik während eines Asthmaanfalls desorganisiert eine gezielte, ruhige
  und überlegte Verhaltenssteuerung und damit auch Krisenbewältigung
  im Sinne einer korrekten Selbstmedikation (Inhalation) und Physio-
  therapie. Eine solche Unter-, Über- oder Fehlbehandlung beeinträchtigt
  wiederum die Symptomkontrolle. Die schmerzliche Bilanzierung eines
  persönlichen Scheiterns bei Asthmakrisen beeinträchtigt wiederum das
  Selbstbild und die Selbstwirksamkeit und damit die psychische Entwicklung insgesamt.
- Operant wirksame Lernerfahrungen in Form einer übertriebenen
  Zuwendung (positive Verstärkung) bzw. Entpflichtung von alters-
  gerechten Anforderungen (negative Verstärkung) durch Eltern oder
  Bezugspersonen kann ein demonstratives Zurschaustellen der Sympto-
  matik triggern sowie die Motivation zur Bekämpfung der Grund-
  erkrankung reduzieren.
- Asthma bronchiale kann verschiedene psychische Komorbiditäten
  bahnen:
  - Angststörungen z. B. im Zuge erlebter Erstickungsangst,
  - Depression in Folge eines sozialen Rückzugs und damit Verstärker-
    verlusts,
  - Somatoforme Störung bei hypochondrischer Fehlinterpretation von
    objektiv harmlosen Veränderungen des Atemflusses als vermeintliche
    Anzeichen eines sich ankündigenden Asthmaanfalls.
- Die Erkrankung erzeugt psychosoziale Folgebelastungen (z. B. Körper-
  und Selbstbild; Verlust von Autonomie) und Einschränkungen der
  Lebensqualität.
- Die Asthmasymptomatik kann eine sekundäre Funktion bei der
  Regulation familiärer Konflikten gewinnen: Die „dramatische"
  (unbewusste bzw. operant verstärkte) Präsentation von Atem-
  beschwerden eines Jugendlichen im Moment eines heftigen Streits

zwischen den Elternteilen (Paarebene) kann diese dazu bringen, diesen abzubrechen und sich gemeinsam in Sorge um ihr krankes Kind zu kümmern (Elternebene). Die Symptomatik kann so belastende Konfliktauseinandersetzungen zumindest vordergründig wieder neutralisieren.

- Psychische Faktoren (z. B. unzureichende Krankheitsakzeptanz) können die Bereitschaft zur Therapiemitarbeit (Adhärenz, Compliance), insbesondere zur prophylaktischen Behandlung im symptomfreien Intervall blockieren. Im Ergebnis droht eine Verschlechterung des Krankheitsverlaufs, der wiederum die Folgebelastungen verstärkt, was wiederum die Krankheitsakzeptanz weiter verschlechtern kann (Teufelskreis).
- Neben den allergischen (z. B. Hausstaubmilbe, Pollen) und infektiösen (verschleimte, entzündete Atemwege) Asthmaauslösern können auf dem Wege der klassischen Konditionierung auch zeitgleich auftretende emotionale Faktoren zum Auslöser für Atemnotzustände (Dyspnoe) werden.

Gesundheitsbezogene Lebensqualität und Wohlbefinden

Im Unterschied zur Erfassung klinischer Komorbidität richtet sich das Paradigma der gesundheitsbezogenen Lebensqualität und des Wohlbefindens auf subklinische Beeinträchtigungen, die also unterhalb einer psychopathologischen Störungswertigkeit liegen. Gesundheitsbezogene Lebensqualität (health related quality of life; HrQoL) umfasst kognitive, emotionale, funktionelle und soziale Einschränkungen (Hall et al. 2019; Hon et al. 2015). Die Hervorhebung auf die *gesundheitsbezogene* Lebensqualität soll den Akzent auf solche Einschränkungen legen, die sich in Folge der gesundheitlichen Einschränkungen, nicht aber in Folge anderer widriger Lebensumstände (Armut, zerrüttete familiäre Verhältnisse, Vernachlässigung etc.) ergeben haben. Beeinträchtigungen der Lebensqualität beim betroffenen Kind und bei den Eltern korrelieren hoch miteinander, beeinträchtigen sich wechselseitig und weisen auf gemeinsam geteilte, ursächliche Belastungs- und Risikofaktoren hin (Barlow und Ellard 2006; Hall et al. 2019; Leeman et al. 2016). Die Übersicht 5 führt physische, psychische und soziale Dimensionen der gesundheitsbezogenen Lebensqualität bei vorliegender chronischer Erkrankung bzw. Behinderung auf.

Übersicht 5:
Physische, psychische und soziale Dimensionen gesundheitsbezogener
Lebensqualität
Physische Funktionsfähigkeit

- Schweregrad der Symptomatik
- Verteilung, Dauer, Intensität, Kontrollierbarkeit von Schmerzen
- Motorische Mobilität, Funktionsniveau, Behinderung
- Sensorische Funktionsbeeinträchtigung, Behinderung

Psychische Funktionsfähigkeit

- Lernen und Intelligenz: normal versus beeinträchtigt
- Stimmung, Affekt, Emotionsregulation
- Akzeptanz von Beeinträchtigungen
- Kommunikation und Sprachkompetenz
- Körperbild
- Selbstwertregulation
- Soziale Selbstsicherheit

Soziale Funktionsfähigkeit

- Sichtbarkeit der Erkrankung in der Öffentlichkeit
- Stigma, Beschämung, Ausgrenzung
- soziale Teilhabe, Partizipation
- schulisch-berufliche Integration

Mittlerweile liegt eine Vielzahl von Inventaren zur Messung der gesundheitsbezogenen Lebensqualität vor (Janssens et al. 2016; Morris et al. 2015; Noeker
2006; Silva et al. 2019). Die Bestimmung der gesundheitsbezogenen Lebensqualität hat sich neben den etablierten medizinischen Outcomeparametern der
Letalität (Sterberate), des Risikos von Folgeerkrankungen (Morbidität, z. B.
Visusbeeinträchtigung bei Diabetes mellitus) sowie der Lebenserwartung zu
einem weiteren, zunehmend wichtigen komplementären Parameter für die
differentielle Indikation bei medizinischen Behandlungsentscheidungen entwickelt. In der pädiatrischen Onkologie wird zum Beispiel das verbesserte
Wissen über die Langzeitrisiken von Amputationen bei Knochentumoren oder

kognitiven Einbußen in Folge einer ZNS-Bestrahlung und damit von signifikanten Bedrohungen einer nachhaltigen gesundheitsbezogenen Lebensqualität als relevantes Entscheidungskriterium in die differentielle Therapieindikation einbezogen (Noeker 2012).

Fragebogeninventare zur Lebensqualität lassen sich in generische versus krankheitsspezifische Verfahren unterteilen. Letztere enthalten Items, die nur beim Vorliegen einer bestimmten Erkrankungsgruppe sinnvoll angewendet werden können. So sind Fragen zur Angst vor einer Hypoglykämie (Unterzuckerung) bei einem individuell vorliegenden Diabetes mellitus, Angst vor Atemnot bei Asthma bronchiale, Angst vor einem Anfallsereignis bei Epilepsie sinnvoll anwendbar. Solche Items zu krankheitsspezifischen Symptomen und deren emotionale Folgen haben den Vorteil einer besonders hohen Sensitivität für die Messung des Spektrums und der Intensität von Lebensqualitätseinbußen, weil sie die persönlich im Vordergrund stehenden Beschwerden und Belastungsquellen sehr gut wiederspiegeln. Krankheitsspezifische Fragebogenitems haben jedoch in methodischer Hinsicht den Nachteil, dass sie keinen Vergleich zwischen unterschiedlichen Krankheitsentitäten erlauben. Würde man in einer Vergleichsstudie unter Beteiligung von Jugendlichen mit Diabetes, Asthma und Epilepsie Items zu Unterzuckerung, Atemnot oder zerebralen Anfällen aufnehmen, so würden die Fragen bei den jeweils nicht betroffenen Personen keinen Sinn ergeben. Die Anwendung solcher Fragen würde also reine Artefakte erzeugen. In Studien, die die „Wucht" der Einbußen an Lebensqualität bei verschiedenen chronischen Erkrankungen vergleichen möchten, können daher nur generische Instrumente verwendet werden. Generische Verfahren enthalten nur krankheitsübergreifende Items, die die Folgewirkungen der jeweiligen Krankheitsbilder auf einer übergeordneten Ebene aggregieren. Fragen wie „In Folge meiner Erkrankung fühle ich mich beim Sport/bei sozialen Kontakten/in meiner Zufriedenheit mit meinem Körper usw. eingeschränkt" erlauben es, eine Vergleichbarkeit zwischen verschiedenen Krankheitsbildern herzustellen. Bei der Auswahl von geeigneten Fragebogeninstrumenten ergibt sich daher regelmäßig ein Zielkonflikt zwischen der besseren Sensitivität der krankheitsspezifischen Verfahren und der Option auf quantitative und qualitative Vergleichbarkeit der Belastungswirkungen bei unterschiedlichen Krankheitsbildern. Vielfach ist in Studien eine Kombination von generischen und spezifischen Verfahren angezeigt, um sowohl Sensitivität wie Vergleichbarkeit zu gewährleisten.

Einen fließenden Übergang zu Dimensionen der gesundheitsbezogenen Lebensqualität bietet das Konstrukt des (selbst berichteten) Wohlbefindens (Blackwell et al. 2019). Wohlbefinden korrespondiert weitgehend mit der psychischen (emotionalen und kognitiven) Subdimension der gesundheits-

bezogenen Lebensqualität. Dieses Konstrukt eignet sich für generisch angelegte
Fragestellungen. Es erlaubt nicht nur den Vergleich zwischen Erkrankungs-
gruppen, sondern auch den Vergleich zwischen chronisch kranken und gesunden
Personen. Dies gilt zumindest, wenn die Fragebogenitems ohne unmittelbaren
Bezug zum Vorliegen einer Erkrankung formuliert sind.

Studienergebnisse zur Lebensqualität und zum Wohlbefinden können mitunter irritierende Befunde liefern. Es ist nicht selten, dass sie nämlich nur geringe
oder auch gar keine signifikanten Unterschiede zwischen kranken und gesunden
Personen identifizieren (z. B. Blackwell et al. 2019). Solche Befunde wirken
kontraintuitiv, weil aus der Perspektive des Außenbeobachters dramatische Einschränkungen infolge Krankheit und Behandlung so offensichtlich nachvollziehbar und einfühlbar sind, diese sich aber erstaunlicherweise in den Daten nicht
abbilden. Wie muss man solche empirischen Befunde interpretieren, wenn man
die Daten ernst nehmen und nicht vorschnell als methodische Artefakte abquali-
fizieren will?

Eine wesentliche Antwort dazu findet sich in der Psychologie der Stress-
regulation und Adaptation an chronische Gesundheitsbelastungen (Noeker 2011b,
2012). Demnach ist stets zu beachten, dass Einschränkungen in Lebensqualität
und Wohlbefinden keine unmittelbare, lineare Folge der Erkrankung sind (vgl.
Abb. 1), sondern durch zwischengeschaltete, transaktionale kognitiv-emotionale
Prozesse der stetigen Neubewertung und des (mehr oder weniger erfolgreichen)
Bewältigungsverhaltens moduliert werden. Fragebogeninventare erfassen nicht
die objektiven Belastungen, sondern immer die schon mehr oder weniger gut
bewältigten Belastungen. Viele chronisch kranke Jugendliche, die zum Beispiel in Folge einer körperlichen Beeinträchtigung bei sportlichen Aktivitäten
objektiv stark beeinträchtigt sind, passen über den Krankheitsverlauf schrittweise
ihr Anspruchsniveau und ihr Bedürfnis nach sportlicher Betätigung an und ver-
lagern ihre Interessen möglicherweise auf andere Interessen und Hobbys. Nach
einer längeren Anpassungszeit vermissen sie Sport nicht mehr. Werden sie dann
zu ihrer Lebensqualität im Bereich Sport befragt, geben sie keine bedeutsamen
Einbußen mehr an, weil sie diese nicht mehr spüren.

7   Biopsychosoziales Modell der psychischen Adaptation an chronische Erkrankung

Die Abb. 2 zeigt ein integratives Entwicklungsmodell, das die relevanten
Bedingungsfaktoren der Herausbildung der individuellen psychischen Gesundheit bei chronischer Erkrankung als weitere Ausdifferenzierung von Abb. 1 noch

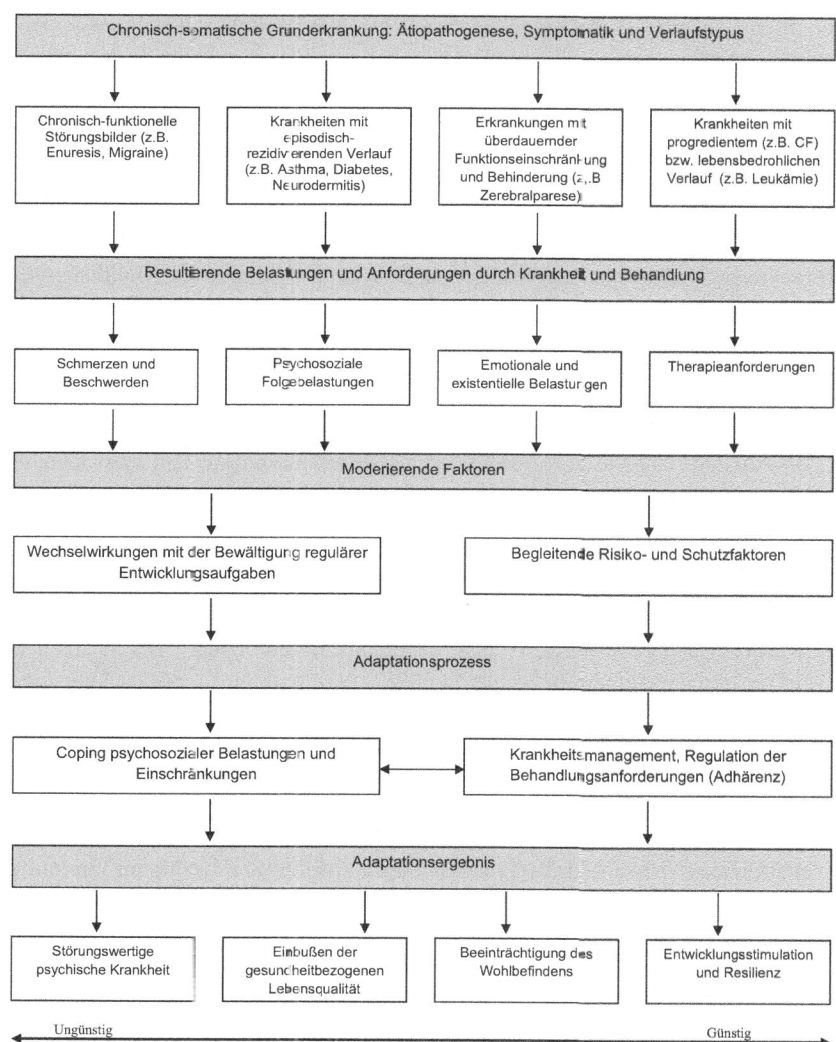

Abb. 2 Prozessmodell zur Adaptation an chronisch-somatische Erkrankung. (Quelle: Eigene Abbildung)

detaillierter aufschlüsselt (vgl. Noeker 2019b). Das Modell soll nicht nur konzeptuell die entscheidenden Determinanten in ihrem Zusammenwirken benennen,
sondern kann auch klinisch-diagnostisch genutzt werden. Erfasst man via
Anamnese und Befunderhebung schrittweise die einzelnen aufgeführten Faktoren
in ihrer jeweiligen Ausgestaltung, so kann man die Genese der individuellen
psychischen Gesundheit rekonstruieren. Daraus können sich auch vielfältige
Hinweise für die psychotherapeutische bzw. psychosoziale Intervention ergeben
zum Beispiel in Form einer Familienberatung zur Reduktion spezifisch erfasster
erkrankungs- und behandlungsbezogener Belastungsfaktoren, zur Mobilisierung
von Ressourcen, zur kognitiven Verhaltenstherapie oder zum Krankheits-
und Selbstmanagement (Noeker 2013; 2019a, b). Folgende Etappenschritte
charakterisieren entsprechend der Abb. 2 den Adaptationsprozess:

- **Erkrankungsmerkmale:** Das medizinische Verlaufsmuster der chronischen
  Erkrankung (episodisch-rezidivierend, persistierend, progredient bzw. lebens-
  bedrohlich) hat stresspsychologisch relevante Implikationen für die erlebte
  Vorhersagbarkeit und Kontrollierbarkeit des Erkrankungsverlaufs durch den
  Patienten.
- **Resultierende Belastungen und Anforderungen:** Vier Arten von Stressoren
  ergeben sich: Schmerzen und Beschwerden, Funktionseinschränkungen,
  psychosoziale Belastungen und Therapieanforderungen. Bei manchen
  Erkrankungen kann die Belastung in Folge mühseliger und aversiver Therapie-
  anforderungen die Belastungswirkung der Grunderkrankung übersteigen
  (Noeker und Petermann 2020a). Wenn jemand stärker an der Behandlung
  als an der Erkrankung leidet, so kann die Motivation zur Therapiemitarbeit
  und zum Krankheitsmanagement leiden. Stresspsychologisch sind nicht der
  Schweregrad aus einer Beobachterperspektive, sondern das empfundene
  Bedrohungserleben und die Einschätzung vorhandener Bewältigungsoptionen
  für das Bewältigungsverhalten entscheidend.
- **Moderierende Faktoren des Bewältigungsprozesses** sind der individuelle
  kognitive und emotionale Entwicklungsstand sowie die krankheitsunabhängigen und krankheitsabhängigen Risiko- und Schutzfaktoren, die die
  Bewältigungsleistung erschweren oder erleichtern. Kinder mit überwiegend
  protektiven Merkmalen (soziale Schicht, Intelligenz, soziale Kompetenz, gute
  Integration in die Gleichaltrigengruppe, familiäre Kohäsion u. a.) können auch
  eine sehr bedrohliche und belastende Grunderkrankung ohne Entwicklung
  einer psychischen Störung überstehen. Umgekehrt können Kinder mit einer
  hohen primären Vulnerabilität (z. B. im Sinne der fünften Achse des ICD-10)
  schon an der Bewältigung einer relativ harmlosen Erkrankung scheitern, wenn

der Erkrankungsausbruch zu einer Vielzahl vorbestehender Belastungsfaktoren hinzutritt (Compas et al. 2012; Noeker und Petermann 2003; 2008a, b).

- **Der Adaptationsprozess** des Kindes richtet sich zum einen auf die Regulation der Erkrankungssymptomatik im engeren Sinne (Krankheitsmanagement) und zum anderen auf die Bewältigung der sekundären psychosozialen Belastungen (Coping). Beide Aspekte interagieren über den Erkrankungs- und Entwicklungsverlauf miteinander.
- **Das Adaptationsergebnis** ergibt sich aus dem Wechselspiel der genannten biologischen, psychischen und sozial-familiären Faktoren. Das Adaptationsergebnis ist nicht statisch, sondern dynamisch zu verstehen. Wenn sich im Rahmen einer unzureichenden Krankheitsverarbeitung eine psychische Störung herausbildet, so erhöht dies rekursiv die Vulnerabilität und das Stresserleben des Kindes und beeinträchtigt die Qualität der weiteren Bewältigungsversuche. Die Manifestation einer psychischen Störung kann aber auch kompensatorische Unterstützungsmaßnamen der Familie, des sozialen Netzwerkes und professioneller Therapeuten mobilisieren, die zu einer neuen Stabilität und einem höheren Adaptationsniveau verhelfen. Das Adaptationsergebnis lässt sich, wie schon in Abb. 1 dargestellt, über vier Kategorien von ungünstigen zu günstigen Ausgängen Manifestation einer psychischen Störung, subklinische Einschränkungen des Wohlbefindens und der gesundheitsbezogenen Lebensqualität, unauffällige Normalentwicklung bis hin zu einem Entwicklungsgewinn und Resilienz abstufen.

Über den weiteren Textverlauf sollen diese Etappenschritte weiter ausdifferenziert dargestellt werden.

8   Resultierende Belastungen und Anforderungen durch Krankheit und Behandlung

Aus der Erkrankung und ihrer Behandlung resultieren für betroffene Kinder und Jugendliche vielschichtige Belastungen und Bewältigungsanforderungen. Die Eltern bzw. die Gesamtfamilie sind ebenfalls betroffen: mittelbar durch die Mitverantwortung für das Wohlergehen des Kindes, aber auch unmittelbar persönlich, etwa durch verengte Spielräume für eigene Unternehmungen, Berufstätigkeit, Hobbys und Kontakte. Übersicht 6 führt Belastungen des betroffenen Kindes und der Familienmitglieder integriert auf.

Übersicht 6:
Belastungen des Patienten und der Familie infolge einer chronischen Erkrankung

Beschwerden und Schmerzen

- Schmerzen und Beschwerden aufgrund der Erkrankung. Beispiele: Schmerz bei rheumatischer Arthritis, Luftnot bei Asthma bronchiale, Hyper- oder Hypoglykämie bei Diabetes mellitus
- Schmerzen und Beschwerden aufgrund der Behandlung. Beispiele: Übelkeit und Erbrechen bei Chemotherapie im Rahmen onkologischer Therapie, Schmerzen bei invasiven Prozeduren wie Spritzen und Punktionen, Nebenwirkungsreaktionen zum Beispiel bei systemischer Steroidgabe bei chronisch-entzündlicher Darmerkrankung (Colitis ulcerosa; Morbus Crohn) oder Rheuma

Psychosoziale Belastungen

- Verringerte Planbarkeit im Alltag infolge nicht vorhersehbarer Erkrankungskrisen
- Verengte Spielräume und erhöhter Koordinationsbedarf bei Urlaubsgestaltung und Freizeitaktivitäten
- Erhöhter, eventuell konfliktbehafteter innerfamiliärer Abstimmungsbedarf
- Reduzierte Zeit für sich selbst
- Zurückstellen eigener Zukunftsentwürfe (z. B. Berufstätigkeit der Mutter)
- Finanzielle Einbußen (z. B. durch reduzierten Stundenumfang im Beruf) bzw. Mehraufwendungen
- Erschwerte Gleichbehandlung der Geschwister bei gleichzeitiger Berücksichtigung der legitimen Bedürfnisse des erkrankten Kindes
- Erziehungsschwierigkeiten
- Geschwisterrivalität
- Überwiegen der Elternfunktion gegenüber der Partnerschaftsrolle
- Aufklärung eines manchmal unverständigen sozialen Umfeldes über die Erkrankung
- Stigmatisierungserfahrungen

Emotionale und existenzielle Belastungen (Anforderungen primär der Emotionsregulation)

- Unvorhersagbarkeit des Erkrankungsverlaufs
- Akzeptanz der Erkrankung und ihrer Chronizität
- Verarbeitung der enttäuschten Hoffnung auf ein gesundes Kind, Gefühle tiefer Kränkung, mitunter auch Scham oder Wut
- Schuldgefühle bezüglich einer (vermeintlichen) Krankheitsverursachung bzw. bezüglich eines vermeintlich unzureichenden Einsatzes für die Belange des Kindes
- Existenzielle Sinnfrage und evtl. Glaubenskrise („warum unser Kind?"; „warum ein unschuldiges Kind?")
- Entwicklung neuer Wertehierarchien
- Veränderte Perspektiven bei erneutem Kinderwunsch (Genetisches Wiederholungsrisiko? Grenzen familiärer Belastbarkeit?)

Therapieanforderungen

- Organisation und Koordination von Behandlungsterminen
- Informationen einholen und aufnehmen zu Krankheitsbild und Therapiemöglichkeiten
- Durchführung pflegerischer oder ko-therapeutischer Maßnahmen
- Zubereitung von Mahlzeiten nach Diätregeln
- Überwachung des Gesundheitszustandes und verstärkte Beaufsichtigung des Kindes
- Motivieren und Anhalten des Kindes zur Therapiemitarbeit bei gleichzeitigem Respekt vor seiner Autonomie
- Disziplin aufbringen bei immer wiederkehrenden Behandlungsmaßnahmen
- Übernahme von Letztverantwortung bei unsicheren Therapieentscheidungen

Die Wirkung in der Übersicht 6 dargestellten Belastungen und Herausforderungen auf die psychische Gesundheit wird moduliert durch verschiedene kognitive Einschätzungen zu deren weiterer Veränderung in der Zukunft bzw.

Veränderbarkeit durch eigene Bewältigungsanstrengungen (Selbstwirksamkeit). Kognitive Belastungs- und Bedrohungseinschätzungen richten sich u. a. auf die

- *Valenz:* Wie stark ist die erlebte Belastung und Bedrohung und ihre Wirkung auf das persönliche Wohlbefinden?
- *Veränderlichkeit:* Wie hoch ist die Wahrscheinlichkeit, dass die Situation sich von selbst verändern wird?
- *Voraussagbarkeit und Ambiguität:* Wie hoch ist das Ausmaß von Unklarheit und Uneindeutigkeit in der Belastungssituation?
- *Wiederauftreten:* wie hoch ist die Wahrscheinlichkeit, dass die gleiche Belastungssituation wiederholt auftreten wird (zum Beispiel erneut erzwungene längere Schulabwesenheit)?
- *Kontrollierbarkeit:* Welche Möglichkeiten sind erkennbar zur Minimierung der Bedrohung?
- *Verfügbarkeit eigener Bewältigungsressourcen (sekundäre Einschätzungen).*

Wenn zum Beispiel die Mutter eines chronisch kranken Jugendlichen wegen ihrer starken zeitlichen und emotionalen Beanspruchung auf eine eigene Berufstätigkeit verzichtet, so kann diese Einschränkung leichter ertragen werden, wenn eine zeitliche Begrenzung absehbar ist, etwa, weil die Großmutter des Kindes in die Nähe der Familie ziehen und Betreuungsleistungen übernehmen wird. Andererseits kann eine solche Problemlösung indirekt neue Folgeprobleme herausbeschwören, etwa eine zu eng empfundene Nähe zu den Großeltern oder die Befürchtung, dass diese sich zu stark in die Erziehung in nicht gewünschter Form einmischen werden.

9 Wechselwirkungen mit der Bewältigung regulärer Entwicklungsaufgaben

Chronisch kranke Kinder und Jugendliche müssen Anpassungsleistungen in zwei Richtungen erbringen. Sie sind nicht nur gefordert, die Vielzahl der in Übersicht 6 dargestellten, nicht-normativen Belastungsfolgen zu bewältigen, die sich aus der Erkrankung ergeben. Sie müssen ebenfalls – wie alle gleichaltrigen gesunden Kinder und Jugendlichen auch – alterstypische, normative Entwicklungsaufgaben bewältigen (vgl. Abb. 3 und 4).

Abb. 3 Verlauf der Adaptation im Schnittfeld des Verlaufs der chronischen Erkrankung und der Bewältigung ihrer nicht-normativen Belastungen und Anforderungen einerseits und den allgemeinen Entwicklungsverlauf und der Bewältigung der normativen Entwicklungsaufgaben und Alltagsstressoren andererseits. (Quelle: Eigene Abbildung)

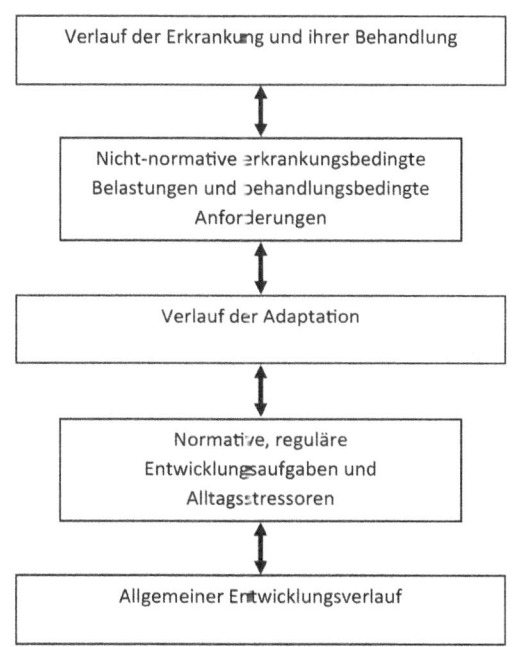

Verlauf der Erkrankung und ihrer Behandlung

↕

Nicht-normative erkrankungsbedingte Belastungen und behandlungsbedingte Anforderungen

↕

Verlauf der Adaptation

↕

Normative, reguläre Entwicklungsaufgaben und Alltagsstressoren

↕

Allgemeiner Entwicklungsverlauf

Diese treten nicht nur additiv zu den psychosozialen Folgen der Erkrankung hinzu, vielmehr können sich die beiden Bewältigungsleistungen wechselseitig potenzieren und beinträchtigen:

- *Eine defizitäre Krankheitsbewältigung beeinträchtigt sekundär die gesamte Verhaltensentwicklung.* Zum Beispiel können wiederholte Misserfolge beim Diabetes- oder Asthmamanagement insgesamt die Selbstwirksamkeitserwartungen und das Selbstkonzept des Jugendlichen sowie die Beziehung zu den Eltern und die Integration in die Gleichaltrigengruppe beschädigen.
- *Defizite in der allgemeinen Verhaltensentwicklung beeinträchtigen sekundär auch die Krankheitsbewältigung.* Zunächst krankheitsunabhängige Risikofaktoren in der allgemeinen Verhaltensentwicklung erschweren nicht nur die erfolgreiche Bewältigung der normativen Entwicklungsaufgaben, sondern in der Folge zusätzlich auch die spezifische Adaptation an die Erkrankung. Beispiel: Eine allgemein beeinträchtigte Vertrauensbeziehung zu den Eltern verleitet einen Jugendlichen, eigene Schwächen beim Diabetesmanagement vor

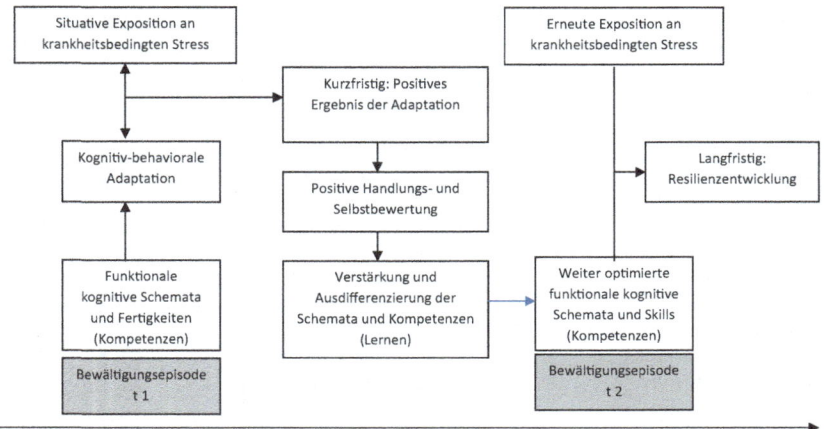

Abb. 4 Entwicklung von Resilienz über die wiederkehrende effektive Adaptation an wiederkehrende Episoden von Stressexposition mit positivem Bewältigungsergebnis. (Quelle: Eigene Abbildung)

diesen zu verheimlichen, weil er Sanktionen befürchtet. Im Ergebnis wird ein so gemeinsam mit den Eltern abgestimmtes Diabetesmanagement blockiert.

Insbesondere im Jugendalter stehen viele alterstypische Entwicklungsaufgaben an (Seiffge-Krenke 1998), die eine erfolgreiche Krankheitsbewältigung in Mitleidenschaft ziehen können:

- Akzeptieren der eigenen körperlichen Erscheinung trotz erkennbarer „Defizite" der körperlichen Funktionsfähigkeit,
- Identifikation mit der eigenen Geschlechtsrolle, der sexuellen Orientierung, Entwickeln erster Beziehungen zu Partnern mit der Herausforderung, diesen die eigene Erkrankung offen zu kommunizieren,
- Graduelle Entwicklung von Unabhängigkeit von den Eltern, obwohl man von diesen in manchen Belangen des Krankheitsmanagements objektiv noch abhängig ist,
- Harmonisierung schulisch-beruflicher Anforderungen (Leistung, Fehlzeiten, soziale Integration) mit Anforderungen aus Krankheit und Behandlung.

Begleitende Risiko- und Schutzfaktoren
Die oben dargestellten Entwicklungsprinzipien der Äqui- und Multifinalität (vgl. Abb. 1) zeigen an, dass die individuelle Ausprägung persönlicher wie familiärer Risiko- wie Schutzfaktoren den Bewältigungserfolg und damit den Adaptationsverlauf nachhaltig sowohl beeinträchtigen wie stabilisieren kann und so die jeweils resultierende psychische Gesundheit prägt. Die Übersicht 7 führt solche Faktoren auf. Da Schutzfaktoren den Verlauf positiv beeinflussen, eignen sich diese auch als Zielvariablen für die therapeutische Behandlungsplanung. Wird zum Beispiel eine eher verschlossene Familie, in der jedes Familienmitglied gewohnt ist, seine Sorgen mit sich selbst auszumachen, ermuntert, Sorgen und Bedürfnisse im Zusammenhang mit dem Krankheitsgeschehen offener in der Familie mitzuteilen, so kann in der Regel erwartet werden, dass dies sich positiv auf das psychische Wohlbefinden und die Lebensqualität auswirkt.

Übersicht 7:
Ressourcen zur erfolgreichen familiären Krankheitsbewältigung
(vgl. Petermann et al. 1987; Noeker 2002b)

1. Strukturelle Ressourcen

- hoher Bildungsgrad
- ökonomische Reserven
- Abwesenheit weiterer chronischer Stressoren und Anforderungen (z. B. pflegebedürftige Großeltern im gleichen Haushalt)

2. Individuelle Bewältigungskompetenzen und Ressourcen einzelner Familienmitglieder

- Hoher Informationsstand bezüglich Erkrankung und Therapie
- Bereitschaft zur eigenverantwortlichen Therapiemitarbeit
- Realistische Behandlungsmotivation
- Fähigkeit zu eindeutiger und offener Kommunikation, freies Äußern eigener Bedürfnisse
- Fähigkeit zu engagiertem, aktivem Problemlösen
- Regenerationsfähigkeit, sinnvolles Freizeitverhalten und innere Erlaubnis zu Phasen des Abschaltens und Genießens ohne Schuldgefühle
- Selbstsicherheit

3. Intrafamiliäre Ressourcen: Interaktion, Aufgabenverteilung, Kommunikation und Werteorientierungen

- Rollenflexibilität bei der Aufgabenwahrnehmung innerhalb der Familie
- Wechselseitiger Respekt gegenüber individuell verschiedenartigen Stilen der (emotionalen) Krankheitsverarbeitung
- Empathie, Bedürfnisse des Patienten unverzerrt wahrzunehmen
- Liebevolles, konsequentes, Orientierung vermittelndes Erziehungsverhalten
- Warmherzige Eltern-Kind-Beziehung
- Ausgewogene Balance halten zwischen Belangen der chronischen Krankheit und anderen familiären Bedürfnissen und Anliegen
- Positive Geschwisterbeziehungen
- Aufrechterhaltung der Generationsgrenzen
- Zufriedenheit mit der Partnerschaftsbeziehung
- Hohes Verpflichtungsgefühl gegenüber der Familie („commitment")
- Wahrnehmung eines positiven Sinns der Erkrankung und weltanschauliche Verankerung in haltgebender Werteorientierung (z. B. Religion, Spiritualität)
- Fähigkeit, um Unterstützung bitten und annehmen zu können

4. Extrafamiliäre Ressourcen

- Aufrechterhaltung der sozialen Integration in außerfamiliäre Netzwerke (Nachbarschaft, Verwandtschaft, Freunde) und gegebenenfalls Selbsthilfegruppen
- Konstruktive, kooperative, vertrauensvolle Beziehungen zu Behandlungspersonal

10 Resilienz trotz widriger Krankheitserfahrungen: Ein Entwicklungsmodell

Das Konzept der Resilienz hat über die letzten Jahrzehnte eine breite Popularität gewonnen. Angesichts einer langen Tradition einer akzentuierten Defizitorientierung in der entwicklungspsycho(patho)logischen Forschung zur

Exposition von Kindern und Jugendlichen an die unterschiedlichsten bio-psychosozialen Risikokonstellationen hat dieser Begriff wesentlich dazu bei-getragen, die interindividuelle Variabilität und intraindividuelle Dynamik von Entwicklungsverläufen und hier insbesondere günstige Ausgänge in den Blick zu rücken. Auf der anderen Seite muss man kritisch konstatieren, dass ins-besondere bei der Anwendung des Begriffs in Studiendesigns nicht immer klar definiert wurde, ob Resilienz als disponierender, trait-analoger Eigenschafts-begriff oder als Prozessmerkmal im Sinne funktionaler Copingstrategien oder aber als Outcomeparameter im Sinne eines Adaptationsergebnisses zu verstehen und zu operationalisieren ist. Gerade bei langzeitig wirksamen, adversen Risiko-bedingungen (Armut, psychisch kranke Eltern, chronische Vernachlässigung etc.) ist Resilienz als dynamischer Prozess zu konzipieren (Rutter 2012), bei dem sich über die transaktionale Interaktion von Person und Umwelt von Bewältigungs-episode zu Bewältigungsepisode je nach Funktionalität des Bewältigungsver-haltens konsekutive Risikomaximierungen versus Risikominimierungen auf den Langzeitoutcome ergeben können.

So hat auch im Bereich der Forschung zur Adaptation an chronische Erkrankung eine Reihe von Studien und Übersichtsarbeiten belegen können, dass es einer Teilmenge von Patientinnen und Patienten gelingt, aus der Konfrontation mit den Belastungserfahrungen sogar persönliche Wachstums- und Entwicklungs-gewinne zu ziehen. Dieses Phänomen ist nicht zuletzt für die weitere Theorie-entwicklung zum Zusammenhang zwischen körperlicher und psychischer Gesundheit aufschlussreich. Solche Resilienzentwicklungen (Noeker und Peter-mann 2008b) belegen, dass die Vorstellung einer linearen, korrelativen Beziehung zwischen körperlicher und psychischer Gesundheit zu kurz greift. Das Phänomen möglicher Entwicklungsgewinne und Resilienzverläufe unterstreicht para-digmatisch die breite Heterogenität der psychischen Entwicklungsprozesse und -ausgänge in Abhängigkeit von den individuellen Krankheitsmerkmalen, den Belastungen und Anforderungen, den interagierenden Entwicklungsaufgaben sowie den moderierenden Risiko- und Schutzfaktoren sowie Bewältigungs-kompetenzen (vgl. Abb. 1 und 2).

Gegenüber Betroffenen und deren Familien kann der Verweis auf mögliche Resilienzentwicklungen die breiten Spielräume aufzeigen, die im Zuge eines Aufbaus von funktionalen Bewältigungsstrategien und Selbstmanagement-kompetenzen sowie die Aktivierung von Ressourcen zur Stabilisierung des eigenen Wohlbefindens trotz der großen Herausforderungen einer chronischen Erkrankung erreichbar bleiben. Eine solche Ermutigung ist mit Respekt und gebotenen Vorsicht zum Ausdruck zu bringen. Sie ist mit einer Validierung der erlebten Leidenserfahrungen zu begleiten und in Einklang zu bringen. Sie sollte nicht die Botschaft transportieren, nun selbst an psychischen Beein-trächtigungen Schuld zu sein, da andere Personen es ja augenscheinlich schaffen, die Belastungen leicht zu überwinden und sogar noch dadurch stärker zu werden. Das Phänomen der Resilienzentwicklung konnte exemplarisch bei Über-lebenden einer lebensbedrohlichen Krebserkrankung aufgezeigt werden (Noeker 2002b, 2008, 2012; Noeker und Petermann 2015). Dies darf als Hin-weis gewertet werden, dass einem Entwicklungsgewinn regelhaft eine besonders außergewöhnliche Bedrohung vorausgeht, deren glückliche Wendung dann aber als besonders stabilisierend für zukünftige Krisensituationen verarbeitet wird.

In der Abb. 1 wurde die Entstehung dieser Variabilität über die vier Abstufungen hergeleitet aus einer Interaktion der erkrankungs- und behandlungs-bedingten Faktoren mit den psychologischen Merkmalen des Patienten. Bei den letzteren wird die Wichtigkeit schon prämorbide vorliegender kognitiv-emotionaler Schemata und verhaltensbezogener Kompetenzen für den Langzeit-verlauf herausgestellt. Abb. 4 differenziert diese Konzeption weiter aus. Leitend ist die Vorstellung, dass prämorbide funktionale Schemata auch zu einer funktionaleren und kompetenteren Integration der bedrohlichen Krankheits-erfahrungen disponieren. Dies mündet wiederum in erfolgreichere Bewältigungs-ergebnisse, die internal mit Erfahrung von Selbstwirksamkeit und Stolz attribuiert werden können oder als Beleg für hilfreiche Glaubenssysteme im Sinne einer letztlich doch Sicherheit und Geborgenheit vermittelnden Welt gewertet werden. Prämorbide vulnerable Personen, die in Familien mit niedrigem Funktions-niveau aufwachsen, tragen ein hohes Risiko, Fehlschläge und traumatisch wirksame Erfahrungen im Zuge der Auseinandersetzung beispielsweise mit einer Krebserkrankung zu kumulieren und damit wiederum das Risiko für eine psychopathologische Dekompensation und Symptombildung weiter zu erhöhen. Umgekehrt gilt der gleiche Verlauf mit umgekehrten Vorzeichen: Prämorbide schon kompetent verarbeitende und bewältigende Personen haben gute Chancen zu einer auch erfolgreichen Lösung der erkrankungsbedingten Herausforderungen und damit weiterer Stärkung positiver, optimistischer Glaubenssysteme. Über die Erfahrung eigener erfolgreicher Bewältigungsleistungen wird das Kind zum eigenständigen Akteur seiner Resilienzentwicklung. Eine realistische und stolze Handlungs- und Selbstbewertung von Bewältigungsleistungen stärkt trotz und mitunter sogar gerade wegen der wiederkehrenden Exposition an belastende Umgebungsbedingungen die zunehmende Ausdifferenzierung und hierarchische Integration von Fähigkeiten zur effektiven Problemlösung und Emotions-regulation.

Literatur

Bal, M.I., Sattoe, J.N., Roelofs, P.D., Bal, R., van Staa, A. & Miedema, H.S. (2016). Exploring effectiveness and effective components of self-management interventions for young people with chronic physical conditions: A systematic review. *Patient Education and Counselling, 99,* 1293–1309.

Barker, M.M., Beresford, B., Bland, M. & Fraser, L.K. (2019). Prevalence and Incidence of Anxiety and Depression Among Children, Adolescents, and Young Adults With Life-Limiting Conditions. A Systematic Review and Meta-analysis *JAMA Pediatrics, 173,* 835–844.

Barlow, J.H. & Ellard, D.R. (2006). The psychosocial well-being of children with chronic disease, their parents and siblings: An overview of the research evidence base. *Child, Care, Health and Development, 32,* 19–31.

Bennett, S., Shafran, R., Coughtrey, A., Walker, S. & Heyman, I. (2015). Psychological interventions for mental health disorders in children with chronic physical illness: a systematic review. *Archives of Diseases in Childhood, 100,* 308–316.

Blackwell, C. B., Elliott, A. J., Ganiban, J., Herbstman, J. Hunt, K., Forrest, C. B., Camargo Jr, B.A. (2019). Program collaborators for Environmental influences on Child Health Outcomes. General Health and Life Satisfaction in Children With Chronic Illness. *Pediatrics, 143.*

Buchberg, B, Huppertz, H., Krabbe, L., Lux, B., Mattiv, J.T. & Siafarikas, A. (2016). Symptoms of Depression and Anxiety in Youth With Type 1 Diabetes: A Systematic Review and Meta-Analysis. *Psychoneuroendocrinology, 70,* 70–84.

Chernyshov, P.V. (2016). Stigmatization and self-perception in children with atopic dermatitis. *Clinical Cosmetics Investigation and Dermatology, 9,* 159–166.

Compas, B.E., Jaser, S.S., Dunn, M.J. & Rodriguez EM. (2012). Coping with chronic illness in childhood and adolescence. *Annual Review of Clinical Psychology, 8,* 455–480.

Didsbury, M.S. et al. (2016). Socio-economic status and quality of life in children with chronic disease: A systematic review. *Journal of Paediatric Child Health, 52,* 1062–1069

Eccleston, C., Fisher, E., Law, E., Bartlett, J. & Palermo, T.M. (2015). Psychological interventions for parents of children and adolescents with chronic illness. *Cochrane Database Systematic Reviews, Apr 15;4:CD009660.*

Gontard, A. von (2018). *Enuresis* (3., überarb. Aufl.). Göttingen Hogrefe.

Gonzalez, J.S., Tanenbaum, M.L. & Commissariat, P.V. (2016). Psychosocial factors in medication adherence and diabetes self-management: Implications for research and practice. *American Psychologist, 71,* 539–551.

Härter, M., Baumeister, H. & Bengel, J. (Herausgeber) (2007) Psychische Störungen bei körperlichen Erkrankungen. Heidelberg: Springer.

Hall, C.A., Donza, C., McGinn, S., Rimmer, A., Skomial, S., Todd, E. & Vaccaro, F. (2019). Health-Related Quality of Life in Children With Chronic Illness Compared to Parents: A Systematic Review. *Pediatric Physical Therapy, 31,* 315–322.

Heinz, A., Catunda, C., van Duin, C. & Willems, H. (2020). Suicide prevention: Using the number of health complaints as an indirect alternative for screening suicidal adolescents. *Journal of Affective Disorders, 260,* 61–66.

Holtmann, M. (2007). *Psychiatrische Syndrome nach Hirnfunktionsstörungen*. Göttingen: Hogrefe.

Hon, K.L., Pong, N.H., Poon, T.C., Chan, D.F., Leung, T.F., Lai, K.Y., Wing, Y.K. & Luk, N.M. (2015). Quality of life and psychosocial issues are important outcome measures in eczema treatment. *Journal of Dermatological Treatment, 26*, 83–89.

Hood, K.K., Huestis, S., Maher, A., Butler, D., Volkening, L. & Laffel, M.B. (2006). Depressive Symptoms in Children and Adolescents With Type 1 Diabetes: Association With Diabetes-Specific Characteristics. *Diabetes Care, 29*, 1389–1391.

Hurrelmann, K., Richter, M., Klotz, T. & Stock, S. (2018). *Referenzwerk Prävention und Gesundheitsförderung: Grundlagen, Konzepte und Umsetzungsstrategien. (5. Auflage)*. Göttingen: Hogrefe.

Hurrelmann, K. & Richter, M. (2013). *Gesundheits- und Medizinsoziologie. Eine Einführung in sozialwissenschaftliche Gesundheitsforschung*. Weinheim: Beltz Juventa.

Janssens, A., Rogers, M., Thompson Coon, J., Allen, K., Green, C., Jenkinson, C., Tennant, A., Logan, S. & Morris, C. (2016). A Systematic Review of Generic Multidimensional Patient-Reported Outcome Measures for Children, Part II: Evaluation of Psychometric Performance of English-language Versions in a General Population. *Value Health, 18*, 334–345.

Jaser, S.S., Patel, N., Xu, M., Tamborlane, W.V. & Grey, M. (2017). Stress and Coping Predicts Adjustment and Glycemic Control in Adolescents with Type 1 Diabetes. *Annals of Behavioral Medicine, 51*, 30–38.

Kern, M.R., Heinz, A. & Willems H. (2020). School-Class Co-Ethnic and Immigrant Density and Current Smoking among Immigrant Adolescents. *International Journal of Environmental Research and Public Health, 17* (2) E598.

Kirk, S., Beatty, S., Callery, P., Gellatly, J., Milnes, L. & Pryjmachuk, S. (2012). The effectiveness of self-care support interventions for children and young people with long-term conditions: a systematic review. *Child, Care, Health and Development, 39*, 305–324.

Klauber, J. Günster, C., Gerste, B. & Robra, B.-P. (Hrsg.). (2016). *Versorgungs-Report 2015/2016: Schwerpunkt: Kinder und Jugendliche*. Stuttgart: Schattauer.

Kompetenznetz Patientenschulung im Kindes- und Jugendalter e.V. (2016). *Modulares Schulungsprogramm für chronisch kranke Kinder und Jugendliche sowie deren Familien „ModuS". Band 1: Modulare Patientenschulung* (3., überarb. Aufl.). Lengerich: Pabst (vgl. www.kompetenznetz-patientenschulung.de).

Kroll, K.H. (2020). *Pediatric Psychology in Clinical Practice: Empirically Supported Interventions*. New York: Cambridge University Press.

Leeman, J., Crandell, J.L., Lee, A. Jinbing, B., Sandelowski, M. & Knafl, K. (2016). Family Functioning and the Well-Being of Children With Chronic Conditions: A Meta-Analysis. *Research in Nursing Health, 39*, 229–343.

Legenbauer, T., Radix, A.K., Augustat, N. & Schütt-Strömel, S. (2018). Power of Cognition: How Dysfunctional Cognitions and Schemas Influence Eating Behavior in Daily Life Among Individuals With Eating Disorders. *Frontiers of Psychology, 9*, 2138, eCollection.

Lindsay, S., Kingsnorth, S., McDougall, C. & Keating, H. (2014). A systematic review of self-management interventions for children and youth with physical disabilities. *Disability and Rehabilitation, 36*, 276–288.

Mitchell, A.E. (2018). Bidirectional relationships between psychological health and dermatological conditions in children. *Psychological Research on Behavioral Management, 11,* 289–298.

Mitchell, A.E., Fraser, J.A., Ramsbotham, J., Morawska, A, & Yates, P. (2015). Childhood atopic dermatitis: a cross-sectional study of relationships between child and parent factors, atopic dermatitis management, and disease severity. *International Journal of Nursing Studies, 52,* 216–228.

Morris, C. et al. (2015). Meaningful Health Outcomes for Paediatric Neurodisability: Stakeholder Prioritisation and Appropriateness of Patient Reported Outcome Measures. *Health Qual Life Outcomes, 13,* 87.

Noeker, M. & Petermann, F. (2003). Entwicklungsorientierte Betrachtung chronischer Krankheiten im Kindes- und Jugendalter. *Zeitschrift für Klinische Psychologie, Psychopathologie und Psychotherapie, 51,* 191–229.

Noeker, M. & Petermann, F. (2008a). Chronische Erkrankungen. In F. Petermann & S. Schneider (Hrsg.). *Angewandte Entwicklungspsychologie* (S. 635–676). Göttingen: Hogrefe.

Noeker, M. & Petermann, F. (2008b). Resilienz: Funktionale Adaptation an widrige Umgebungsbedingungen. *Zeitschrift für Psychiatrie, Psychologie und Psychotherapie, 56,* 255–263.

Noeker, M. & Petermann, F. (2013). Chronisch-körperliche Erkrankungen. In F. Petermann (Hrsg.) *Lehrbuch der Klinischen Kinderpsychologie* (7., veränd. Aufl., S. 535–552). Göttingen: Hogrefe.

Noeker, M. & Petermann, F. (2015). Childhood Cancer: Psychological Aspects. In J. D. Wright (Ed.). *International Encyclopedia of Social and Behavioral Sciences* (pp. 459–464) (sec. ed.; vol. 3). Oxford: Elsevier.

Noeker, M. & Petermann, F. (2020). Schmerz bei invasiven Behandlungen. In F. Petermann (Hrsg.). *Entspannungsverfahren: Das Praxishandbuch* (6. überarb. Aufl., im Druck). Weinheim: Beltz.

Noeker, M. (2002a). Biopsychosoziale Leitprinzipien für die psychosoziale Arbeit bei chronisch-pädiatrischen Erkrankungen. *Psychotherapie im Dialog, 3,* 26–32.

Noeker, M. (2002b). Praxis behavioral-systemischer Familienberatung bei Tumor- und Leukämieerkrankungen im Kindes- und Jugendalter. *Psychotherapie im Dialog, 3,* 53–60.

Noeker, M. (2005). Lernstörungen bei chronischer Erkrankung. *Monatsschrift für Kinderheilkunde, 153,* 630–639.

Noeker, M. (2006). Psychologische Diagnostik bei chronischer Erkrankung. *Monatsschrift für Kinderheilkunde, 154,* 326–337.

Noeker, M. & Petermann, F. (2008). Resilienz: Funktionale Adaptation an widrige Umgebungsbedingungen. *Zeitschrift für Psychiatrie, Psychologie und Psychotherapie, 56,* 255–263.

Noeker, M. (2008a). Das Gemeinsame im Speziellen: Krankheitsübergreifende Module und Lernziele der Patientenschulung. *Prävention und Rehabilitation, 20,* 2–11.

Noeker, M. (2008b). *Funktionelle und somatoforme Störungen im Kindes- und Jugendalter.* Göttingen: Hogrefe.

Noeker, M. (2011a). Selbstmanagement bei Diabetes mellitus. In C. von Hagen & H.-P. Schwarz (Hrsg.). *Selbstmanagement bei chronischer Erkrankung* (S. 189–207). Stuttgart: Kohlhammer.

Noeker, M. (2011b). Motivations- und gesundheitspsychologische Grundlagen des Selbst-
managements bei chronischer Krankheit. In Cornelia von Hagen & Hans-Peter Schwarz
(Hrsg.), *Selbstmanagement bei chronischer Erkrankung* (S. 46–61). Stuttgart: Kohlhammer.

Noeker, M. (2012). Überlebende von Krebserkrankungen des Kindes-und Jugendalters:
Entwicklungsverläufe zwischen Traumatisierung und Resilienz. *Bundesgesundheitsblatt –
Gesundheitsforschung - Gesundheitsschutz, 55,* 481–492.

Noeker, M. (2013). Kindzentrierte Interventionen bei chronischen Erkrankungen. In M.
Pinquart (Hrsg.). *Wenn Kinder und Jugendliche körperlich chronisch krank sind.
Psychische und soziale Entwicklung* (S. 151–165). Berlin: Springer.

Noeker, M. (2019a). Verhaltenstherapie in der Kinderheilkunde. In F. Petermann (Hrsg.).
(2019). *Kinderverhaltenstherapie. Grundlagen, Methoden und Anwendungen* (6., vollständig überarbeitete Auflage). Göttingen: Hogrefe.

Noeker, M. (2019b). Verhaltenstherapie in der Pädiatrie. In S. Schneider & J. Margraf
(Hrsg.), *Lehrbuch der Verhaltenstherapie, Band 3: Störungen im Kindes- und Jugendalter.* Berlin: Springer.

Noeker, M. (2020). *Konversionsstörungen und Störungen mit funktionellen neurologischen
Symptomen* (Leitfaden der Kinder- und Jugendpsychotherapie; im Druck). Göttingen:
Hogrefe.

Noeker, M., Haverkamp-Krois, A. & Haverkamp, F. (2005). Development of mental health
dysfunction in childhood epilepsy. *Brain & Development, 27,* 5–16.

Noeker, M., Mußhoff, F., Franke, I. & Madea, B. (2010). Münchhausen-by-proxy-
Syndrom. *Rechtsmedizin, 20,* 223–235.

Nolte, S. & Osborne, R.H. (2013). A systematic review of outcomes of chronic disease self
management interventions. *Quality of Life Research, 22,* 1805–1816.

Petermann, F., Noeker, U. & Bode, U. (1987). *Psychologie chronischer Krankheiten im
Kindes- und Jugendalter.* München: Psychologie Verlags Union.

Petermann, U, Petermann, F. & Ulrich, F. (2020). Risikofamilien. *Kindheit und Entwicklung, 29,* 1–4.

Richter. M. & Hurrelmann, K. (2016). Soziologie von Gesundheit und Krankheit. Weinheim: Juventa Beltz.

Roberts, M. C. & Steele, R.G. (2018). Handbook of Pediatric Psychology (Fifth Edition).
New York: Guilford Press.

Rutter, M. (2012). Resilience as a dynamic concept. Developmental Psychopathology, 24,
335–344.

Sarimski, K. (2019). *Psychosoziale Entwicklung von Kindern und Jugendlichen mit
Behinderung. Prävention, Intervention und Inklusion.* Göttingen: Hogrefe.

Seiffge-Krenke, I. (1998). Chronic Disease and Perceived Developmental Progression in
Adolescence. *Developmental Psychology, 34,* 1073–1084.

Shapiro, M.C., Henderson, C.M., Hutton, N. & Boss, R.D. (2017). Defining Pediatric
Chronic Critical Illness for Clinical Care, Research, and Policy. *Hospital Pediatrics, 7,*
236–244.

Silva, N., Pereira, M., Otto, C., Ravens-Sieberer, U., Canavarro, M.C. & Bullinger,
M. (2019). Do 8- to 18-year-old children/adolescents with chronic physical health
conditions have worse health-related quality of life than their healthy peers? a meta-

analysis of studies using the KIDSCREEN questionnaires. *Quality of Life Research,28,* 1725–1750.

Suryavanshi, M, S. & Yang, Y. (2016). Clinical and economic burden of mental disorders among children with chronic physical conditions, United States, 2008–2013. *Preventing Chronic Disease 13.*

Trivedi, D. (2013). Cochrane review summary: psychological interventions for parents of children and adolescents with chronic illness. *Primary Health Care Research Development, 14,* 224–228.

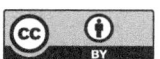

Bedeutung von Peerbeziehungen im Zusammenhang mit der Entwicklung von Gesundheit und Wohlbefinden von Jugendlichen

Heike Eschenbeck und Arnold Lohaus

1 Entwicklungsanforderungen im Jugendalter

Ausgehend von den vielfältigen Entwicklungsanforderungen, die sich Jugendlichen stellen, wird in diesem Kapitel darauf eingegangen, welche Rolle Peerbeziehungen bei der Bewältigung von Entwicklungsanforderungen spielen und auf welche Entwicklungsdimensionen sie Einfluss nehmen. Daran anschließend wird auf bedeutsame Mechanismen eingegangen, über die Gleichaltrige die Entwicklung von Jugendlichen beeinflussen. Abschließend wird auf die Rolle Gleichaltriger für das Wohlbefinden und die Gesundheit von Jugendlichen eingegangen.

1.1 Entwicklungsaufgaben, kritische Lebensereignisse und Alltagsprobleme

Jugendliche sind mit vielen neuen Anforderungen konfrontiert, die sich einerseits aus den pubertär bedingten körperlichen Veränderungen und andererseits durch vielfältige neue soziale Herausforderungen ergeben, da auch die soziale Umwelt veränderte Erwartungen an Jugendliche heranträgt. Hinzu kommt die

H. Eschenbeck (✉)
Abteilung Pädagogische Psychologie und Gesundheitspsychologie, Pädagogische Hochschule Schwäbisch Gmünd, Schwäbisch Gmünd, Deutschland
E-Mail: heike.eschenbeck@ph-gmuend.de

A. Lohaus
Fakultät für Psychologie und Sportwissenschaft, Universität Bielefeld, Bielefeld, Deutschland
E-Mail: arnold.lohaus@uni-bielefeld.de

© Der/die Autor(en) 2022

A. Heinen et al. (Hrsg.), *Wohlbefinden und Gesundheit im Jugendalter*,
https://doi.org/10.1007/978-3-658-35744-3_6

101

zunehmende Fähigkeit zur Selbstreflektion und damit verbunden zum Aufbau des Selbstkonzepts und einer eigenständigen Identität.

Wie schon Havighurst (1953, 1972) konstatierte, gehört zu den typischen Entwicklungsaufgaben im Jugendalter unter anderem (a) die Akzeptanz und der effektive Umgang mit dem eigenen Körper, (b) die Findung und Übernahme von Geschlechtsrollen, (c) der Aufbau neuer und reifer Beziehungen zu Gleichaltrigen des eigenen und des anderen Geschlechts sowie (d) die Loslösung und emotionale Unabhängigkeit von den Eltern und anderen Erwachsenen (s. auch Eschenbeck und Knauf 2018). Neben den Entwicklungsaufgaben stellen sich vielen Jugendlichen weitere Anforderungen durch kritische Lebensereignisse (wie chronische Erkrankungen oder Verlust von Bezugspersonen) sowie durch alltägliche Probleme (wie Streitereien mit Mitschülern oder Klausuren und Hausaufgaben). Dem großen Spektrum an potenziellen Anforderungen steht auf der anderen Seite häufig ein noch unzureichendes Bewältigungspotenzial gegenüber, um die Anforderungen erfolgreich meistern zu können. Aus den Entwicklungsaufgaben, aus kritischen Lebensereignissen und alltäglichen Problemen kann also eine Überlast entstehen, wenn gleichzeitig ein Mangel an personalen und sozialen Bewältigungsressourcen besteht. Dies kann wiederum mit erhöhten Entwicklungsrisiken für betroffene Jugendliche verbunden sein.

1.2 Aufbau von Beziehungen zu Gleichaltrigen als Entwicklungsaufgabe

In dem Maße, in dem Jugendliche ihre Eltern de-idealisieren und die Werte und Normen der Elterngeneration in Frage stellen (Lohaus und Vierhaus 2019), wenden sie sich vielfach Gleichaltrigen zu, die ihnen in vielerlei Hinsicht ähnlicher sind (z. B. im Hinblick auf Kleidungsstil, Sprache, Musikgeschmack, Einstellungen etc.). Hinzu kommt, dass Beziehungen zu anderen Jugendlichen nach eigenen Präferenzen gezielt hergestellt und gestaltet werden können, während dies bei den Beziehungen innerhalb der Familie deutlich schwieriger ist, weil diese Beziehungen nicht frei wählbar sind und über lange Zeiträume entstanden sind, was gleichzeitig bedeutet, dass sie sich bereits weitgehend stabilisiert haben (Laursen und Adams 2018). Hier Veränderungen herbeizuführen, bedeutet Konflikte und Auseinandersetzungen, die im Jugendalter ebenfalls nicht untypisch sind und insbesondere im Übergang zwischen früher und mittlerer Adoleszenz häufig auftreten (Koepke und Denissen 2012). Der Aufbau von Beziehungen zu Gleichaltrigen schafft hier oftmals ein Gegengewicht, um zur Kompensation von Problemen in der Familie (und auch in anderen Sozial-

settings wie der Schule) beizutragen (Cooper und Cooper 1992). Der Beziehungsaufbau zu Gleichaltrigen ist (somit) nicht nur eine Entwicklungsaufgabe, die
eigene Anforderungen an die Jugendlichen stellt, sondern ebenso eine Ressource,
die dazu beitragen kann, Anforderungen in anderen Bereichen zu kompensieren.

1.3 Beziehungen zu Gleichaltrigen als Schutz- und Risikofaktoren

Im Allgemeinen können Beziehungen zu Gleichaltrigen als Schutzfaktoren
aufgefasst werden, weil sie durch soziale und emotionale Unterstützung zur
Anforderungsbewältigung (z. B. beim Umgang mit Entwicklungsaufgaben) sowie
auch zum allgemeinen Wohlbefinden im Jugendalter beitragen können. Dies setzt
allerdings in der Regel eine hinreichende soziale Kompetenz voraus, da dadurch
ein Beziehungsaufbau leichter gelingen kann (Wentzel und Erdley 1993). Neben
mangelnden sozialen Kompetenzen kann es auch weitere biopsychosoziale
Charakteristika geben, die es manchen Jugendlichen erschweren, Beziehungen
zu Gleichaltrigen aufzubauen. Insgesamt ist der Anteil der Jugendlichen, die
angeben, über keinerlei enge Beziehungen zu Gleichaltrigen zu verfügen, eher
gering (Claes 1992). Da in diesen Fällen jedoch andere Jugendliche als Quelle
sozialer und emotionaler Unterstützung ausfallen, erhöht dies die Gefahr von
Entwicklungsrisiken, die gegebenenfalls auf anderen Wegen auszugleichen sind
(z. B. durch familiären Rückhalt).

In der Regel ist allerdings davon auszugehen, dass Jugendliche einen großen
Teil ihrer freien Zeit mit Gleichaltrigen verbringen und dass sie mehr als andere
Altersgruppen um soziale Akzeptanz in der Gleichaltrigengruppe bemüht sind
(Brown 2011; Reitz et al. 2014). Es hängt dabei vor allem von der Ausrichtung
der präferierten Gleichaltrigen ab, ob der Schutz- oder Risikocharakter der
Gleichaltrigenbeziehungen überwiegt. Man kann davon ausgehen, dass prosozial orientierte Gleichaltrige eher Schutzeffekte erzeugen, während antisozial
eingestellte Gleichaltrige eher mit einer Intensivierung von Entwicklungsrisiken
(im Sinne von aggressivem Verhalten, Alkohol- und Drogenkonsum, frühem
Einsetzen sexueller Aktivitäten und niedrigeren Bildungsabschlüssen) assoziiert
sind (Sanders et al. 2017). Wenn Gleichaltrigenbeziehungen bestehen, können
sie demnach eine ambivalente Wirkung (in die positive und negative Richtung)
erzielen (Müller und Minger 2013).

Ob Beziehungen zu anderen Jugendlichen als Schutz- bzw. Risikofaktor
wirken können, hängt nicht nur von der sozialen Ausrichtung der Gleichaltrigen
ab, sondern auch von der Intensität der Einbindung in ein Gleichaltrigen-Netz-

werk. Nach Fussan (2006; s. auch Röhrle 1994) sind dabei als Parameter die Größe des Netzwerks, die Zentralität der Position eines Jugendlichen in einem Gleichaltrigen-Netzwerk sowie die Kontakthäufigkeit zu nennen. So ist die Chance einer Beeinflussung, im positiven wie im negativen Sinn, größer bei einem kleinen bis mittleren Netzwerk, in dem bei hoher Kontakthäufigkeit eine zentrale Position eingenommen wird. Umgekehrt wird der Einfluss in der Regel geringer sein bei einem sehr großen Netzwerk, in dem eine randständige Position bei geringer Kontakthäufigkeit eingenommen wird.

Man kann also zusammenfassend festhalten, dass Jugendliche mit hohen Anforderungen durch Entwicklungsaufgaben, kritische Lebensereignisse und alltägliche Probleme konfrontiert sein können. Angesichts eines häufig noch geringen Erfahrungsschatzes im Umgang mit Anforderungen und Problemen können sich aus Beziehungen zu Gleichaltrigen im positiven Sinne Ressourcen zur Problembewältigung, aber auch Entwicklungsrisiken ergeben. Gleichzeitig ist der Aufbau von Gleichaltrigen-Beziehungen eine Entwicklungsaufgabe für Jugendliche, die ihrerseits Anforderungen an sie stellt, die zu bewältigen sind.

2   Formen von Peerbeziehungen

2.1   Gleichaltrige, Freunde, Cliquen und Subkulturen

Gleichaltrigenbeziehungen sind durch Reziprozität und Gleichberechtigung charakterisiert, wodurch sie sich im Regelfall von Erwachsenen-Kind-Beziehungen (wie Eltern-Kind-Beziehungen) unterscheiden. Sie bieten damit gleichzeitig einen Lernraum zum Aufbau, zur Aufrechterhaltung und gegebenenfalls auch zur Beendigung von Sozialbeziehungen. Das Alter der „Gleichaltrigen" kann dabei durchaus variieren, entscheidend ist, wer als gleichaltrig wahrgenommen wird. Insgesamt nehmen Gleichaltrigenbeziehungen im Jugendalter an Bedeutung zu, was daran zu erkennen ist, dass mehr Zeit mit Gleichaltrigen verbracht wird und dass die Erwartungen und Meinungen von Gleichaltrigen zunehmend wichtiger werden (Brown und Larson 2009).

Ein Spezialfall der Gleichaltrigenbeziehungen sind Freundschaftsbeziehungen, die nicht nur durch Reziprozität, Gleichberechtigung und Freiwilligkeit, sondern auch ein hohes Ausmaß an Intimität und gegenseitigem Vertrauen charakterisiert sind. Nach Brown und Larson (2009) basieren Freundschaften häufig auf dem Prinzip der Ähnlichkeit (von Interessen, Einstellungen, Werten etc.), wobei jedoch auch Ergänzungseffekte zu beobachten sind. Dies bedeutet, dass Freunde gewählt werden, die über Kompetenzen verfügen, von denen man lernen kann und die die eigene Entwicklung fördern. Freunde stellen eine wichtige (und in der Regel verlässliche) Ressource da, um soziale, emotionale und instrumentelle Unterstützung bei der Bewältigung von Anforderungen zu erhalten. Andererseits können sich Freundschaften eher als familiäre Bindungen wieder auflösen, sodass sich aus den Freundschaftsbindungen auch Entwicklungsrisiken ergeben können (Poulin und Chan 2010). Besondere Probleme können sich vor allem dann ergeben, wenn Jugendliche in nur wenige, aber sehr intensive Freundschaften involviert sind, die dann jedoch zerbrechen.

Von engen Freundschaftsbeziehungen sind Cliquenbildungen unter Jugendlichen zu unterscheiden, die in der Regel größere Gruppen umfassen, zwischen denen enge Kontakte bestehen. Die emotionalen Bindungen zwischen den Gruppenmitgliedern sind weniger eng als bei Freundschaften, wobei jedoch zwischen einzelnen Mitgliedern auch emotionale Bindungen im Sinne von Freundschaften bestehen können. Insgesamt sind die sozialen Beziehungen innerhalb von Cliquen häufig über die Zeit weniger stabil als Freundschaftsbeziehungen (Brown 2004). Cliquen sind für Jugendliche nicht nur eine Ressource zum Erhalt von Hilfe und Unterstützung, sondern schaffen auch eine Möglichkeit, sich Gleichaltrigen mit ähnlichen Interessen und Präferenzen anzuschließen. Gleichzeitig können sich aus den Cliquen gleich- und gegengeschlechtliche Freundschaften entwickeln. Entwicklungsrisiken können sich hier – ähnlich wie bei Freundschaften – aus Konflikten innerhalb von Cliquen ergeben, die zur Auflösung einer Clique oder zum Ausschluss einzelner Mitglieder führen. Während enge Freundschaftsbeziehungen häufiger von Mädchen berichtet werden, sind Jungen häufiger in Cliquen organisiert (Buhrmester 1990).

Subkulturen kennzeichnen Jugendlichen-Gruppierungen mit gemeinsamen Werten, Einstellungen und Lebensstilen (Bobakova et al. 2015), denen sich einzelne Jugendliche zugehörig fühlen, wobei das Zugehörigkeitsgefühl beispielsweise durch einen ähnlichen Kleidungsstil, einen ähnlichen Musikgeschmack oder ähnliche Werte zum Ausdruck gebracht werden kann. Im Unterschied zu Cliquen bestehen nicht notwendigerweise direkte Interaktionen zwischen den Subkulturmitgliedern. Die empfundene Zugehörigkeit zu einer Subkultur kann insofern eine Ressource sein, als sie die Identitätsbildung sowie das Affiliationsbedürfnis Jugendlicher unterstützt.

2.2 Offline- und Online-Beziehungen

Da Internetverbindungen mittlerweile für Jugendliche praktisch flächendeckend und täglich verfügbar sind (z. B. über Smartphones), finden viele Kontakte

zwischen Jugendlichen nicht mehr nur in unmittelbaren Face-to-Face-Inter-
aktionen, sondern auch über soziale Online-Netzwerke statt. Vergleicht man
Freundschaftsbeziehungen, die ausschließlich offline stattfinden, mit Online-
Freundschaften, dann lässt sich konstatieren, dass reine Online-Freundschaften
als weniger eng und unterstützend beschrieben werden als reine Offline-Freund-
schaften (Glüer und Lohaus 2016; Mesch und Talmund 2006). Auch Online-
Beziehungen werden (wie Offline-Beziehungen) von Mädchen häufig als enger
beschrieben als von Jungen (Valkenburg und Peter 2007), während auf der
anderen Seite Jungen wiederum in Online-Beziehungen eine größere Bereitschaft zeigen, über eigene Probleme ins Gespräch zu kommen (Schouten et al.
2007). Während die Kommunikation in sozialen Online-Netzwerken in der Regel
verbal unter Zuhilfenahme von Symbolen oder Bildern erfolgt, steht in Offline-
Kommunikationen zusätzlich das gesamte Spektrum an Mimik und Gestik zur
Verfügung. Dies mag dazu beitragen, dass die Beziehungsqualität bei reinen
Offline- und Online-Beziehungen teilweise als unterschiedlich beschrieben wird
(Glüer und Lohaus 2016).

Tatsächlich sind reine Offline- bzw. Online-Beziehungen im Alltag allerdings
wohl eher die Ausnahme. Deutlich verbreiteter sind gemischte Beziehungen
mit Offline- und Online-Anteilen. Hier kann vermutet werden, dass eine Off-
line-Beziehung durch zusätzliche Online-Interaktionen in sozialen Online-Netzwerken eher gewinnt (Khan et al. 2016). Dadurch steigt einerseits die gemeinsam
verbrachte Zeit und andererseits können leichter auch Themen angesprochen
werden, die man im direkten Face-to-Face-Kontext vielleicht nicht anzusprechen
gewagt hätte.

Mit Online-Kontakten können nicht nur bestehende Beziehungen intensiviert
werden, sondern es können auch neue Kontakte aufgebaut werden. Insofern
bieten sich über soziale Online-Netzwerke vielfältige Gelegenheiten für Jugendliche, eigene soziale Netzwerke aufzubauen und auszubauen und dadurch
zusätzliche soziale Kompetenzen zu erwerben. Mit der Partizipation an sozialen
Online-Netzwerken sind jedoch nicht nur Ressourcen, sondern auch Risiken verbunden. In diesem Zusammenhang ist insbesondere das Cyberbullying zu nennen,
da mit sozialen Online-Netzwerken auch die Möglichkeit verbunden ist, den
Teilnehmenden Schaden zuzufügen (z. B. durch die Verbreitung von Gerüchten,
durch Identitätsdiebstahl oder durch das Blocken von Teilnehmern; Glüer und
Lohaus 2015).

2.3   Romantische Beziehungen

Eine Sonderform der Freundschaftsbeziehung ist in der Aufnahme einer romantischen Beziehung zu sehen. Während Freundschaftsbeziehungen zu mehreren Freunden bestehen können, sind romantische Beziehungen in der Regel auf einen Partner gerichtet. Nach der Shell-Jugendstudie 2019 gehört es zu den wichtigsten Werten für Jugendliche, über gute Freunde und über eine vertrauensvolle Partnerschaft zu verfügen. In einer festen Partnerschaft sehen sich 5 % der 12- bis 14-Jährigen, 24 % der 15- bis 17-Jährigen, 34 % der 18- bis 21-Jährigen sowie 52 % der 22- bis 25-Jährigen. Es fällt dabei auf, dass die Angaben beim weiblichen Geschlecht höher ausfallen als beim männlichen Geschlecht (Albert et al. 2019). Als Grund für diesen Geschlechtsunterschied wird unter anderem die frühere körperliche Reife von Mädchen diskutiert, die die Wahrscheinlichkeit von Kontakten zu älteren Gleichaltrigen und damit der Aufnahme einer Partnerschaft erhöht (Vierhaus und Wendt 2018). Nach Seiffge-Krenke (2003) steigt die Partnerschaftsdauer mit dem Alter und liegt im Alter von 13 Jahren bei vier Monaten, mit 15 Jahren bei fünf Monaten, mit 17 Jahren bei 12 Monaten und mit 21 Jahren bei 21 Monaten. Ähnliche Daten werden auch von Wendt und Walper (2013) berichtet (s. zusammenfassend Vierhaus und Wendt 2018). Partnerschaften sind damit im Jugendalter vielfach nicht über lange Zeiten hinweg stabil, bieten aber ein wichtiges Lernfeld für den Aufbau sozialer und emotionaler Kompetenzen in engen Beziehungen, wobei auch die Bewältigung der Auflösung einer engen Beziehung dazu gehören kann.

Häufig eng verknüpft mit dem Aufbau von Partnerschaften ist der Aufbau sexueller Beziehungen. Nach einer repräsentativen Befragung zur Jugendsexualität der Bundeszentrale für gesundheitliche Aufklärung (BZgA, Bode und Heßling 2015) gaben 6 % der 14-Jährigen an, über Geschlechtsverkehr-Erfahrungen zu verfügen. Die Werte steigen auf 19 %, 39 %, 58 % und 59 % im Alter von 15 bis 18 Jahren an. Da die Werte höher liegen als die Angaben zu den festen Partnerschaften, spricht dies dafür, dass sexuelle Erfahrungen teilweise auch außerhalb fester Partnerschaften gesammelt werden. Insgesamt ist das Jugendalter ein wichtiges Experimentierfeld zum Sammeln erster sexueller Erfahrungen, die die weiteren Einstellungen und Verhaltensweisen im Bereich der Sexualität prägen können und zur Findung einer eigenen sexuellen Identität und Orientierung beitragen (Lohaus und Vierhaus 2019).

2.4   Soziometrischer Status

Das Ausmaß, in dem Jugendliche in Sozialbeziehungen involviert sind und von Gleichaltrigen akzeptiert werden, wird im soziometrischen Status abgebildet. Typischerweise wird der soziometrische Status auf der Grundlage der Häufigkeit, mit der ein Jugendlicher von der Gleichaltrigengruppe als guter Freund benannt wird, bestimmt. Umgekehrt kann ebenso berücksichtigt werden, wie häufig ein Jugendlicher von der Gruppe abgelehnt wird (Wentzel 2003).

Viele Freundschaftsnominierungen bei gleichzeitig wenig Ablehnungen weisen auf einen hohen soziometrischen Status hin, während sich das umgekehrte Muster bei schlecht integrierten Jugendlichen zeigt. Auch kann es sein, dass ein Gruppenmitglied zugleich viele positive als auch viele negative Nominierungen erhält, also einen kontroversen Status in der Gruppe innehat. Wird ein Jugendlicher nicht als Freund genannt, jedoch auch nicht abgelehnt, ist dies ein Indiz dafür, dass er oder sie in der Gruppe wenig beachtet wird. Der soziometrische Status verdeutlicht also die soziale Position eines Jugendlichen in seiner Bezugsgruppe und kann als Maß für den sozialen Rückhalt, den ein Jugendlicher in einer Gleichaltrigengruppe genießt, dienen.

Es gibt viele Hinweise darauf, dass der soziometrische Status als Maß für die soziale Integration mit einer Reihe von Entwicklungsparametern assoziiert ist. So ließ sich beispielsweise zeigen, dass nicht nur zu sozial-emotionalen, sondern auch zu kognitiv-leistungsbezogenen Parametern Bezüge bestehen (Gallardo et al. 2016). Unter den abgelehnten Jugendlichen lässt sich eine Teilgruppe identifizieren, die durch feindliches, störendes oder aggressives Verhalten charakterisiert ist, und weiterhin eine Teilgruppe, die sich sehr zurückgezogen verhält und deswegen von der Gleichaltrigengruppe abgelehnt wird. Die erste Teilgruppe schließt sich nicht selten antisozialen Cliquen an, während die zweite Teilgruppe eher internalisierende Symptome (wie depressive Symptome) entwickelt (Vierhaus und Wendt 2018). Umgekehrt legen Jugendliche mit einem positiven soziometrischen Status häufiger prosoziales Verhalten und hohe soziale Kompetenz an den Tag. Nicht selten ist diese Gruppe auch durch bessere Schulleistungen charakterisiert (Wentzel 2003).

Allgemein lässt sich festhalten, dass die Sozialbeziehungen im Jugendalter viele verschiedene Formen annehmen können. Der soziometrische Status kann dabei ein Indikator für die soziale Integration eines Jugendlichen sein. Er indiziert jedoch nur die Integration in eine spezifische Jugendlichengruppe und vernachlässigt dabei, dass es häufig viele weitere Bezugsgruppen (online und offline, familiäre Beziehungen etc.) geben kann, in denen Jugendliche agieren und die gegebenenfalls ergänzende oder ausgleichende Ressourcen bereitstellen können. Die Gleichaltrigengruppe ist damit eine sehr wichtige, aber nicht unbedingt alles entscheidende Ressource für das Wohlbefinden im Jugendalter.

3 Bedeutsame Entwicklungsdimensionen, auf die Peerbeziehungen Einfluss nehmen

3.1 Selbstkonzept

Im Folgenden soll auf einige wichtige Entwicklungsdimensionen eingegangen werden, bei denen Peerbeziehungen einen großen Stellenwert haben können. Im Gegensatz zu den Entwicklungsaufgaben geht es hier nicht um normative, entwicklungsbezogene Anforderungen, die von einem Individuum typischerweise in einem bestimmten Zeitfenster zu bewältigen sind. Es handelt sich vielmehr um Entwicklungsdimensionen, bei denen sich im Jugendalter (aber auch in anderen Lebensabschnitten) wichtige Veränderungen ergeben können.

Zu den Entwicklungsdimensionen, auf die Gleichaltrigenbeziehungen Einfluss nehmen können, gehört unter anderem das Selbstkonzept, womit die eigene Selbstwahrnehmung bzw. das selbstbezogene Wissen angesprochen ist (Thomsen et al. 2018). Im Jugendalter wird das Selbstkonzept durch die Ausweitung der Informationsquellen sowie zunehmende Fähigkeiten zu Selbstreflexion und Perspektivenübernahme differenzierter und vielschichtiger. Man kann davon ausgehen, dass Jugendliche aus Gleichaltrigenbeziehungen vielfältige Informationen gewinnen, die sie zum eigenen Selbstkonzeptaufbau nutzen. Sie sind dementsprechend stark damit befasst, die Meinungen und das Verhalten anderer Jugendlicher zu analysieren, um dadurch Rückschlüsse über sich selbst und das eigene Verhalten zu ziehen. Viele Jugendliche sehen sich von einem imaginären Publikum umgeben, das sie beobachtet und bewertet (Elkind 1985). Eigene Fehler werden dadurch häufig überdramatisiert, weil davon ausgegangen wird, dass sie das eigene Ansehen in der Gleichaltrigengruppe nachhaltig beschädigt haben können. Insgesamt ist die Aufmerksamkeit stark auf das eigene Selbst gerichtet, wobei gleichzeitig eine starke Vulnerabilität für die Einflüsse von Gleichaltrigen besteht, die eine zentrale Informationsquelle für die Selbstkonzeptentwicklung darstellen (Sebastian et al. 2008).

3.2   Werte und Normen

Aus der Forschung zur Moralentwicklung ist bekannt, dass beim moralischen
Urteil deutliche Entwicklungsfortschritte vom Kindesalter zum Jugendalter
erkennbar sind. Jugendliche sind in der Regel kognitiv dazu in der Lage, verschiedene Bedürfnisse und Interessen gegeneinander abzuwägen und ihren
Urteilen auch allgemeine Regeln und Prinzipien zugrunde zu legen (Lohaus
und Vierhaus 2019). Neben Werten, die das moralische Handeln leiten können,
kennen sie auch sozial-konventionelle Normen (Turiel 1998), die der Regulation
sozialer Interaktionen dienen (z. B. Normen, die im Umgang mit Gleichaltrigen gelten). Allerdings ist aus der Forschung zur Moralentwicklung ebenfalls bekannt, dass keine eindeutigen Beziehungen zwischen der Fähigkeit zur
moralischen Urteilsbildung und dem tatsächlichen moralischen Handeln bestehen
(Blasi 1980). Nach Blasi (1983) ist von zentraler Bedeutung, dass Werte und
Normen in das eigene Selbstkonzept integriert werden, um handlungswirksam
zu werden (s. auch Hardy und Carlo 2005). Als Teil des Selbstkonzepts steigt
wiederum ihre subjektive Bedeutsamkeit, sodass eine Nicht-Beachtung im tatsächlichen Handeln dazu führen könnte, dass das eigene Selbstkonzept hinterfragt
werden müsste. Es ist auch denkbar, dass durch die wahrgenommene Diskrepanz
zwischen Selbstkonzept und eigenem Handeln negative Emotionen (wie Scham-
gefühle) ausgelöst werden (Bandura 1991). Tatsächlich weist auch Krettenauer
(2017) darauf hin, dass antizipierte Emotionen das antisoziale und prosoziale Verhalten im Kindes- und Jugendalter vorhersagen. Dies gilt für negative Emotionen
(wie Scham oder Schuld) ebenso wie für positive Emotionen (wie Freude oder
Stolz). Sowohl die Integration von Werten und Normen in das Selbstkonzept als
auch antizipierte Emotionen können also dazu beitragen, dass ein stärkerer Bezug
zum tatsächlichen Handeln erfolgt. Der Aufbau von Werten und Normen wird im
Jugendalter durch Gleichaltrige beeinflusst, während die Integration in das Selbstkonzept eine Entwicklungsaufgabe des jeweiligen Jugendlichen ist.

3.3   Soziale Kompetenzen und soziale Integration

Nach Hinsch und Pfingsten (2015) bestehen soziale Kompetenzen aus mehreren
Komponenten. Dazu gehören (a) berechtigte Interessen anmelden oder
unberechtigte Forderungen ablehnen zu können, (b) eigene Gefühle, Bedürfnisse
und Wünsche wahrnehmen und angemessen zum Ausdruck bringen zu können
sowie (c) erwünschte Kontakte zu anderen aufnehmen und aktiv mitgestalten zu

können (s. auch Pfingsten 2020). Hinzu kommt die Fähigkeit, auch die Gefühle und das Verhalten anderer zu verstehen und angemessen darauf reagieren zu können (Booker und Dunsmore 2017). Soziale Kompetenzen sind assoziiert mit einer positiven psychosozialen Anpassung, während als niedrig wahrgenommene soziale Kompetenzen unter anderem mit depressiven Symptomatiken verbunden sind (Lee et al. 2010). Weiterhin finden sich Bezüge zu quantitativen (wie Größe des sozialen Netzwerks) und qualitativen Parametern der Interaktion mit anderen Sozialpartnern. Soziale Kompetenzen werden bereits im Kindesalter aufgebaut, sie erweitern sich jedoch noch einmal wesentlich im Umgang mit Gleichaltrigen in der Adoleszenz. Sie sind ein wichtiger Schlüssel zur sozialen Integration, wobei eine gute soziale Integration zum weiteren Aufbau sozialer Kompetenzen beiträgt. Umgekehrt erschweren geringe soziale Kompetenzen die soziale Integration, wodurch wenig zum weiteren Aufbau sozialer Kompetenzen beigetragen wird. In beide Richtungen sind damit sich aufschaukelnde Kreisläufe denkbar.

Man kann also zusammenfassen, dass Gleichaltrigenbeziehungen vielfältige Effekte auf die weitere Entwicklung von Jugendlichen haben können, wobei hier vor allem auf das Selbstkonzept, auf Werte und Normen sowie auf Sozialkompetenzen und soziale Integration als wesentliche Entwicklungsparameter Bezug genommen wurde. Aus Gleichaltrigenbeziehungen können sich diesbezüglich Ressourcen, aber auch Entwicklungsrisiken ergeben.

4   Bedeutsame Mechanismen, über die Peerbeziehungen Einfluss nehmen

4.1   Modelllernen und soziale Verstärkung

Die sozial-kognitive Lerntheorie nach Bandura (1977) betont die Bedeutung sozialer Einflüsse für das Lernen: Peers beeinflussen sich durch Modelllernen. Durch das Beobachten einer anderen, der Person hinreichend ähnlichen Person, und Nachahmen können komplexe Verhaltensmuster gelernt werden. Hierzu zählen aggressives und prosoziales Verhalten oder auch gesundheitsrelevante Verhaltensweisen wie Rauchen und Alkoholkonsum. Beispielsweise beeinflussen vorgelebte Konsumgewohnheiten von Eltern, Gleichaltrigen, Freunden oder in Medien (als sog. Modelle) die Entwicklung eigener Konsummuster (z. B. Wellman et al. 2016) Der Beobachter kann dabei gänzlich neues, bislang noch nicht gezeigtes Verhalten lernen oder es können nach Beobachten der Verhaltensfolgen bereits gelernte Verhaltensweisen zukünftig seltener bzw.

häufiger auftreten (zusammenfassend Edelmann und Wittmann 2019). Das Modell wird die Aufmerksamkeit eines Beobachters eher auf sich lenken, wenn es sozial anerkannt und dem Beobachter ähnlich ist. Das später möglicherweise gezeigte Verhalten wird durch Motivations- und Verstärkungsprozesse mitbestimmt. Unter Jugendlichen ist hier insbesondere auch die soziale Verstärkung relevant. Personen mit einem hohen sozialen Status werden eher nachgeahmt. Förderlich wirkt ebenfalls, wenn das Modell für sein Verhalten positive soziale Konsequenzen erhält (z. B. Prestige, Bewunderung durch andere) bzw. der Jugendliche Aufmerksamkeit, Anerkennung und Wertschätzung durch andere für sich selbst infolge des neu gelernten Verhaltens antizipiert.

4.2 Soziale Einflüsse und Gruppendruck

Wie jeder Mensch suchen auch Jugendliche Kontakt und Nähe zu anderen und möchten oftmals zu einer Gruppe Gleichgesinnter dazugehören. Dabei wählen sie eher andere, die ihnen ähnlich sind (hinsichtlich z. B. Alter, Bildungsniveau, Ethnie, Geschlecht, aber auch gesundheitsrelevanter Verhaltensweisen wie z. B. Rauchen; sog. Freundschaftshomophilie, McPherson et al. 2001). Konformität bezeichnet ferner die Tendenz des Individuums mit den Normen der Gruppe übereinzustimmen. Die Werte und Normen, die Einstellungen und das Verhalten der Gruppe haben dann Einfluss auf das Individuum. Zwei Arten von Einflüssen der Gruppe auf das Individuum werden unterschieden: informative und normative (z. B. Kessels und Hannover 2015). Beim sozialen Informationseinfluss dienen andere als Informationsquelle. Meinung und Verhalten der anderen Gruppenmitglieder werden als Standard für die eigene Meinung und das eigene Verhalten übernommen (Sherif 1935). Dies passiert insbesondere, wenn die Situation unklar und mehrdeutig ist, die Gruppenmitglieder als Experten wahrgenommen werden, die Person sich selbst hingegen als inkompetent wahrnimmt. In Gleichaltrigengruppen werden Jugendliche mit z. B. einem hohen sozialen Status oder mit Vorerfahrungen in einem (für andere noch unsicheren) Bereich wie Umgang mit Alkohol, Zigaretten oder Sexualität als wahrgenommene Experten die übrigen Gruppenmitglieder stärker beeinflussen.

Ferner spielen in Peergruppen auch normative soziale Einflüsse eine Rolle. Menschen passen sich an und verhalten sich konform, um in der eigenen Gruppe gemocht und akzeptiert zu sein (Asch 1956). Dies passiert insbesondere, wenn es für die Person sehr wichtig ist, ein Gruppenmitglied zu sein, sie davon ausgeht, dass abweichendes Verhalten sanktioniert würde und die Mitglieder die Gruppenmeinung konsistent äußern. Soziale Einflüsse (meist normativer Art) können ferner auch über Online-Interaktionen (z. B. Likes, Follower) wirksam werden (Nesi und Prinstein 2019). Da Gleichaltrigenbeziehungen im Jugendalter sehr an Bedeutung z. B. für die eigene Identität gewinnen, ist davon auszugehen, dass Jugendliche häufig eher konform mit den Normen ihrer Gruppe sind (z. B. hinsichtlich ihres Äußeren, ihrer Einstellungen, aber auch hinsichtlich gesundheitsrelevanter Verhaltensweisen wie Rauchen, Alkoholkonsum, Nutzung digitaler Medien. So zeigte am Beispiel des Rauchens eine Meta-Analyse für den Rauchbeginn einen stärkeren Einfluss durch enge Freunde (mit einem größeren Potenzial sozialer Einflussnahme) als durch Peers (Liu et al. 2017). Zudem wurden Kultureffekte deutlich: Der Einfluss durch Gleichaltrige auf das Rauchverhalten war stärker ausgeprägt in kollektivistisch geprägten Kulturen mit einer Betonung von sozialen Beziehungen und Zugehörigkeit (im Unterschied zu individualistisch geprägten Kulturen mit einem stärkeren Fokus auf das Individuum).

4.3   Soziale und emotionale Unterstützung

Andere Menschen wie Familie, Lehrer, aber auch Gleichaltrige und gute Freunde können helfen, Anforderungen zu bewältigen. Bei der sozialen Unterstützung wird zwischen wahrgenommener, erhaltener und gegebener sozialer Unterstützung unterschieden. Subjektiv wahrgenommene Unterstützung bezeichnet die Überzeugung einer Person, bei Bedarf Unterstützung aus ihrem sozialen Netzwerk erhalten zu können. Studien beziehen sich meist auf diese Form der sozialen Unterstützung. Erhaltene Unterstützung umfasst demgegenüber die tatsächlich erhaltene Unterstützung aus Sicht der Person, die unterstützt wurde. Gegebene Unterstützung umfasst die Perspektive der Person, die Unterstützung geleistet hat (s. Knoll et al. 2017). Dabei kann die (wahrgenommene, erhaltene bzw. gegebene) soziale Unterstützung emotional, instrumentell oder informationell sein. Beispielsweise kann Trost oder Zuneigung ausgedrückt werden, beim Lösen des Problems geholfen werden und relevante Information geteilt oder ein Rat gegeben werden.

Positive Zusammenhänge von sozialer Unterstützung (insbesondere wahrgenommener sozialer Unterstützung) mit Wohlbefinden und Gesundheit sind mittlerweile auch für die Altersgruppe von Kindern und Jugendlichen gut dokumentiert (s. die Meta-Analysen von Chu et al. 2010; Rueger et al. 2016). Es werden unterschiedliche Wirkmechanismen diskutiert. Soziale Unterstützung kann sich generell günstig auswirken über z. B. die Stärkung positiver Emotionen, Zugehörigkeit und Wertschätzung. Soziale Unterstützung kann demgegenüber aber auch speziell in Belastungssituationen als Ressource die ungünstigen Effekte von Stress abpuffern (Cohen und Wills 1985). Empirische Belege liegen für beide Wirkannahmen vor (Rueger et al. 2016). Auch ist denkbar, dass soziale Unterstützung über gesundheitsrelevante Verhaltensweisen einen Einfluss hat. Beispielsweise können Familie und auch Freunde dabei unterstützen, sportlich aktiv zu sein (Gill et al. 2018), was wiederum Gesundheit und Wohlbefinden fördert. Mit Blick auf die möglichen Quellen sozialer Unterstützung zeigten sich – für Jungen wie für Mädchen – günstige Effekte für die Unterstützung durch Familie, Gleichaltrige, Lehrkräfte sowie enge Freunde (Rueger et al. 2016). In Abhängigkeit von der Unterstützungsquelle kann soziale Unterstützung aber auch ungünstige Effekte haben. Hierauf verweisen beispielsweise Brezina und Azimi (2018) im Zusammenhang mit der sozialen Unterstützung durch Peers mit deviantem, antisozialem Verhalten.

4.4   Ausgrenzung und (Cyber-)Bullying

Bullying ist ein durch Ausgrenzung und Schikane geprägtes Interaktionsmuster in sozialen Gruppen wie z. B. Schulklassen. Die aggressiven Angriffe erfolgen wiederholt und über einen längeren Zeitraum und richten sich gegen schwächere Schülerinnen oder Schüler, die sich nicht wehren können. Zentrale Definitionskriterien von Bullying sind die Schädigungsintention, der Wiederholungscharakter und das ungleiche Kräfteverhältnis zwischen Täter und Opfer (Olweus 1993, 2013). Letzteres kann aus Unterschieden in körperlicher Stärke, verbaler Gewandtheit oder der sozialen Position in der Peergruppe resultieren. So können auch die Schikanen unterschiedlicher Art sein: physisch (z. B. verprügeln), verbal (z. B. beleidigen) oder relational (z. B. ausgrenzen; Scheithauer et al. 2003). Zudem können die Schikanen über digitale Medien erfolgen (z. B. per Handy, Chat, soziale Netzwerke). Beispiele sind die Verbreitung von Gerüchten oder das Ausschließen aus Online-Gruppen. Bullying über digitale Medien wird als Cyberbullying bezeichnet. Mit Blick auf die Zusammenhänge über die beiden Kontexte (traditionelles Bullying und Cyberbullying) dokumentiert eine Meta-Analyse eine hohe Korrespondenz für die Opfer und die Täter (Modecki et al. 2014).

Bei der Entstehung und Aufrechterhaltung von Bullying hat die gesamte Gruppe einen wichtigen Anteil, nicht nur Täter und Opfer. Nach dem Participant-Role-Ansatz (Salmivalli et al. 1996) sind so gut wie alle Mitglieder einer Schulklasse in irgendeiner Weise involviert. Die Reaktionen der Klassenkameraden können Bullying verstärken (z. B. lachen), passiv sein (z. B. wegsehen) oder

Bullying entgegenwirken (z. B. Opfer verteidigen). Bullying ist weit verbreitet. In einer deutschsprachigen Stichprobe mit 198 Schulklassen der 6. und 9. Stufe waren (basierend auf den Angaben von Peers) ein Drittel der Schülerinnen und Schüler als Pro-Bullying-Akteur (Täter, Assistenten, Verstärker), als Opfer oder als Bully-Opfer involviert. Nur etwa 10 % setzten sich als Verteidiger für die Opfer ein (Knauf et al. 2017).

Wichtige Angriffspunkte zum Stoppen von Bullying in Schulklassen sind die Etablierung Gewalt ächtender sozialer Normen, eine Stärkung der Klassengemeinschaft sowie die Mobilisierung bislang untätiger Klassenkameraden (Knauf et al. 2018; s. auch Ma et al. 2019). Nach Zych et al. (2019) zählte (basierend auf Meta-Analysen) zu den Schutzfaktoren ein Schulklima, das positive Interaktionen unter Gleichaltrigen stärkt. Zudem erwiesen sich Peer-Einflüsse (z. B. prosoziale Gleichaltrige, sozialer Status) neben elterlicher Erziehung und persönlichen Kompetenzen als protektiv gegenüber Bullying.

Zusammenfassend können sich Gleichaltrige über unterschiedliche Mechanismen beeinflussen. Vorgestellt wurden Modelllernen und soziale Verstärkung, Gruppendruck und sozialer Einfluss, soziale und emotionale Unterstützung sowie Ausgrenzung und Bullying. Hieraus können – je nach Gruppe – günstige wie auch eher ungünstige Wirkungen auf Wohlbefinden und Gesundheit resultieren.

5   Peerbeziehungen und ihr Einfluss auf Wohlbefinden und Gesundheit

5.1   Psychisches Wohlbefinden

Nach den Daten des Kinder- und Jugendgesundheitssurveys KiGGS kann die Mehrheit der Kinder und Jugendlichen (etwa 80 %) in Deutschland als psychisch gesund bezeichnet werden; d. h. sie zeigen keine Anhaltspunkte für psychische Auffälligkeiten (Baumgarten et al. 2018). Meta-Analysen oder Überblicksarbeiten zu Assoziationen zwischen Peerbeziehungen und explizit Wohlbefinden oder psychischer Gesundheit liegen unseres Wissens nach nicht vor. Mit Blick auf einzelne Studien zeigte sich z. B. erwartungskonform eine positive Assoziation für Wohlbefinden mit einem unterstützenden Freundschaftsnetzwerk (Almquist et al. 2014). Bereits Havighurst (1972) postulierte, dass eine gelungene Bewältigung alterstypischer Entwicklungsaufgaben mit Wohlbefinden und Lebenszufriedenheit einhergeht. Demnach sollten soziale Beziehungen mit Gleichaltrigen (als relevante Entwicklungsaufgabe Jugendlicher) einflussreich für Gesundheit und Wohlbefinden sein (s. Roisman et al. 2004).

5.2   Internalisierende Symptomatiken

Internalisierende Auffälligkeiten wie Angst oder Depression nehmen ins-
besondere für Mädchen im Jugendalter zu (Baumgarten et al. 2018). Die
Ursachen sind multifaktoriell und berücksichtigen bio-psycho-soziale Faktoren.
So kann eine Überforderung in der Bewältigung alterstypischer Entwicklungsaufgaben (z. B. Aufbau von Beziehungen zu Gleichaltrigen) mit internalisierenden
Problemen einhergehen (s. Heinrichs und Lohaus 2011). Zum Einfluss von
Freunden und Gleichaltrigenbeziehungen für internalisierende Symptome
liegen umfangreiche Studien vor. Im Kindes- und Jugendalter mindestens einen
Freund zu haben, erwies sich – für Mädchen wie für Jungen – als protektiv gegen
internalisierende Symptome im jungen Erwachsenenalter (nach Kontrolle für
kindliche Symptomatik und elterliche Depression; Sakyi et al. 2015). Vertrauensvolle und sichere Peerbeziehungen waren in einer Meta-Analyse mit weniger
internalisierenden Symptomen assoziiert, hingegen unsichere Beziehungen
(charakterisiert durch Gefühle wie Ärger und Distanz) mit depressiven
Symptomen (Gorrese 2016).

Für Ausgrenzung durch Peers und Bullying-Viktimisierung dokumentierten
Schoeler et al. (2018) in ihrer Meta-Analyse negative Auswirkungen auf
internalisierende und externalisierende Probleme wie auch für akademische
Schwierigkeiten. Die Kausaleffekte waren insgesamt niedrig und mit $d = .27$
am stärksten für internalisierende Symptome. Mit zeitlichem Abstand zum
Bullying-Geschehen nahmen die schädlichen Effekte ab. Reijntjes et al. (2010)
zeigten in ihrer Meta-Analyse auf der Basis von Längsschnittdaten Wechselbeziehungen zwischen Viktimisierung und internalisierenden Problemen.
Demnach festigen internalisierende Symptome den Status der Kinder und
Jugendlichen als Bullying-Opfer und sind nicht allein Folge der Schikanen. Mit
einem Fokus auf Cyberviktimisierung bestätigt die Meta-Analyse von Fisher
et al. (2016) negative Assoziationen mit internalisierenden und externalisierenden
Symptomen. Peers können somit ein Risikofaktor für internalisierende Symptome
sein. Dies zeigte sich deutlich im Zusammenhang mit Viktimisierung. Jedoch
können sich z. B. auch in innigen Freundschaften insbesondere Mädchen
beim gemeinsamen Grübeln über Probleme (als Risikofaktor für Depressivi-
tät) gegenseitig „anstecken" (Felton et al. 2019). Freunde und Peers gehen aber
auch als Ressource mit einer günstigen Anpassung einher. Als protektiv diskutieren die Autoren (z. B. Gorrese 2016; Sakyi et al. 2015) die Stärkung sozialer
und emotionaler Unterstützung, sozialer Kompetenzen und des Selbstwerts.
Ähnlich waren gute schulische Leistungen, soziale Kompetenzen, eine gute

Eltern-Kind-Beziehung und prosoziale Freunde protektiv beim Durchbrechen der Assoziation von Bullying-Viktimisierung mit internalisierenden Problemen (Ttofi et al. 2014).

5.3　Externalisierendes Problemverhalten

Unter externalisierendem Problemverhalten werden antisoziale Verhaltensweisen wie Aggression und Delinquenz, aber auch selbstverletzendes Verhalten, riskantes Sexualverhalten oder Substanzkonsum subsummiert (z. B. Fisher et al. 2016). Dieser Abschnitt fokussiert antisoziales Verhalten. Aggression ist ein Verhalten, das mit der Absicht ausgeführt wird, Personen oder Sachen zu schädigen, und geht meistens mit einer Verletzung von Normen und Regeln einher. Verstoßen Jugendliche mit ihrem Verhalten gegen strafrechtliche Normen des Landes, ist dies delinquent (z. B. Körperverletzung, Sachbeschädigung). Nach dem Deutschen Jugendinstitut (DJI 2019) ist Jugendgewalt häufig ein vorübergehendes Phänomen, entsteht situativ in der Gruppe und vollzieht sich dabei meist in der zugehörigen Alters- und Geschlechtergruppe, was auf die Bedeutung sozialer Bindungen und devianter Peergruppen als Risikofaktoren hinweist (s. auch Beelmann 2018, für ein kumulatives Entwicklungsmodell).

Kinder und Jugendliche mit externalisierendem Verhalten haben keine generellen Schwierigkeiten, Freundschaften zu schließen. Nach Ackermann et al. (2018) ist jedoch die Form aggressiven Verhaltens einflussreich: offen aggressives Verhalten (z. B. physischer Angriff) ging eher mit einer negativen Freundschaftsqualität (konfliktreich, weniger intim und unterstützend) einher, relational aggressives Verhalten (z. B. andere ausgrenzen) eher mit positiveren Freundschaften (trotz vieler Konflikte). Auch für externalisierendes Problemverhalten resultierten (vergleichbar mit Längsschnittstudien zu internalisierenden Auffälligkeiten) in einer Meta-Analyse Wechselbeziehungen mit Peer-Viktimisierung und Ausgrenzung (Reijntjes et al. 2011). So können externalisierende Verhaltensprobleme wie Aggression der Viktimisierung vorausgehen oder folgen. Basierend auf Querschnittsdaten zeigen sich ähnliche Zusammenhänge mit Cyberviktimisierung (Fisher et al. 2016). Als Schutzfaktoren gut belegt sind Freundschaftsbeziehungen zu prosozialen Gleichaltrigen (z. B. Brumley und Jaffee 2016; Ttofi et al. 2014).

5.4   Gesundheitsverhaltensweisen

In Kindheit und Jugend werden gesundheitsrelevante Verhaltensweisen erlernt und stabilisiert. Hierzu zählen z. B. Ernährung, körperliche Aktivität, Alkohol- und Tabakkonsum oder Sexualverhalten. Dabei sind verschiedene Gesundheitsverhaltensweisen miteinander assoziiert. Beispielsweise identifizierten Busch et al. (2013) bei Jugendlichen vier Bereiche: (a) Risikoverhalten (z. B. Rauchen, Alkoholkonsum, Sexualverhalten), (b) Bullying (Täter, Opfer), (c) problematischer Medienkonsum (z. B. exzessives Videospielen) und (d) körperliche Inaktivität und ungesunde Ernährung. Als Einflussfaktoren sind neben individuellen Faktoren (z. B. Selbstwirksamkeit) auch soziale Faktoren seitens der Familie (z. B. gute Beziehung zu den Eltern, elterliches Monitoring) oder der Gleichaltrigen (z. B. deren Einstellungen, Normen oder Verhaltensweisen) relevant (s. Lohaus et al. 2006). In einem umfangreichen Review sind Montgomery und Kollegen (2020) dem Einfluss sozialer Peer-Netzwerke im schulischen Umfeld auf gesundheitsrelevantes Verhalten wie Alkoholkonsum, Rauchen, körperliche Aktivität und Ernährung nachgegangen. Über alle Gesundheitsverhaltensweisen hinweg zeigten sich Hinweise auf soziale Homophilie (Jugendliche wählten Freunde mit ähnlichen Gesundheitsverhaltensweisen) und/ oder sozialen Einfluss (Jugendliche übernahmen Verhaltensweisen ihrer Freunde oder passten ihr Verhalten dem ihrer Freunde an). Für Jugendliche mit günstigen gesundheitsrelevanten Verhaltensmustern wirken demnach Freunde mit ebenfalls günstigem Verhalten (z. B. Nichtrauchen) gesundheitsverhaltensverstärkend. Anders ist die Lage bei Jugendlichen mit gesundheitlichem Risikoverhalten: Hier verstärken (rauchende) Freunde das riskante Verhaltensmuster. Ferner zeigten sich Assoziationen zwischen Beliebtheit in der Gleichaltrigengruppe und Gesundheitsverhaltensweisen. Die Wirkrichtung ist bislang offen: ein Anstieg der Popularität kann Folge bestimmter (Risiko)Verhaltensweisen sein. Auch kann Popularität zu Veränderungen gesundheitsrelevanter Verhaltensweisen führen.

5.5   Schulleistung und Schulerfolg

Gesundheit und Schulerfolg sind wechselseitig assoziiert (Dadaczynski 2012), auch über die Bewältigung alterstypischer Entwicklungsaufgaben Jugendlicher. Rahmenmodelle zu schulischen Leistungen berücksichtigen zahlreiche Einflussfaktoren und beinhalten als Facetten der schulischen Lernumwelt auch peerbezogene Einflüsse (z. B. Tarelli und Zylowski 2012). Empirisch zeigte eine Meta-Analyse einen schwach positiven Zusammenhang zwischen dem Vorhandensein von Freundschaften in der Schule und der Schulleistung (Schulnoten oder Leistungstests; Wentzel et al. 2018). Als Vermittlungspfade diskutieren die Autoren Möglichkeiten vertiefter kognitiver Verarbeitung, Modelllernen und soziale Verstärkung beim gemeinsamen Lösen schwieriger Aufgaben, Aspekte sozialer und emotionaler Unterstützung, gemeinsame leistungsbezogene Normen und Werte wie auch generell die Assoziation von prosozialem Verhalten mit Selbstkontrolle. Dabei wählten Jugendliche bevorzugt Freunde, die ihnen hinsichtlich ihrer schulischen Leistung ähnlich waren – mit einer Ausnahme: Galt in der Klasse Leistung als uncool, vermieden leistungsstarke Schüler Freundschaften untereinander. Generell vermieden Leistungsstarke jedoch leistungsschwache Peers als Freunde und umgekehrt Leistungsschwache leistungsstarke Peers (Laninga-Wijnen et al. 2019). Freunde können somit insbesondere unter leistungsschwächeren Mitschülern Motivation und Schulerfolg negativ beeinflussen.

Eine weitere Meta-Analyse der Autorengruppe (Wentzel et al. 2020) fand einen mittleren Zusammenhang zwischen sozialem Status und Schulleistung. Sozial akzeptierte und gemochte Klassenkameraden zeigten eine bessere akademische Leistung. Der Zusammenhang war (unabhängig vom Geschlecht der Kinder) stärker für jüngere Schülerinnen und Schüler wie auch für Schülerinnen und Schüler asiatischer Länder (als stärker kollektivistisch geprägte Kultur) im Vergleich zu Schülerinnen und Schülern aus Nordamerika oder Europa. Als Mediatoren waren höhere leistungsbezogene Überzeugungen (wie akademisches Selbstkonzept oder Selbstwirksamkeit), ein stärkeres Engagement (wie Anstrengung oder Kooperation) und weniger negative Emotionen relevant. Mikami et al. (2017) verdeutlichen die Relevanz von Zugehörigkeit und Verbundenheit mit den Klassenkameraden für die Schulleistung. Schüler, die sich ihren Klassenkameraden verbunden und zugehörig fühlten, engagierten sich im Schuljahresverlauf stärker im Unterricht, was wiederum das Gefühl der Zugehörigkeit stärkte, und auch mit einer besseren Leistung am Schuljahresende einherging. Nach den Autoren ermöglicht ein unterstützendes Klassenklima das Suchen von Hilfe und sozialer Unterstützung. Fühlen sich hingegen Schülerinnen und Schüler sozial ausgegrenzt, führt dies eher zu Schwierigkeiten bei der Konzentration und Bearbeitung der schulischen Aufgaben. So zeigten sich Hinweise auf schwach negative Effekte von Bullying-Viktimisierung auf die Schulleistung (Schoeler et al. 2013).

6   Ausblick

6.1   Reziproke Effekte

Gleichaltrige beeinflussen die Entwicklung Jugendlicher. Für alle betrachteten Aspekte zu Gesundheit und Wohlbefinden (internalisierende und externalisierende Auffälligkeiten, diverse Gesundheitsverhaltensweisen und Schulleistung) liegen zahlreiche empirische Befunde zu förderlichen wie auch problematischen Einflüssen durch Peers vor. Wenn auch mehrere Längsschnitt-studien existieren, sind Aussagen über die Kausalrichtung der Befunde nicht einfach. Vielmehr ist von komplexen, multikausalen Wechselwirkungen auszugehen (z. B. Reijntjes et al. 2010). Weiter berücksichtigten unterschiedliche Studien unterschiedliche Arten jugendlicher Peerbeziehungen (z. B. Freunde, soziale Peernetzwerke) selten in ihrer Kombination. Jedoch ist auch hier von Wechsel-wirkungsprozessen und komplexeren Einflüssen auszugehen (z. B. Liu et al. 2017 für enge Freunde im Vergleich zu Peers).

Wie können nun Peerbeziehungen Gesundheit und Wohlbefinden beeinflussen? Mit ihrem Einfluss auf Selbstwert, Selbstkonzept, soziale Kompetenz, soziale Integration oder soziale Unterstützung wurden als Entwicklungsdimensionen empirisch gesicherte Schutzfaktoren für die Entwicklung von Kindern und Jugendlichen angesprochen (Bengel und Rottmann 2009). Ergänzend zu den Gleichaltrigen sind mit Blick auf die soziale Umwelt weitere soziokulturelle Ein-flussfaktoren mit ihren wechselseitigen Beziehungen für die Entwicklung relevant (Bronfenbrenner und Morris 2006). Beispielsweise zeigten sich Hinweise auf kulturspezifische Zusammenhänge (Liu et al. 2017). Auch Faktoren bezogen auf die Schule (z. B. Schulklima), die Nachbarschaft (z. B. Wohngegend, Kriminali-tät) oder die Familie (z. B. Eltern-Kind-Beziehung) können eher protektive oder auch schädliche Effekte für die Anpassung Jugendlicher haben (Brumley und Jaffee 2016).

6.2   Eltern-Kind-Beziehung

Für den Aufbau von Gleichaltrigenbeziehungen wie auch für Gesundheit und Wohlbefinden kommt der Familie, speziell der Eltern-Kind-Beziehung, eine besondere Bedeutung zu (s. Walper et al. 2018). So können die Beziehungs-, Bindungs- und Erziehungsqualität, wie sie Familie und Eltern bieten, als Ressourcen oder Entwicklungsrisiken Effekte auf die kindliche Entwicklung und die Bewältigung alterstypischer Entwicklungsaufgaben zeigen (Bengel et al. 2009). Zudem sind die Beziehungen Jugendlicher zu ihren Eltern und auch der Aufbau von Peerbeziehungen vor dem Hintergrund bisheriger Bindungserfahrungen zu sehen (Grossmann und Grossmann 2012). Eine sichere Eltern-Kind-Bindung in der frühen Kindheit kann als Schutzfaktor wirken und Gleichaltrigenbeziehungen im Jugendalter positiv beeinflussen. Ferner schwindet mit der Umgestaltung der Eltern-Kind-Beziehung und dem zunehmenden Einfluss Gleichaltriger im Jugendalter der elterliche Einfluss nicht gänzlich; vielmehr wird der Einfluss Gleichaltriger durch das elterliche Erziehungsverhalten mitbestimmt (Laursen et al. 2015).

6.3 Prävention und Gesundheitsförderung

Im Rahmen von (schulischer) Prävention und Gesundheitsförderung sind Ansätze zur Förderung von Lebenskompetenzen etabliert (s. Knauf et al. 2018). So hat die WHO (1994, 2003) zentrale Kompetenzen beschrieben, die neben kognitiven (z. B. kritisches Denken) und persönlichen Kompetenzen (z. B. Selbstkonzept, Selbstregulation) auch interpersonale, soziale Kompetenzen ansprechen. Zu Letzteren zählen Beziehungsgestaltung, Kommunikation, Empathie, Kooperation und Selbstbehauptung. Aufbau und Stärkung der Lebenskompetenzen (als Ressourcen) unterstützen Jugendliche, mit alltäglichen und entwicklungsbezogenen Anforderungen kompetent umzugehen, gesundheitsförderliches Verhalten zu zeigen und riskantes, gesundheitsschädliches Verhalten zu unterlassen. Lebenskompetenzansätze sind häufig individuumsbezogen und zielen auf die Beeinflussung des Verhaltens (z. B. Übungen zum Ablehnen einer Zigarette). Ergänzend kann eine Berücksichtigung verhältnispräventiver Maßnahmen mit Einbezug der Umwelt Jugendlicher (Schule, Freizeit, Familie) hilfreich sein. Vor dem Hintergrund der starken Bedeutung Gleichaltriger für Gesundheit und Wohlbefinden sollten entwicklungssensitive Präventionsmaßnahmen im Jugendalter Peerbeziehungen und Freundschaften explizit berücksichtigen. Beispiele sind die Stärkung individueller sozialer Kompetenzen, die Förderung prosozialer Peerbeziehungen (z. B. soziale Unterstützung, kooperative Arbeitsformen) oder das Abschwächen negativer Peereinflüsse (z. B. Umgang mit Gruppendruck).

Literatur

Ackermann, K., Büttner, G., Bernhard, A., Martinelli, A., Freitag, C. M. & Schwenck, C. (2018). Freundschaftsqualitäten und unterschiedliche Formen aggressiven Verhaltens bei Jungen und Mädchen im späten Kindes- und Jugendalter. *Kindheit und Entwicklung, 27,* 81-90.

Albert, M., Hurrelmann, K., Quenzel, G. & Kantar (2019). *Jugend 2019 – Eine Generation meldet sich zu Wort.* Weinheim: Beltz.

Almquist, Y. B., Östberg, V., Rostila, M., Edling, C. & Rydgren, J. (2014). Friendship network characteristics and psychological well-being in late adolescence: Exploring differences by gender and gender composition. *Scandinavian Journal of Public Health, 42,* 146–154.

Asch, S. E. (1956). Studies in independence and conformity: A minority of one against a unanimous majority. *Psychological Monographs, 70,* 416.

Bandura, A. (1977). *Social learning theory.* Englewood Cliffs: Prentice Hall.

Bandura, A. (1991). Social cognitive theory of moral thought and action. In W. M. Kurtines & J. L. Gewirtz (Hrsg.), *Handbook of moral behavior and development. Volume 1: Theory* (S. 45–103). Hillsdale, N.J.: Lawrence Erlbaum.

Baumgarten, F., Klipker, K., Göbel, K., Janitza, S. & Hölling, H. (2018). Der Verlauf psychischer Auffälligkeiten bei Kindern und Jugendlichen – Ergebnisse der KiGGS-Kohorte. *Journal of Health Monitoring, 3,* 60–65.

Beelmann, A. (2018). Dissoziales Verhalten. In B. Gniewosz & P. T. Titzmann (Hrsg.), *Handbuch Jugend: Psychologische Sichtweisen auf Veränderungen in der Adoleszenz* (S. 472–489). Stuttgart: Kohlhammer.

Bengel, J., Meinders-Lücking, F. &. & Rottmann, N. (2009*). Schutzfaktoren bei Kindern und Jugendlichen – Stand der Forschung zu psychosozialen Schutzfaktoren für Gesundheit.* Köln: BZgA.

Blasi, A. (1980). Bridging moral cognition and moral action: A critical review of the literature. *Psychological Bulletin, 88,* 1–45.

Blasi, A. (1983). Moral cognition and moral action: A theoretical perspective. *Developmental Review, 3,* 178–210.

Bobakova, D., Geckova, A. M., Klein, D., van Dijk, J. P. & Reijneveld, S. A. (2015). Fighting, truancy and low academic achievement in youth subcultures. *Young, 23,* 357–372.

Bode, H. & Heßling, A. (2015). *Jugendsexualität 2015. Die Perspektive der 14- bis 25-Jährigen. Ergebnisse einer aktuellen Repräsentativen Wiederholungsbefragung.* Köln: Bundeszentrale für gesundheitliche Aufklärung.

Booker, J. A. & Dunsmore, J. C. (2017). Affective social competence in adolescence: Current findings and future directions. *Social Development, 26,* 3–20.

Brezina, T. & Azimi, A. M. (2018). Social support, loyalty to delinquent peers, and offending: An elaboration and test of the differential social support hypothesis. *Deviant Behavior, 39,* 648–663.

Bronfenbrenner, U. & Morris, P. A. (2006). The bioecological model of human development. In R. M. Lerner & W. Damon (Eds.), *Handbook of child psychology: Theoretical models of human development* (6th Ed., pp. 793–828). New York: Wiley.

Brown, B. B. (2004). Adolescents' relationships with peers. In R. M. Lerner & L. Steinberg (Eds.), *Handbook of adolescent psychology* (2nd Ed., pp. 363–394). New York: Wiley.

Brown, B. B. (2011). Popularity in peer group perspective: The role of status in adolescent peer systems. In A. H. N. Cillessen, D. Schwartz & L. Mayeux (Eds.), *Popularity in the peer system* (pp. 165–192). New York, NY: Guilford Press.

Brown, B. B. & Larson, J. (2009). Peer relationships in adolescence. In R. M. Lerner & L. Steinberg (Eds.), *Handbook of adolescent psychology: Contextual influences on adolescent development* (p. 74–103). New York: Wiley.

Brumley, L. D. & Jaffee, S. R. (2016). Defining and distinguishing promotive and protective effects for childhood externalizing psychopathology: A systematic review. *International Journal for Research in Social and Genetic Epidemiology and Mental Health Services, 51*, 803–8.15.

Buhrmester, D. (1990). Intimacy of friendship, interpersonal competence, and adjustment during preadolescence and adolescence. *Child Development 61*, 1101–1111.

Busch, V., Van Stel. H. F., Schrijvers, A. J. & De Leeuw, J. R. J. (2013). Clustering of health-related behaviors, health outcomes and demographics in Dutch adolescents: a cross-sectional study. *BMW Public Health, 13,* 1118.

Chu, P. S., Saucier, D. A. & Hafner, E. (2010). Meta-analysis of the relationships between social support and well-being in children and adolescents. *Journal of Social and Clinical Psychology, 29*, 624–645.

Claes, M.E. (1992). Friendship and personal adjustment during adolescence. *Journal of Adolescence, 15*, 39–55.

Cohen, S., & Wills. T. A. (1985). Stress, social support, and the buffering hypothesis. *Psychological Bulletin, 98*, 310–357.

Cooper, C. R. & Cooper, R. G. (1992). Links between adolescents' relationships with their parents and peers: Models, evidence, and mechanisms. In R. D. Parke & G. W. Ladd (Eds.), *Family–peer relationships: Modes of linkage* (p. 135–158). Lawrence Erlbaum Associates, Inc.

Dadaczynski, K. (2012). Stand der Forschung zum Zusammenhang von Gesundheit und Bildung: Überblick und Implikationen für die schulische Gesundheitsförderung. *Zeitschrift Für Gesundheitspsychologie, 20*, 141–153.

DJI (2019). *Zahlen, Daten, Fakten: Jugendgewalt.* http://www.dji.de/jugendkriminalitaet

Edelmann, W. & Wittmann, S. (2019). *Lernpsychologie* (8. Aufl). Weinheim: Beltz.

Elkind, D. (1985). Egocentrism redux. *Developmental Review, 5*, 218–226.

Eschenbeck, H. & Knauf, Rh.-K. (2018). Entwicklungsaufgaben und ihre Bewältigung. In A. Lohaus (Hrsg), *Entwicklungspsychologie des Jugendalters* (S. 23–50). Heidelberg: Springer.

Felton, J. W., Cole, D. A., Havewala, M., Kurdziel, G. & Brown, V. (2019). Talking together, thinking alone: Relations among co-rumination, peer relationships, and rumination. *Journal of Youth and Adolescence, 48*, 731–743.

Fisher, B. W., Gardella, J. H. & Teurbe-Tolon, A. R. (2016). Peer cybervictimization among adolescents and the associated internalizing and externalizing problems: A meta-analysis. *Journal of Youth and Adolescence, 45*, 1727–1743.

Fussan, N. (2006). Einbindung Jugendlicher in Peer-Netzwerke. Welche Integrationsvorteile erbringt die Mitgliedschaft in Sportvereinen? *Zeitschrift für Soziologie der Erziehung Sozialisation, 26*, 383–402.

Gallardo, L. O., Barrasa, A. & Guevara-Viejo, F. (2016). Positive peer relationships and academic achievement across early and midadolescence. *Social Behavior and Personality, 44*, 1637–1648.

Gill, M., Chan-Golston, A. M., Rice, L. N., Roth, S. E., Crespi, C. M., Cole, B. L., Koniak-Griffin, D. & Prelip, M. L. (2018). Correlates of social support and its association with physical activity among young adolescents. *Health Education & Behavior, 45*, 207–216.

Glüer, M. & Lohaus, A. (2015). Frequency of victimization experiences and well-being among online, offline and combined victims on social online network sites of German children and adolescents. *Frontiers in Public Health, 3*, 274.

Glüer, M. & Lohaus, A. (2016). Participation in social network sites: Associations with the quality of offline and online friendships in preadolescents and adolescents. *Cyberpsychology: Journal of Psychosocial Research on Cyberspace, 10*, 1.

Gorrese, A. (2016). Peer attachment and youth internalizing problems: A meta-analysis. *Child & Youth Care Forum, 45*, 177–204.

Grossmann, K. & Grossmann, K. E. (2012). *Bindungen. Das Gefüge psychischer Sicherheit*. Stuttgart: Klett-Cotta.

Hardy, S. A. & Carlo, G. (2005). Identity as a source of moral motivation. *Human Development, 48*, 232–256.

Havighurst, R. J. (1953). *Human development and education*. New York: David McKay.

Havighurst, R. J. (1972). *Developmental tasks and education* (3rd edition). New York: Longman.

Heinrichs, N. & Lohaus, A. (2011). *Klinische Entwicklungspsychologie kompakt: Psychische Störungen im Kindes- und Jugendalter*. Weinheim: Beltz.

Hinsch, R. & Pfingsten, U. (Hrsg.) (2015). *Gruppentraining sozialer Kompetenzen GSK*. Weinheim: Beltz.

Kessels, U. & Hannover, B. (2015). Gleichaltrige. In E. Wild & J. Möller (Hrsg.), *Pädagogische Psychologie* (S. 283–302). Berlin: Springer.

Khan, S., Gagné, M., Yang, L. & Shapka, J. (2016). Exploring the relationship between adolescents' self-concept and their offline and online social worlds. *Computers in Human Behavior, 55*, 940–945.

Knauf, Rh.-K., Eschenbeck, H. & Hock, M. (2018). Bystanders of bullying: Social-cognitive and affective reactions to school bullying and cyberbullying. *Cyberpsychology: Journal of Psychosocial Research on Cyberspace, 12*, 3.

Knauf, Rh.-K., Eschenbeck, H. & Käser, U. (2017). Bullying im Klassenverband. Prävalenz, soziometrische und leistungsbezogene Merkmale der Participant Roles. *Zeitschrift für Entwicklungspsychologie und Pädagogische Psychologie, 49*, 186–196.

Knauf, Rh.-K., Hofmann, H. & Eschenbeck, H. (2018). Förderung von Lebenskompetenzen. In C.-W. Kohlmann, C. Salewski & M. A. Wirtz (Hrsg.), *Psychologie in der Gesundheitsförderung* (S. 355–368). Bern: Huber.

Knoll, N., Scholz, U. & Rieckmann, N. (2017). *Einführung in die Gesundheitspsychologie* (4. Aufl.). München: Ernst Reinhardt.

Koepke, S. & Denissen, J. J. (2012). Dynamics of identity development and separation–individuation in parent–child relationships during adolescence and emerging adulthood – A conceptual integration. *Developmental Review, 32*, 67–88.

Krettenauer, T. (2017). Pro-environmental behavior and adolescent moral development. *Journal of Research on Adolescence, 27*, 581–593.

Laninga-Wijnen, L., Gremmen, M. C., Dijkstra, J. K., Veenstra, R., Vollebergh, W. A. M. & Harakeh, Z. (2019). The role of academic status norms in friendship selection and influence processes related to academic achievement. *Developmental Psychology, 55*, 337–350.

Laursen, B. & Adams, R. (2018). Conflict between peers. In W.M. Bukowski, B. Laursen & K.H. Rubin (Eds.), *Handbook of peer interactions, relationships, and groups* (pp. 265–283). New York, NY: Guilford Press.

Laursen, B., Žukauskienė, R., Raižienė, S., Hiatt, C. & Dickson, D. J. (2015). Perceived parental protectiveness promotes positive friend influence. *Infant and Child Development, 24*, 452–468.

Lee, A., Hankin, B. L. & Mermelstein, R. J. (2010). Perceived social competence, negative social interactions, and negative cognitive style predict depressive symptoms during adolescence. *Journal of Clinical Child & Adolescent Psychology, 39*, 603–615.

Liu, J., Zhao, S., Chen, X., Falk, E. & Albarracín, D. (2017). The influence of peer behavior as a function of social and cultural closeness: A meta-analysis of normative influence on adolescent smoking initiation and continuation. *Psychological Bulletin, 143*, 1082–1115.

Lohaus, A., Jerusalem, M. & Klein-Heßling, J. (2006). *Gesundheitsförderung im Kindes- und Jugendalter.* Göttingen: Hogrefe.

Lohaus, A. & Vierhaus, M. (2019). *Entwicklungspsychologie des Kindes- und Jugendalters* (4. Aufl.). Heidelberg: Springer.

Ma, T.-L., Meter, D. J., Chen, W.-T. & Lee, Y. (2019). Defending behavior of peer victimization in school and cyber context during childhood and adolescence: A meta-analytic review of individual and peer-relational characteristics. *Psychological Bulletin, 145*, 891–928.

McPherson, M., Smith-Lovin, L. & Cook, J. M. (2001). Birds of a feather: Homophily in social networks. *Annual Review of Sociology, 27*, 415–444.

Mesch, G. & Talmud, I. (2006). The quality of online and offline relationships: The role of multiplexity and duration of social relationships. *Information Society, 22*, 137–148.

Mikami, A. Y., Ruzek, E. A., Hafen, C. A., Gregory, A. & Allen, J. P. (2017). Perceptions of relatedness with classroom peers promote adolescents' behavioral engagement and achievement in secondary school. *Journal of Youth and Adolescence, 46*, 2341–2354.

Modecki, K. L., Minchin, J., Harbaugh, A. G., Guerra, N. G. & Runions, K. C. (2014). Bullying prevalence across contexts: A meta-analysis measuring cyber and traditional bullying. *Journal of Adolescent Health, 55*, 602–611.

Montgomery, S. C., Donnelly, M., Bhatnagar, P., Carlin, A., Kee, F. & Hunter, R. F. (2020). Peer social network processes and adolescent health behaviors: A systematic review. *Preventive Medicine, 130*, 105900.

Müller, C. & Minger, M. (2013). Which children and adolescents are most susceptible to peer influence? A systematic review regarding antisocial behavior. *Empirische Sonderpädagogik, 2*, 107–129.

Nesi, J. & Prinstein M. J. (2019). In search of likes: Longitudinal associations between adolescents' digital status seeking and health-risk behaviors. *Journal of Clinical Child & Adolescent Psychology, 48*, 740–748.

Olweus, D. (1993). *Bullying at school. What we know and what we can do.* Oxford: Blackwell Publishers.

Olweus, D. (2013). School bullying: Development and some important challenges. *Annual Review of Clinical Psychology, 9*, 751–780.

Pfingsten, U. (2020). Soziale Kompetenzen. In A. Lohaus & H. Domsch (Hrsg.), *Psychologische Förder- und Interventionsprogramme für das Kindes- und Jugendalter* (2. Aufl.). Heidelberg: Springer (in Vorbereitung).

Poulin, F. & Chan, A. (2010). Friendship stability and change in childhood and adolescence. *Developmental Review, 30,* 257–272.

Reijntjes, A., Kamphuis, J. H., Prinzie, P., Boelen, P. A., van der Schoot, M. & Telch, M. J. (2011). Prospective linkages between peer victimization and externalizing problems in children: A meta-analysis. *Aggressive Behavior, 37,* 215–222.

Reijntjes, A., Kamphuis, J. H., Prinzie, P. & Telch, M. J. (2010). Peer victimization and internalizing problems in children: A meta-analysis of longitudinal studies. *Child Abuse & Neglect, 34,* 244–252.

Reitz, A. K., Zimmermann, J., Hutteman, R., Specht, J. & Neyer, F. J. (2014). How peers make a difference: The role of peer groups and peer relationships in personality development. *European Journal of Personality, 28,* 279–288.

Röhrle, B. (1994). *Soziale Netzwerke und soziale Unterstützung.* Weinheim: Beltz.

Roisman, G. I., Masten, A. S., Coatsworth, J. D. &. & Tellegen, A. (2004). Salient and emerging developmental tasks in the transition to adulthood. *Child Development, 75,* 123–133.

Rueger, S. Y., Malecki, C. K., Pyun, Y., Aycock, C. & Coyle, S. (2016). A meta-analytic review of the association between perceived social support and depression in childhood and adolescence. *Psychological Bulletin, 142,* 1017–1067.

Sakyi, K. S., Surkan, P. J., Fombonne, E., Chollet, A. & Melchior, M. (2015). Childhood friendships and psychological difficulties in young adulthood: An 18-year follow-up study. *European Child & Adolescent Psychiatry, 24,* 815–826.

Salmivalli, C., Lagerspetz, K., Björkqvist, K., Österman, K. & Kaukiainen, A. (1996). Bullying as a group process. Participant roles and their relations to social status within the group. *Aggressive Behavior, 22,* 1–15.

Sanders, J., Munford, R., Liebenberg, L. & Ungar, M. (2017). Peer paradox: The tensions that peer relationships raise for vulnerable youth. *Child & Family Social Work, 22,* 3–14.

Scheithauer, H., Hayer, T. & Petermann, F. (2003). *Bullying unter Schülern: Erscheinungsformen, Risikobedingungen und Interventionskonzepte.* Göttingen: Hogrefe.

Schoeler, T., Duncan, L., Cecil, C. M., Ploubidis, G. B. & Pingault, J.-B. (2018). Quasi-experimental evidence on short- and long-term consequences of bullying victimization: A meta-analysis. *Psychological Bulletin, 144,* 1229–1246.

Schouten, A. P., Valkenburg, P. M. & Peter, J. (2007). Precursors and underlying processes of adolescents' online self-disclosure: Developing and testing an "Internet-Attribute-Perception" model. *Media Psychology, 10,* 292–315.

Sebastian, C., Burnett, S. & Blakemore, S.-J. (2008). Development of the self-concept during adolescence. *Trends in Cognitive Sciences, 12,* 441–446.

Seiffge-Krenke, I. (2003). Testing theories of romantic development from adolescence to young adulthood: Evidence of a developmental sequence. *International Journal of Behavioral Development, 27,* 519–531.

Sherif, M. (1935). A study of some social factors in perception. *Archives of Psychology, 27,* 1–60.

Tarelli, I., Wendt, H., Bos, W. & Zylowski, A. (2012). Ziele, Anlage und Durchführung der Internationalen Grundschul-Lese-Untersuchung (IGLU 2011). In W. Bos, T. Tarelli, A. Bremerich-Vos & K. Schwippert (Hrsg.), *IGLU 2011 Lesekompetenzen von Grundschulkindern in Deutschland und im internationalen Vergleich* (S. 27–68). Münster: Waxmann.

Thomsen, T., Lessing, N., Greve, W. & Dresbach, S. (2018). Selbstkonzept und Selbstwert. In A. Lohaus (Hrsg.), *Entwicklung im Jugendalter* (S. 91–111). Heidelberg: Springer.

Ttofi, M. M., Bowes, L., Farrington, D. P. & Lösel, F. (2014). Protective factors interrupting the continuity from school bullying to later internalizing and externalizing problems: A systematic review of prospective longitudinal studies. *Journal of School Violence, 13*, 5–38.

Turiel, E. (1998). The development of morality. In W. Damon (Series Ed.) und N. Eisenberg (Vol. Ed.) *Handbook of child psychology. Vol. 3. Social, emotional, and personality development* (pp. 863–932). New York: Wiley.

Valkenburg, P. M. & Peter, J. (2007). Preadolescents' and adolescents' online communication and their closeness to friends. *Developmental Psychology, 43*, 267–277.

Vierhaus, M. & Wendt, E.-V. (2018). Sozialbeziehungen zu Gleichaltrigen. In A. Lohaus (Hrsg.), *Entwicklung im Jugendalter* (S. 139–167). Heidelberg: Springer.

Walper, S., Lux, U. & Witte, S. (2018). Sozialbeziehungen zur Herkunftsfamilie. In A. Lohaus (Hrsg.), *Entwicklungspsychologie des Jugendalters* (S. 113–137). Heidelberg: Springer.

Wellman, R. J., Dugas, E. N., Dutczak, H., O'Loughlin, E. K., Datta, G. D., Lauzon, B. & O'Loughlin, J. (2016). Predictors of the onset of cigarette smoking: A systematic review of longitudinal population-based studies in youth. *American Journal of Preventive Medicine, 51*, 767–778.

Wendt, E.-V. & Walper, S. (2013). Sexualentwicklung und Partnerschaften Jugendlicher: Ergebnisse einer repräsentativen Befragung von 15- bis 17-Jährigen. *Zeitschrift für Soziologie der Erziehung und Sozialisation, 33*, 62–81.

Wentzel, K. R. (2003). Sociometric status and adjustment in middle school: A longitudinal study. *Journal of Early Adolescence, 23*, 5–28.

Wentzel, K. R. & Erdley, C.A. (1993). Strategies for making friends: Relations to social behavior and peer acceptance in early adolescence. *Developmental Psychology, 29*, 819–826.

Wentzel, K. R., Jablansky, S. & Scalise, N. R. (2018). Do friendships afford academic benefits? A meta-analytic study. *Educational Psychology Review, 30*, 1241–1267.

Wentzel, K. R., Jablansky, S. & Scalise, N. R. (2020). Peer social acceptance and academic achievement: A meta-analytic study. *Journal of Educational Psychology*, online first.

WHO (1994). *Life skills education in schools: Programs on mental health*. Genf: WHO.

WHO (2003). *Skills for health. Skills-based health education including life skills: An important component of a child-friendly/health-promoting school* (Information Series on School Health, Document 9).

Zych, I., Farrington, D. P. & Ttofi, M. M. (2019). Protective factors against bullying and cyberbullying: A systematic review of meta-analyses. *Aggression and Violent Behavior, 45*, 4–19.

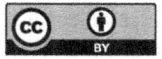

Mental Health and Well-Being in Adolescence: The Role of Child Attachment and Parental Reflective Functioning

Alessandro Decarli, Blaise Pierrehumbert, André Schulz und Claus Vögele

1   Introduction

During the last 60 years, attachment theory has acquired an important role in the conceptualization of emotional and social development, and it has become one of the most influential and investigated models in Developmental Psychology.

At the core of attachment theory are the dynamics that occur in the parent–child relationship and how these affect the future development of the child. More precisely, attachment can be defined as an innate disposition to seek proximity to and contact with a specific figure (usually parents or more generally caregivers) and to do so in situations where they experience distress: a child could smile or vocalize to express his interest in interacting, or he could cry and cling if

A. Decarli (✉)
Division of Youth Psychiatry, CHNP, Ettelbruck, Luxembourg
E-Mail: s1aldeca@uni-trier.de

B. Pierrehumbert
SUPEA, University of Lausanne, Lausanne, Switzerland
E-Mail: blapier@gmail.com

A. Schulz · C. Vögele
Department of Behavioural and Cognitive Sciences,
University of Luxembourg, Esch-sur-Alzette, Luxembourg
E-Mail: Andre.schulz@uni.lu

C. Vögele
E-Mail: Claus.voegele@uni.lu

© Der/die Autor(en) 2022
A. Heinen et al. (Hrsg.), *Wohlbefinden und Gesundheit im Jugendalter,*
https://doi.org/10.1007/978-3-658-35744-3_7

129

he perceives some kind of risk. It is extremely important to respond to these signals, especially in times when the child is distressed, as the availability of the parental figure is the factor that creates a difference in the development of a secure attachment (Bowlby 1969/1982; Cassidy 2016). For example, if the child feels that the parent is present both physically and emotionally in case of need, he can slowly move away to explore the surrounding environment, aware that if something should happen (a loud noise, or a small accident in the game) he can always return to the caregiver to be comforted. For this reason the parent acts as "a secure base from which to explore" (Ainsworth 1970, p. 61). The need to be comforted and the need to explore can be expressed in various ways, thus leading to the formation of different attachment patterns. Attachment security represents a good balance between the attachment and exploration systems, and is also the natural theoretical outcome, as well as the most desirable one (Solomon and George 2016). The most important factor for the development of a secure attachment is to make sure that the child acquires the feeling that the parent is present and available, because in this way he will internalize this representation, adapt this model, and generalize it to other relationships (Bretherton 1985).

2   Theoretical Framework

2.1   Attachment in Adolescence

Adolescence is often seen as a sensitive developmental period, which is characterized by "storm and stress", as many changes occur at a biological, cognitive, affective and social level (Arnett 1999; Moretti and Peled 2004). Emotional development in adolescence should lead to a realistic and coherent sense of identity that allows a person to learn how to cope with stress and manage emotions as well as to relate to others (Santrock 2001). As evidenced by several studies (e.g., Lee et al. 2014), adolescence is also a vulnerable period for the onset of serious mental disorders, which then tend to persist into adulthood. While there is ample evidence concerning risk factors for mental disorders in adolescence, less is known about protective factors, although one important protective factor to have emerged from recent research concerns attachment security (Moretti 2016).

According to Rice (1990), the quality of the attachment bond is strictly implicated in the adolescents' development of identity and in their emotional and social adjustment. Bowlby (1969/1982) sustained that during adolescence most children still have a strong attachment toward their parents, even if the child-parent relationship is changing and the adolescent also develops significant bonds with other people. This change has been described as "a realignment and redefinition of family ties" (Steinberg 2001, p. 255) and consists in a process of individuation, characterized in terms of autonomy, independence and detachment from family members (Ryan and Lynch 1989). According to Kobak and Duemmler (1994), the relationship between adolescents and parents becomes increasingly goal-corrected: while in infancy this goal-corrected partnership was more "coordinated", in adolescence it should be considered more as "negotiated" (Allen and Tan 2016). During the previous operations of the attachment system, the child became used to "habitual patterns of responding" (Allen and Tan 2016, p. 400) while in this new stage of life, this pattern does not fit anymore with the adolescent's need for autonomy. Therefore, to accomplish social development, which is a major task in adolescence, the adolescent has to develop a new balance between his attachment behaviors and his exploration urges; to do so, he or she has to decrease their need for dependence on parental attachment figures to satisfy the need for exploration. Despite this disengagement and transformation of family interactions, it is important to emphasize that adolescents still feel that it is important to be connected with their parental figures, even if they share less time and activities (Larson et al. 1996). Furthermore, Liebermann Doyle and Markiewicz (1999) found that, during adolescence, the perception of parental availability is still as important as in childhood, but the need for parental help and support decreases as children grow up. Nevertheless according to Fraley and Davis (1997) and Trinke and Bartholomew (1997), adolescents still seek parents, and in particular mothers, more than friends when they need a secure base (Doyle and Moretti 2000; Kerns et al. 2015).

2.2   Parental Reflective Function

Several studies acknowledge the influence of parents' representations about their children on their development. There is evidence that parental representations of their children are linked to children's emotional, social and cognitive development, and attachment security (Fonagy et al. 2002; Rosenblum et al. 2009; Slade 2005). The characteristics of the parents' representations also seem related to later affect regulation, and social relationships (Slade 2005), and mental health in adolescence (Fonagy and Gergely 2000). Studies have highlighted the link between parental reflective functioning (PRF), i.e. the ability to think about one's own thoughts and feelings and those of the child, and quality of child attachment, and the role of PRF in protecting adolescents from psychopathology (Fonagy et al. 2002).

The concept of reflective functioning (RF) or mentalization was first introduced in the context of the "London Parent–Child Project", which investigated the intergenerational transmission of attachment security (Steele and Steele 2008). RF has been defined as the capacity to understand one's own and others' mental states in terms of thoughts, feelings and desires. It is a very specific human feature that allows for emotion regulation and providing meaning to social interactions (Bateman and Fonagy 2016). RF has been proposed to be the missing link in the transmission of attachment security (Fonagy and Target 2005). Fonagy and colleagues (1991a, b), in their very first study on RF using the Adult Attachment Interview (AAI; George and Main 1984), could not only show that there was a high concordance between parent and child attachment, but also that the ability to reflect upon one's own history of attachment was significantly correlated with the child's attachment security. They concluded that the development of mentalizing ability originates within the parent–child relationship, where the child experiences the caregiver as being able to recognize and understand her or his mental states. Several years later, this idea was confirmed, by expanding it into a new line of research, i.e., by applying it to the Parent Development Interview – Revised (PDI-R; Slade et al. 2012), designed to evaluate parents' mental representations of their child, of the relationship with him or her and of themselves as a parent. Instead of assessing a person's ability to understand mental states with regard to his or her parents, this interview focuses on the capacity of parents to keep their child in mind, defined as parental reflective function (PRF). The caregivers' capacity to hold in mind that their children have feelings, desires and intentions, allows children to discover their internal experience through the parents' representation (Slade 2005). When children experience a change in their own mental state, parents need to be able to understand this moment by representing it and acknowledging this change through gestures, actions, words and play. The sensitization and the understanding of self-states occur through parental affect mirroring (Gergely and Watson 1996), where the caregiver produces an exaggerated version of realistic emotion expression, mirroring the infant's state. The parent's ability to observe changes in the child's mental states lays the foundations for the development of secure attachment, which, in turn, provides the psychological basis in the acquisition of mentalizing abilities (Fonagy and Target 1997). The intersubjective process of reflectiveness allows the child to understand the caregivers' behavior and to perceive an image of him- or her-self as mentalizing, desiring and believing. Lastly, sensitive parenting also implies that parents are aware of their own mental states, so that they are able to differentiate between their own internal experience, and the one of their child (Slade 2005). Studies over the last decades have shown that PRF does not only affect children's attachment security (Fonagy et al. 2002; Slade 2005) but parents' emotion regulation as well (Schultheis et al. 2019).

Despite the growing evidence of the importance of PRF for the emotional development of children, most studies have focused on parents of infants, neglecting the role of PRF during adolescence. To our knowledge, only five studies have explored PRF in parents of older children. In the first study of this kind, Benbassat and Priel (2012) assessed PRF with the PDI in a group of mothers and fathers of adolescents and found that there was a positive association between PRF and the adolescents' socio-emotional adjustment. A second study investigated a sample of clinically anxious children, including both mothers and fathers who completed the AAI (Esbjørn et al. 2013). The results showed that lower levels of maternal but not paternal reflective functioning (RF) were associated with higher child anxiety. A third study on a group of adopted adolescents, showed a strong relation between maternal RF, assessed with the PDI and child's attachment (Molina et al. 2015). In a fourth study, researchers administered the PDI to a sample of parents, which mainly included mothers (Borelli et al. 2016). The results show that child-focused RF was significantly associated with child attachment security. Finally, the last study highlighted that mothers with higher levels of PRF would exhibit less overcontrolling behaviors with their children (Borelli et al. 2017). In summary, the results of these studies suggest that PRF is significantly associated with outcomes concerning the socioemotional adjustment and the well-being of children during middle childhood and adolescence.

2.3   The Project "ATTACH": Studies and Methodology

More recently, we conducted a project ("Mental health and well-being during adolescence: The role of child attachment and parents' representations of their children – ATTACH") at the University of Luxembourg, which included families of adolescents from Luxembourg and Germany and which took place between October 2015 and November 2019. The project aimed to shed light on some of the potential factors that can affect attachment, mental health and well-being in adolescence. We assessed adolescents as part of a family system and, therefore, investigated the role of parental influence on adolescents' psychological adjustment, and explored psychological and psychophysiological processes that are associated with attachment and parenting. The project involved three studies:

- In the first study, we investigated the relationship of PRF with parental gender, parental cortisol responses and parenting behaviors (Decarli, Schulz, Pierrehumbert & Vögele, in press);
- In the second study, we examined the factors that are associated with different attachment classifications and the association between attachment and internalizing and externalizing behavioral problems (Decarli, Pierrehumbert, Schulz & Vögele, in press);
- In the third study, we tested whether adolescents with different attachment classifications show different patterns of emotion regulation strategies, both from a behavioral and physiological perspective, during two attachment relevant situations: an attachment interview and a parent–child conflict interaction task (Decarli et al. 2022).

After receiving ethics approval, we recruited participants in the German speaking area of the Greater Region of Luxembourg. Exclusion criteria were mental health problems of adolescents or parents, and participants needed to be fluent in either German, English, or French. Participants were 49 adolescents and their mothers and fathers. Not all fathers took part in the study. Adolescents had a mean age of 14.2 years and had different family backgrounds: 23 were living in their biological families, 19 had divorced or separated parents, and 7 had been adopted. The study design included three separate visits. During the first meeting we met with parent(s) on their own (consent form, interview and questionnaires), while the second meeting took place with the adolescents alone (consent form, attachment interview, questionnaires). These meetings took place at the family home, while the third meeting was scheduled with the whole family at the Clinical Psychophysiology Laboratory of the University of Luxembourg (for a detailed overview see Decarli et al. 2022, in press).

We used a multi-method approach with interviews, the observation of parent–child interactions, questionnaires and the assessment of psychophysiological stress responses during attachment-related situations. Concerning interviews and questionnaires, both parents were administered an interview to assess their RF capacities (PDI-R; Slade et al. 2012), then one of them took part in an interview to assess possible attachment difficulties of the child during childhood, and both parents (if possible) completed a questionnaire to evaluate their child's behavioral problems. The adolescents were administered an interview to assess their attachment representations (Friends and Family Interview – FFI; Steele and Steele 2014) and then completed a self-reported questionnaire to evaluate behavioral problems. Concerning the parent–child interaction (Family Interaction Task – FIT; Allen et al. 2012), mothers and fathers took part separately in a conflict interaction task with their child and were asked to discuss a disagreement and to try to reach a solution. The interaction task allowed for the assessment of the adolescents' ability to express their own opinions with confidence while maintaining an engaged and amicable connectedness with their parents. Parenting behaviors were operationalized as sensitive autonomy support and psychological control. We monitored heart rate and electrodermal activity as physiological indicators of stress and arousal from the adolescents both during the attachment interview, selecting the most attachment-relevant questions, and during the interaction task, focusing on the first 4 min, since some dyads after this time started discussing non-problematic issues. For analyses a reactivity score was calculated, by subtracting baseline means from the respective means of the selected questions during the FFI and means during the 1-min periods of the FIT. Concerning the parents, we collected 5 salivary cortisol samples during the FIT and calculated a reactivity score in terms of total hormone concentration over a period of reactivity.

3 Results

3.1 PRF, Parenting Behaviors and Attachment

We could show that PRF plays an important role in regulating the parents' own stress responses in the context of parenting (operationalized in terms of cortisol reactivity). However, parental physiological reactivity alone did not predict parenting behaviors. The findings showed that parents who display higher mentalizing capacities show lower cortisol reactivity (i.e., stress in the context of parenting) and at the same time, thanks to their RF abilities, better caregiving behaviors, with higher levels of sensitive autonomy support and lower levels of psychological control. Current research has shown that emotional arousal and psychosocial stress are factors that can cause a reduction of the capacity to understand someone else's mental states (Nolte et al. 2013). This is particularly true in the context of attachment relationships. There is evidence that when emotional arousal is high, the capacity to mentalize in a conscious, controlled and reflective way switches to an automatic, non-conscious and unreflective mode (e.g., Fonagy and Luyten 2018). During adolescence, the intensity and the frequency of conflicts between parents and children increase, and although these conflicts are also considered to be a means to negotiate relational changes, they can also enhance parenting stress (e.g., Branje 2018).

High levels of RF in both mother and fathers were the best predictors of secure attachment, confirming previous studies on infant samples (e.g., Steele and Steele 2008) and adding new important information about its role in adolescence. We would however have expected that parenting behaviors predicted attachment security as well, which occurred only in the case of attachment disorganization. Unexpectedly, its best predictor were indeed maternal behaviors undermining relatedness (but not the paternal ones), which also might explain the relation between disorganized attachment and maternal RF. Therefore, in the case of disorganization, maternal hostile and threatening behaviors seem to be the primary mechanism through which mothers' RF is translated and communicated in the relationship with their adolescent children. These results might be explained as a consequence of the task we used to measure parental sensitivity and parenting behaviors, in that it might lacked ecological validity. The FIT is mainly designed around the notions of autonomy and relatedness, and more connected to the concept of "secure base" (Allen et al. 2003). Therefore, on the one hand, we might not have been able to capture sensitive behaviors that a highly reflective parent may use in other contexts, as for instance when the child is upset. On the other hand, an interaction task that challenges autonomy negotiations, which is conflictual by nature, might have maximized the opportunity for mothers with low RF capacities to display more often and at a higher extent hostile and threatening behaviors, since they might have felt more helpless and frustrated (Borelli et al. 2017; Hennighausen et al. 2011). Future research on parents' sensitivity towards their adolescent children should include also other problem-solving situations that might be encountered by these dyads, as for example helping with a difficult task (Borelli et al. 2017), planning a vacation together (Becker-Stoll et al. 2008) or offering emotional support after a stressful task as the Trier Social Stress Test for Children (Buske-Kirschbaum et al. 1997).

Of significant interest are also the results concerning differences between mothers and fathers in the RF capacities. This finding was somewhat surprising, since research has shown that women usually have higher or at least similar RF levels as men (e.g., Steele and Steele 2008; Cooke et al. 2017). However, there may be several reasons for this result: (1) the possible presence of an assortative mating effect among intact and adoptive families (Borelli et al. 2017), (2) the possible influence of a divorced family status on maternal RF (Amato 2014), (3) the missing information concerning most of the fathers in the divorced families, and (4) the sociocultural changes concerning the role of fathers in

families of western societies over the last fifty years (Cowan and Cowan 2019).
It is important to note that these results (i.e., gender differences in RF levels and
maternal behaviors predicting disorganized attachment) may have been possibly
influenced at most by the fact that the data of the fathers were not randomly
missing. Their participation could have explained more variance in the regression
models, especially for what concerns autonomy support, and could serve as one
of the possible interpretations as to why only maternal RF and behaviors were
associated with disorganization. Recent studies have indeed shown that paternal
sensitive support of autonomy is linked to attachment security and better psychological adjustment both in infancy and adolescence (Benbassat and Priel 2015;
Grossmann et al. 2002). It remains entirely speculative, of course, whether or not
the inclusion of fathers from divorced couples would have changed our findings
and future studies should try to involve both parents, to better understand how
each of them can uniquely contribute to the psychological adjustment of their
children.

3.2   Attachment, Emotion Regulation and Mental Health

The most important results of the project ATTACH concern the converging
evidence that disorganized attachment is linked to (1) more behavioral
withdrawal during parent–child interactions, (2) heightened stress reactivity
during attachment relevant situations and (3) more internalizing behavioral
problems as compared to organized categories. With regard to the FIT, the lack of
affect and engagement suggests that especially the interactions with the mothers
were dominated by fear or by dissociative processes, which resulted in the full
withdrawal of the adolescent (Allen et al. 2012; Duschinsky 2018). Concerning
psychophysiological responses, our findings are in line with previous results
from studies on infant samples, which showed that disorganized children during
the SSP had higher heart rate responses when alone in the room (Spangler
and Grossmann 1993), and increased heart rate during separation from and a
decrease during reunion with the caregiver (Willemsen-Swinkels et al. 2000).
However, our findings also differed from those of Beijersbergen, Bakermans-
Kranenburg, van IJzendoorn and Juffer (2008), who did not find any differences
between adolescents with resolved and unresolved attachment representation,
but the authors argued that this might be due to how they measured physiological reactivity concerning loss, abuse and trauma experiences. Studies on
adult samples have also shown that disorganized individuals displayed enhanced

psychophysiological reactions during attachment related tasks (e.g., De Rubeis et al. 2016; Reijman et al. 2016). Finally, our results concerning the relation of attachment disorganization and internalizing behavioral problems were consistent with previous research (Brumariu and Kerns 2010; Madigan et al. 2016), further indicating its negative effects also on mental health. The pervasive negative influence that disorganized attachment has on the psychological, behavioral and physiological systems and its repeatedly demonstrated associations with maladjustment and psychopathology, has led to a call for disorganization to be included in psychiatric diagnostic systems as a developmental disorder (see Lyons-Ruth and Jacobvitz 2016). More recent reviews have pointed out, however, that disorganized attachment only shows modest stability over time, giving room for interventions with children and their parents (Granqvist et al. 2017).

The findings concerning dismissing attachment support the notion that during conflict interactions dismissing individuals tend to employ a fight or flight strategy, as evidenced by their display of behaviors undermining autonomy and relatedness at a higher extent and frequency than secure and preoccupied adolescents. It also appears that dismissing individuals experienced more stress than secure and preoccupied ones during the FFI suggesting that the attachment interview was able to activate their attachment-related defensive processes (Mikulincer et al. 2009) both from a narrative perspective (i.e., using idealization or derogation) as well as from a physiological one (i.e., using ineffectively a deactivating strategy). Our results are in line with previous findings from Dozier and Kobak (1992) and Roisman et al. (2004), who found that deactivation is associated with increased stress reactivity. In contrast, our findings differ from those of Beijersbergen and colleagues (2008) who found that dismissing individuals seemed to be less stressed than secure and preoccupied ones during the AAI. These contrasting results might be due to differences in the task that we used. We would argue that the questions of the FFI were better able to trigger attachment-related physiological responses in dismissing adolescents, because the interview is not focused on their early attachment experiences, but on current ones (Steele and Steele 2005). Our results concerning the psychophysiological responses during the FIT are also different from the ones of Beijersbergen and colleagues (2008) and this might be due to the different setting were the inter-action took place (home vs. laboratory in our study). Moreover, the sample of Beijersbergen et al.'s study was only composed of adopted adolescents, and studies have shown that interactions between adopted children and their parents are more intense than those that occur in other families (Rueter et al. 2009). Future studies should therefore focus on different family types to find possible similarities and differences. Finally, our results are also consistent with the literature on problem behaviors (e.g. Madigan et al. 2016), since dismissing individuals reported higher externalizing symptoms and were judged by their mothers as having more externalizing difficulties.

In conclusion, it seems plausible that dismissing individuals might have developed some self-regulatory abilities that help them to deal physiologically with stressful circumstances (as for instance an interaction). Adolescents with disorganized attachment may not have this capacity, because their fear system is continuously activated, leading simultaneously to an excessive deactivation of the vagal system (freezing) and to the activation of the sympathetic nervous system (fight or flight), which does not allow for any response strategies. This process is reminiscent of what has been described in the literature on disorganized attachment as "fright without solution" (Hesse und Main 1999. p. 484).

4   Limitations and Future Research

Limitations of the current project concern, for example, the sample size, which was small in statistical terms and which might have led to insufficient statistical power to detect further differences between different attachment representations. Furthermore, the high rates of insecurity and, in particular of disorganization, present in our (non-clinical) sample might suggest that participant recruitment might have been biased. Families were mostly self-selected and the possible presence of an assortative mating effect might suggest that we have recruited in a way that maximized the possibility of finding thoughtful, reflective and sensitive parents among intact and adoptive families, whereas parents of the divorced group were probably more motivated by personal reasons (e.g., they felt that they struggled more in their parenting role or that their son or daughter had difficulties). Furthermore, the complexity of data collection, as for instance the inclusion of both parents, the fact of being interviewed and video-recorded, and last but not least the collection of physiological data might have limited participations. The selection of a bigger sample would probably bypass this "selection bias" and it would allow for better generalizability of the results. It is also important to point out that we did not assess other factors that might affect child attachment, PRF, parenting behaviors and parenting stress, and parents' own attachment representations and parenting alliance. Therefore, some important information was missing from this project that might have added further explanatory power to our model. We can only hypothesize that parents with lower reflective capacities had an insecure (or unresolved) state of mind with respect to attachment, which is amply supported by the literature (Steele and Steele 2008).

In this case, however, this remains speculative. The same applies to parenting alliance, since assessing how cooperative, communicative and mutually respectful parents are with regard to caring for their children has important effects on the parenting behaviors and this might have been especially important to explore in families with divorced parents (Becher et al. 2019). Future studies should assess both these variables when investigating PRF, parenting behaviors, parenting stress and the child's psychological outcomes.

In our study on physiological responses during attachment relevant situations, we examined the physiological reactivity of the adolescents during an attachment interview and during a conflict interaction with their mothers and fathers. However, we used different methods to assess the physiological responses (heart rate and electrodermal activity for the adolescents and cortisol for the parents). It would be interesting in future research to examine the same indicators of physiological reactivity in all participants. Cortisol is widely used in research but also carries some limitations, as it can be imprecise and influenced by other factors (Nicolson 2007). Therefore, the assessment of heart rate and electrodermal activity could have provided greater time-specificity for their associations with PRF and parenting behaviors. Furthermore, future research may also focus on the concordance of physiological responses of parents and adolescents during a conflict interaction task in relation to attachment representation. In a previous study, Zelenko et al. (2005) reported that heart rate changes during the SSP were more consistent in secure mother-infant dyads than in insecure dyads. Other studies have also shown the powerful impact of maternal-infant social contact on the infant's physiological systems and the results evidenced that the concordance between maternal and infant biological rhythms increased significantly during episodes of affect and vocal synchrony compared to non-synchronous moments (Feldman et al. 2011). This focus would give more insight into the importance of attachment representations for psychophysiological attunement also during adolescence. Moreover, another area that needs to be further explored concern peer relationships during adolescence. Although parents are still the main attachment figures in the life of adolescents, close friends and romantic acquire new significant importance (Allen and Tan 2016). Future studies should also investigate whether adolescents with different attachment representations would show the same physiological patterns of activation during conflict interactions with close friends as with their parents. This has been previously done with adult couples and the results showed that adults classified as insecure showed more physiological reactivity during interactions with romantic partners than secure adults (Roisman 2007). Future research should also focus on other factors that might influence attachment, as for instance neural mechanism behind attachment and parenting, and child temperament and genetics (Verhage et al. 2016).

A final important consideration concerns the impact that divorce has on the well-being of family members. In our study a divorced family status was significantly associated with lower maternal RF capacities, lower sensitivity and higher levels of adolescents' disorganization. Previous research has shown that divorce increases the probability of developing insecure attachment, since there is less parental availability, more conflicts between parents and more parent–child negative interactions (Howes and Markman 1989; Waters et al. 1993). Divorce, however, can also cause discontinuity of attachment: individuals who experienced divorce during their childhood are more at risk of displaying insecure attachment in adolescence, although they had been assessed as secure in infancy (Lewis et al. 2000). However, the relationship between divorce and quality of attachment has been predominantly investigated in infancy/childhood (Solomon and George 1999; Page and Bretherton 2001) whereas only two studies have addressed this topic in an adolescent sample (Lewis et al. 2000; Hamilton 2000). We would argue that divorced mothers often do not have the possibility to rely on someone else in situations of (parenting) stress and this might activate feelings of helplessness, which in turn would activate their attachment system and might induce the use of automatic mentalization and display subsequently less sensitive behaviors and more psychological control (Fauber et al. 1990; Fonagy and Luyten 2009). Nevertheless it is probably not divorce per se that causes parents to show more psychologically controlling behaviors but the sequelae of stressful factors that divorce brings with it. These findings advance our understanding of stress in the context of parenting as influencing the parental ability to cope with the daily challenges that child rearing brings with it, especially during the sensitive period of adolescence, and on the effects that these factors have on the quality of their children's attachment. Therefore, more longitudinal studies are needed in order to infer causality and to understand what are the different factors that influence the developmental trajectories of an individual in one direction rather than in another, leading to significant differences in their psychological and social adjustment.

5   Clinical Implications and Concluding Remarks

The results of this project are particularly innovative and relevant for Luxembourg and Germany, since they highlight the importance of secure attachment representations during adolescence. The study can also provide significant guidance for the services that are involved in mental-health interventions, indicating the factors that enhance attachment-related security in families, to prompt the development of targeted interventions, both preventive and rehabilitative. Furthermore, the study of the attachment representations of adolescents with divorced parents could support clinical services in the establishment of interventions that can also help parents in better understanding the children's needs and difficulties, thus improving their well-being.

Therefore, clinical interventions should help parents in developing their reflective skills, which can then be translated in more sensitive parenting behaviors, and adolescents in better integrating their attachment representations, to develop a more coherent and reflective state of mind. Attachment-based interventions (for an overview see Kobak and Kerig 2015; Slade 2007) are receiving increasing attention and might be a first choice, given their efficacy in helping parents to better understand their children's thoughts, feelings and needs, and adolescents in better regulating their emotions (e.g., Attachment-Based Family Therapy; Connect Program; Mentalization-Based Treatment for Adolescents; Reflective Parenting Program). Other interventions could aim at involving more the paternal figures, mediating parental conflicts, and socially and financially supporting single mothers, who most often after a divorce might face social isolation and financial challenges. Moreover, it would be also important to train professional figures who are in close contact with families, as pediatricians or general practitioners, to recognize possible difficulties at an early stage, in order to promptly activate appropriate measures to support the child and his or her parents (Cohen and Weitzman 2016).

References

Ainsworth, M. D. S., & Bell, S. M. (1970). Attachment, exploration and separation: Illustratedby the behavior of one-year-olds in a Strange Situation. *Child Development, 41*, 49–67. doi: https://doi.org/10.2307/1127388.

Allen, J. P., Hauser, S. T., Bell, K. L., McElhaney, K. B., Tate, D. C., Insabella, G. M., & Schlatter, A. K.W. (2012). *Autonomy and Relatedness Coding System, Manual Version 2.15*. Unpublished manuscript. University of Virginia.

Allen, J. P., McElhaney, K. B., Land, D. J., Kuperminc, G. P., Moore, C. W., O'Beirne-Kelly, H., & Kilmer, S. L. (2003). A secure base in adolescence: Markers of Attachment security in the mother-adolescent Relationship. *Child Development, 74*, 292–307. doi:https://doi.org/10.1111/1467-8624.t01-1-00536.

Allen, J. P., & Tan, J. S. (2016). The multiple facets of attachment in adolescence. In J. Cassidy & P. R. Shaver (Eds.), *Handbook of Attachment: Theory, Research and Clinical Applications* (pp. 399–415). New York: The Guilford Press.

Amato, P. R. (2014). The consequences of divorce for adults and children: An update. *Drustvena Istrazivanja, 23,* 5–24. doi:https://doi.org/10.5559/di.23.1.01.

Arnett, J. J. (1999). Adolescent storm and stress, reconsidered. *American Psychologist, 54,* 317–326. doi:https://doi.org/10.1037//0003-066x.54.5.317.

Bateman, A., & Fonagy, P. (2016). *Mentalization-based treatment for personality disorders: A practical guide.* New York, NY, US: Oxford University Press. doi:https://doi.org/10.1093/med:psych/9780199680375.001.0001.

Becher, E. H., Kim, H., Cronin, S. E., Deenanath, V., McGuire, J. K., McCann, E. M., & Powell, S. (2019). Positive parenting and parental conflict: Contributions to resilient coparenting during divorce. *Family Relations, 68,* 150–164 doi:https://doi.org/10.1111/fare.12349.

Becker-Stoll, F., Fremmer-Bombik, E., Wartner, U., Zimmermann, P., & Grossmann, K. E. (2008). Is attachment at ages 1, 6 and 16 related to autonomy and relatedness behavior of adolescents in interaction towards their mothers? *International Journal of Behavioral Development, 32,* 372–380 doi:https://doi.org/10.1177/0165025408093654.

Beijersbergen, M. D., Bakermans-Kranenburg, M. J., van IJzendoorn, M. H., & Juffer, F. (2008). Stress regulation in adolescents: Physiological reactivity during the Adult Attachment Interview and conflict interaction. *Child Development, 79,* 1707–1720. doi:https://doi.org/10.1111/j.1467-8624.2008.01220.x.

Benbassat, N., & Priel, B. (2012). Parenting and adolescent adjustment: The role of parental reflective function. *Journal of Adolescence, 35,* 163–174. doi:https://doi.org/10.1016/j.adolescence.2011.03.004.

Benbassat, N., & Priel, B. (2015). Why is fathers' reflective function important? *Psychoanalytic Psychology, 32,* 1–22. doi:https://doi.org/10.1037/a0038022.

Borelli, J. L., Hong K., Rasmussen, H. F., & Smiley, P. A. (2017). Reflective functioning, physiological reactivity, and overcontrol in mothers: Links with school-aged children's reflective functioning. *Developmental Psychology, 53,* 1680–1693. doi:https://doi.org/10.1037/dev0000371.

Borelli, J. L., St. John, H. K., Cho, E., & Suchman, N. E. (2016). Reflective functioning in parents of school-aged children. *American Journal of Orthopsychiatry, 86,* 24–36. doi:https://doi.org/10.1037/ort0000141.

Bowlby, J. (1969/1982). *Attachment and Loss: Vol. 1. Attachment.* New York: Basic Books.

Branje, S. (2018). Development of parent-adolescent relationships: Conflict interactions as a mechanism of change. *Child Development Perspectives, 12,* 171–176. doi:https://doi.org/10.1111/cdep.12278.

Bretherton, I. (1985). Attachment theory: Retrospect and prospect. *Monographs of the Society for Research in Child Development, 50,* 3-35. doi:https://doi.org/10.2307/3333824.

Brumariu, L. E., & Kerns, K. A. (2010). Parent–child attachment and internalizing symptoms in childhood and adolescence: A review of empirical findings and future directions. *Development and Psychopathology, 22,* 177–203. doi:https://doi.org/10.1017/s0954579409990344.

Buske-Kirschbaum, A., Jobst, S., Wustmans, A., Kirschbaum, C., Rauh, W., & Hellhammer, D. (1997). Attenuated free cortisol response to psychosocial stress in children with atopic dermatitis. *Psychosomatic Medicine, 59,* 419–426. doi:https://doi.org/10.1097/00006842-199707000-00012.

Cassidy, J. (2016). The nature of the child's ties. In J. Cassidy & P. R. Shaver (Eds.), *Handbook of Attachment: Theory, Research and Clinical Applications* (pp. 3–24). New York: TheGuilford Press.

Cohen, G. J., & Weitzman, C. C. (2016). Helping children and families deal with divorce and separation. *Pediatrics, 138*, e20163020–e20163020. doi:https://doi.org/10.1542/peds.2016-3020.

Cooke, D., Priddis, L., Luyten, P., Kendall, G., & Cavanagh, R. (2017). Paternal and maternal reflective functioning in the western Australian Peel Child Health Study. *Infant Mental Health Journal, 38*, 561–574. doi:https://doi.org/10.1002/imhj.21664.

Cowan, P. A., & Cowan, C. P. (2019). Introduction: Bringing dads into the family. *Attachment and Human Development, 21*, 419–426. doi:https://doi.org/10.1080/14616734.2019.1582594.

Decarli, A., Pierrehumbert, B., Schulz, A., Schaan, V. K., & Vögele, C. (2022). Disorganized attachment in adolescence: Emotional and physiological dysregulation during the Friends and Family Interview and a conflict interaction. *Development and Psychopathology, 34*, 431–445. https://doi.org/10.1017/S0954579420001352.

Decarli, A., Schulz, A., Pierrehumbert, B., & Vögele, C. (in press). Mothers' and fathers' reflective functioning and its association with parenting behaviors and cortisol reactivity during a conflict interaction with their adolescent children. *Emotion*.

De Rubeis, J., Sütterlin, S., Lange, D., Pawelzik, M., van Randenborgh, A., Victor, D., & Vögele, C. (2016). Attachment status affects heart rate responses to experimental ostracism in inpatients with depression. *PLoS ONE, 11*, e0150375. doi:https://doi.org/10.1371/journal.pone.0150375.

Doyle, A. B., & Moretti, M. M. (2000). *Attachment to parents and adjustment in adolescence: Literature review and policy implications*. Report to Childhood and Youth Division Health Canada. Ottawa, Canada.

Dozier, M., & Kobak, R. R. (1992). Psychophysiology in attachment interviews: Converging evidence for deactivating strategies. *Child Development, 63*, 1473–1480. doi:https://doi.org/10.1111/j.1467-8624.1992.tb01708.x.

Duschinsky, R. (2018). Disorganization, fear and attachment: Working towards clarification. *Infant Mental Health Journal, 39*, 17–29. doi:https://doi.org/10.1002/imhj.21689.

Esbjørn, B. H., Pedersen, S. H., Daniel, S. I. F., Hald, H. H., Holm, J. M., & Steele, H. (2013). Anxiety levels in clinically referred children and their parents: Examining the unique influence of self-reported attachment styles and interview-based reflective functioning in mothers and fathers. *British Journal of Clinical Psychology, 52*, 394–407. doi:https://doi.org/10.1111/bjc.12024.

Fauber, R., Forehand, R., Thomas, A. M., & Wierson, M. (1990). A mediational model of the impact of marital conflict on adolescent adjustment in intact and divorced families: The role of disrupted parenting. *Child Development, 61*, 1112. doi:https://doi.org/10.2307/1130879.

Feldman, R., Magori-Cohen, R., Galili, G., Singer, M., & Louzoun, Y. (2011). Mother and infant coordinate heart rhythms through episodes of interaction synchrony. *Infant Behavior and Development, 34*, 569–577. doi:https://doi.org/10.1016/j.infbeh.2011.06.008.

Fonagy, P., Gergely, G., Jurist, E. L., & Target, M. (2002). *Affect Regulation, Mentalization, and the Development of the Self*. New York, NY, US: Other Press.

Fonagy, P., & Luyten, P. (2009). A developmental, mentalization-based approach to the understanding and treatment of borderline personality disorder. *Development and Psychopathology, 21*, 1355–1381. doi:https://doi.org/10.1017/s0954579409990198.

Fonagy, P., & Luyten, P. (2018). Attachment, mentalizing, and the self. In W. J. Livesley & R. Larstone (Eds.), *Handbook of Personality Disorders: Theory, Research, and Treatment* (pp. 123–140). New York, NY, US: The Guilford Press.

Fonagy, P., Steele, H., Moran, G., Steele, M., & Higgitt, A. (1991a). The capacity for understanding mental states: The reflective self in parent and child and its significance for security of attachment. *Infant Mental Health Journal, 13*, 200–217. doi:https://doi.org/10.1017/S0954579497001399.

Fonagy, P., Steele, H., & Steele, M. (1991b). Maternal representations of attachment during pregnancy predict the organization of infant-mother attachment at one year of age. *Child Development, 62*, 891–905. doi:https://doi.org/10.2307/1131141.

Fonagy, P., & Target, M. (1997). Attachment and reflective function: Their role in self-organization. *Development and Psychopathology, 9*, 679–700. doi:https://doi.org/10.1017/s0954579497001399.

Fonagy, P., & Target, M. (2005). Bridging the transmission gap: An end to an important mystery of attachment research? *Attachment & Human Development, 7*, 333–343. doi: https://doi.org/10.1002/1097-0355(199123)12:3<201::aid-imhj2280120307>3.0.co;2-7.

Fonagy, P., Target, M., & Gergely, G. (2000). Attachment and borderline personality disorder. A theory and some evidence. *Psychiatric Clinics of North America, 23*, 103–122.

Fraley, R. C., & Davis, K. E. (1997). Attachment formation and transfer in young adults' close friendships and romantic relationships. *Personal Relationships, 4*, 131–144. doi:https://doi.org/10.1111/j.1475-6811.1997.tb00135.x.

George, C., Kaplan, N., & Main, M. (1984). *Adult Attachment Interview Protocol* (Unpublished manuscript). University of California: Berkeley.

Gergely, G., & Watson, J. S. (1996). The social biofeedback theory of parental affect-mirroring: The development of emotional self-awareness and self-control in infancy. *The International Journal of Psychoanalysis, 77*, 1181–1212.

Granqvist, P., Sroufe, L. A., Dozier, M., Hesse, E., Steele, M., van Ijzendoorn, M., ... & Duschinsky, R. (2017). Disorganized attachment in infancy: A review of the phenomenon and its implications for clinicians and policy-makers. *Attachment & Human Development, 19*, 534–558. doi:https://doi.org/10.1080/14616734.2017.1354040.

Grossmann, K., Grossmann, K. E., Fremmer-Bombik, E., Kindler, H., & Scheuerer-Englisch, H. (2002). The uniqueness of the child–father attachment relationship: Fathers' sensitive and challenging play as a pivotal variable in a 16-year longitudinal study. *Social Development, 11*, 301–337. doi: https://doi.org/10.1111/1467-9507.00202.

Hamilton, C. E. (2000). Continuity and discontinuity of attachment from infancy through adolescence. *Child Development, 71*, 690–694. doi:https://doi.org/10.1111/1467-8624.00177.

Hennighausen, K. H., Bureau, J.-F., David, D. H., Holmes, B. M., & Lyons-Ruth, K. (2011). Disorganized attachment behavior observed in adolescence: Validation in relation to adult attachment interview classifications at age 25. In J. Solomon & C.

George (Eds.), *Disorganized Attachment and Caregiving* (pp. 207–244). New York, NY, US: The Guilford Press.

Hesse, E., & Main, M. (1999). Second-generation effects of unresolved trauma in nonmaltreating parents: Dissociated, frightened, and threatening parental behavior. *Psychoanalytic Inquiry, 19*, 481–540. doi:https://doi.org/10.1080/07351699909534265.

Howes, P., & Markman, H. J. (1989). Marital quality and child functioning: A longitudinal investigation. *Child Development, 60,* 1044–1051. doi:https://doi.org/10.1111/j.1467-8624.1989.tb03535.x.

Kerns, K. A., Mathews, B. L., Koehn, A. J., Williams, C. T., & Siener-Ciesla, S. (2015) Assessing both safe haven and secure base support in parent-child relationships. *Attachment and Human Development, 17*, 337–353. doi:https://doi.org/10.1080/14616734.2015.1042487.

Kobak, R. R., & Duemmler, S. (1994). Attachment and conversation: Toward a discourse analysis of adolescent and adult security. In K. Bartholomew & D. Perlman (Eds.), *Advances in Personal Relationships: Vol. 5. Attachment processes in adulthood* (pp. 121–149). London: Jessica Kingsely.

Kobak, R. R., & Kerig, P. K. (2015). Introduction to the special issue: attachment-based treatments for adolescents. *Attachment & Human Development, 17,* 111–118. doi:https://doi.org/10.1080/14616734.2015.1006382.

Larson, R. W., Richards, M. H., Moneta, G., Holmbeck, G., & Duckett, E. (1996). Changes in adolescents' daily interactions with their family from ages 10 to 18: Disengagement and transformation. *Developmental Psychology, 32,* 744–754. doi:https://doi.org/10.1037//0012-1649.32.4.744.

Lee, F. S., Heimer, H., Giedd, J. N., Lein, E. S., Šestan, N., Weinberger, D. R., & Casey, B. J.(2014). Adolescent mental health - Opportunity and obligation. *Science, 346*, 547–549.doi:https://doi.org/10.1126/science.1260497.

Lewis, M., Feiring, C., & Rosenthal, S. (2000). Attachment over Time. *Child Development, 71,* 707–720. doi:https://doi.org/10.1111/1467-8624.00180.

Liebermann, M., Doyle, A.-B., & Markiewicz, D. (1999). Developmental patterns in security of attachment to mother and father in late childhood and early adolescence: Associations with peer relations. *Child Development, 70,* 202–213. doi:https://doi.org/10.1111/1467-8624.00015.

Lyons-Ruth, K., & Jacobvitz, D. (2016). Attachment disorganization from infancy to adulthood: Neurobiological correlates, parenting contexts, and pathways to disorder. In: J. Cassidy & P. R. Shaver (Eds.), *Handbook of Attachment: Theory, Research, and Clinical Applications* (pp. 667–695). New York: Guilford.

Madigan, S., Brumariu, L. E., Villani, V., Atkinson, L., & Lyons-Ruth, K. (2016). Representational and questionnaire measures of attachment: A meta-analysis of relations to child internalizing and externalizing problems. *Psychological Bulletin, 142,* 367–399. doi:https://doi.org/10.1037/bul0000029.

Mikulincer, M., Shaver, P. R., Cassidy, J., & Berant, E. (2009). Attachment-related defensive processes. In J. H. Obegi & E. Berant (Eds.), *Attachment Theory and Research in Clinical Work with Adults* (pp. 293–327). New York, NY, US: The Guilford Press.

Molina, P., Casonato, M., Ongari, B., & Decarli, A. (2015). Les représentations d'attachement chez les adolescents adoptés et leurs parents. *Neuropsychiatrie de l'Enfance et de l'Adolescence, 63*, 376–384. doi:https://doi.org/10.1016/j. neurenf.2015.04.004.

Moretti, M. M. (2016). *Adolescence, attachment and mental health: Translating knowledgeinto evidence based practice. [Conference presentation].* International WinterTraining School (*3rd Edition): Evidence Based Interventions to preventDevelopmental Risk Outcomes in Youth and Adolescence, Pavia, Italy.*

Moretti, M. M., & Peled, M. (2004). Adolescent-parent attachment: Bonds that support healthydevelopment. *Paediatrics & Child Health, 9*, 551–555. doi:https://doi. org/10.1093/pch/9.8.551.

Nicolson, N. A. (2007). Measurement of cortisol. In L. J. Luecken & L. C. Gallo (Eds.), *Handbook of Physiological Research Methods in Health Psychology* (pp. 37–74). Thousand Oaks, CA, US: Sage Publications, Inc. doi:https://doi. org/10.4135/9781412976244.n3.

Nolte, T., Bolling, D. Z., Hudac, C. M., Fonagy, P., Mayes, L., & Pelphrey, K. A. (2013). Brain mechanisms underlying the impact of attachment-related stress on social cognition. *Frontiers in Human Neuroscience, 7*. doi:https://doi.org/10.3389/ fnhum.2013.00816.

Page, T., & Bretherton, I. (2001). Mother- and father-child attachment themes in the story completions of pre-schoolers from post-divorce families: Do they predict relationships with peers and teachers? *Attachment & Human Development, 3*, 1–29. doi:https://doi. org/10.1080/14616730122749.

Reijman, S., Alink, L. R. A., Compier-De Block, L. H. C. G., Werner, C. D., Maras, A., Rijnberk, C., van IJzendoorn, M. H., & Bakermans-Kranenburg, M. J. (2016). Attachment representations and autonomic regulation in maltreating and nonmaltreating mothers. *Development and Psychopathology, 29*, 1075–1087. doi:https://doi. org/10.1017/s0954579416001036.

Rice, K. G. (1990). Attachment in adolescence: A narrative and meta-analytic review. *Journal of Youth and Adolescence, 19*, 511–538. doi:https://doi.org/10.1007/ bf01537478.

Roisman, G. I. (2007). The psychophysiology of adult attachment relationships: Autonomic reactivity in marital and premarital interactions. *Developmental Psychology, 43*, 39–53. doi:https://doi.org/10.1037/0012-1649.43.1.39.

Roisman, G. I., Tsai, J. L., & Chiang, K. S. (2004). The emotional integration of childhood experiences: Physiological. facial expressive, and self-reported emotional response during the Adult Attachment Interview. *Developmental Psychology, 40*, 776–789. doi:https://doi.org/10.1037/0012-1649.40.5.776.

Rosenblum, K. L., Dayton, C. J., & Muzik, M. (2009). Infant social and emotional development: Emerging competence in a relational context In C. H. Zeanah, Jr. (Ed.), *Handbook of Infant Mental Health* (pp. 80–103). New York, NY, US: The Guilford Press.

Rueter, M. A., Keyes, M. A., Iacono, W. G., & McGue, M. (2009). Family interactions in adoptive compared to nonadoptive families. *Journal of Family Psychology, 23*, 58–66. doi:https://doi.org/10.1037/a0014091.

Ryan, R. M., & Lynch, J. H. (1989). Emotional autonomy versus detachment: Revisiting the vicissitudes of adolescence and young adulthood. *Child Development, 60*, 340–356. doi:https://doi.org/10.2307/1130981.

Santrock, J. W. (2001). *Adolescence*. New York: McGraw-Hill.

Schultheis, A. M., Mayes, L. C., & Rutherford, H. J. V. (2019). Associations between emotion regulation and parental reflective functioning. *Journal of Child and Family Studies, 28,* 1094–1104. doi:https://doi.org/10.1007/s10826-018-01326-z.

Slade, A. (2005). Parental reflective functioning: An introduction. *Attachment & Human Development, 7,* 269–281. doi:https://doi.org/10.1080/14616730500245906.

Slade, A. (2007). Reflective parenting programs: Theory and development. *Psychoanalytic Inquiry, 26,* 640–657. doi:https://doi.org/10.1080/07351690701310698.

Slade, A., Aber, J., Bresgi, I., Berger, B., & Kaplan, M. (2012). *The Parent Development Interview Revised - Short Version.* Unpublished protocol. The City University of New York.

Solomon, J., & George, C. (1999). The development of attachment in separated and divorced families. *Attachment & Human Development, 1,* 2–33. doi:https://doi.org/10.1080/14616739900134011.

Solomon, J., & George, C. (2016). The measurement of attachment security and relatedconstructs in infancy and early childhood. In J. Cassidy & P. R. Shaver (Eds.),*Handbook of Attachment: Theory, Research, and Clinical Applications* (pp. 383–416).New York: The Guilford Press.

Spangler, G., & Grossmann, K. E. (1993). Biobehavioral organization in securely and insecurely attached infants. *Child Development, 64,* 1439–1450. doi:https://doi.org/10.2307/1131544.

Steele, H., & Steele, M. (2005). The construct of coherence as an indicator of attachment security in middle childhood: The Friends and Family Interview. In K. Kerns & R. Richardson (Eds.), *Attachment in Middle Childhood* (pp. 137–160). New York: Guilford Press.

Steele, H., & Steele, M. (2008). On the origins of reflective functioning. In F. N. Busch (Ed.), *Psychoanalytic Inquiry Book Series. Mentalization: Theoretical Considerations, Research Findings, and Clinical Implications* (pp. 133–158). Mahwah, NJ, US: Analytic Press.

Steele, H., & Steele, M. (2014). *The Friends and Family Interview.* Unpublished protocol, New York: Department of Psychology, New School for Social Research.

Steinberg, L. (2001). We know some things: Parent-adolescent relationships in retrospect and prospect. *Journal of Research on Adolescence, 11,* 1–19. doi:https://doi.org/10.1111/1532-7795.00001.

Trinke, S. J., & Bartholomew, K. (1997). Hierarchies of attachment relationships in young adulthood. *Journal of Social and Personal Relationships, 14,* 603–625. doi:https://doi.org/10.1177/0265407597145002.

Verhage, M. L., Schuengel, C., Madigan, S., Fearon, R. M. P., Oosterman, M., Cassibba, R., Bakermans-Kranenburg, M. J., & van IJzendoorn, M. H. (2016). Narrowing the transmission gap: A synthesis of three decades of research on intergenerational transmission of attachment. *Psychological Bulletin, 142,* 337–366. doi:https://doi.org/10.1037/bul0000038.

Waters, E., Posada, G., Crowell, J., & Lay, K.-L. (1993). Is attachment theory ready to contribute to our understanding of disruptive behavior problems? *Development and Psychopathology, 5,* 215–224. doi:https://doi.org/10.1017/s0954579400004351.

Willemsen-Swinkels, S. H. N., Bakermans-Kranenburg, M. J., Buitelaar, J. K., van IJzendoorn, M. H., & van Engeland, H. (2000). Insecure and disorganized attachment in children with a pervasive developmental disorder: Relationship with social interaction and heart rate. *Journal of Child Psychology and Psychiatry, 41,* 759–767. doi:https://doi.org/10.1111/1469-7610.00663.

Zelenko, M., Kraemer, H., Huffman, L., Gschwendt, M., Pageler, N., & Steiner, H. (2005). Heart rate correlates of attachment status in young mothers and their infants. *Journal of the American Academy of Child & Adolescent Psychiatry, 44,* 470–476. doi:https://doi.org/10.1097/01.chi.0000157325.10232.b1.

It's a Family Affair: Family Health and Child Well-being

Liyousew Borga, Conchita D'Ambrosio
und Anthony Lepinteur

1   Introduction

Health is one of the most important predictors of subjective well-being (Clark et al. 2019).[1] A large literature shows that both physical health and mental health matter (Ferrer-i Carbonell and Van Praag 2002; Shields and Price 2005). While adverse health outcomes immediately affect well-being, they also have long-lasting effects in terms of happiness (Oswald and Powdthavee 2008).

---

[1] As standard practice in Economics, we will use the terms "subjective well-being" and "happiness" interchangeably in this chapter. Subjective well-being is generally measured by variables such as self-assessed satisfaction with own job, or own life. See Chap. 1 (Borga, D'Ambrosio & Lepinteur) for more details about those concepts in Economics.

The data used in this publication come from Young Lives, a 20-year study of childhood poverty and transitions to adulthood in Ethiopia, India, Peru and Vietnam (www.younglives.org.uk). Young Lives is funded by UK aid from the Foreign, Commonwealth & Development Office and a number of further funders. The views expressed here are those of the author(s). They are not necessarily those of Young Lives, the University of Oxford, FCDO or other funders.

L. Borga (✉) · C. D'Ambrosio A. Lepinteur
Department of Behavioural and Cognitive Sciences, University of Luxembourg,
Esch-sur-Alzette, Luxembourg
E-Mail: Liyousew.Borga@uni.lu

C. D'Ambrosio
E-Mail: Conchita.Dambrosio@uni.lu

A. Lepinteur
E-Mail: Anthony.Lepinteur@uni.lu

A. Heinen et al. (Hrsg.), *Wohlbefinden und Gesundheit im Jugendalter,*
https://doi.org/10.1007/978-3-658-35744-3_8

151

Subjective well-being is also known to be relative. Clark and Oswald (1996) use the British Panel Household Survey to show that job satisfaction increases with own wage but diminishes with the wage level of colleagues. Using a quasi-natural experiment, Card et al. (2012) demonstrate that disclosing information on peers' salaries lowers job satisfaction of workers below the median of their pay unit. However, there is also evidence that the relationship between one's own well-being and other's incomes can be positive. Using the Russian Longitudinal Monitoring Survey, Senik (2004) shows that the reference group's income exerts a positive influence on individual life satisfaction. Similarly, D'Ambrosio et al. (2020) find that relative wealth increases life satisfaction in German data. This latter phenomenon has come to be known in the literature as the information effect: the presence of richer or wealthier individuals signals that there is a possibility for oneself to get richer in the future, which increases own well-being even before any actual enrichment takes place (Hirschman and Rothschild 1973).

The aforementioned articles often consider individuals with common characteristics (for instance age, gender, and education) as the reference group at the basis of these relative comparisons. However, one can also postulate that subjective well-being may be influenced by family members' outcomes and behaviours. This is the case in Clark (2003) where life satisfaction of the unemployed is higher when they live with an unemployed partner. Powdthavee (2009) and Wunder and Heineck (2013) demonstrate that empathetic (or altruistic) reactions affect well-being to the extent that one's life satisfaction is a direct function of the partner's life satisfaction.

Very little is known about the link between the health of relatives and life satisfaction. Much of the related literature is limited to investigating partners' health and find negative effects on subjective well-being (Van den Berg et al. 2014; Clark et al. 2019). Using the 1970 British Cohort Study and the Malaise score to measure mental health, Layard et al. (2014) and Clark and Lepinteur (2019) show that mothers' mental health status in 1980 still affects subjective well-being of their children in 2000. To the best of our knowledge, only Powdthavee and Vignoles (2008) specifically address the question of whether parents' mental distress influence their child's life satisfaction. Using British data, they show that lower levels of paternal mental health reduces life satisfaction of children. Maternal mental health only affects that of daughters.

We here take advantage of a longitudinal birth-cohort data from four developing countries (i.e. Ethiopia, India, Peru, and Vietnam) and investigate the consequences of relatives' health on subjective well-being of children. Our study's contribution to the literature is twofold. First, we account simultaneously for the effect of the health of the father, the mother and the siblings on own life satisfaction. To the best of our knowledge our work is the first contribution addressing this point. Our approach paints a better picture of the key pathways through which parental and sibling health translates into child well-being. Siblings spend considerable time together, and siblings' characteristics and sibling dynamics substantially influence developmental trajectories and outcomes. Second, most of the extant literature focused on developed countries and we here provide what we believe to be the first evidence from developing countries. This is particularly important since families in developing countries are likely to be further affected by potential health disparities, persistent poverty, and poor access to health services. The dataset we use allows us to explore how patterns are similar or different across those countries and make comparisons that are relevant for other countries with similar circumstances.

We first show that the health of the parents and the siblings are strongly correlated with the life satisfaction of the children of our estimation sample. We find that the effect of the health of siblings is more important than the effect of parental health. We then explore whether the underlying transmission mechanism of the observed correlation is due to objective causes, namely the shared environment and the parental investment decisions affecting the intra-household time allocation, or to psychological factors such as the information effect or empathy. We find that the health of the parents have little impact beyond the shared environment. This is particularly true for mothers. While having ill siblings reduces the probability of attending school and increases the time spent on paid and housework, the drop in life satisfaction due to the sibling's illness seems to be mainly driven by psychological factors.

The remainder of the chapter is organised as follows. In Sect. 2 we outline a brief conceptual framework. Section 3 describes the data, and the empirical strategy appears in Sect. 4. Results are presented in Sect. 5. We conclude in Sect. 6.

2   Conceptual Framework

Several studies in Developmental Psychology have found that child well-being is predicted by family well-being and parenting quality (see Newland 2015, for an extended review). Studies in Economics that focuses on the effect of parental health, however, have a narrow scope and are limited mostly to school enrolment outcomes (Gertler et al. 2004; Sun and Yao 2010; Bratti and Mendola 2014). Recent models of human capital formation (Heckman 2007) link human development to the stability of the home and to parental (mental) health. The home environment has notable impacts on child well-being that may affect the stock of human capital in adulthood (Knudsen et al. 2006; Heckman 2007). The extant literature heavily focused on measuring child well-being by cognitive/non-cognitive standardized test scores. Conti and Heckman (2014) stress that well-being indicators must incorporate dynamic processes such as self-realization and the degree to which a person is fully functioning in society. We contribute to these strands of literature by asking if there is a robust relationship between the health of family members (e.g. parents, siblings) and subjective well-being (SWB) of adolescents.

Our conceptual framework is set-up in the spirit of Todd and Wolpin (2003) and Cunha and Heckman (2008), but we focus on the role of family circumstances in producing a child's subjective well-being. The framework has several important characteristics. It models how environments and investments joined with own characteristics affect the evolution of well-being; it accounts for the preferences of the parents which help shape the investments in children; and it factors in the constraints that the families face (see Conti and Heckman 2014, for a comprehensive review of a human capital model).

In Fig. 1 we outline the basic conceptual framework for how we specify the empirical model of the relationship between family health shocks and child well-being outcomes. We consider key pathways from family health to child well-being: both the direct pathways, and the indirect pathways through parental investment decisions and the shared environment.

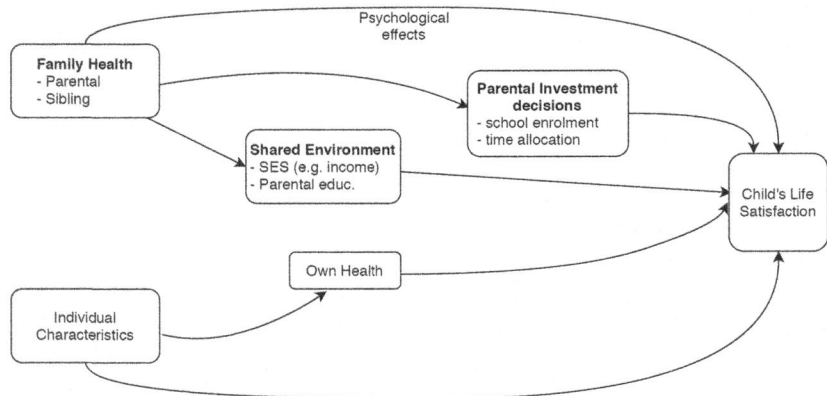

Fig. 1 Conceptual framework

2.1   The Effects of Parental Investment and the Shared Environment on Child's Life Satisfaction

The literature in the Economics of Happiness mostly explored the determinants of adult life satisfaction in developed countries. Little is comparatively known about the causes of life satisfaction of children and adolescents living in developing countries. However, several hypotheses can be formulated based on the extant literature.

Children with parents investing in their education are expected to have higher levels of life satisfaction for at least two reasons. According to Kahneman et al. (2004), housework and working time are the activities associated with the lowest levels of pleasures. In developing countries, children might be asked to quit school and spend more time in housework or on the labour market. Consequently, parental investments in education make children spending relatively less time in activities that would reduce their life satisfaction. Beyond its impact on current time allocation, education is expected to give children better expectations regarding their future life; and positive expectations about future outcomes are associated with higher contemporaneous life satisfaction (Senik 2008).

Gaps in human capital development of children across different socioeconomic groups have counterparts in gaps in family environments. Francesconi and Heckman (2016) review the related empirical literature and conclude that disadvantaged children have compromised early environments as measured on a variety of dimensions. For example, children from disadvantaged environments are exposed to a substantially less rich vocabulary than children from more advantaged families. Cunha et al. (2013) also documents the lack of parenting knowledge among disadvantaged parents. Parenting styles are important determinants of early child development (Fiorini and Keane 2014; Del Bono et al. 2016). Consequently, a shared environment where resources (monetary and time) are scarce is expected to inhibit child development and happiness.

2.2   The Effect of Family Health on Child's Life Satisfaction

2.2.1 Through Parental Investment

Health shocks to parents might reduce the time they invest in the education of their children; for instance, parental involvement in the child's education and care-giving may reduce when one or both parents face serious illness (Dhanaraj

2016). Parents may also force children to participate in home/market work, or they may decide to take children out of school as the opportunity cost of children's time increases. Bratti and Mendola (2014) study the effect of parental morbidity on child school enrolment and find that a young adult (age 15–24) with an ill mother but healthy father is significantly less likely to be enrolled in school. Alam (2015) use longitudinal data from Tanzania and shows that father's illness reduces children's education by decreasing their attendance.

2.2.2 Through the Shared Environment

Parental health shocks (in the absence of insurance) affect elements shared by the household by constraining its income (and consumption).[2] The usual mechanisms of consumption smoothing are often limited for resource constrained households in low and middle income countries due to the absence of well-developed credit and insurance markets (Jensen 2000). In this situation, households optimize by investing less in children (Becker and Tomes 1986). Luca and Bloom (2018) show that, regardless of gender, each parent's health is significantly associated with his or her own labour market activity and earnings, as well as intrinsically linked to their spouse's labour market status and earnings. They find paternal health to be associated with child schooling outcomes, especially for girls. However, child schooling outcomes are substantially and negatively affected when both parents suffer health shocks. The latter in the case of the father negatively affect aggregate household consumption, particularly food and education expenditures.

2.2.3 Direct Psychological Effects

Family illness could cause stress that may affect the well-being of children. There is some evidence about emotional and psychological transmissions of negative emotions and mental distress from one family member to the other (Powdthavee

---

[2]While it is not the focus of our analysis, it is important to stress that elements composing the shared environment (e.g. income, parental education) are also known to affect health. There is a well documented evidence that across countries, within countries at a point in time, and over time with economic growth, wealthy people live longer and have lower morbidity, on average, than poor people (Case et al. 2002). This disparity in health across socio-economic status (SES) groups is often known as the SES-health gradient. A number of SES measures have been proposed, other than income, such as wealth, education, employment status, and race/ethnicity.The SES-health gradient is also remarkably similar between countries with relatively low levels of social protection from loss of work and health risks, such as the US, and those with stronger welfare systems, such as the Netherlands (Galama and Van Kippersluis 2019).

and Vignoles 2003). Consequently, a lower level of family health might directly translate into a lower level of life satisfaction. The information effect (Hirschman and Rothschild 1973) can have a similar effect: the presence of ill individuals in the same household signals that there is a possibility for oneself to get ill in the future, which decreases own happiness even before any actual change in health takes place. Along the same line, one might postulate that children have altruistic preferences and might value having a family in good health.

Siblings' rivalry might also play an ambiguous role in the relationship between life satisfaction and siblings' health. Knowing that parents make decisions on how to allocate investments across different siblings and might compensate for or reinforce initial differences among them (Behrman et al. 1982), children may become rivals in the face of labour and capital constraints. Hence, a sibling in relatively poor health might be a source of lower or higher happiness if parents invest their resources to respectively compensate or reinforce differences in health between siblings.

3   Data

The data for this study are from the *Young Lives* survey, a study tracking the lives of children in four countries: Ethiopia, India (in the states of Andhra Pradesh and Telangana), Peru and Vietnam over 15 years. In each study country, the Young Lives surveys involve tracking 3000 children in two cohorts. The younger cohort consists of 2000 children who were born between January 2001 and May 2002. The older cohort consists of approximately 1000 children from each country born in 1994–1995.

Currently, five survey waves are available: the baseline round in 2002 and four follow-up waves in 2006, 2009, 2013 and 2016. The data are clustered and cover 20 sites in each country across rural and urban areas. The objectives of Young Lives project is to study the causes and consequences of childhood poverty. Hence, the sample was designed to include a high proportion of poor children, while at the same time including other children with whom their experiences could be compared Study sites in each country were selected non-randomly, with rich areas excluded from the sample and poor areas over-sampled. Children in the right age group in the selected sites were then sampled randomly. For the younger cohort the children were aged between 6 and 18 months, while they were aged 7 to 8 years for the older cohort sample.[3]

Even though the study sites were chosen purposely to reflect the diverse socioeconomic conditions within the study countries and therefore are not statistically representative for the country, comparisons with representative datasets like the Demographic and Health Survey (DHS) samples do show that the data contain a similar range of variation as nationally representative datasets in each of the countries.

The Young Lives survey consists of three main sources of data: a child questionnaire, a household questionnaire, and a community questionnaire. Our variables are from the household and child questionnaires. From the household questionnaire we obtain data on parental background, household and child education, the number of household members by sex and age groups, the size of the household, urban/rural location, and indicators of household socio-economic status.

From the child questionnaire, we obtain data on a wide range of child well-being indicators such as schooling, time-use, health, social networks, feelings and attitudes, anthropometry, as well as cognitive and non-cognitive tests. Subjective well-being is measured with a Cantrill ladder question that seeks to capture a child's view on where she places herself on a ladder ranging from 1 to 9 reflecting worst to best possible life. A picture of the ladder is shown to the child by the survey enumerator as the question is asked.

The survey records detailed information about the history of illness and injury suffered by members of the household. Health shocks are defined such that the respondent perceives the illness of the household member to have affected the welfare of the household negatively.

Last, the time use diary documents all of the activities of the children over a 24 h period on one randomly chosen weekday. These activities are then grouped into the following eight major categories: Caring for others (younger siblings, the elderly, ill household members); domestic chores (fetching water, firewood, cleaning, cooking, shopping); tasks at the family business (farm, cattle herding, other family business); activities for pay outside of household; at school; studying outside of school (including extra tutorship, and studying at home); play time/ general leisure, and sleep.

---

[3] See the survey documentation at https://www.younglives.org.uk/ for further details.

4   Empirical Strategy

We first estimate how the health of relatives affects the life satisfaction of Young Lives respondents via the following OLS regression:

$$LS_{ijt} = \alpha_0 + \alpha_1 FatherIll_{ijt} + \alpha_2 MotherIll_{ijt} + \alpha_3 SiblingIll_{ijt} + \alpha_4 OwnHealth_{ijt} + \alpha_5 SE_{ijt} + \delta_i + \lambda_t + \epsilon_{it}. \quad (1)$$

where LS_{ijt} is the life satisfaction reported by the Young Lives respondent i from household j in wave t on a 9-point scale. The other variables are described below.[4]

The validity and reliability of responses to well-being questions can be a source of concern. We have discussed in details some facts in favour of its use in Chapter 1 (Borga, D'Ambrosio & Lepinteur). We know, for example, that responses to subjective well-being questions and physiological expressions of emotions or brain activity are strongly correlated (Urry et al. 2004). In addition, life satisfaction is a good predictor of future behaviours, such as marital break-up (Guven et al. 2012) or job quits (Clark 2001). This evidence shows that subjective measures of well-being reveal useful information about individual preferences and thus behaviour, even after controlling for a wide range of objective variables. As these findings are also based on pooled regressions, it seems that survey respondents share a common understanding of life-satisfaction scales and it supports its use for interpersonal comparisons.

FatherIll$_{ijt}$, *MotherIll$_{ijt}$* and *SiblingIll$_{ijt}$* are dummies equal one when respectively the father, the mother or any of the child's siblings were ill between wave t and $t-1$. The households were asked to identify which among a predefined list of events/shocks had a negative consequence on them. Illness of a family member (father, mother, and siblings) is among these predefined events asked to every household. These shock-related variables are binary (the variable equals 1 when shock was reported during the period in between rounds, and 0 otherwise). Note that answers are based on perceptions; that is, they do not show whether a negative event has occurred, rather they show whether the respondent considers the event has affected the welfare of the household negatively.

OwnHealth$_{ijt}$ is self-reported health ranging from 1 to 5 (i.e., "very poor health" to "very good health"). It is reported by the main caregiver of the child.

---

[4]While we lack statistical power to convincingly correct for the Nickell bias, a dynamic panel model yields similar estimates. Results are available upon requests.

Regarding the different concerns about the interpretation and reporting biases of self-assessed health, Doiron et al. (2015) illustrate its predictive power on mortality, risk of coronary heart diseases and chronic diseases using an Australian survey data linked to administrative individual medical records. They find that self-assessed health predicts future health such as hospitalizations and prescription drugs. According to Doiron et al. (2015), the predictive power of self-assessed health is even more precise in cases of serious and chronic diseases.

δ_i and λ_t represent individual fixed effects and survey-round fixed effects. The former captures the influence of time-invariant characteristics of the respondents, such as personality traits or genes. Survey-round fixed effects neutralize the influence of elements that are shared by all respondents in a given survey round, e.g. macroeconomic environment, design of the questionnaire, etc.

SE_{ijt} is a set of control variables capturing the impact of the shared environment (the parental education, the household size, a wealth index and an urban dummy). We will present in our main results two versions of Eq. 1 where we will respectively not control for and then control for SE_{ijt}. In the first version, α_1, α_2, α_3 can be considered as the net effects of the health of the different family members on the life satisfaction of the Young Lives respondents. In the second version of Eq. 1, α_1, α_2, α_3 will measure the effect of the various measures of health net of the shared environment. The comparison of the different vectors of estimates will give us the opportunity to evaluate the relative importance of the shared environment in explaining the relationship between family health and own life satisfaction.

However, this exercise does not allow to quantify to what extent the effect of family members' health is due to objective detrimental changes due to parental investment decisions (i.e. higher probability to quit school and to work) or psychological reasons. This is why we estimate this second regression via OLS:

$$LS_{ijt} = \beta_0 + \beta_1 FatherIll_{ijt} + \beta_2 MotherIll_{ijt} + \beta_3 SiblingIll_{ijt} +$$
$$\beta_4 OwnHealth_{ijt} + \beta_5 SE_{ijt} + \beta_6 PI_{ijt} + \delta_i + \lambda_t + \varepsilon_{it}.$$

PI_{ijt} is a vector of parental investments that may mediate the relationship between family members' health and life satisfaction as outlined in Sect. 2 (and summarized in Fig. 1). We include the probability to be enrolled at school, the share of time spent on paid work outside of the home as well as the share of time spent in housework. We believe that these variables capture the influence of the most important objective channels that may explain a potential objective relationship between family members' health and life satisfaction. If this is true, β_1, β_2

and β_3 should respectively be significantly lower than α_1, α_2 and α_3. If β_1, β_2 and β_3 remain significantly different from zero, it would mean that family illness affects life satisfaction beyond objective reasons. This would imply that a part of the relationship between family illness and happiness is based on psychological factors such as the information effect or empathy.

Each regression we report here is carried out using all of the survey members who have non-missing values for the dependent variable and independent variables. This produces an estimation sample of 22,352 observations. The children from our estimation sample are on average 14 years old and their average life satisfaction is 5.71 (on a scale from 1 to 9). They report a level of health of 3.71 on average (on a scale from 1 to 5). The probability of having a father ill is 9 %. The same figure applies to mother and siblings. The complete descriptive statistics appear in Table 1.

Table 1 Descriptive statistics – estimation sample

	Mean	SD	Min	Max
Life Satisfaction	5.71	1.78	1	9
Own Health	3.71	0.78	1	5
Father ill	0.09		0	1
Mother ill	0.10		0	1
Siblings ill	0.10		0	1
Age	14.08	4.19	6.75	25.58
Female	0.48		0	1
Father Education	6.74	4.29	0	16
Mother Education	5.56	4.33	0	16
Household Size	5.10	1.84	1	26
Urban	0.40		0	1
Wealth Index	0.57	0.19	0	3.69
School Enrollment	0.82		0	1
Daily time on the Labour Market (in minutes)	24.28	24.86	0	140
Daily time in Housework (in minutes)	13.38	13.65	0	126

Notes: Pooled data (average for all waves). Number of observations for the four countries is: 4,747 in Ethiopia, 4,875 in India, 5,336 in Peru, and 7,394 in Vietnam

5   Results

5.1   Family Health and Subjective Well-being

Table 2 shows how life satisfaction is correlated with the measures of health status of the different household members. The first column presents the estimation results that only include dummies for illness of the father, mother and siblings. The second column adds own health and the third includes all of the other family outcomes. The last column introduces individual fixed-effects. All specifications control for the gender and age of the respondent as well wave and region fixed effects.

Column (1) of Table 2 reports the association between life satisfaction and family health. We find a significant negative correlation between household members' health and the child's life satisfaction. Pairwise Wald tests confirm that the effect of father and mother illness are not significantly different while the negative impact of siblings' illness is significantly larger.

Table 2 Effect of family illness on children's subjective wellbeing: pooled OLS and panel results controlling for the influence of the shared environment

	Life Satisfaction [1–9]			
	(1)	(2)	(3)	(4)
Father ill	-0.137^{***}	-0.123^{***}	-0.092^{**}	-0.087^{*}
	(0.041)	(0.040)	(0.039)	(0.051)
Mother ill	-0.147^{***}	-0.128^{***}	-0.096^{**}	-0.055
	(0.041)	(0.041)	(0.040)	(0.053)
Siblings ill	-0.216^{***}	-0.173^{***}	-0.182^{***}	-0.242^{***}
	(0.040)	(0.040)	(0.039)	(0.051)
Own Health		0.231^{***}	0.199^{***}	0.118^{***}
		(0.017)	(0.017)	(0.022)
Observations	22.352	22.352	22.352	22.352
Shared Environment	-	-	✓	✓
Individual FE	-	-	-	✓

Notes: These are linear regressions. Robust standard errors clustered at the household level in parentheses. Each estimation controls for the survey-round and region fixed effects. Family variables are maternal and paternal education, household size, wealth index, and an urban dummy. We control for the child gender and age when we do not control for individual fixed-effects. * p < 0.10, ** p < 0.05, *** p < 0.01

The estimates from column (1) might confound the effect of unobserved variables that may simultaneously affect life satisfaction and household members' health. To account for this, we first control for own health in Column (2). Consistent with the literature on health and subjective well-being (Clark et al. 2019), we find that health is an important predictor of happiness. Own health attracts a positive and precise estimate. Note that one cannot directly compare the magnitude of the effect of own health to the effect family illness as they do not share a common scale. However, the most precisely estimated coefficient is unsurprisingly the one associated with own health. Controlling for own health also lowers the magnitudes of family health estimates (but they remain significantly different from zero at 1 % level).

We control for the effect of the shared environment in column (3). The parents' health variables still attract positive estimates but their significance is reduced. Standard errors remain the same implying that the loss in significance is only due to the lower magnitude of the estimates. The effect of siblings' health remains unchanged and still highly significant. The effect of own health is still positive and significantly different from zero at 1 % level albeit its magnitude is slightly reduced. The introduction of household characteristics aims at capturing the influence of the common shared environment. Regarding the evolution of our estimates, it seems that it partially explains the effect of parental health.

Last, we introduce individual fixed-effects in column (4). This allows controlling for the influence of all time invariant factors (such as genetics and personality traits) that may affect the relationship between life satisfaction and family illness. Maternal health is now no longer significantly different from zero. Paternal health remains a negative predictor of life satisfaction but only at the 10 % significance level. This result suggests that most of the effect of parental health observed in column (1) transits via the objective living conditions, i.e. the common shared environment, and the time invariant characteristics we controlled for. However, the effect of siblings' health is remarkably stable across specifications and, as such, relatively insensitive to the influence of the effects of aforementioned objective living conditions. We explore more deeply the mechanisms that might explain our results in the next sub-section.

5.2   Parental Investment or Psychological Factors?

We now ask whether the negative effects of the father's and siblings health are explained by objective and detrimental changes in parental investments or by psychological factors. To do so, we first check whether lower levels of health of the relatives reduce the probability of the main respondent attending school. We also verify how the time a child spends on the market work and on household chores reacts to changes in the health of the relatives.

We replicate our main model but use the probability of school enrolment, the time spent on the market work, and the time spent in housework as dependent variables. Results are shown in Table 3. The probability of school enrolment is unsurprisingly lower when the father is ill but also when the siblings are ill. This might be explained by the results in column (2). A sick father is also less likely to work and it might create the need for the other household members to spend a larger share of their time on the labour market. This is consistent with a mechanism of intra-household compensation in working time. Furthermore, we find that when the mother or the siblings are sick, the time spent in housework also increases (see the last column of Table 3). As expected from countries where the adherence to conservative gender norms is still high, we do not find any substitution mechanism between the cohort members and the fathers' health when we consider the time spent in housework.

As suggested by Table 3, children who grew up with sick family members in our estimation sample are less likely to go to school and more likely to devote time in the labour market and on housework. Such changes in the time allocation

Table 3 Effect of family illness on children's time allocation: Panel results

	School Enrollment	Time on Market Work	Time in Housework
	(1)	(2)	(3)
Father ill	-0.040^{***}	1.113^{*}	0.130
	(0.011)	(0.594)	(0.349)
Mother ill	-0.016	1.060^{*}	1.001^{***}
	(0.010)	(0.551)	(0.324)
Siblings ill	-0.036^{***}	1.022^{*}	0.786^{**}
	(0.010)	(0.550)	(0.350)
Own Health	0.019^{***}	-0.549^{**}	-0.221
	(0.004)	(0.233)	(0.148)
Observations	22.352	22.352	22.352

Notes: These are linear regressions. Robust standard errors clustered at the household level in parentheses. Each estimation controls for maternal and paternal education, household size, wealth index, an urban dummy, and individual, survey-round and region fixed effects.
* $p < 0.10$, ** $p < 0.05$, *** $p < 0.01$

of the cohort members would explain the estimates we found in column (4) of Table 2 if well-being is positively correlated with school enrolment and negatively correlated with the time spent on the labour market and housework.

We formally test this hypothesis in Table 4. The first column replicates our baseline estimates. The results in the next three columns are in line with our expectations: schooling is positively associated with well-being and the time spent on the labour market and in housework reduces life satisfaction. We may then expect the detrimental effect of father and sibling's sickness to be potentially driven by the reduction in the probability to be enrolled and the increase in the time spent on the labour market and in housework. However, none of the health estimates appears to be affected by the inclusion of these different variables. The

Table 4 Effect of family illness on children's subjective wellbeing: Panel results controlling for the influence of parental investment decisions

	Life Satisfaction [1–9]				
	(1)	(2)	(3)	(4)	(5)
Father ill	-0.087^*	-0.081	-0.084^*	-0.086^*	-0.081
	(0.051)	(0.051)	(0.051)	(0.051)	(0.051)
Mother ill	-0.055	-0.053	-0.052	-0.050	-0.048
	(0.053)	(0.053)	(0.053)	(0.053)	(0.053)
Siblings ill	-0.242^{***}	-0.237^{***}	-0.240^{***}	-0.238^{***}	-0.234^{***}
	(0.051)	(0.051)	(0.051)	(0.051)	(0.051)
Own Health	0.118^{***}	0.115^{***}	0.117^{***}	0.117^{***}	0.115^{***}
	(0.022)	(0.022)	(0.022)	(0.022)	(0.022)
School enrollment		0.141^{***}			0.124^{**}
		(0.045)			(0.053)
Time in market work			-0.002^{***}		0.000
			(0.001)		(0.001)
Time in housework				-0.005^{***}	-0.005^{***}
				(0.001)	(0.001)
Observations	22.352	22.352	22.352	22.352	22.352

Notes: These are linear regressions. Robust standard errors clustered at the household level in parentheses. Each estimation controls for maternal and paternal education, household size, wealth index, an urban dummy, and individual, survey-round and region fixed effects. $^*\,p < 0.10$, $^{**}\,p < 0.05$, $^{***}\,p < 0.01$

effect of a father's illness is no longer significantly different from zero in column (2) but it is not significantly lower than the baseline estimate in column (1). We finally follow a "horse race" approach in the last column, i.e. we control for all the potential channels in a single regression. Both school enrolment and the time spent doing housework remain significant predictors of well-being. The effect of the siblings' health remains negative and highly significant while the effect of the father illness is no longer different from zero.

These results suggest that the well-being effect of the health of the parents is mostly explained by the control variables we used in the columns (3) and (4) of Table 2, i.e. the shared environment. However, the reduction in well-being caused by sibling's illness is neither explained by the shared environment nor objective changes in parental investment (school enrolment, time on the labour market, time in housework). As none of the objective factors we controlled for in our empirical analysis influenced the well-being effect of the health of the siblings, we suspect the relationship between life satisfaction and sibling's illness to be mostly driven by psychological factors such as the information effect or empathy.

5.3   Heterogeneity

Table 2 shows the average effect of family illness on the whole estimation sample. One may then argue that certain individuals are more affected by the health of their relatives than others. For instance, it is shown in the related literature that the determinants of happiness differ across gender (Fugl-Meyer et al. 2002). We account for this concern by splitting the sample by gender and re-estimating our main model. These results are shown in the first two columns of Table 5 and we do not find significant differences between boys and girls.

We then split our sample between "poor" and "non-poor" household. As there is no measure of income in our dataset, we use the median of the wealth index computed by the data provider as the poverty threshold. Results are displayed in columns (3) and (4). The effect of own health in both cases is positive and significant. The effects of the illness of the siblings are always negative and comparable in magnitude across samples. Note that the effect of having an ill father is only negative and significant for children from poor households. However, the estimate is only significant at 10 % level.

We next consider rural and urban households separately in columns (5) and (6). While most of the estimates are comparable across samples, a noticeable element here is that the health of mothers is significantly different from zero in rural households only.

Table 5 Effect of family illness on children's subjective wellbeing – Heterogeneity analysis

	Life Satisfaction [1–9]							
	Boys	Girls	Poor	Non-poor	Rural	Urban	Old Cohort	Young Cohort
	(1)	(2)	(3)	(4)	(5)	(6)	(7)	(8)
Father ill	−0.055	−0.118	−0.153*	0.009	−0.061	−0.056	−0.040	−0.119*
	(0.067)	(0.077)	(0.081)	(0.076)	(0.066)	(0.083)	(0.082)	(0.063)
Mother ill	−0.010	−0.102	−0.089	0.063	−0.139**	0.072	−0.065	−0.043
	(0.071)	(0.079)	(0.080)	(0.084)	(0.069)	(0.087)	(0.085)	(0.065)
Siblings ill	−0.220***	−0.266***	−0.250***	−0.239***	−0.224***	−0.252***	−0.257***	−0.228***
	(0.069)	(0.076)	(0.075)	(0.082)	(0.068)	(0.080)	(0.081)	(0.064)
Own Health	0.085***	0.151***	0.107***	0.117***	0.133***	0.102***	0.158***	0.113***
	(0.030)	(0.032)	(0.033)	(0.034)	(0.029)	(0.035)	(0.037)	(0.027)
Observations	11.651	10.701	11.268	11.084	13.501	8851	6414	15.938
Shared Environment	✓	✓	✓	✓	✓	✓	✓	✓
Individual FE	✓	✓	✓	✓	✓	✓	✓	✓

Notes: These are linear regression. Robust standard errors clustered at the household level in parentheses. Each estimation controls for maternal and paternal education, household size, wealth index, child gender, child age, an urban dummy, and individual, survey-round and region fixed effects. * $p < 0.10$, ** $p < 0.05$, *** $p < 0.01$

One might finally wonder whether the effect of the health of relatives depends on the age of the respondents. We here take advantage of the particular setting of the Young Lives Study as two different cohorts are surveyed at the same time: the *Older* cohort and the *Younger* cohort. The former is on average 19 years old in our estimation sample while the latter is on average 12.6 years old. Once again, we find few differences between the two categories as revealed by columns (7) and (8). The most important factors are own health and the health of siblings while the health of the parents attract estimates that are hardly significantly different from zero.[5]

6   Conclusion

The role of the health of parents and siblings have so far received scant attention in the literature. Our contribution aimed to fill this gap.

Family health is a strong predictor of child well-being through its potential impact on parental investment decisions and family interactions. Health shocks entail both economic and psychological costs to children and may alter their time allocation patterns. Resource constrained families living in underdeveloped communities with limited access to health services are further affected by this. Hence, understanding the impact of health shocks and their transmission mechanisms helps inform public policy.

Using a dataset covering four developing countries (namely Ethiopia, India, Peru and Vietnam), we show that having parents and siblings in poor health significantly reduces own life satisfaction. We then find that the loss in well-being produced by the poor health of parents is mostly explained by the shared environment (education level of the parents, level of wealth). The health of the parent's matters more in terms of well-being for children who grew up in poor and rural households.

---

[5]We considered here individual sources of heterogeneity. One may argue that heterogeneity may arise from the institutional context and that we should analyse separately the four countries from our estimation sample. When we do so, we find very similar results in Ethiopia, Peru and Vietnam. We do not find any effect of health (own and relative) on life satisfaction in India. This is not surprising as we have less observations and less within-variability in this country: we then attribute the absence of significant estimates to the limited statistical power.

Having at least one sibling in poor health has a stronger effect on life satisfaction than a sick parent. Keeping constant the shared environment and accounting for time-invariant characteristics does not explain the effect. While we show that a sick sibling decreases the probability to be enrolled at school and increases the time on market and domestic work, none of these channels explain the negative effect of a sick sibling.

As none of the objective factors we considered could explain the loss in wellbeing induced by the poor health of siblings, we postulate that it may be caused by psychological processes in line with the information effect or empathic behaviour. We know from the Economics of Happiness literature that individuals tend to compare to persons they consider as peers to have a better understanding of what the future might bring to them (i.e. the information effect). But we also know that individuals genuinely care about their relatives (i.e. empathic behaviours). Future research should determine whether our estimates reflect a "pure" empathy or if it reflects a "tunnel effect". Are the children of our estimation sample simply worrying for the health of their siblings or are they concerned for themselves? Note also that our conclusion regarding the psychological nature of the association between sibling's health and own life satisfaction holds under the assumption that the influence of all objective channels is kept constant.

There are some limitations and potential weaknesses in our study. The empirical implementation of our research questions is problematic for a number of reasons. First, not all the determinants of subjective well-being (and their histories) are observable; second, there may be some endogeneity effects with respect to unobserved endowments and prior realizations of outcome (for example, indirect effects caused by parental behavioural responses or other confounding factors); and third, our outcome and main explanatory variables could be measured with error. Our study overcomes some of these limitations. We control for time invariant omitted variables through the inclusion of the child fixed effect, and account for correlated omitted variables that are shared by all respondents in a given survey round (such as macroeconomic environment) thanks to the survey-round-fixed effect. Despite our attempt to demonstrate as close to a causal relationship between family health and child life satisfaction, we are aware of the fact that our results cannot be interpreted as completely causal. There is still ample room for future research to find an appropriate identification strategy that purges the issues of omitted variables and endogeneity and establish the causal impact of family health on child's subjective well-being.

Our results are important for policy makers. The benefits of health policies would be underestimated if one only accounts for the better health of the targeted individuals. This means that cost–benefit analyses would be more accurate if they were likely to consider the potential positive spillover effects of any health policy.

References

Alam, S. A. (2015). "Parental health shocks, child labor and educational outcomes: Evidence from Tanzania." *Journal of Health Economics*, 44, 161–175.

Becker, G. S., & Tomes, N. (1986). "Human capital and the rise and fall of families." *Journal of Labor Economics*, 4, S1–S39.

Behrman, J. R., Pollak, R. A., & Taubman, P. (1982). "Parental preferences and provision for progeny." *Journal of Political Economy*, 90, 52–73.

Bratti, M., & Mendola, M. (2014). "Parental health and child schooling." *Journal of Health Economics*, 35, 94–108.

Card, D., Mas, A., Moretti, E., & Saez, E. (2012). "Inequality at work: The effect of peer salaries on job satisfaction." *American Economic Review*, 102, 2981–3003.

Case, A., Lubotsky, D., & Paxson, C. (2002). "Economic status and health in childhood: The origins of the gradient." *American Economic Review*, 92, 1308-1334.

Clark, A. E. (2001). "What really matters in a job? Hedonic measurement using quit data." *Labour Economics*, 8, 223–242.

Clark, A. E. (2003). "Unemployment as a social norm: Psychological evidence from panel data." *Journal of Labor Economics*, 21, 323–351.

Clark, A. E., Flèche, S., Layard, R., Powdthavee, N., & Ward, G. (2019). *The origins of happiness: The science of well-being over the life course.* Princeton University Press.

Clark, A. E., & Lepinteur, A. (2019). "The causes and consequences of early-adult unemployment: Evidence from cohort data." *Journal of Economic Behavior and Organization*, 166, 107–124.

Clark, A. E., & Oswald, A. J. (1996). "Satisfaction and comparison income." *Journal of Public Economics*, 61, 359–381.

Conti, G., & Heckman, J. (2014). "The economics of child well-being." In A. Ben-Arieh, F. Casas, I. Frønes, & J. Korbin (Eds.), *Handbook of child well-being*, 363–401.

Cunha, F., Elo, I., & Culhane, J. (2013). *Eliciting maternal expectations about the technology of cognitive skill formation.* NBER Working Paper N. 19144.

Cunha, F., & Heckman, J. J. (2008). "Formulating, identifying and estimating the technology of cognitive and non-cognitive skill formation." *Journal of Human Resources*, 43, 738-782.

D'Ambrosio, C., Jäntti, M., & Lepinteur, A. (2020). "Money and happiness: Income, wealth and subjective well-being." *Social Indicators Research*, 148, 47–66.

Del Bono, E., Francesconi, M., Kelly, Y., & Sacker, A. (2016). "Early maternal time investment and early child outcomes." *Economic Journal*, 126, F96–F135.

Dhanaraj, S. (2016) "Effects of parental health shocks on children's schooling: Evidence from Andhra Pradesh, India." *International Journal of Educational Development*, 49, 115–125.

Doiron, D., Fiebig, D. G., Johar, M., & Suziedelyte, A. (2015). "Does self-assessed health measure health?" *Applied Economics*, 47, 180–194.

Ferrer-i Carbonell, A., & Van Praag, B. M. (2002). "The subjective costs of health losses due to chronic diseases: An alternative model for monetary appraisal." *Health Economics*, 11, 709–722.

Fiorini, M., & Keane, M. P. (2014). "How the allocation of children's time affects cognitive and noncognitive development." *Journal of Labor Economics*, 32, 787–836.

Francesconi, M., & Heckman, J. J. (2016). "Child development and parental investment: Introduction." *Economic Journal*, 126, F1–F27.

Fugl-Meyer, A. R., Melin, R., & Fugl-Meyer, K. S. (2002). "Life satisfaction in 18-to 64-year-old swedes: In relation to gender, age, partner and immigrant status." *Journal of Rehabilitation Medicine*, 34, 239–246.

Galama, T. J., & Van Kippersluis, H. (2019). "A theory of socio-economic disparities in health over the life cycle." *Economic Journal*, 129, 338–374.

Gertler, P., Levine, D. I., & Ames, M. (2004). "Schooling and parental death." *Review of Economics and Statistics*, 86, 211–225.

Guven, C., Senik, C., & Stichnoth, H. (2012). "You can't be happ er than your wife. Happiness gaps and divorce." *Journal of Economic Behavior & Organization*, 82, 110–130.

Heckman, J. J. (2007). "The economics, technology, and neuroscience of human capability formation." *Proceedings of the National Academy of Sciences*, 104, 13250–13255.

Hirschman, A. O., & Rothschild, M. (1973). "The changing tolerance for income inequality in the course of economic development: With a mathematical appendix." *Quarterly Journal of Economics*, 87, 544–566.

Jensen, R. (2000). "Agricultural volatility and investments in children." *American Economic Review*, 90, 399–404.

Kahneman, D., Krueger, A. B , Schkade, D. A., Schwarz, N., & Stone, A. A. (2004). "A survey method for characterizing daily life experience: The day reconstruction method." *Science*, 306, 1776–1780.

Knudsen, E. I., Heckman, J. J., Cameron, J. L., & Shonkoff, J. P. (2006). "Economic, neurobiological, and behavioral perspectives on building America's future workforce." *Proceedings of the National Academy of Sciences*, 103, 10155–10162.

Layard, R., Clark, A. E., Cornaglia, F., Powdthavee, N., & Vernoit, J. (2014). "What predicts a successful life? A life-course model of well-being." *Economic Journal*, 124, F720–F738.

Luca, D. L., & Bloom, D. E. (2018). *The returns to parental health: Evidence from Indonesia*. NBER Working Paper N. 25304.

Newland, L. A. (2015). "Family well-being, parenting, and child well-being: Pathways to healthy adjustment." *Clinical Psychologist*, 19, 3–14.

Oswald, A. J., & Powdthavee, N. (2008). "Does happiness adapt? A longitudinal study of disability with implications for economists and judges." *Journal of Public Economics*, 92, 1061–1077.

Powdthavee, N. (2009). "I can't smile without you: Spousal correlation in life satisfaction." *Journal of Economic Psychology*, 30, 675–689.

Powdthavee, N., & Vignoles, A. (2008). "Mental health of parents and life satisfaction of children: A within-family analysis of intergenerational transmission of well-being." *Social Indicators Research*, 88, 397–422.

Senik, C. (2004). "When information dominates comparison: Learning from Russian subjective panel data." *Journal of Public Economics*, 88, 2099–2123.

Senik, C. (2008). "Is man doomed to progress?" *Journal of Economic Behavior & Organization*, 68, 140–152.

Shields, M. A., & Price, S. W. (2005). "Exploring the economic and social determinants of psychological well-being and perceived social support in England." *Journal of the Royal Statistical Society: Series A (Statistics in Society)*, 168, 513–537.

Sun, A., & Yao, Y. (2010). "Health shocks and children's school attainments in rural China." *Economics of Education Review*, 29, 375–382.

Todd, P. E., & Wolpin, K. I. (2003). "On the specification and estimation of the production function for cognitive achievement." *Economic Journal*, 113, F3-F33.

Urry, H. L., Nitschke, J. B., Dolski, I., Jackson, D. C., Dalton, K. M., Mueller, C. J., ... Davidson, R. J. (2004). "Making a life worth living: Neural correlates of well-being." *Psychological Science*, 15, 367–372.

Van den Berg, B., Fiebig, D. G., & Hall, J. (2014). "Well-being losses due to care-giving." *Journal of Health Economics*, 35, 123–131.

Wunder, C., & Heineck, G. (2013). "Working time preferences, hours mismatch and well-being of couples: Are there spillovers?" *Labour Economics*, 24, 244–252.

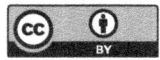

Child Deprivation and Well-being in Luxembourg

Anne-Catherine Guio

1 Introduction

Combating child poverty and investing in child well-being has featured on the agenda of the European Union (EU) for many years. In February 2013, a new milestone was reached when the European Commission published a recommendation entitled 'Investing in children: breaking the cycle of disadvantage' (European Commission, 2013), which was then adopted by the EU Council of Ministers. One key element of the EU recommendation is the fact that it calls on Member States to '(reinforce) statistical capacity where needed and feasible, particularly concerning child deprivation'.

The best way to provide accurate information on the actual living conditions of children in the EU, without making assumptions about the sharing of resources within the household, is to develop child-specific deprivation indicators – i.e. indicators based on information on the specific situation of children, which may differ from that of their parents. Children's needs and standards of living may differ from those of adults, even within the same household (Gordon und Nandy

Anne-Catherine Guio is a researcher at the Luxembourg Institute of Socio-Economic Research (LISER, Luxembourg).

This work has been supported by the Third Network for the Analysis of EU-SILC (Net-SILC3), funded by Eurostat. The European Commission bears no responsibility for the analyses and conclusions, which are solely those of the authors.

A.-C. Guio (✉)
Luxembourg Institute of Socio-Economic Research (LISER), Esch-sur-Alzette, Luxembourg
E-Mail: anne-catherine.guio@liser.lu

© Der/die Autor(en) 2022   173
A. Heinen et al. (Hrsg.), *Wohlbefinden und Gesundheit im Jugendalter,*
https://doi.org/10.1007/978-3-658-35744-3_9

2012; Main und Besemer 2013; Dermott und Pomati 2016; Main und Bradshaw 2016), meaning that data specific to the children themselves is required.

Understanding and measuring child deprivation is crucial, as it can have both a direct and an indirect impact on well-being. Children experience direct and immediate suffering due to elements they are lacking in terms of food, clothing, comfort and activities. However, they also suffer indirectly as result of the consequences of these deprivations for their health and emotional well-being. Some forms of deprivation (nutrition, housing comfort[1], lack of protection and care) may have an impact on short-term and long-term physical health (Repka 2013). Children may also experience feelings of shame and stigmatisation relative to their peers. Qualitative studies have also shown that children in households suffering from deprivation often do not ask their parents for things they need that cost money, in an attempt to protect their parents from stress and feelings of guilt (Ridge 2002 and 2011). In general terms, it has been shown that growing up in poverty increases the risk of experiencing poverty as an adult via numerous mechanisms relating to education, health, self-worth and so on (Pascoe et al. 2016; Gregg et al. 1999; Bellani and Bia 2017).

The EU's 2009 statistical survey on income and living conditions (EU-SILC) included for the first time an ad-hoc module designed to collect this information. The first in-depth analysis of this data, performed by Guio et al. (2012), identified an optimal set of deprivation items specific to children and proposed an aggregated index. These items were then collected in the EU-SILC 2014 ad-hoc module, enabling supplementary analysis by Guio et al. (2018). The final list of items proposed by these authors was adopted at a European level in March 2018, in order to measure child deprivation on a comparable basis across the entire Union. This list is made up of 17 items covering both the material and the social aspects of deprivation, which have been put together to form a child deprivation scale.

This chapter analyses the determinants of child deprivation in Luxembourg, using this new child deprivation indicator adopted at European Union level in March 2018. It serves as an extension to the econometric analyses performed by Guio et al. (2020), which sought to identify micro-level and macro-level risk factors in child deprivation across 31 European countries[2]. Section 2 presents the

---

[1] Marsh et al. 2000.

[2] A similar analysis of deprivation in Belgium is available in Guio und Vandenbroucke 2018.

indicators used. The third section discusses the drivers of child deprivation. The subsequent section presents the results of econometric tests in Luxembourg, and the final section offers a conclusion.

2 Child poverty and deprivation: what indicator(s) should be used?

Income can be taken into account when measuring child poverty: the members of a household (children and adults) are considered 'poor' if their income is below a threshold set at 60 % of the national median income. The income poverty rate commonly used in Europe therefore depends on each country's income level. It is a relative indicator.

To study more 'absolute' differences between countries, material deprivation indicators are also used on a European level. The conceptual approach used was inspired by the research conducted by Peter Townsend into relative deprivation during the 1960 s, which he succinctly described as follows in 1979:

> 'Poverty can be defined objectively and applied consistently only in terms of the concept of relative deprivation. [...] Individuals, families and groups in the population can be said to be in poverty when they lack the resources to obtain the type of diet, participate in the activities and have the living conditions and amenities which are customary, or at least widely encouraged or approved, in the societies to which they belong. Their resources are so seriously below those commanded by the average individual or family that they are, in effect, excluded from ordinary living patterns, customs or activities.' (Townsend 1979, p. 31).

Until 2018, European deprivation indicators were based on information relating to a household as a whole, or to the adults within it. To measure the everyday difficulties experienced by children, which may differ from those of their parents, researchers developed an additional European-level indicator: the **child-specific deprivation indicator**[3]. This indicator measures **access to the same set of 17 items considered as socially perceived necessities for all children living in Europe:** Does the child eat fruit and vegetables every day? Do they sometimes invite friends round to their home? Can they participate in school trips and events? Do they live in an adequately warmth home? Do they go on holiday for at

---

[3] For more information about this indicator, see Guio et al. 2018.

least one week per year? **A child is considered to be experiencing deprivation if they are deprived of at least three of the 17 items** (*see complete list below*). The higher the number of items lacked, the more severe the deprivation. Only deprivation resulting from unaffordability (and not life choices) is included in the calculation.

List of 17 items used to measure child deprivation
1. Child: Some new (not second-hand) clothes
2. Children: Two pairs of properly fitting shoes
3. Children: Fresh fruit and vegetables daily
4. Children: Meat, chicken, fish or vegetarian equivalent daily
5. Children: Books at home suitable for the children's age
6. Children: Outdoor leisure equipment
7. Children: Indoor games
8. Children: Regular leisure activities
9. Children: Celebrations on special occasions (birthday etc.)
10. Children: Invitation of friends to play and eat from time to time
11. Children: Participation in school trips and school events
12. Children: Holiday (one week per year)
13. Household: Replace worn-out furniture
14. Household: No payment arrears
15. Adults in household: Access to internet
16. Household: Home adequately warm
17. Household: Access to a care for private use

Table 1 presents the proportion of children in this situation for each item for every country in the EU, and the average for the EU-27. This data was collected as part of EU-SILC 2014.[4]

The table uses colours to highlight the countries with systematically high deprivation levels for different items (in orange/red), such as Bulgaria or Romania, and conversely those with low levels (in green: Nordic countries, Austria, the Netherlands and **Luxembourg**). It also shows the countries that have

---

[4] See https://statistiques.public.lu/en/surveys/espace-households/EU-SILC/index.html for more information about this survey in Luxembourg. The sample covers 3800 households in Luxembourg. For information about all EU countries, see the Eurostat website (https://ec.europa.eu/eurostat/web/income-and-living-conditions/overview).

Table 1 'Heat map' showing the proportion of deprived children in the country for each item, population of children aged 1 to 15, EU countries, 2014, %

	Fruit & vegetables	Books	Shoes	Indoor games	Protein	Internet	Celebrations	Outdoor leisure	Clothing	School trips	Friends	Car	Warm home	Recreation	Arrears	Holidays	Furniture
Sweden	0.1	0.6	0.3	0.3	0.0	0.4	1.3	0.8	0.9	0.8	0.7	3.1	0.9	2.6	0.0	5.5	3.0
Finland	0.3	0.5	0.8	0.2	0.2	0.4	0.3	0.3	3.5	0.6	0.1	3.6	0.7	1.3	16.5	7.2	11.6
Denmark	0.5	2.5	1.1	0.8	0.6	0.6	1.3	2.2	2.0	1.4	1.5	5.1	2.5	3.3	9.5	9.1	14.6
Austria	0.5	1.3	1.1	1.1	1.8	1.0	1.8	3.1	1.9	2.5	3.6	7.4	4.3	10.2	10.6	17.8	15.7
Netherlands	0.6	0.5	3.6	0.4	2.5	0.2	1.9	1.6	1.6	1.4	1.2	6.5	2.8	6.4	9.5	16.2	25.2
Luxembourg	0.8	0.8	1.0	1.5	1.1	1.4	1.9	1.7	2.0	3.6	2.3	2.1	1.0	2.7	6.3	9.4	20.9
Slovenia	1.0	1.1	1.2	1.3	1.4	1.3	2.5	2.0	5.9	2.3	3.4	3.3	4.0	10.7	28.0	7.2	15.8
Spain	1.7	2.3	3.0	3.5	2.9	13.5	11.4	5.8	7.7	10.6	12.8	6.6	12.0	13.1	17.8	34.5	46.4
Germany	1.8	0.7	2.2	0.6	3.6	0.9	1.5	1.3	2.1	0.6	1.7	4.4	5.3	6.2	9.7	17.4	17.8
Malta	1.9	2.0	5.9	2.1	6.9	4.4	4.9	4.1	6.1	2.7	4.9	4.5	21.6	6.0	22.0	34.9	29.7
Cyprus	2.1	5.4	1.3	3.6	2.4	8.7	10.8	7.7	5.4	2.5	12.3	1.4	25.4	21.2	41.7	40.2	60.9
Belgium	2.3	4.4	3.6	2.5	2.7	3.8	5.8	4.2	8.2	3.8	6.0	7.4	4.8	9.0	12.1	19.2	18.4
Italy	2.6	7.7	2.9	5.6	5.7	10.8	7.1	6.0	8.5	9.5	7.5	2.3	18.4	13.7	20.6	29.5	38.8
Ireland	2.6	1.0	6.5	1.4	3.1	4.8	3.0	1.7	12.3	3.3	3.2	6.6	9.4	7.3	25.6	53.1	28.6
France	2.7	1.2	5.2	1.0	2.3	1.8	5.2	1.7	8.9	4.8	2.4	2.8	5.1	6.2	15.0	11.6	28.0
Portugal	2.9	6.4	3.6	5.4	1.2	11.5	8.3	4.6	14.4	9.1	13.6	9.9	25.2	23.4	17.7	36.7	57.5
Czechia	3.0	2.0	3.0	2.8	4.7	4.0	3.6	7.8	6.3	5.0	2.4	11.8	6.0	8.5	10.4	8.7	47.8
Poland	3.5	2.9	1.4	2.3	3.0	3.1	9.7	4.3	3.2	8.5	8.7	7.5	7.9	18.8	19.3	26.2	31.5
EU-27	4.1	4.4	4.7	4.7	5.2	6.9	7.2	7.1	7.5	7.4	8.2	8.7	10.0	12.6	18.3	26.3	33.8
Croatia	4.5	7.2	3.2	5.7	6.2	4.9	5.6	5.9	5.3	7.8	7.4	7.0	9.1	8.9	35.9	29.2	32.3
Greece	5.4	0.6	1.6	1.6	0.2	0.3	18.5	3.7	1.8	21.2	14.1	8.6	30.5	15.8	54.2	41.3	57.5
Estonia	6.7	2.3	0.4	2.8	6.3	5.3	5.0	6.6	13.0	5.8	4.9	9.7	1.4	4.1	16.2	10.3	27.4
Lithuania	7.8	10.4	6.6	7.6	12.9	9.1	12.0	11.0	14.0	9.1	9.9	12.0	25.6	18.8	17.8	19.2	50.1
Slovakia	9.8	6.6	1.6	2.8	8.2	9.1	10.3	16.4	24.5	7.6	15.3	13.9	7.8	11.0	10.8	15.5	45.3
Latvia	10.0	11.0	11.7	8.7	22.0	8.1	10.3	55.5	24.5	7.6	11.3	23.4	18.2	16.2	31.6	27.6	57.7
Romania	14.8	24.8	28.0	42.4	21.6	36.7	33.2	17.0	26.6	30.3	40.1	45.3	15.4	60.1	29.3	61.4	67.3
Hungary	22.8	15.5	7.8	13.7	22.0	18.2	15.4	52.0	27.2	15.2	30.6	31.1	12.5	20.9	36.2	51.1	52.9
Bulgaria	40.2	43.2	49.0	38.4	42.4	26.9	32.3	52.0	36.2	42.5	41.4	30.2	40.2	52.3	43.9	54.6	72.1

Source: Guio, Marlier, Vandenbroucke und Verbunt (2020).

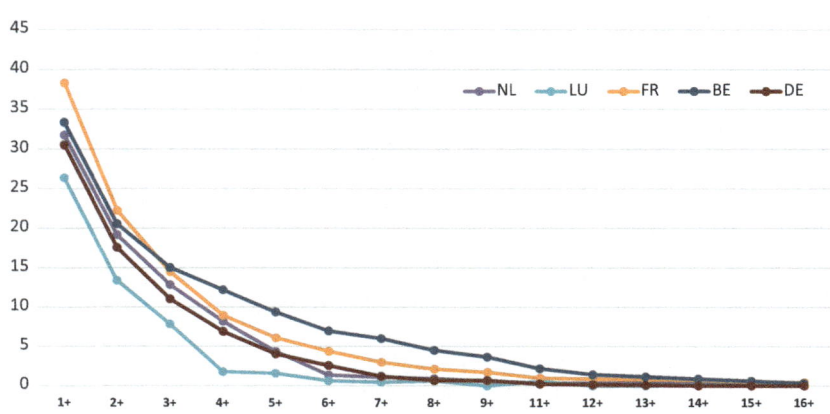

Fig. 1 Child distribution (aged 1 to 15) by the number of items of which they are deprived, Belgium, France, Germany, the Netherlands and Luxembourg, 2014, %. Source: Guio and Vandenbroucke (2018), op. cit.

a more nuanced picture depending on the item, i.e. countries that are at a relative disadvantage for some items and a relative advantage for others.

Despite Luxembourg's overall enviable results, child deprivation is not non-existent here. 9 % of children live in a household that does not have the resources to offer them a week of holiday per year. More than 20 % of children in Luxembourg live in a household that is not able to replace worn-out furniture. Some children suffer from the lack of the most severe items: 3–4 % of children are unable to buy new clothes or pay for school trips.

This table shows the percentage of children deprived of *each item taken separately*. We will now examine the extent to which children accumulate these 17 items. Figure 1 shows child distribution by the number of items of which they are deprived, for Luxembourg and for neighbouring countries (the Netherlands, France, Germany and Belgium).

This chart shows that Luxembourg has the best relative position among neighbouring countries: Luxembourg is the best-positioned country, whatever the deprivation threshold (i.e. the 'severity' of the deprivation). Using the threshold of three items lacked (the threshold used on a European level), Luxembourg has a child deprivation rate of 8 % compared with 15 % in Belgium and France, 13 % in the Netherlands and 11 % in Germany.

If the threshold is set at four or more items lacking (i.e. for more severe forms of deprivation): 12 % of children are deprived of at least four items in Belgium,

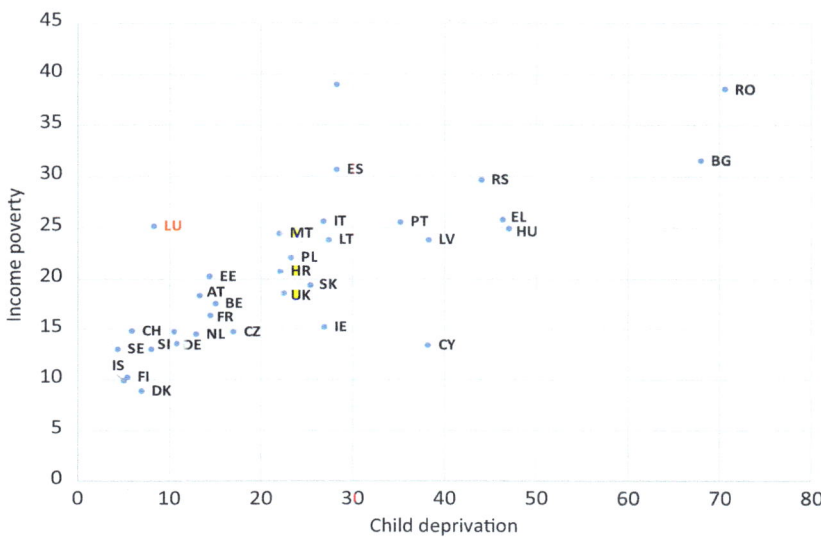

Fig. 2 The proportion of children (aged 1 to 15) deprived of at least three items (of the 17) and the proportion of children suffering from income poverty. EU 27 countries and non-EU countries covered by the EU-SILC, 2014, % *NB:* For a list of country abbreviations, see Appendix 1. Source: Guio Marlier, Vandenbroucke und Verbunt (2020), using cross-sectional data from the EU-SILC 2014 study

whilst this proportion is extremely low in Luxembourg (2 %) and at 7–9 % in the Netherlands, Germany and France.

These figures illustrate that this child-specific deprivation indicator sheds new light on the situation of children in Luxembourg. Until this point, it was traditionally thought that a quarter of children in Luxembourg were living below the poverty threshold. This new indicator pinpoints 8 % of the child population as suffering from deprivation. Figure 2 compared the child poverty rate with the child-specific deprivation rate in all EU countries. The European indicator for **child poverty** is defined as being the proportion of children living in households with an income below 60 % of the equivalent national median household

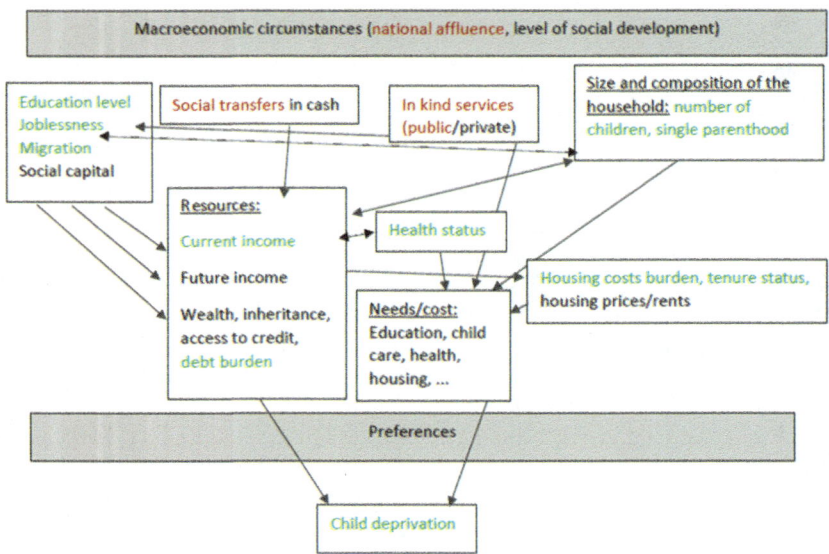

Diagram 1 Determinants of child deprivation. Source: Guio und Vandenbroucke, 2018, op. cit

income[5]. This is a relative income poverty indicator (given that the poverty threshold varies from one country to another).

This chart confirms that in comparison to the rest of Europe, Luxembourg has a higher child poverty level (25 %) but a lower child deprivation level (8 %).

---

[5] A household's equivalent income is the net (disposable) income. It is calculated in three stages: a) all monetary income received from any source by each member of the household or by the household itself is added up (including labour and capital income, social benefits in cash, and cash transfers between households), deducting any taxes and social contributions paid; b) to reflect differences in household size and composition, the total (net) income of the household is divided by the number of 'equivalent adults' using the 'modified OECD equivalence scale' which applies a weighting to all household members (1 to the first adult, 0.5 to the second and all subsequent people aged over 14, and 0.3 to each child aged under 14); and c) the final result, the equivalent disposable income, is assigned equally to each member of the household (adults and children).

This chart is based on *aggregate* data on a macro level. It shows the position occupied by Luxembourg within the European rankings, and the wide variety of national situations within the EU. But what are the specific risk factors for deprivation in the EU and Luxembourg? In order to better understand these factors at household level and institutional level, the following sections continue this analysis at the *individual (child)* level, using econometric analysis to highlight which household/ parent characteristics play a significant role in explaining child deprivation.

3   Child deprivation drivers in EU countries and Luxembourg

This section presents the conceptual framework of Guio et al. (2020), who used various models to analyse risk factors for child deprivation in the EU.

From a theoretical perspective, the authors identified three sets of factors that could explain the probability and/or intensity of child deprivation[6] as shown in Diagram 1:

1) the longer-term command over resources;
2) the needs and costs;
3) the size and composition of the household.

The relationships between these different types of determinants are also set out in Diagram 1.

First of all, the authors explain that children's material well-being depends on how much the household is able to consume, which, in turn, depends on its **'longer-term command over resources'**[7].

Although current (disposable) household income as measured by the survey is usually used as a proxy for 'command over resources', this is only one element in a household's resources, which are also affected by its previous, current and future income, its wealth and its ability to borrow. However, these elements are difficult to collect and are not available in the EU-SILC survey. There are variables that offer a way to approximate them: level of education, position on the labour market, and migration background. These factors act as follows:

---

[5] For a review of the determinants of material deprivation, see Perry, 2002; Bárcena-Martin et al. 2014, 2017 and 2018; Boarini and Mira d'Ercole 2006.
[7] See also Fusco et al. 2011 for a similar frame of reference.

- Level of education offers a more enviable position on the labour market and relatively easy access to credit institutions to overcome potential liquidity problems. Level of education is also an indicator of future income (especially for young people) according to investment in human capital. In the same way that highly qualified individuals are often the offspring of highly qualified individuals, we can also presume that they often benefit from larger inheritances, which will contribute to their wealth.
- *Ceteris paribus,* a non-EU migration background often correlates with a more vulnerable position on the labour market, a smaller inheritance, and less easy access to credit institutions.
- Similarly, joblessness within the household is a probable indicator of a precarious position on the labour market for working-age members of the household, which is a predictor of future risk of unemployment and can also hinder access to credit institutions in order to overcome liquidity problems. If joblessness is due to long-term unemployment, it can also result in the household's wealth and savings being eroded and ultimately lead to debt.

Furthermore, available resources are affected by social transfers in cash (which are included in the available income variable used). However, the type and design of social transfers can also be important for combating child deprivation. For similar aggregate transfers between two countries, we can assume that the country that best targets its transfers towards the poorest and where replacement transfers are the most appropriately used will be the most effective at combating child deprivation.

Secondly, the authors argue that deprivation is also affected by **costs and needs;** households with the same resources may have different needs and may be facing different costs. Needs in particular depend on the health of the people in the household, home ownership, housing costs and cost of public services such as education or childcare. The link between health and deprivation has been widely documented (see for example Marsh et al. 2000).

The third set of explanatory factors mentioned above (**size and composition of household**) affects the level of resources, the probability of joblessness, and the costs faced by the household. For example, single-parent households are more economically vulnerable (because they have a reduced ability to pool the risk of unemployment between multiple adults in the household). Single parents also find it harder to reconcile their professional and family life, and are therefore more likely to opt for part-time work or no work. In terms of needs/costs, they are facing fixed costs (housing, education, etc.) that generally represent a higher proportion of their resources than would be the case in households with multiple adults.

Furthermore, similar levels of resources and needs do not necessarily imply similar levels of deprivation. **Individual preferences** also play a role and affect consumption (it could be argued that to a certain extent, preferences are shaped by the level of resources, education, cultural context, etc.).

Diagram 1 also shows that certain relationships go both ways. For example, it can be assumed that there are interactions between parents' level of education, professional status and cultural context on the one hand, and the size and composition of the household on the other. Health affects employment and wage level, and is affected by the general level of resources.

Applying this model to the available data, it is difficult to analyse the impact of each determinant given the lack of information for certain variables. The variables in green in Diagram 1 are available at individual (child) level in the data sample. Some important factors affecting both the household's command over resources and its costs are not available: for example, in-kind support provided by family/friends or a direct measurement of inheritance. Data in this field is limited to the national total for this social spending in-kind (the volume received by each household is ignored in the sample). In Diagram 1, the variables shown in red are available at macro level. Those in black are not available at all.

Diagram 1 does not include one element that can affect econometric results: the difficulty of measuring income and deprivation (and potentially other explanatory variables) equally well. For example, it is difficult to measure income from self-employment or capital. Similarly, it is not always easy to collect reliable information on child deprivation due to parents' potentially feeling ashamed to admit that their children are deprived of essential items. As for people living in long-term poverty, it is known that preferences can be adaptive (such people may lower their expectations and claim that they do not need an item that they cannot afford to purchase). Some of these difficulties are incorporated into the empirical model.

4 What Factors Cause Deprivation in Luxembourg?

4.1 Econometric Strategy

To evaluate the *specific risks of deprivation* in Luxembourg, we have chosen an econometric model designed to test the relationships highlighted in Diagram 1 by grouping together Luxembourg, Belgium and the Netherlands. This enables us to shed new light on whether determinants in Luxembourg are different from the other two countries. The dependant variable varies from 0 to 17 (deprivation

Table 2 Results of negative binomial model, Luxembourg, Belgium and the Netherlands, 2014

	Coef	Impact	Different in Luxembourg?	Different in the Netherlands?
Self-employment (reference: no member of household self-employed)	−0.3***	Mitigating	No	No
Income	−0.1***	Mitigating	Yes, more mitigating	Yes, less mitigating
Jobless household (ref: with job)	0.4***	Aggravating	No	Yes, less aggravating
Single parent (ref: other households with children)	0.2***	Aggravating	Yes, more aggravating	No
Primary, lower secondary education (ref: tertiary education)	0.7***	Aggravating	Yes, less aggravating	No
Upper secondary education (ref: tertiary education)	0.5***	Aggravating	Yes, less aggravating	Yes, less aggravating
Very heavy housing burden (ref: light burden)	16.8***	Aggravating	No	No
Slightly heavy housing burden (ref: light burden)	1.0***	Aggravating	No	No
Number of children	0.0	No	No	No
Non-EU migrant (ref: Lux or EU)	0.2***	Aggravating	No	No
Renting (ref: owners or free housing)	0.7***	Aggravating	No	No
Heavy debt burden (ref: light debt burden)	0.4***	Aggravating	No	Yes, more aggravating

NB: ***Coefficient significantly different from zero, Significant at *1 %* level. *Reading note:* Children living in single parent households are at a greater risk of deprivation than others, this risk is higher in Luxembourg than in the other two countries. *Source:* EU-SILC 2014 cross-sectional data, author's computation.

items) and has a high level of over-dispersion, a variance that is higher than average. Using a negative binomial model is therefore recommended. By grouping together data from Luxembourg, Belgium and the Netherlands, we are able to perform tests to estimate if the impact of each variable differs between the different countries.

4.2   Results

Table 2 presents the results of the (negative binomial) model, explaining the *number* of deprivations experienced by a child based on the characteristics of the household in which they live. Essentially, a model of this type helps enable an understanding of *each* characteristic's impact on the number of deprivations suffered by a child, once the impact of other characteristics has been taken into account (in other words, 'all other things being equal'). Traditionally, the impact of each characteristic is measured by comparing the difference in deprivation risk between a group suffering from a risk factor (e.g. those living in a jobless household) and a reference group (e.g. those living in a household with employment). The results shown in the first column demonstrate the impact of these explanatory factors for the three countries. We then test the differences between Luxembourg and the other two countries (second column) or between the Netherlands and the other two countries (third column).

The results confirm the impact of variables linked to 'longer-term command over resources' and to 'household needs', as implied in Diagram 1. In particular, they show that:

Household income has a significant impact on child deprivation in the three countries, but this impact is even higher in Luxembourg. Living in a (quasi-) jobless household increases child deprivation, even if income is already taken into account by the model. However, living in a jobless household in the Netherlands increases deprivation by a smaller amount than in the other two countries. Parents' level of education also has a significant impact on the intensity of child deprivation, even once other household characteristics are taken into account. People with lower qualifications are more likely to suffer deprivation than those with higher levels of education. Nevertheless, this negative impact is less pronounced in Luxembourg (and in the Netherlands for the intermediate category), which is doubtless due to the fact that there are more employment opportunities for less skilled people than in Belgium, where unemployment levels are very high. For similar income level, households with one or more self-employed members tend to suffer from fewer deprivations. As explained above,

Table 3 Deprivation rate for all children compared with those living in a single-parent household (in %), and risk ratio, Population of children aged 1 to 15, EU countries covered by EU-SILC, 2014

Country	All children	Single parent	Risk ratio
IT	27	30	1.1
BG	68	82	1.2
RO	70	89	1.3
ES	29	36	1.3
PT	36	48	1.3
EL	46	64	1.4
LV	38	56	1.5
HU	47	77	1.6
EE	14	24	1.6
HR	21	36	1.7
CY	38	66	1.8
LT	27	49	1.8
DK	7	13	1.9
SK	25	49	1.9
IE	27	52	2.0
PL	23	46	2.0
UK	22	44	2.0
SI	10	21	2.1
FR	14	30	2.1
CZ	17	36	2.1
DE	11	26	2.3
AT	14	32	2.3
FI	6	14	2.4
MT	22	54	2.5
SE	4	11	2.5
BE	15	38	2.5
NL	13	33	2.6
LU	8	30	3.5

NB: For a list of country abbreviations, see Appendix 1. Source Own computations using cross-sectional data from the EU-SILC 2014 study

this may be partly due to the difficulty of correctly measuring income from self-employment in surveys such as EU-SILC, or of drawing a distinction between personal and professional assets and costs for the self-employed.

Variables relating to debt or housing costs prove to be important predictors of child deprivation. Renters are at a greater risk of deprivation than homeowners, even when other variables are taken into account. Non-EU migrants are at risk of greater deprivation than native or EU migrants, once other characteristics are taken into account.

Finally, living in a single-parent household significantly increases child deprivation, even once other differences are accounted for. Living alone with children is a risk factor in itself. As explained above, this may be due to higher fixed costs (housing, education, childcare etc.) that generally represent a higher proportion of the household's resources than would be the case in households with multiple adults. Where income levels are comparable, single-parent households can also suffer from greater income volatility (because they do not have the income of another adult to rely on). It should be noted that this risk is even higher in Luxembourg. Table 3 illustrates the extent to which single-parent households are at a very high relative disadvantage in Luxembourg. This table presents the child deprivation rates in all European countries, both for the total child population and for those living with a single parent. The ratio between these two figures is then calculated. A ratio above 1 means a higher risk for single-parent households. This table shows that Luxembourg is the European champion, with the deprivation risk three times higher for children living with a single parent than it is for children as a whole.

5   Conclusions

What conclusions can be drawn from this analysis in order to understand child deprivation in Luxembourg? Our analysis has shown that children in Luxembourg are better protected from deprivation than those in neighbouring countries. Nevertheless, this good performance on a national level hides some disparities among children living in Luxembourg. Those living with a single parent are particularly at risk: nearly a third of such children suffer from deprivation in their daily lives, 3.5 times higher than for the general population of children.

There are also other factors affecting the risk of deprivation. The most powerful predictors are housing costs, household income, household joblessness, and parents' level of education. However, our results also clearly show that the explanatory power of the different variables affecting households differs from one country to another, even between neighbouring countries such as Belgium, Luxembourg or the Netherlands. This means that countries differ in terms of how each variable relates to the risk of child deprivation, in other words that household income, unemployment, the burden of single parenthood, housing costs, and debt level have a different impact on child deprivation in each country.

This could be due to differences that are not measured in the data, such as in-kind transfers or the quality and cost of public services (education, childcare, public transport, etc.). These elements can substantially increase permanent income and/or reduce household needs and the related costs in countries where they are provided for free or at low cost.

These analyses show that it is important to measure child-specific deprivation and to understand its determinants in order to remedy them by putting in place appropriate public measures. Every child growing up in a situation of deprivation has a higher probability of suffering from poverty in adulthood. This is therefore an acute problem right now, with repercussions for the future. In Luxembourg, our study shows the importance and urgency of remedying the heightened risk and difficulties experienced by single-parent households, households in debt, and those facing high housing costs.

Appendix 1 List of country abbreviations

BE Belgium	LT Lithuania
BG Bulgaria	LU Luxembourg
CZ Czechia	HU Hungary
DK Denmark	MT Malta
DE Germany	NL Netherlands
EE Estonia	AT Austria
IE Ireland	PL Poland
EL Greece	PT Portugal
ES Spain	RO Romania
FR France	SI Slovenia
HR Croatia	SK Slovakia
IT Italy	FI Finland
CY Cyprus	SE Sweden
LV Latvia	

References

Bárcena-Martín, E., Lacomba, B., Moro-Egido, A. I. & Pérez-Moreno, S. (2014). Country Differences in Material Deprivation in Europe. *Review of Income and Wealth*, 60(4), 802-820.

Bárcena-Martín, E., Blasquez, M., Budria, S. & Moro-Egido, A. (2017). Child deprivation and social benefits: Europe in cross-national perspective. *Socio-Economic Review*, 15(4), 717-744.

Bárcena-Martin, E., Blanco-Arana, M. C. & Perez-Moreno, S. (2018). Social Transfers and Child Poverty in European Countries: Pro-poor Targeting or Pro-child Targeting?. *Journal of Social Policy*, 47(4), 739–758.

Bellani, L. and Bia, M. (2017), 'The impact of growing up poor in Europe'. In: AAtkinson, A. B., Guio, A.-C. & Marlier, E. (Eds.). Monitoring Social Inclusion in Europe. Luxembourg: Eurostat.

Boarini, R. and d'Ercole, M. M. (2006). Measures of material deprivation in OECD countries. In: *Social, Employment and Migration Working Papers*, No. 37. Paris: OECD.

Dermott, E. and Pomati, M. (2016). The parenting and economising practices of lone parents: Policy and evidence. *Critical Social Policy*, 2016, 36(1): 62–81.

European Commission (2013), *Investing in Children: breaking the cycle of disadvantage*, Commission Recommendation 2013/112/EU. Brussels: European Commission

Fusco, A. Guio, A.-C. & Marlier, E. (2011). Characterising the income poor and the materially deprived in European countries. In: Atkinson, A.B. and Marlier, E. (Eds.). *Income and living conditions in Europe*. Luxembourg: Publications Office of the European Union, pp. 132-153.

Gordon, D. and Nandy, S. (2012). Measuring child poverty and deprivation. In: Minujin, A. and Nandy, S. (Eds.). Global child poverty and well-being: Measurement, concepts, policy and action. Bristol: Policy Press, pp. 57–101.

Gregg, P., Harkness, S. & Machin, S. (1999). Child Poverty and its Consequences. Joseph Rowntree Foundation.

Guio, A-C., Gordon, D. & Marlier, E. (2012). Measuring Material Deprivation in the EU. Indicators for the whole Population and Child-Specific Indicators. *Eurostat Methodologies and working papers*. Luxembourg: Publications Office of the European Union.

Guio, A. C., Gordon, D., Marlier, E., Najera, H. & Pomati, M. (2018). Towards an EU measure of child deprivation. *Child indicators research*, 11(3), 835-860.

Guio, A.-C. and Vandenbroucke, F. (2018). La pauvreté et la déprivation des enfants en Belgique. Comparaison des facteurs de risque dans les trois Régions et les pays voisin. *Fondation Roi Baudouin*.

Guio, A.-C., Marlier, E., Vanderbroucke, F. & Verbunt, P. (2020). Micro- and macro-drivers of child deprivation in 31 European countries. *Eurostat Statistical Working Papers*. Luxembourg: Publications Office of the European Union.

Main, G. and Besemer, K. (2013). Children's material living standards in rich countries. In: Ben-Arieh, A., Casas, F., Frones, I. & Korbin, J. (Eds.). Handbook of child well-being. New York: Springer.

Main, G. and Bradshaw, J. (2016). Child poverty in the UK: Measures, prevalence and intra-household sharing. *Critical Social Policy*, 2016, 36(1), 1–24.

Marsh, A., Gordon, D., Pantazis, C. & Heslop, P. (2000). Housing deprivation and health: A longitudinal analysis. *Housing Studies*, 15(3), 411–428.

Pascoe, J. M., Wood, D. L., Duffee, J. H. & Kuo, A. (2016). 'Mediators and adverse effects of child poverty in the United States'. Paediatrics, April 2016, 137 (4).

Perry, B. (2002). The mismatch between income measures and direct outcome measures of poverty. *Social Policy Journal of New Zealand*, 19, 101–127.

Repka, M. (2013). 'Enduring damage: the effects of childhood poverty on adult health'. *Chicago Policy Review* (27 November 2013).

Ridge, T. (2002) Childhood poverty and social exclusion: From a child's perspective. Bristol: The Policy Press.

Ridge, T. (2011). The everyday costs of poverty in childhood: A review of qualitative research exploring the lives and experiences of low-income children in the UK. *Children and Society*, 25(1), 73–84.

Townsend, P. (1979). Poverty in the United Kingdom. Hardmonsworth: Penguin Books.

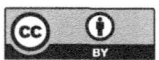

Academic Achievement and Subjective Well-being: A Representative Cross-sectional Study

Rachel Wollschläger, Pascale Esch, Ulrich Keller, Antoine Fischbach und Ineke M. Pit-ten Cate

1 Introduction

Beyond cognitive outcomes, such as academic achievement, that have traditionally been used to evaluate learning objectives and the quality of an educational system, non-cognitive outcomes, such as student well-being, should be considered as a specific, distinctive and yet complementary aim of education (Hascher et al. 2018; Opdenakker and Van Damme 2000). Benjamin Bloom in the mid-70 s already emphasized the importance of student well-being in regards to educational success (Bloom 1976), yet the concept has only been considered by educational policies in recent years. Such policies recognize the (reciprocal) relationship between student well-being and academic achievement, whereby

R. Wollschläger (✉) · P. Esch · U. Keller · A. Fischbach · I. M. Pit-ten Cate
Luxembourg Centre for Educational Testing I LUCET, University of Luxembourg, Esch-sur-Alzette, Luxembourg
E-Mail: rachel.wollschlaeger@uni.lu

P. Esch
E-Mail: pascale.esch@uni.lu

U. Keller
E-Mail: ulrich.keller@uni.lu

A. Fischbach
E-Mail: antoine.fischbach@uni.lu

I. M. Pit-ten Cate
E-Mail: ineke.pit@uni.lu

© Der/die Autor(en) 2022
A. Heinen et al. (Hrsg.), *Wohlbefinden und Gesundheit im Jugendalter,*
https://doi.org/10.1007/978-3-658-35744-3_10

student well-being has been considered both as an indicator of the quality of the educational system and as an outcome. Notable endeavours to integrate student well-being as an indicator of quality in education were launched by the United Nations Educational, Scientific and Cultural Organization (UNESCO) Happy Schools Project in 2014. This international project focuses on the need for education systems to go beyond strictly academic outcomes by providing a framework of definition and strategies to foster and measure well-being in the school context (UNESCO 2016)[1]. In the same spirit, the Organization for Economic Co-operation and Development (OECD) first introduced the concept of student well-being in their Programme for International Student Assessment (PISA) in 2015. More specifically, PISA 2015 included a comprehensive set of well-being indicators that covered both negative factors (e.g., anxiety, low performance) and positive impulses (e.g., interest, engagement, motivation to achieve) that promote educational success (OECD 2017). At the national level, the Luxembourg School Monitoring Programme Épreuves Standardisées (Martin et al. 2015) consists of written (partly computer-based) tests and questionnaires. ÉpStan combines cognitive outcomes (i.e., a standardized record of competences in key school areas) and non-cognitive aspects, such as social inclusion, anxiety, motivation to learn as well as school and class climate for Grades 1, 3, 5, 7 and 9. Although the ÉpStan mainly aims to monitor the quality of the Luxembourgish educational system, data can be used to investigate relationships between the measured cognitive and non-cognitive outcome variables.

2 Theoretical Background

2.1 Subjective Well-being in School

In educational research, subjective well-being (SWB) has gained increasing interest as specific research has advanced the importance of emotional and affective factors when it comes to achieving learning objectives (Hascher et al. 2018; Pekrun 2005). According to Hascher (2008), who focused her research on SWB in the specific context of school, SWB can be considered an enhancer of academic achievement as it fosters the fulfilment of academic and social goals

---

[1]A national counterpart of the Happy Schools Project is "CARAT", which focuses on the school climate and was launched in 2014 by the division of pedagogical innovation within the ministry of education (Niles et al. 2016).

in positively experienced learning environments. As a consequence of growing interest, a challenge in addressing SWB in educational research occurs from the diversity or imprecision of related definitions and methods (Bücker et al. 2018; Hascher and Edlinger 2009). However, despite the heterogeneity of conceptual frameworks to model SWB, there is growing consensus that SWB is a complex, multi-dimensional phenomenon which combines affective and cognitive facets. The emotional dimension reflects the presence of positive feelings such as satisfaction and pleasure and the absence of negative feelings such as anxiety. The social dimension includes relationships with teachers and peers and class climate, whereas the cognitive dimension refers to academic self-concept and attitudes towards school (Bücker et al. 2018; Diener 1984; Hascher and Edlinger 2009). These three dimensions are also reflected in conceptions of perceived inclusion (Venetz et al. 2014).

In his theory of wellbeing, Seligman (2011) conceives wellbeing as a construct composed of five components: positive emotion, engagement, relationships, meaning and accomplishment. The so-called Positive Emotion, Engagement, Relationships, Meaning, and Accomplishment (PERMA) model puts a strong focus on the inclusion of both hedonic (i.e., living a life of pleasure) and eudaimonic (i.e., living a purposeful life) components. In comparison, Hascher and colleagues (Hascher 2004; Hascher and Hagenauer 2011; Hascher and Lobsang 2004) proposed a multidimensional model of SWB representing a state of feeling induced by a combination of predominantly positive emotions and cognitions towards school and learning objectives as well as towards teacher – and peer relationships. Their model advances a stronger focus on hedonic components by including positive attitudes towards school, feelings of pleasure or happiness when in school as well as the extent of anxiety related to achievement. In comparison to the PERMA model, the conceptual framework of Hascher may be more appropriate to model SWB in preadolescent children, as preadolescents tend to be more responsive and thus more aware of hedonic aspects when self-evaluating their wellbeing. Eudaimonic aspects of SWB would require capacities of abstract reasoning and metacognition which start around age 8 and progress through adolescence reaching maturity in early adulthood (Rosso et al. 2004). Thus, concepts relating to human flourishing, purpose and community engagement may be more poorly understood by preadolescent children (Ravens-Sieberer et al. 2014).

2.2   Academic Achievement in the Luxembourgish Education System

In Luxembourg, school attendance is compulsory for students aged four to sixteen years (for a detailed description of the Luxembourgish school system, see Lenz and Heinz 2018). Primary education consists of four learning cycles, with each cycle lasting two years (i.e., students attend primary school for a minimum of six and a maximum of eight years). If learning objectives have not been reached within the 2-year period, an extension of a learning cycle is a common intervention to cope with academic failure or developmental immaturity. By the end of primary education, 20.5 % of students have at some stage been retained in a learning cycle (MENJE 2018). From the age of 12 years, students enter secondary level, education, which is hierarchically structured in three levels: Enseignement secondaire classique (ESC), Enseignement secondaire général (ESG) and Enseignement secondaire général – voie de preparation (ESG-P). Successful completion of the highest academic track (ESC; seven school years), will give the student access to university. Within the middle track (ESG) there are options to complete a technical stream (eight school years), which prepares the student for the technical baccalaureate; a technician's stream (seven school years) that prepares the students for the technician certificate; and a vocational stream (six school years), which prepares students for a professional qualification. The technical and technician streams will provide access to higher education, whilst completion of the vocational stream allows direct access to professional life. Passage through the lowest track (ESG-P, three school years) is integrated in the ESG and designed for students who experience significant educational difficulties. The preparatory system will allow these students to attend classes in the lower levels of the ESG or to enter the vocational stream (Lenz and Heinz 2018).

In secondary education, grade retention varies with school tracks (Klapproth and Schaltz 2015; MENJE 2018). In the school year 2016/2017, 16.9 % of students within the ESC had repeated at least one grade, whereas within the ESG track 62.4 % of the students had fallen behind (MENJE 2018). Grade repetitions seem relatively common for students within the ESG track, but may be most pronounced for students in ESG-P track (Klapproth and Schaltz 2015). Considering these figures, grade retention is a more common practice in Luxembourg in comparison to other European countries (Eurydice 2011) and can be considered a salient indicator of academic achievement. However, there is consistent empirical evidence that grade retention does not provide positive outcomes in the mid- and long-term, but rather has a negative and even harmful effect on several school-related behaviours such as psychosocial adjustment (Hattie 2009; Holmes 1989; Jimerson 2001). Retained students are reported to skip more classes and show more negative attitudes toward school in general than their promoted peers. Furthermore, retained students were reported to be more likely to drop out of school (Jimerson 1999; Roderick 1994).

2.3 Luxembourg School Monitoring Programme: Épreuves Standardisées

The Luxembourg School Monitoring Programme Épreuves Standardisées (ÉpStan) assess students' academic competencies, learning motivation and attitudes towards school at the beginning of each learning cycle of compulsory education (i.e., at the beginning of grade levels 1, 3, 5, 7 and 9). Thus, in primary school, the ÉpStan are administered three times (in the first term of cycles 2, 3 and 4 or Grade 1, 3 and 5 respectively) and twice in secondary school (i.e., in Grade 7 and 9). The tests are developed in accordance with the Luxembourgish curriculum by experienced elementary and secondary school teachers under the methodological guidance of scientific staff from the Luxembourgish Centre for Educational Testing (LUCET). In the frame of ÉpStan all students enrolled in public schools following the national curriculum take part, meaning that the ÉpStan are not conducted in private schools or public international schools. The ÉpStan aims at evaluating students' academic achievement against predefined competence standards and as such assess if educational goals from the previous learning cycles have been met. The tests are developed in accordance with the Luxembourgish curriculum by experienced elementary and secondary school teachers under the methodological guidance of scientific staff from the Luxembourgish Centre for Educational Testing (LUCET) (further details may be found on www.epstan.lu). In the grades of interest in the current research, namely Grades 5 and 9, the educational goals defined for the previous learning cycles – cycle 3 for Grade 5 and school years 7 and 8 for Grade 9 – are tested to see whether and to what extent they have been achieved in three areas of competence: German reading comprehension, French reading comprehension and mathematics (Martin et al. 2015).

2.4   Relationship Between Subjective Well-being and Academic Achievement

Results of experimental mood-induction research indicate that positive and negative mood significantly affects how much interest children show for a given task and how they rate the level of difficulty as well as the expected effort they need to apply to solve the task (Edlinger and Hascher 2008; Pekrun 2005). Consequently, academic achievement can be affected by these variables with a potentially different impact at distinct stages of development. A longitudinal study by Gutman und Vorhaus (2012) identified small to medium correlations between dimensions of well-being (emotional, behavioural, social and school well-being) and concurrent and future academic achievement in a cohort of children followed from age 7 to age 13. For example, the authors reported that emotional well-being was predictive of academic achievement in younger children, whereas in secondary education no significant association was found (Gutman and Vorhaus 2012). Kirkcaldy and colleagues (2004) focused on secondary education and explored data issued from 30 countries. They identified a significantly positive association between SWB and PISA competence scores with the strongest correlation being reported for reading literacy ($r = 0.63$).

Considering the reported diversity of definitions and methods when exploring SWB in school, conclusions about the magnitude of the relationship between SWB and academic achievement are mixed. A recent meta-analysis targeted this issue and synthesized 151 effect sizes from 47 studies including 38.946 participants (Bücker et al. 2018). Results indicated a statistically significant small mean effect size (average $r = 0.16$, 95 % CI [0.11, 0.23]), thus confirming the impact of socio-emotional factors on academic achievement. The correlation was stable across various levels of demographic variables (age, gender, country and level of education), different domains of SWB (e.g., academic vs. life in general), different components of SWB (emotional vs. cognitive well-being) as well as alternative measures of academic achievement or SWB. Even though these findings appear robust, the authors concluded that future research should aim to further explore the impact of different dimensions of SWB and to include other potentially relevant moderator variables such as ability level, socioeconomic status and migration background. Furthermore, most of the included studies had focused on secondary and tertiary education, with only 3 % of effect sizes coming from primary school. Considering these limitations and recommendations, the present contribution aims to investigate the relationship between SWB and academic achievement in relation to demographic characteristics, educational level and pathways.

3   Research Question

This contribution investigated the relationship between four distinct dimensions of subjective well-being in school and standardized competence test scores at two different time-points of compulsory education (i.e., Grade 5 – primary education and Grade 9 – secondary education). Grades 5 and 9 were chosen based on the assumption that in these grades, students had been taught in relatively stable class compositions within the same educational setting for at least two years. Additionally, based on developmental perspectives and empirical evidence, we assumed self-perceptions of students in Grade 5 would be more reliable and stable than in earlier grades (Guay et al. 2003; Marsh 1989). Targeted dimensions of SWB included academic self-concept, school anxiety, social inclusion, and emotional inclusion. General academic self-concept and school anxiety have been identified as key components of school related affect and motivation (Gogol et al. 2017), whereas social and emotional inclusion reflect the extent to which students feel accepted and embedded in their classes and school (Venetz et al. 2014). The research aims of the study are twofold:

1. The first aim concerns the levels of SWB in relation to the specificities of the Luxembourgish school system with a high rate of grade retention (Eurydice 2011) and a strongly segmented secondary school system (MENJE 2020). More specifically, the following questions will be addressed:
   - *To what extent do the four dimensions of SWB differ as a function of grade (Grade 5 vs. Grade 9)?*
   - *To what extent does SWB vary between students who did or did not experience grade retention?*
   - *For Grade 9, to what extent does SWB differ between students the different secondary school tracks (ESC vs. ESG vs. ESG-P)?*
2. The second aim of the study concerns the relationship between SWB and academic achievement. In this context the following questions will be addressed:
   - *To what extent do the four dimensions of SWB predict academic achievement after controlling for students' sociodemographic characteristics (gender, migration background socioeconomic status)?*

Both research questions consider the relationship between academic achievement and SWB. For research question 1, we consider indirect measures of academic achievement (i.e., grade retention and school tracking), whereas for research question 2, we used actual student performance. Based on research indicating a positive association between academic achievement and SWB (for a review see Bücker et al. 2018), we expected that students that experienced grade retention would report lower levels of SWB, especially in the domain of academic self-concept and school anxiety, than students that did not experience grade retention. Similarly, we expected the SWB of Grade 9 students to be associated with school track, whereby students in the higher tracks would report higher levels of SWB than students in lower tracks.

4   Methods

4.1   Sample

Data was retrieved from the Luxembourgish School Monitoring Programme (Martin et al. 2015) in November 2018, which comprised of an entire cohort of 5th and 9th graders. More specifically, 5159 Grade 5 students and 6279 Grade 9 students were assessed. It is important to note, that this data is of cross-sectional nature (i.e., students in Grade 5 are not the same as in Grade 9). In Grade 9, 28.5 % of the students attended the highest academic track (ESC), 61.6 % attended the intermediary track (ESG), and 9.9 % attended the lowest track (ESG-P). See Table 1 for additional sample characteristics.

For both grades, we identified the group of students that were on regular or advanced paths within the school system and the group of students that was delayed (i.e., students with irregular pathways who experienced grade retention). The student's birth year was used as a proxy for educational path. More specifically, students attending Grade 5, who were born in 2008, were considered to be on regular or advanced pathways, whereas students born in or before 2006 were classified as on irregular pathways. For students born in

Table 1 Sample characteristics by grade for ÉpStan 2018 (own illustration)

	Female	Migration Background	Age		HISEI*
			min–max	M (SD)	M (SD)
Grade 5	49.6 %	55.3 %	9–13	10.61 (0.69)	47.92 (16.46)
Grade 9	48.0 %	56.9 %	13–18	14.99 (0.97)	43.87 (17.31)

Note. *Highest International Socio-Economic Index of Occupational Status (Ganzeboom 2010; Ganzeboom and Treiman 1996)

2007, no classification was applied as the dataset only included birth year, which did not allow us to determine if the student was delayed (when born before September 2007) or on a regular path (when born on or after September 1st, 2007). This procedure resulted in the identification of 521 (10 %) Grade 5 students on irregular pathways, with at least one year of grade retention, 2541 students (49 %) on regular or advanced pathways, and 2097 students unclassified (i.e., born in 2007; 41 %). A similar approach was followed for Grade 9, whereby 1637 students (26 %) were identified to be on irregular pathways, with up to three grade retentions, 2223 students (35 %) on regular pathways and 2419 students unclassified (39 %).

4.2 Instruments

4.2.1 Subjective Well-Being
Four indicators of subjective well-being were used (i.e., general academic self-concept, school anxiety, social- and emotional inclusion). Given the extent of the ÉpStan assessment, long forms of scales cannot be considered and hence all constructs were measured on single item scales (for an empirical foundation see Gogol et al. 2014). General academic self-concept, reflecting students' mental representation of their academic abilities (Brunner et al. 2010) was measured with the item: "I am good at most school subjects". To measure experiences of anxiety across school subjects, the item "I am afraid of most school subjects" was used (Gogol et al. 2017). Emotional and social inclusion were measured on the items "I like going to school", and "In my class, we get along well", respectively. Students rated all questions on a 4-point Likert scale ranging from 1 "not at all true" to 4 "certainly true", whereby we used a visual scale in Grade 5 and a verbal scale in Grade 9. Missing responses on these items were recorded for between 2 and 3 % of students in Grade 5, and between 1 and 5 % in Grade 9.

4.2.2 Achievement
The ÉpStan was used to assess students' academic competencies, learning motivation and attitudes towards school. For both Grade 5 and Grade 9, French reading comprehension, German reading comprehension as well as mathematics are assessed. Language tests comprise continuous (i.e., literary or factual texts) and discontinuous text forms (i.e., tables, illustrations or assembly instructions) and focus on the sub-skills of identifying and understanding information presented in a text as well as analyzing texts. The Mathematical tests comprises tasks, which are presented in a decontextualized and/or contextualized way

and designed to be as language free as possible. In Grade 9 three different test versions with different difficulty levels are available depending on the academic track students are enrolled in. Tests in different tracks were equated using common items and Rasch parameters were jointly estimated for all tracks. This means that test scores from students in different tracks are on the same scale and can be compared directly even though they completed partially different tests (Martin et al. 2015).

4.2.3 Student Background Variables

Within the ÉpStan assessment, students (in Grades 5 and 9) and parents (only in Grade 5) were asked to complete a questionnaire concerning the students' socioeconomic family background among other variables. The parental occupational status is defined by the International Socio-Economic Index of Occupational Status (Ganzeboom 2010; Ganzeboom and Treiman 1996). The values of this index vary from 10 to 89 (ISCO-08) or 16 to 90 (ISCO-88) and are based on information regarding the professional occupation of parents. The higher the value of these variables, the higher the socioeconomic status of the family. For each student, the occupation of either mother or father was used, whichever reflected the highest status. Regarding migration background, students whose parents were both born in a country other than Luxembourg were considered having a migration background, regardless of their own country of birth.

4.3   Data Preparation and Analysis

To compare students' subjective well-being across grades, educational paths (regular vs. irregular) and secondary school tracks (ESC vs. ESG vs. ESG-P), two mixed model analyses were conducted. This type of analysis allows for the comparison of means of different groups on multiple outcome variables at the same time (akin to a multivariate analysis of variance or MANOVA) while accounting for the fact that the observations of students belonging to the same class may not be independent in the statistical sense. Academic self-concept, school anxiety, social inclusion, and emotional inclusion were included as related dependent variables whereby we investigated mean differences based on grade and educational path (Model 1) or secondary school track (Model 2). To test for group differences in detail, we then employed multiple comparisons based on the estimated models. To address our second research question, investigating the relationship between SWB and school achievement, we first modelled a latent factor of academic achievement through confirmatory factor analyses (CFA) using the ÉpStan scores of the three competency tests (German and French reading comprehension, mathematical ability). Using this procedure, one achievement factor was detected explaining 65 % of the shared variance in Grade 5 (factor loadings ranging from 0.74–0.85) and 69 % in Grade 9 (factor loadings ranging from 0.80–0.85). We calculated factor scores that capture this common variance for each student and used these scores as the measure for academic achievement. For this variable, 3 % of students had missing data in Grade 5 vs. 8 % in Grade 9. The latter, comparatively high, number is explained by the fact that not all tests were administered to all students in all domains in Grade 9. We then used step-wise regression analyses, which is a statistical procedure that identifies the relationship between variables after controlling for others and allows for the estimation of one (criterion) variable based on different levels (or values) of the other (predictor) variables. More specifically, we used step-wise regression to predict academic achievement by academic self-concept, school anxiety, social inclusion, and emotional inclusion after controlling for student background variables (gender, parents' occupational status and migration background). As in the analyses discussed above, the lack of statistical independence resulting from the clustered data had to be considered. In this case, we corrected the standard errors estimated in the step-wise regression.

For all analyses we employed multiple imputation under a mixed model in order to deal with missing data. In this procedure, a statistical model is estimated that quantifies the relationships between all variables. Based on this model missing data points are filled in with "plausible" values – not once, but multiple times, creating multiple mostly identical datasets that differ only where previously data was missing. The analyses are then performed using each of these datasets and the results are combined in a way that considers the added insecurity introduced by the missing data.

The analyses described above were performed using R version 4.0.3 (R Core Team 2020) with the packages mitml (Grund et al. 2019), mitools (Lumley 2019), jomo (Quartagno and Carpenter 2020), lme4 (Bates et al. 2015), jtools (Long 2020), multcomp (Hothorn et al. 2008), emmeans (Lenth 2020), and survey (Lumley 2004).

5   Results

5.1   Differences in Subjective Well-being in Relation to Specificities in the School System

To test for differences in SWB in relation to grade and educational pathways, Grade (5 vs. 9) and educational pathway (regular vs. irregular) were entered as factors to compare the four dimensions of SWB. Mixed model results showed statistically significant differences in SWB based on grade, $F(8, 121,164) = 180.61$, $p < .001$, as well as educational pathway, $F(8, 63,989) = 17.75$, $p < .001$. The interaction of grade × path was significant as well, $F(7, 94,621) = 189.10$, $p < .001$ (see Table 2 for descriptive statistics). Post-hoc tests revealed significant main effects for grade on all dimensions of SWB (academic self-concept, $z = 17.50$, $p < .001$; school anxiety, $z = -16.90$, $p < .001$; social inclusion, $z = 7.60$, $p < .001$, and emotional inclusion: $z = 17.50$, $p < .001$). For all four dimensions, students in Grade 5 reported higher SWB than students in Grade 9. More specifically, students in Grade 5 reported significantly higher levels of perceived academic self-concept, social- and emotional inclusion and lower levels of school anxiety compared to students in Grade 9 (see Fig. 1).

Similarly, univariate results for educational pathway indicated significant differences for all dimensions of SWB. More specifically, students on regular pathways reported significantly higher levels of academic self-concept ($z = 7.30$, $p < .001$), as social inclusion ($z = 3.71$, $p = .001$), and emotional inclusion ($z = 2.54$, $p = .006$, and lower levels of school anxiety ($z = -6.97$, $p < .001$) compared to students that had repeated one or more grades (see Fig. 2).

In the second mixed model analysis, secondary school track (ESC vs. ESG vs. ESG-P) was entered as factor and the four dimensions of SWB as dependent variable. Results of this analysis, including students in Grade 9 only, showed that SWB varied as a function of school track, $F(2, 40,219) = 15.71$, $p < 0.001$ (see Table 2 for descriptive statistics). The interaction term between dimension and school track was significant, indicating that the school track effect was not uniform across SWB dimensions, $F(6, 14,339) = 34.29$, $p < .001$. Post hoc analyses (Tukey) revealed that perceived SWB decreased with school track. That is, for all four dimensions, students in ESC reported significantly higher levels of SWB compared to students in other tracks ($p = .001$ for all comparisons). Furthermore, students in ESG reported significantly higher levels of SWB compared to students in ESG-P (p ranging from < .001 to .019; see Fig. 3).

Table 2 Descriptive statistics for the dimensions of subjective well-being as a function of grade, educational pathway and school track (own illustration)

		Self-concept			Anxiety			Social Inclusion			Emotional Inclusion		
Model 1	N	Grade 5	Grade 9	Total	Grade 5	Grade 9	Total	Grade 5	Grade 9	Total	Grade 5	Grade 9	Total
		M (SD)	M (SD)	M (SD)	M (SD)	M (SD)	M (SD)	M (SD)	M (SD)	M (SD)	M (SD)	M (SD)	M (SD)
Regular Path	4596	3.44 (0.61)	2.99 (0.69)	3.23 (0.69)	1.32 (0.70)	1.80 (0.87)	1.54 (0.82)	3.31 (0.77)	3.14 (0.83)	3.23 (0.81)	3.19 (0.90)	2.77 (0.95)	3.00 (0.94)
Irregular Path	1997	3.25 (0.72)	2.82 (0.73)	2.93 (0.75)	1.52 (0.84)	1.95 (0.93)	1.84 (.93)	3.24 (0.86)	3.01 (0.86)	3.07 (0.86)	3.17 (0.96)	2.70 (1.00)	2.82 (1.01)
Total	6693	3.41 (0.63)	2.92 (0.71)	3.14 (0.72)	1.36 (0.73)	1.86 (0.90)	1.63 (0.87)	3.30 (0.79)	3.01 (0.84)	3.18 (0.83)	3.19 (0.91)	2.75 (0.97)	2.94 (0.97)
Model 2													
ESC	1734		3.00 (0.67)			1.72 (0.81)			3.23 (0.76)			2.88 (0.89)	
ESG	3643		2.89 (0.71)			1.89 (0.90)			3.05 (0.85)			2.69 (0.98)	
ESG-P	526		2.80 (0.06)			2.01 (1.02)			2.84 (0.99)			2.56 (1.00)	
Total	5903		2.91 (0.72)			1.85 (0.89)			3.09 (0.84)			2.74 (0.97)	

Note. Data in grey reflect non-significant differences between groups.

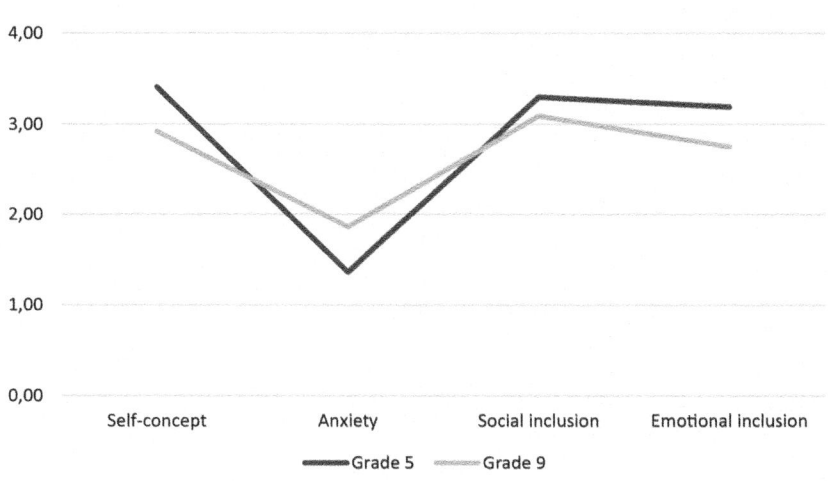

Fig. 1 Dimensions of SWB in relation to school grade (Grade 5 vs. Grade 9) (own illustration)

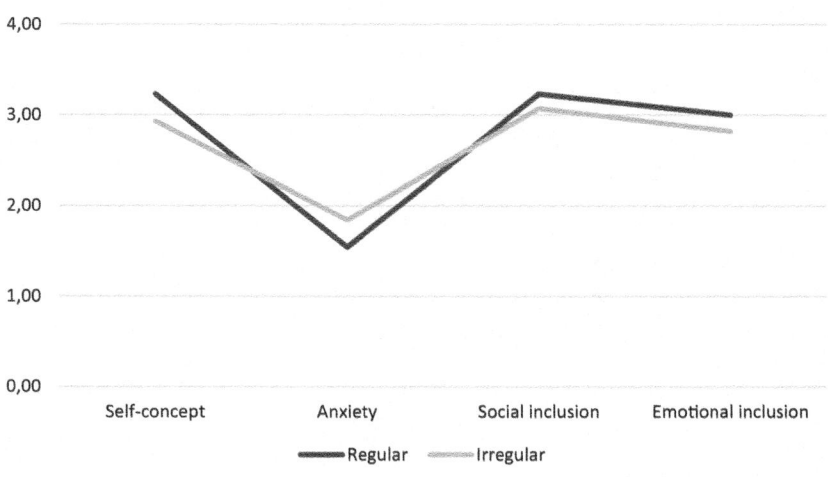

Fig. 2 Dimensions of SWB in relation to educational pathway (regular vs. irregular) (own illustration)

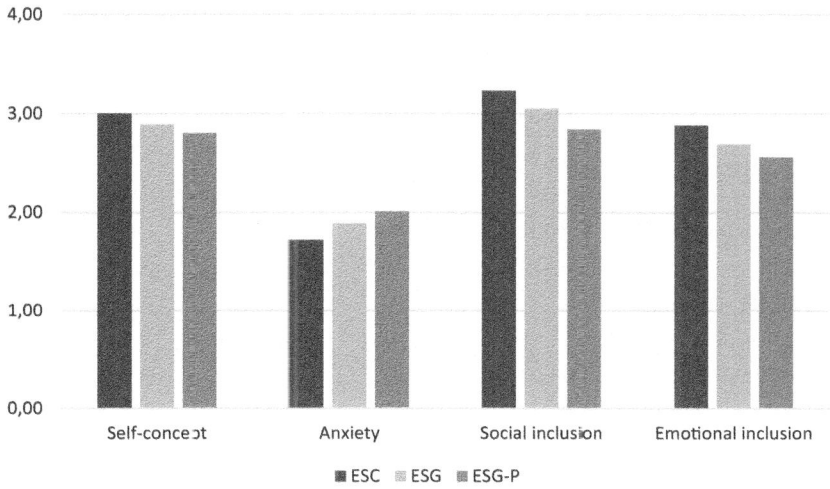

Fig. 3 Dimensions of SWB in relation to school track (ESC vs. ESG vs. ESG-P) (own illustration)

5.2   Predictive Value of Subjective Well-being

To test the relationship between SWB and academic achievement we conducted a step-wise regression analysis for each grade. In the first step, we entered demographic characteristics (i.e., gender, migration background and HISEI) as predictor variables (Model 1). In a second step, we added the four dimensions of SWB (Model 2). Results indicated that 14 % and 18 % of variance in academic achievement in Grade 5 and Grade 9 respectively, could be predicted by demographic characteristics. For both grades, the four dimensions of SWB explained a significant additional proportion of variance. In Grade 5, only the dimensions school anxiety and academic self-concept significantly contributed to the prediction, whereas in Grade 9 all four SWB dimension did (see Table 3).

Table 3 Results from predicting academic achievement through subjective well-being
(own illustration)

Variables	Grade 5 ($N = 4990$)		Grade 9 ($N = 5783$)	
	Model 1	Model 2	Model 1	Model 2
	β	β	β	β
Gender	0.08^{**}	0.10^{***}	0.07	0.08
Migration Background	-0.14^{***}	-0.07^{*}	-0.17^{***}	-0.15^{***}
HISEI	0.34^{***}	0.30^{***}	0.40^{***}	0.37^{***}
Academic self-concept		0.20^{***}		0.12^{***}
School anxiety		-0.10^{***}		-0.11^{***}
Social inclusion		0.01		0.04^{*}
Emotional inclusion		0.01		0.06^{***}

Note. For Grade 5, $R^2 = .13$ for Step 1 ($p < .001$); $\Delta R^2 = 0.06$ for Step 2 ($p < .001$);
For Grade 9, $R^2 = .19$ for Step 1 ($p < .001$); $\Delta R^2 = .04$ for Step 2 ($p < .001$); $^{*} p < .05$;
$^{**} p < .01$; $^{***} p < .001$

---

6   Discussion

This contribution aimed at investigating dimensions of subjective well-being in
relation to students' educational pathways and academic achievement. Drawing
on representative full cohort data from the Luxembourg School Monitoring
Programme "Épreuves Standardisées" 2018, results indicated subjective well-being
to be higher in Grade 5 than in Grade 9, to be lower when students experience
grade retention as well as in less prestigious secondary school tracks, and to predict
a significant amount of variance in academic achievement.

Grade 5 students reported significantly higher levels of perceived academic
self-concept, social- and emotional inclusion and lower levels of school anxiety
compared to Grade 9 students. These results are in line with the conclusions
by Hascher und Edlinger (2009), that SWB varies per school setting and that
initial positive feelings toward school may decrease over time (i.e., the longer
students are in the school system). In combination with the results of our
hierarchical regression analyses, which suggest the relationship between SWB
and achievement remains relatively constant between grades, the decrease of
SWB appears worrisome. The absence of the moderating effect of grade is in line
with the results of the meta-analysis of Bücker and colleagues (2018). However,
although the meta-analysis also failed to detect a moderating effect of SWB

dimensions, our results suggest differential effects of SWB dimensions between grades. Although in Grade 5, only academic self-concept and school anxiety were related to achievement, in Grade 9 all four dimensions of SWB significantly contributed to the explanation of variance in achievement. Hence, whilst SWB decreases with age, the impact of the different dimensions on achievement becomes more visible. It should be noted however, that in the meta-analysis, the vast majority of effect sizes came from secondary and higher education with (much) older students, with only a small percentage of studies conducted in primary. This may have resulted in a different comparative framework as in the current study.

Students, who experienced grade retention, reported lower academic self-concept and social inclusion, as well as higher school anxiety, replicating previous findings that demonstrated a rather negative effect of grade retention (Hattie 2009). In the present study, retained students gave lower ratings of social inclusion, indicating that they perceived the students within their class to get along less well than students on a regular pathway. As students may experience grade retention repeatedly (up to three years by Grade 9), social inclusion may become increasingly challenging given the widering of the age gap and associated differences in developmental maturity in relation to their peers (A. J. Martin 2009). Consequently, the current study contributes to the growing body of evidence showing an association between grade retention and SWB. In line with previous findings, our results indicate that lower achieving students may develop negative attitudes toward school (e.g., Gogol et al. 2017; Van Houtte 2006), which in turn may affect their school engagement and hence long term educational success (Jimerson and Ferguson 2007; A. J. Martin 2011; Roderick 1994).

Results further showed that for Grade 9 students perceived SWB decreases with school track. Students attending the more prestigious ESC track reported significantly higher levels of SWB compared to students in other tracks. Especially students registered with the preparatory scheme (ESG-P) may be vulnerable when it comes to academic and socio-emotional wellbeing as they provided significantly lower ratings for all four dimensions of SWB. In line with the conclusions by Belfi and colleagues (2012), who reported that ability-grouped classes had a positive impact on the school well-being of high-performing students, whereas the contrary was observed for weaker students, our results also imply that there is a cumulative (dis)advantage (i.e., high performance leads to more opportunities for future success and increased SWB, whereas lower performance relates to reduced opportunities and in turn less change of future success and decreased SWB). In line with prior (national) research on performance differences between academic tracks (see e.g., Keller et al. 2012, 2013), the present study thus provides further evidence for the presence of a so-called Matthew effect (Merton 1968) in the national secondary educational system.

7   Limitations and Implications

This research drew on cross-sectional data from large-scale assessment in 2018. Therefore, when comparing Grade 5 and Grade 9, it is important to note that these are not the same students followed longitudinally, but rather two different cohorts. An implicit assumption of the present paper is, that Grade 5 anno 2018 and Grade 9 anno 2018 are identical in their functioning and composition, and thus comparable. This assumption is supported by the fact that we are working with population data, and that the birth years of both cohorts remain relatively close. In addition, due to the lack of students' birth month, several students remained unclassified regarding their school path. Whilst this approach increased certainty in correct classification and contrasted the groups of interest, for future research, a replication and extension of the present findings with longitudinal data seems desirable. Longitudinal data may also allow for a more comprehensive comparison to further elaborate the decline in SWB to a finer distinction and considering an even more precise level of retention.

Future research should also consider the relationship between students and teachers as it was reported to influence students' sense of belonging at school (OECD 2017). In general, current educational research (in Luxembourg) is very much input/output-focused. To gain a better understanding of the educational processes and the students' educational paths, research should also focus on the interaction processes between students, their peers, and their teachers and their impact on their academic and non-academic development (Jennings and Greenberg 2009).

8   Conclusion

From an international perspective, the results of the present study contribute to the growing empirical body of knowledge on grade retention and early tracking as prominent yet questionable pedagogical interventions to target students in need of support. Whereas most studies on the aforementioned educational mechanisms focus on academic outcomes (i.e., school grades, diploma, results in standardized achievement tests) the current study shows their impact on socio-emotional well-being is considerable and should not be neglected. From a national perspective, the results of this study are critical new pieces of information, which could inform an already ongoing discussion on how to complement or replace existing, generic mechanisms of diversity management (i.e., performance grouping and grade retention) through more specific, genuinely pedagogical interventions (Fischbach et al. 2016; Martin et al. 2015; Wrobel et al 2013). Such discussion could lead to the adaptation of school and education to an increasingly heterogeneous student population in a continued attempt to ultimately reduce educational inequalities.

References

Bates, D., Mächler, M., Bolker, B., & Walker, S. (2015). Fitting Linear Mixed-Effects Models Using me4. *Journal of Statistical Software, 67*(1), 1–48. https://doi.org/10.18637/jss.v067.i01

Belfi, B., Goos, M., De Fraine, B., & Van Damme, J. (2012). The effect of class composition by gender and ability on secondary school students' school well-being and academic self-concept: A literature review. *Educational Research Review, 7*, 62–74. https://doi.org/10.1016/j.edurev.2011.09.002

Bloom, B. (1976). *Human characteristics and school learning*. New York NY, USA: McGraw-Hill.

Brunner, M., Keller, U., Dierendonck, C., Reichert, M., Ugen, S., Fischbach, A., & Martin, R. (2010). The structure of academic self-concepts revisited: The nested Marsh/Shavelson model. *Journal of Educational Psychology, 102*(4), 964–981. https://doi.org/10.1037/a0019644

Bücker, S., Nuraydin, S., Simonsmeier, B. A., Schneider, M., & Luhmann, M. (2018). Subjective well-being and academic achievement: A meta-analysis. *Journal of Research in Personality, 74* 83–94. https://doi.org/10.1016/j.jrp.2018.02.007

Diener, E. (1984). Subjective Well-Being. *Psychological Bulletin, 95*, 542–575.

Edlinger, H., & Hascher, T. (2008). Von der Stimmungs- zur Unterrichtsforschung: Überlegungen zur Wirkung von Emotionen auf schulisches Lernen und Leisten. *Unterrichtswissenschaft, 36*(1), 55–70.

Eurydice. (2011). *Grade retention during compulsory education in Europe: Regulations and statistics*. Brussels, Belgium: EACEA; Eurydice. https://doi.org/10.2797/50570

Fischbach, A., Ugen, S., & Martin, R. (2016). Bilanz nach zwei vollen Erhebungszyklen [Taking stock after two full assessment cycles]. In SCRIPT & LUCET (Eds.), *PISA 2015—Nationaler Bericht Luxemburg*. Luxembourg: MENJE.

Ganzeboom, H. B. G. (2010). *International standard classification of occupations ISCO-08 with ISEI-08 scores*. Retrieved from http://www.ilo.org/public/english/bureau/stat/isco/index.htm

Ganzeboom, H. B. G., & Treiman, D. J. (1996). Internationally Comparable Measures of Occupational Status for the 1988 International Standard Classification of Occupations. *Social Science Research*, *25*(3), 201–239. https://doi.org/https://doi.org/10.1006/ssre.1996.0010

Gogol, K., Brunner, M., Goetz, T., Martin, R., Ugen, S., Keller, U., ... Preckel, F. (2014). 'My Questionnaire is Too Long!' The assessments of motivational-affective constructs with three-item and single-item measures. *Contemporary Educational Psychology*, *39*(3), 188–205. https://doi.org/10.1016/j.cedpsych.2014.04.002

Gogol, K., Brunner, M., Martin, R., Preckel, F., & Goetz, T. (2017). Affect and motivation within and between school subjects: Development and validation of an integrative structural model of academic self-concept, interest, and anxiety. *Contemporary Educational Psychology*, *49*, 46–65. https://doi.org/10.1016/j.cedpsych.2016.11.003

Grund, S., Robitzsch, A., & Luedtke, O. (2019). *mitml: Tools for Multiple Imputation in Multilevel Modeling*. Retrieved from https://CRAN.R-project.org/package=mitml

Guay, F., Marsh, H. W., & Boivin, M. (2003). Academic self-concept and academic achievement: Developmental perspectives on their causal ordering. *Journal of Educational Psychology*, *95*, 124–136. https://doi.org/10.1037/0022-0663.95.1.124

Gutman, L. M., & Vorhaus, J. (2012). The Impact of Pupil Behaviour and Wellbeing on Educational Outcomes. *Childhood Wellbeing Research Centre*, 3–42. https://doi.org/10.1016/S2213-8587(14)70016-6

Hascher, T. (2004). *Wohlbefinden in der Schule*. Münster, Germany: Waxmann.

Hascher, T. (2008). Quantitative and qualitative research approaches to assess student well-being. *International Journal of Educational Research*, *47*(2), 84–96. https://doi.org/10.1016/j.ijer.2007.11.016

Hascher, T., & Edlinger, H. (2009). Positive Emotionen und Wohlbefinden in der Schule – ein Überblick über Forschungszugänge und Erkenntnisse [Positive emotions and well-being in school – an overview of methods and results]. *Psychologie in Erziehung Und Unterricht*, *56*, 105–122.

Hascher, T., & Hagenauer, G. (2011). Wohlbefinden und Emotionen in der Schule als zentrale Elemente des Schulerfolgs unter der Perspektive geschlechtsspezifischer Ungleichheiten. In *Geschlechtsspezifische Bildungsungleichheiten* (pp. 285–308). Wiesbaden: VS Verlag für Sozialwissenschaften. https://doi.org/10.1007/978-3-531-92779-4_12

Hascher, T., & Lobsang, K. (2004). Das Wohlbefinden von SchülerInnen. In T. Hascher (Ed.), *Schule positiv erleben: Ergebnisse und Erkenntnisse zum Wohlbefinden von Schülerinnen und Schülern* (pp. 203–228). Bern: Haupt.

Hascher, T., Morinaj, J., & Waber, J. (2018). Schulisches Wohlbefinden. Eine Einführung in Konzept und Forschungsstand. In K. Rathmann & K. Hurrelmann (Eds.), *Leistung und Wohlbefinden in der Schule: Herausforderung Inklusion* (pp. 66–82). Weinheim: Beltz Juventa.

Hattie, J. (2009). *Visible learning: A synthesis of over 800 meta-analyses relating to achievement*. Abingdon, UK: Routledge.

Holmes, C. T. (1989). Grade level retention effects: A meta-analysis of research studies. In L. A. Shepard & M. L. Smith (Eds.), *Flunking grades: Research and Policies on Retention* (pp. 16–33). London, UK: Falmer Press.

Hothorn, T., Bretz, F., & Westfa l, P. (2008). Simultaneous Infe-ence in General Parametric Models. *Biometrical Journal*, *50*(3), 346–363.

Jennings, P. A., & Greenberg, M. T. (2009). The Prosocial Classroom: Teacher Social and Emotional Competence in Relation to Student and Classroom Outcomes. *Review of Educational Research*, *79*(1) 491–525. https://doi.org/10.3102/0034654308325693

Jimerson, S. R. (1999). On the failure of failure: Examining the association between early grade retention and education and employment outcomes during late adolescence. *Journal of School Psychology*, *37*, 243–272. https://doi.org/10.1016/S0022-4405(99)00005-9

Jimerson, S. R. (2001). Meta-analysis of grade retention research: Implications for practice in the 21st century. *School Psychology Review*, *30*, 420–437.

Jimerson, S. R., & Ferguson, P. (2007). A longitudinal study of grade retention: Academic and behavioral outcomes of retained students through adolescence. *School Psychology Quarterly*, *22*, 314–339. https://doi.org/10.1037/1045-3830.22.3.314

Keller, U., Lorphelir, D., Muller, C., Fischbach, A., & Martin, R. (2012). Unterschiede zwischen Schulformen [Differences between educational tracks]. In Romain Martin & M. Brunner (Eds., *Épreuves Standardisées. Nationaler Bericht 2011–2012* (pp. 88–97). Luxembourg: University of Luxembourg, EMACS.

Keller, U., Sonnleitner, P., Villányi, D., Fischbach, A., Lorphelin, D., Ugen, S., ... Martin, R. (2013). Unterschiede zwischen Schulformen und das Pilotprojekt PROCI [Differences between educational tracks and the PROCI project]. In SCRIPT & EMACS (Eds.), *Zusammenfassung der Ergebnisse von Pisa 2012 [Summary of the PISA 2012 results]* (pp. 88–99). Luxembourg: MENFP.

Kirkcaldy, B., Furnham, A., & S efen, G. (2004). The relationship between health efficacy, educational attainment, and well-being among 30 nations. *European Psychologist*, *9*, 107–119. https://doi.org/10.1027/1016-9040.9.2.107

Klapproth, F., & Schaltz, P. (2015). Klassenwiederholungen in Luxemburg. In T. Lenz & J. Bertemes (Eds.), *Bildungsbericht Luxembourg 2015: Band 2 Analysen und Befunde* (pp. 76–83). Esch-sur-Alzette, LU: MENJE & University of Luxembourg

Lenth, R. (2020). *emmeans: Estimated Marginal Means, aka Least-Squares Means*. Retrieved from https://CRAN R-project.org/package=emmeans

Lenz, Thomas, & Heinz, A. (2018). Le système scolaire luxembourgeois: Aperçu et tendances. In LUCET & SCRIPT (Eds.), *Rapport national sur l'éducation au Luxembourg 2018* (pp. 23–34). Esch-sur-Alzette, LU: University of Luxembourg.

Long, J. A. (2020). *jtools: Analysis and Presentation of Social Scientific Data*. Retrieved from https://cran.r-project.org/package=jtools

Lumley, T. (2004). Analysis of complex survey samples. *Journal of Statistical Software*, *9*(1), 1–19.

Lumley, T. (2019). *mitools: Tools for Multiple Imputation of Missing Data*. Retrieved from https://CRAN.R-project.org/package=mitools

Marsh, H. W. (1989). Age and sex effects in multiple dimensions of self-concept: Preadolescence to early adulthood. *Journal of Educational Psychology*, *81*(3), 417–430. https://doi.org/10.1037/0022-0663.81.3.417

Martin, A. J. (2009). Age appropriateness and motivation, engagement, and performance in High School: Effects of age within cohort, grade retention, and delayed school entry. *Journal of Educational Psychology*, *101*, 101–114. https://doi org/10.1037/a0013100

Martin, A. J. (2011). Holding back and holding behind: Grade retention and students' non-academic and academic outcomes. *British Educational Research Journal, 37,* 739–763. https://doi.org/10.1080/01411926.2010.490874

Martin, R., Ugen, S., & Fischbach, A. (2015). *Épreuves Standardisées: Bildungsmonitoring für Luxemburg. Nationaler Bericht 2011 bis 2013.* Esch/Alzette, LU: University of Luxembourg, LUCET.

MENJE (Ed.). (2018). *The key figures of the national education: Statistics and indicators 2016/2017.* Luexmbourg: MENJE/Service des Statistiques et Analyses.

MENJE (Ed.). (2020). *Das luxemburgische Bildungssystem.* Luxembourg: MENJE/Service presse et communication.

Merton, R. K. (1968). *Social theory and social structure.* New York, NY, USA: Free Press.

Nilles, J.-P., Tholl, L., & Schorn, A. (2016). *CARAT – Ein Schulklimamodell für Luxemburger Schulen.* Luxembourg: SCRIPT.

OECD. (2017). *PISA 2015 Results (Volume III): Students' Well-Being.* Paris, France: OECD Publishing. https://doi.org/10.1787/9789264273856-en

Opdenakker, M. C., & Van Damme, J. (2000). Effects of schools, teaching staff and classes on achievement and well-being in secondary education: Similarities and differences between school outcomes. *School Effectiveness and School Improvement, 11*(2), 165–196. https://doi.org/10.1076/0924-3453(200006)11:2;1-Q;FT165

Pekrun, R. (2005). Progress and open problems in educational emotion research. *Learning and Instruction, 15,* 497–506. https://doi.org/10.1016/j.learninstruc.2005.07.014

Quartagno, M., & Carpenter, J. (2020). *jomo: A package for Multilevel Joint Modelling Multiple Imputation.* Retrieved from https://CRAN.R-project.org/package=jomo

R Core Team. (2020). *R: A Language and Environment for Statistical Computing.* Vienna, Austria: R Foundation for Statistical Computing. Retrieved from http://www.R-project.org/

Ravens-Sieberer, U., Devine, J., Bevans, K., Riley, A. W., Moon, J., Salsman, J. M., & Forrest, C. B. (2014). Subjective well-being measures for children were developed within the PROMIS project: Presentation of first results. *Journal of Clinical Epidemiology, 67*(2), 207–218. https://doi.org/10.1016/j.jclinepi.2013.08.018

Roderick, M. (1994). Grade Retention and school dropout: Investigating the association. *American Educational Research Journal, 31,* 729–759.

Rosso, I. M., Young, A. D., Femia, L. A., & Yurgelun-Todd, D. A. (2004). Cognitive and emotional components of frontal lobe functioning in childhood and adolescence. *Annals of the New York Academy of Sciences, 1021,* 355–362. https://doi.org/10.1196/annals.1308.045

Seligman, M. E. P. (2011). *Flourish: A visionary new understanding of happiness and well-being* (1. Free Press hardcover ed). New York, NY: Free Press.

UNESCO. (2016). *Happy schools: A framework for learner well-being in the Asia-Pacific.* Paris, France.

Van Houtte, M. (2006). School type and academic culture: Evidence for the differentiation–polarization theory. *Journal of Curriculum Studies, 38*(3), 273–292. https://doi.org/10.1080/00220270500363661

Venetz, M., Zurbriggen, C., & Eckhart, M. (2014). Entwicklung und erste Validierung einer Kurzversion des „Fragebogens zur Erfassung von Dimensionen der Integration von Schülern (FDI 4-6)" von Haeberlin, Moser, Bless und Klaghofer. *Empirische Sonderpädagogik*, (2), 99–113.

Wrobel, G., Dierendonck, C., Fischbach, A., Ugen, S., Hoffmann, D., Hornung, C., Gamo, S., Böhm, B., & Martin, R. (2013). Zusammenfassung der Ergebnisse von Pisa 2012 [Summary of the PISA 2012 results]. In SCRIPT & EMACS (Eds.), *PISA 2012. Nationaler Bericht Luxemburg [PISA 2012. National report Luxembourg]* (pp. 123–127). Luxembourg: MENFP.

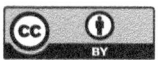

Ungleichheiten in schulischen Gesundheitsproblemen und subjektivem Wohlbefinden bei luxemburgischen Grund- und Sekundarschüler/innen

Andreas Hadjar und Frederick de Moll

1   Einleitung

Wohlbefinden in der Schule ist ein unverzichtbarer Baustein für erfolgreiches Lernen in der Schule, denn es beeinflusst sowohl die Lern- und Leistungsmotivation als auch schulische Leistungen und damit Schulerfolg (Hascher und Hagenauer 2011a, b). Ebenso prägt die physische Gesundheit Lernprozesse. Schüler/innen mit allgemeinen Gesundheitsproblemen werden dadurch in ihrem Lernen behindert (Shaw et al. 2015). Auf der anderen Seite sind die Schulumwelt und Lernen, insbesondere im Hinblick auf Leistungsanforderungen, auch starke Einflussfaktoren von Wohlbefinden von Schülerinnen und Schülern (Gysin 2017; Hascher 2004). Lernen kann auch krank machen im Sinne physischer Gesundheitsprobleme. So kennzeichnet Haub (2007) Schule als pathogenen Ort, wobei Leistungs- und Verhaltenserwartungen   wesentliche   Bestimmungsfaktoren   für   problembehaftete

A. Hadjar (✉) · F. de Moll
Department of Social Sciences, University of Luxembourg, Esch-sur-Alzette, Luxembourg
E-Mail: andreas.hadjar@uni.lu

F. de Moll
E-Mail: frederick.demoll@uni.lu

A. Hadjar
Université de Fribourg, Freiburg, Schweiz
E-Mail: andreas.hadjar@unifr.ch

© Der/die Autor(en) 2022   215
A. Heinen et al. (Hrsg.), *Wohlbefinden und Gesundheit im Jugendalter,*
https://doi.org/10.1007/978-3-658-35744-3_11

Befindlichkeiten von Schüler/innen sind. In Anbetracht dieser Wechselwirkungen zwischen Schule, Lernen und Gesundheit erscheint es sinnvoll, Wohlbefinden als pädagogische Kernaufgabe anzusehen (Fend und Sandmeier 2004).

Wenn Wohlbefinden und Lernen zusammenhängen, kann angenommen werden, dass Bildungsungleichheiten im Sinne systematischer Variationen im Bildungserwerb zwischen verschiedenen Gruppen, die durch askriptive Merkmale wie Sozialschicht, Geschlecht oder Migrationshintergründe definiert sind, mit Ungleichheiten in Wohlbefinden und Gesundheit assoziiert sind. Dahingehend wäre zu untersuchen, inwieweit sogenannte Risikogruppen im Bildungssystem auch durch ein geringeres Wohlbefinden und eine schlechtere Gesundheit gekennzeichnet sind. Zu etwaigen Risikogruppen, d. h. Schüler/innen, die unterdurchschnittliche Leistungen zeigen und ein hohes Risiko haben, die Schule frühzeitig und ohne oder nur mit einem von potenziellen Arbeitgebern als unzureichend stigmatisierten Abschluss zu verlassen (Stichwort: Bildungsverlierer/innen), gehören Arbeiterkinder und Jungen sowie Schüler/innen mit bestimmten Migrationshintergründen (vgl. Hadjar et al. 2010, 2019). Befunde im Nationalen Bildungsbericht Luxemburgs zeigen, dass diese Risikogruppen auch in Luxemburg Benachteiligungen ausgesetzt sind. Arbeiterkinder, Jungen sowie Schüler/innen mit bestimmten Migrationshintergründen (francophone Sprachhintergründe, vor allem portugiesisch sprechende Schüler/innen) zeigen niedrigere Kompetenzniveaus und erhalten schlechtere Schulnoten in der Grund- und in der Sekundarschule. Diese Gruppen sind im *modulaire*-Schulzweig der Sekundarschule, welcher das geringste Anspruchsniveau ausweist und häufig mit einem frühen Verlassen der Schule verbunden ist, überrepräsentiert. Zudem erleben diese Schüler/innen häufigere Klassenwiederholungen (Hadjar et al. 2015).

Im Kern des Beitrags steht zum einen subjektives Wohlbefinden – allgemein und im Hinblick auf die Schule – und schulbezogenes physisches Wohlbefinden im Sinne der Absenz von Gesundheitsproblemen von Schülerinnen und Schülern in der Grund- und Sekundarschulbildung in Luxemburg (Klassen 4/Cycle 3.2. bis Klasse 9). Es wird gefragt, wann bzw. in welcher Klassenstufe diese Gesundheitsprobleme und Wohlbefinden in Schule und Leben vergleichsweise stark ausgeprägt sind und welche Risikogruppen entlang der Ungleichheitsachsen soziale Herkunft, Geschlecht und Migrationshintergrund besonders von einem geringen subjektiven Wohlbefinden und einem geringen physischen Wohlbefinden (Gesundheitsprobleme) betroffen sind. Die Datenbasis geht auf das internationale Projekt SASAL „Schulentfremdung in der Schweiz und in Luxemburg" zurück, welches zwischen 2015 und 2019 an den Universitäten Bern und Luxembourg durchgeführt wurde (zur Studie vgl. u. a. Morinaj et al. 2017; Scharf et al. 2019). Die Analysen basieren auf einem Drei-Wellen-Paneldatensatz, in dem

Informationen zu Luxemburgischen Schülerinnen und Schülern vorhanden sind, die eine Rekonstruktion von Verläufen zwischen Klasse 4/Cycle 3.2 und Klasse 6/Cycle 4.2 in der Grundschule (N = 345) und zwischen Klasse 7 und 9 in der Sekundarschule (N = 387) ermöglichen.

Im folgenden theoretischen Abschnitt wird der Untersuchungsgegenstand des subjektiven Wohlbefindens definiert und konzeptualisiert, wobei zwischen Wohlbefinden in der Schule, allgemeinem Wohlbefinden sowie physischem Wohlbefinden (mit Gesundheitsproblemen als Gegenpol) unterschieden wird. In einem weiterer theoretischen Abschnitt wird der Aspekt der Ungleichheiten eingeführt und es werden allgemeine theoretische Modelle, warum es zwischen verschiedenen Gruppen Unterschiede im Wohlbefinden geben könnte, aufgezeigt. Am Ende des theoretischen Teils wird der Kontext des Luxemburgischen Bildungssystems dargestellt. Auf eine Beschreibung des Untersuchungsdesigns folgt dann die Präsentation der Ergebnisse zu Disparitäten in den drei Wohlbefindensdimensionen in den verschiedenen Gruppen in der Grundschule und in der Sekundarschule, wobei jeweils drei aufeinanderfolgende Schuljahre betrachtet werden. In einem letzten Abschnitt werden die Ergebnisse zusammengefasst und diskutiert.

2   Wohlbefinden von Schülerinnen und Schülern

In diesem Abschnitt geht es zunächst um eine allgemeine Bestimmung dessen, was unter subjektivem Wohlbefinden in Kindheit und Jugend verstanden wird. Dabei wird Wohlbefinden als ein facettenreiches Konstrukt eingeführt, das in unterschiedlichen Disziplinen (z. B. Psychologie, Soziologie, Medizin) und Forschungsfeldern wie der Kindheits-, Jugend- und Bildungsforschung bearbeitet wird. Aufbauend auf eine transdisziplinäre Perspektive werden mentale wie physische bzw. gesundheitliche Komponenten von Wohlbefinden im Kontext Schule in den Blick genommen.

2.1   Allgemeine Definition

Das subjektive Wohlbefinden von Schülerinnen und Schülern wird im Anschluss an Bradshaw et al. (2010, S. 182) verstanden als von jungen Menschen geäußerte evaluierende Einstellungen in Bezug auf ihr persönliches Wohlbefinden sowie ihre Beziehungen zu anderen Menschen und zu ihrer Umwelt. Wir haben es demnach mit den Selbstauskünften von Kindern und Jugendlichen hinsichtlich ihrer „inneren" bzw. mentalen Verfassung in Bezug auf schulische Aspekte, aber auch darüber hinaus zu tun. Eine Definition, die noch stärker auf die Lebenswelt von Kindern und Jugendlichen bezogen ist, formulierten Fattore et al. (2007) auf Basis von Interviews mit Kindern und Jugendlichen. Danach wird Wohlbefinden (bzw. oft auch engl. *Well-being*) von den Befragten als Glück, Fröhlichkeit oder Zufriedenheit definiert und ist mit einem Gefühl der Sicherheit in harmonischen sozialen Beziehungen verbunden. Damit wird der emotionale Aspekt bzw. die affektive Komponente des Wohlbefindens hervorgehoben, wobei aber auch die evaluative Sicht auf Wohlbefinden als Lebenszufriedenheit (im Sinne der kognitiven Komponente) eine Rolle spielt (siehe hierzu z. B. Bradshaw et al. 2013, S. 621). Davon abzugrenzen ist das objektive Wohlbefinden, das über sogenannte harte Faktoren wie den Zugang zu medizinischer Versorgung und Bildung, das elterliche Einkommen und materielle Ressourcen im Leben von Kindern erfasst wird (Axford et al. 2014). Während sich Politik und öffentliche Debatten noch immer vorwiegend an diesen objektiven Maßen für kindliches Wohlbefinden orientieren, finden sich bereits seit einigen Jahren verstärkt Forderungen danach, auch dessen subjektive Seite in bildungs- und sozialpolitischen Initiativen stärker zu berücksichtigen (Ben-Arieh 2005).

Im Folgenden fokussieren wir auf drei zentrale Aspekte kindlichen Wohlbefindens innerhalb und außerhalb der Schule, die vor dem Hintergrund potenzieller sozialer Ungleichheiten besonders relevant und dementsprechend für diesen Beitrag maßgeblich sind.

2.2 Aspekte des Wohlbefindens

Mit Blick auf das Wohlbefinden lassen sich drei Dimensionen als besonders wichtig markieren, insofern diese in der Sozialberichterstattung wie auch in der Forschung regelmäßig besondere Beachtung finden: 1. die allgemeine Lebenszufriedenheit, 2. das schulische Wohlbefinden, das auch als Schulfreude bezeichnet wird und 3. das physische Wohlergehen bzw. Gesundheitsprobleme.

Die allgemeine Lebenszufriedenheit von Kindern und Jugendlichen ist international seit den 1970er Jahren in den Blick der Forschung geraten (Pollard und Lee 2003), nachdem Lebenszufriedenheit zuvor vornehmlich bei Erwachsenen untersucht wurde und hier bereits seit Langem als wichtiger Indikator für Glück und die wahrgenommene Lebensqualität zählt (Gysin 2017; Proctor et al. 2009).

Kinder und Jugendliche verbringen einen großen Teil ihres Alltags in der Schule bzw. mit schulischem Lernen. Das schulische Wohlbefinden deutet somit auch auf ihr Wohlbefinden über den Unterricht hinaus hin, zumal psychische

Probleme von Kindern und Jugendlichen häufig mit schulischen Schwierig-
keiten zusammenhängen. Schulisches Wohlbefinden gilt daher als zentrale
Voraussetzung für erfolgreiche Lernprozesse und Schulerfolg (Hascher und
Hagenauer 2011a) Dies trifft ebenso auf die dritte hier erfasste Dimension von
Wohlbefinden zu, denn bspw. psychosomatische Probleme sind oftmals eine
Begleiterscheinung schulischen Leistungsdrucks (Torsheim und Wold 2001).
Schulfreude und subjektive Gesundheit sind somit potenziell folgenreiche
Facetten des Wohlbefindens. Dennoch werden beide Variablen erst in jüngerer
Zeit verstärkt auch aus einer Ungleichheitsperspektive betrachtet (Currie et al.
2008).

3 Ungleichheiten im Wohlbefinden

Im Folgenden werden einige theoretische Konzepte zu Einflussfaktoren auf das
Wohlbefinden aufgezeigt, die insbesondere auf Bildung und Schule bezogen
werden.

3.1 Theoretischer Rahmen: Die Produktion von Wohlbefinden

Ein allgemeines theoretisches Modell, das sich zur Erklärung von Ungleichheiten im Wohlbefinden eignet, ist die Theorie der sozialen Produktions-
funktionen (Lindenberg 1996; Ormel et al. 1999), welche die Frage ins Zentrum
der Erklärung von Wohlbefinden stellt, inwieweit Individuen bzw. Gruppen über
Ressourcen verfügen, Wohlbefinden herzustellen. Zu den Kernprämissen gehört,
dass alle Menschen physisches Wohlbefinden und soziales Wohlbefinden (auch
als soziale Anerkennung gefasst) als höchste Güter anstreben. Diese Güter bzw.
Ziele werden über instrumentelle Zwischenziele bzw. -güter erreicht: Stimulation,
Komfort, Status, Verhaltensbestätigung und Affekt. Der Aspekt der Stimulation
– d. h. ein bestimmtes Anregungsniveau aufrecht zu erhalten, spannende und
interessante Dinge zu erfahren – und der Aspekt des Komforts – d. h. die Absenz
von physiologischen Mangelerscheinungen wie Durst, Hunger, Unbehagen,
Unsicherheit und damit das Vorhandensein materieller Ressourcen wie von Geld
oder einer angenehmen Wohnumwelt – beziehen sich auf das physische Wohlbefinden. Dem sozialen Wohlbefinden sind folgende instrumentelle Zwischengüter zugeordnet: Status – d. h. einen (prestigereichen) Beruf zu haben bzw. eine
entsprechende Position einzunehmen – Verhaltensbestätigung – d. h. im Einklang

mit sich selbst und den Erwartungen anderer zu denken und zu handeln – sowie Affekt – d. h. emotionale Beziehungen zu anderen zu haben. Um diese Zwischengüter produzieren zu können, sind Ressourcen notwendig. Im Hinblick auf das Leben allgemein und das Schulumfeld lassen sich Ressourcen identifizieren, welche der Erreichung der instrumentellen Ziele und damit der übergeordneten Ziele des Wohlbefindens dienen: Stimulation kann generell über anregende Freizeitaktivitäten produziert werden. Für das konkrete schulische Wohlbefinden sind dies anregende, d. h. spannende und interessante Lerninhalte, -aktivitäten und -methoden oder auch ein anregend gestaltetes Schulumfeld (z. B. mit Posterwänden und Spielen ausgestattete Lernräume). Komfort wird über Essen, Trinken, sicherheitsbezogene Maßnahmen erzeugt. In der Schule können etwa die Bereitstellung eines komfortablen Umfelds mit Schulessen, geregelten Pausenzeiten, angenehmen Sitzgelegenheiten im Unterricht oder auch Couches sowie ein begrünter Schulhof mit Spielelementen für die Pausen wichtige Ressourcen zur Produktion von Komfort darstellen. Der Aspekt des Status, der generell etwa durch das Erreichen entsprechender Bildungszertifikate produziert werden kann, steht bei Schüler/innen wahrscheinlich weniger im Vordergrund, wenngleich sich auch die Schüler/innen bereits bewusst sind, dass das Lernen in der Schule für die spätere Berufswahl von Bedeutung ist (vgl. Scharf et al. 2019). Auch innerhalb der Schule sind jedoch auch statusbezogene Positionen denkbar, etwa die der Schülervertretung oder ein informeller Status als „Klassenbeste/r". Hingegen kann Verhaltensbestätigung durch „die richtigen Dinge tun" erreicht werden, was voraussetzt, dass Wissen über Erwartungen von sich selbst und von anderen besteht und eine Selbstreflexion sowie ein Feedback von anderen das erwartungskonforme Verhalten auch wahrnehmbar macht. Im Hinblick auf die Schule und Lernen können vermutlich das Gefühl der Schüler/in, dass das Verhalten in der Schule im Einklang mit dem Selbstbild ist, ebenso der Produktion von Verhaltensbestätigung dienlich sein wie positive Verstärkungen durch Eltern oder Mitschüler/innen sowie positive Evaluationen und Ermutigungen durch Lehrpersonen und Mitschüler/innen. Affekt als fünftes instrumentelles Zwischenziel wird durch positive soziale Beziehungen produziert. Hinsichtlich Schülerinnen und Schülern sind hier Beziehungen zu Klassenkamerad/innen und Lehrer/innen von besonderer Bedeutung, aber auch positive Beziehungen zu Eltern und Peers außerhalb der Schule (vgl. auch Konzept der Bildungswerte, Scharf et al. 2019).

Die Grundthese hinsichtlich Ungleichheiten im Wohlbefinden ist nun, dass bestimmte Gruppen hinsichtlich der Ressourcen zur Produktion wohlbefindensrelevanter Zwischengüter benachteiligt sind. Diese bedeutsamen Ressourcen lassen sich mittels des Kapitalienkonzepts von Bourdieu

(1983) klassifizieren, welches auch insbesondere auf die Frage des Bildungserwerbs angewendet wurde; Das ökonomische Kapitel bezieht sich auf materielle Ressourcen, die für den Bildungserwerb – oder in unserer Argumentation – für das Wohlbefinden von Bedeutung sind. Im Kern sind das finanzielle Ressourcen, welche genutzt werden können, um Komfort und Status herzustellen, aber auch um soziale Beziehungen (Affekt) oder stimulierende Freizeitaktivitäten (Stimulation) zu finanzieren. Kulturelle Ressourcen – im Sinne objektivierten Kulturkapitals (Bücher), inkorporierten Kulturkapitals (Fähigkeiten, Wissensbestände, internalisierte Motivations- und Verhaltensmuster, Werte, Ziele) oder institutionalisierten Kulturkapitals (Bildungsabschlüsse) – sind ebenso für verschiedene der genannten Zwischengüter sinnvoll: Inkorporiertes und objektiviertes Kulturkapital sind Ressourcen, welche bedeutsam für Stimulation, Affekt und Verhaltensbestätigung sind, denn ein mehr an Wissen und Büchern erleichtert das Aussuchen stimulierender Freizeitaktivitäten, erleichtert soziale Beziehungen und bedeutet auch ein besseres Wissen über eigene und fremde Erwartungen. Institutionalisiertes Kapital in Form von Bildungsabschlüssen ist wiederum besonders von Bedeutung für Statuserwerb (Status) sowie Verhaltensbestätigung (Anerkennung), aber auch – im Hinblick auf Entlohnung – mit besserem Komfort verbunden. Soziales Kapital, definiert als Ressourcen, welche sich aus nützlichen sozialen Beziehungen im Netzwerk ergeben, ist zuallererst ein Produktionsmittel für Affekt, kann aber auch Verhaltensbestätigung (Bestärkungen durch andere), Stimulation (in gemeinsamen Aktivitäten) und Status (Anerkennung durch andere) fördern.

Entsprechend klassischer ungleichheitstheoretischer Ansätze (Bourdieu 1983; Boudon 1974) ist nun anzunehmen, dass Arbeiterkinder gegenüber Kindern aus höheren Sozialschichten (Dienstklassen) über bessere Ressourcen – etwa anregendere Lebensumwelten im Hinblick auf Stimulation, bessere materielle Ausstattung im Hinblick auf Komfort – verfügen, Wohlbefinden herzustellen. Ebenso sollten Schüler/innen mit Migrationshintergrund gegenüber Schüler/innen ohne Migrationshintergrund Ressourcendefizite aufweisen, da sie beispielsweise andere, eher auf der eigenen Ethnie aufbauende, soziale Netzwerke haben, welche im Hinblick auf die Produktion von Wohlbefinden in der Aufnahmegesellschaft und ihren Institutionen (hier: Schule) im geringeren Ausmaß von Nutzen sind. Geschlechterunterschiede in Ressourcen zur Produktion von Wohlbefinden sollten im Generellen nicht bestehen, da entsprechend der tendenziell egalitären Geschlechterbilder Frauen und Männer gleichermaßen Zugang zu Ressourcen haben sollten. Im Hinblick auf einzelne Zwischengüter könnte angenommen werden, dass – entsprechend verbliebener Geschlechterunterschiede – Jungen im

Nachteil bei Stimulation und Mädchen im Nachteil beim Status sind. Hinsichtlich schulischem Wohlbefinden könnten die häufigeren Misserfolgserlebnisse sowie die stärkere Freizeitorientierung (Quenzel und Hurrelmann 2011) von Jungen auch mit einem geringeren schulischen Wohlbefinden einhergehen.

3.2 Ungleichheiten im Wohlbefinden

Obgleich das Wohlbefinden von Kindern aus deren eigener Perspektive etwa im Rahmen der World Vision Studien regelmäßig auf die Agenda gesetzt wird (z. B. Andresen und Schneekloth 2014), standen soziale und ethnische Ungleichheiten im Leben von Kindern über lange Zeit hinweg nicht im Fokus der sozialwissenschaftlichen Kindheitsforschung (Betz 2010, S. 18). Vor allem in qualitativen Studien liegt das Forschungsinteresse meist auf der generationalen Ordnung – und damit auf der unterschiedlichen sozialen Positionierung von Erwachsenen und Kindern im Generationengefüge – sowie auf Differenzen zwischen Jungen und Mädchen. Ansonsten wurden und werden Kinder als weitgehend homogene soziale Gruppe betrachtet und über ihren Status als Kinder konzipiert; Kindheit gerät dabei als sozialstrukturelle Kategorie vornehmlich in *Ergänzung* zu klassischen Ungleichheitsachsen wie Schicht und Migrationshintergrund in den Blick (Qvortrup 2005). Diese Position wurde unter anderem von Betz (2008) in Frage gestellt, die für Deutschland anhand von Daten des DJI-Kinderpanels auf weitreichende Ungleichheiten zwischen Kindern aus unterschiedlichen Milieus und Zuwanderungsgruppen hingewiesen hat. Soziale Disparitäten wurden hier gerade auch im Hinblick auf objektive Maße von Wohlbefinden deutlich, etwa in der Versorgung mit Taschengeld und Lernmaterialen.

In der Sozial- und Bildungsberichterstattung zu Kindern zeigen sich innerhalb und zwischen den wohlhabendsten Ländern der Welt teils erhebliche Unterschiede in Bezug auf materielles Wohlbefinden, schulbezogenes Wohlbefinden und subjektive Gesundheit von 11- bis 15 Jährigen (Adamson 2010). Gerade hinsichtlich selbstberichteter Gesundheitsprobleme der 11- bis 15 Jährigen weist Luxemburg eine vergleichsweise hohe Varianz auf und damit einen erheblichen Abstand zwischen Schülerinnen und Schülern mit geringen Beschwerden und jenen mit stärkeren Problemen, während etwa in Ländern wie den Niederlanden die meisten Kinder und Jugendlichen recht dicht beieinander liegen und generell eher geringe Probleme berichten (Adamson 2010). Allerdings ist die Datenlage mit Blick auf Luxemburg noch keineswegs zufriedenstellend. Bevor sich also über bildungs- und sozialpolitische Implikationen sprechen lässt, sind zunächst grundlegende Analysen zu Ungleichheiten im Wohlbefinden von Kindern und

Jugendlichen vonnöten. Hier lässt die bisherige Forschung aus verschiedenen Disziplinen wie Erziehungswissenschaft, Medizin und pädagogischer Psychologie Ungleichheiten entlang verschiedener Achsen erwarten.

Zum einen liegen bspw. aus Deutschland, der Schweiz und Großbritannien Befunde zu geschlechtsspezifischen Disparitäten vor: So zeigte sich bereits, dass Mädchen häufiger von schulisch bedingten Gesundheitsproblemen berichten als Jungen (Ravens-Sieberer et al. 2004), während Mädchen in der Schule mehr positive Emotionen erfahren als Jungen (Gutman et al. 2010; Hascher und Hagenauer 2011b). Zum anderen beeinflusst der sozioökonomische Hintergrund nachweislich die generelle Lebenszufriedenheit von Kindern (Andresen et al. 2012) ebenso wie deren psychisches Wohlbefinden (McLeod und Owens 2004). Dass soziale und gesundheitliche Lage von Kindern und Jugendlichen stark verschränkt sind, ist mittlerweile empirisch gut belegt; Gesundheit wird wesentlich durch die Lebensumstände wie Armut, materielle Ressourcen der Familie und Schulform mitbestimmt (Jungbauer-Gans und Kriwy 2004; Lampert und Richter 2006). Subjektive Gesundheit wird in der gesundheitssoziologischen Literatur auch unter dem Stichwort psychosoziale Gesundheit behandelt, insofern es hier um die Häufigkeit selbstwahrgenommener psychosomatischer Beschwerden wie Kopfschmerzen und Bauchkrämpfe geht. In der alle vier Jahre von der Weltgesundheitsorganisation (WHO) durchgeführten Studie „Health Behaviour in School-age Children" zeigte sich, dass sich Jugendliche über den Erhebungszeitraum hinweg in beinahe allen untersuchten Staaten in Abhängigkeit von ihrem familiären Wohlstand in ihrer Bewertung des eigenen körperlichen Wohlbefindens unterscheiden (Moor et al. 2015). Jugendliche aus ressourcenschwachen Familien berichten über häufigere Gesundheitsprobleme als sozioökonomisch bessergestellte Jugendliche.

Zusammenfassend können soziale Ungleichheiten *zwischen* Kindern und Jugendlichen trotz dieser Befunde als nach wie vor unterforscht gelten. Gerade in der Bildungsforschung liegt der Fokus zumeist eher auf den Zusammenhängen zwischen schulischem Wohlbefinden und weiteren schulerfolgsrelevanten Variablen.

3.3 Wohlbefinden im Kontext schulbezogener Einstellungen und Schulleistungen

In der erziehungswissenschaftlichen und pädagogisch-psychologischen Forschung wird das subjektive Wohlbefinden von Schülerinnen und Schülern häufig im Kontext der Diskussion um die über die Schullaufbahn abnehmende

Schulfreude diskutiert (z. B. Harazd und Schürer 2006). Fend (1997) versteht Schulfreude als emotionale Bewertung der Schule, die sich in Bildungsmotivation, Wohlbefinden in der Schule und der Identifikation mit der Schule niederschlägt: Eine geringe Schulfreude hat potenziell negative Konsequenzen für das Lernen und kann zu Schulvermeidung führen. Zudem ist bekannt, dass Schülerinnen und Schüler, die sich in der Schule wohlfühlen in geringerem Maße entfremdet vom Lernen sind (z. B. Moreno und de Roda 2003; Rayce et al. 2008). Wohlbefinden hat demnach auch eine protektive Wirkung mit Blick auf Bildungsrisiken und kann über positive Beziehungen in der Schule gefördert werden (Hall-Lande et al. 2007; Hascher und Hagenauer 2010; Rubin et al. 2003). Verlässliche Bindungen zu Lehrkräften und ein als gerecht erlebter Lernkontext sind dabei besonders wichtig (Boekaerts 2001; Hascher 2003).

Mit Blick auf die physische Seite des subjektiven Wohlbefindens zeigte eine schwedische Studie Zusammenhänge mit Schulleistungen, die allerdings für Jungen und Mädchen unterschiedlich stark ausgeprägt waren (Låftman und Modin 2012). Zudem konnten die Autoren positive Korrelationen zwischen subjektiver Gesundheit und Leistungsmotivation und emotionaler Unterstützung durch Lehrkräfte nachweisen. In einer kanadischen Studie konnte eine Beziehung zwischen subjektiver Gesundheit und schulischem Problemverhalten nachgewiesen werden, wobei sich hier auch die Unterscheidung zwischen Individual- und Schulebene als wichtig erwies (Saab und Klinger 2010). Erneut zeigte sich hier die Lernumwelt bzw. die im schulischen Kontext erlebte Unterstützung als maßgeblich für die Gesundheit der Schülerinnen und Schüler; dieser Befund bestätigt sich auch im internationalen Vergleich und gilt gleichermaßen für die generelle Lebenszufriedenheit, wobei Mädchen von einem unterstützenden Umfeld offenbar stärker profitieren (Ravens-Sieberer et al. 2009).

Wenngleich insbesondere das schulische Wohlbefinden von Kindern und Jugendlichen in der Bildungsforschung vielfach diskutiert wird, mangelt es nach wie vor an Studien zu Determinanten der verschiedenen Komponenten von Wohlbefinden.

4   Kontext: Die Luxemburgische Grund- und Sekundarschule

Das Bildungssystem Luxemburgs hat eine lange Tradition der Mehrgliedrigkeit und ist im Vergleich stark stratifiziert (Hadjar und Gross 2016). Es wird zentral gesteuert. Die Schulpflicht setzt mit dem vierten Lebensjahr ein, wenn die Schüler/innen in die verpflichtende Vorschule (Cycle 1.1) eintreten. Die Vor- und

Grundschulzeit ist gesamtschulartig ohne externe Differenzierung/Stratifizierung, wenngleich sich die Schulkomposition aufgrund der räumlichen Lage der Schulen stark unterscheiden kann. So gibt es etwa in Luxemburg Grundschulen, in denen homogene Klassen dominieren, die fast ausschließlich aus Arbeiterkindern mit portugiesischer Herkunft bestehen. Der Sekundarschulbereich ist – wie auch in Deutschland, den Niederlanden, der Schweiz und anderen Ländern stratifiziert – bzw. mehrgliedrig. In Luxemburg werden die Schülerinnen und Schüler in der Regel nach acht Jahren in der Vor-/Grundschule (sechste Grundschulklasse, Cycle 4.2) in einen Sekundarschulzweig selektiert. In Luxemburg werden die Schülerinnen und Schüler von Kommissionen (neuerdings unter einem erweiterten Mitspracherecht der Eltern) auf folgende Sekundarschulzweige orientiert, wobei im Folgenden die Bezeichnungen genutzt werden, welche im Untersuchungszeitraum 2016–2018 der hier präsentierten Analysen galten: Der akademische Sekundarschulzweig, der zu einer uneingeschränkten Hochschulzugangsberichtigung führt, nennt sich *enseignement secondaire* (ES; seit 2019: *enseignement secondaire classique*) und wird in klassischen Gymnasium *(lycée classique)* oder auch in schulischen Mischformen angeboten. Das *enseignement secondaire technique* (EST; seit 2019 *enseignement secondaire générale*), welches in technischen Gymnasien bzw. Lyzeen sowie Mischformen angeboten wird, untergliedert sich in verschiedene Anspruchsniveaus bzw. Schulzweige: Während das EST *théorique* als vergleichsweise höherer Schulzweig ebenso zu einer Hochschulzugangsberechtigung führen kann, sind die technischen Schulzweige des *polyvalente* oder *pratique* stärker berufsbildend. Der niedrigste und kürzeste Schulzweig ist das *modulaire* oder auch *préparatoire,* welches auf eine direkte Transition in das Erwerbsleben vorbereitet und an technischen Gymnasien und Mischformen angeboten wird. Dazu gibt es auch Projektschulen, die von der 7. bis zur 9. Klasse einen gesamtschulartigen technischen Schulzweig durchführen (PROCI), in dem alle technischen Schulzweige vereint sind (Backes und Hadjar 2017). In den mittleren technischen Schulzweigen findet dann nach Klasse 9 ein weiterer Übergang in mittlere und höhere Berufsbildungen und entsprechende Spezialisierungen statt. In den Sekundarschulhäusern in Luxemburg sind oftmals verschiedene Schulzweige beheimatet, wobei eine stärkere räumliche Abtrennung des niedrigsten Schulzweigs, der teilweise in Schulgebäude am Rande der Städte ausgelagert ist, auffällt. Die Schulpflicht endet dem 16. Lebensjahr, wobei die Absolvierung des niedrigsten Pflichtschulzweigs *(modulaire/ préparatoire)* mit einem frühen Verlassen der Schule verbunden ist.

Im Hinblick auf das Wohlbefinden der Schülerinnen und Schüler rückt ein Mechanismus in den Vordergrund: Die verschiedenen parallelen Bildungsinstitutionen (Schulen) oder bildungswegspezifischen Klassenformationen stellen differentielle Sozialisationsumwelten und Entwicklungsmilieus (Baumert et al. 2006) dar. Während gesamtschulartige Systeme durch heterogenere Klassenumwelten geprägt sind, d. h. dass Arbeiter- und Akademikerkinder sowie Schüler und Schülerinnen verschiedener ethnischer Hintergründe in einer Klasse oder Schule zusammen lernen, sind in stratifizierten Systemen homogenere Lernumwelten vorherrschend. In diesen Systemen hat sich – insbesondere im Verlauf der Bildungsexpansion, in dem Kinder aus privilegierten sozialen Schichten zunehmend die neuen höheren Bildungsgelegenheiten in Anspruch nahmen, während benachteiligte Kinder in den niedrigen Sekundarschulformen zurückblieben – eine homogene Schulform mit einem sehr niedrigen Anspruchsniveau herausgebildet. So bestehen mit den *modulaire*-Klassen in Luxemburg distinkte und oftmals räumlich von anderen Lernumwelten getrennte Schulformen, in denen Risikogruppen wie Arbeiterkinder, Jungen und benachteiligten Migrationshintergründe quasi unter sich bleiben (vgl. Hadjar und Becker, 2016; Solga 2007). Gering motivierte Schüler und Schülerinnen mit geringen Leistungen können sich gegenseitig weder hinsichtlich der Motivation noch im Lernen unterstützen und bestärken sich in ihrer Abneigung gegenüber Schule und Lernen (Stichwort: Schulentfremdung; Hascher und Hadjar 2018; Morinaj et al. 2017). Diese Bildungskontexte (Becker und Schulze 2013) sind durch ein geringeres Anspruchsniveau der Lehrpersonen gekennzeichnet. Zudem prägt die Schulkomposition – hier die homogene Zusammensetzung hinsichtlich benachteiligter Schüler/innen – auch Merkmale der Schulorganisation und die didaktischen Konzepte (vgl. Thrupp und Lupton 2006).

5 Forschungsfragen und Hypothesen

Auf Basis der theoretischen Überlegungen und internationalen empirischen Vorbefunde sollen folgende – aufgrund der lückenhaften Forschungslage – eher explorative Hypothesen aufgestellt werden, die vor allem auf Hintergrundannahmen zur Verfügbarkeit von Ressourcen zur Produktion von Wohlbefinden sowie sozialisierter Schulfreude beruhen. In Bezug auf Geschlechterdifferenzen greifen die Hypothesen die komplexere internationale Forschungslage zu den drei betrachteten Aspekten des Wohlbefindens auf.

Hypothese 1: Schülerinnen und Schüler aus sozioökonomisch benachteiligten Verhältnissen zeigen ein geringeres allgemeines, schulisches und physisches Wohlbefinden als sozial privilegierte Schülerinnen und Schüler.

Hypothese 2a: Mädchen sind zufriedener mit ihrem Leben im Allgemeinen als Jungen.
Hypothese 2b: Jungen zeigen ein geringeres Wohlbefinden in der Schule als Mädchen.
Hypothese 2c: Mädchen berichten stärkere gesundheitliche Probleme als Jungen.
Hypothese 3: Schüler/innen mit Migrationshintergrund zeigen ein geringeres Wohlbefinden hinsichtlich der untersuchten Dimensionen als Schüler/innen ohne Migrationshintergrund.

6 Untersuchungsdesign

Die Datengrundlage unserer Untersuchung bildet die SASAL-Studie („Schulentfremdung in der Schweiz und in Luxemburg"), die von 2016 bis 2019 in Luxemburg und der deutschsprachigen Schweiz (Kanton Bern) an Grund- bzw. Primarschulen und Sekundarschulen durchgeführt wurde. Ein wesentliches Merkmal der Studie ist ihr längsschnittliches, sequenzielles Kohortendesign; das heißt, dass dieselben Schülerinnen und Schüler jeweils zu drei Messzeitpunkten befragt wurden. In Luxemburg lagen abschließend Daten von $N = 338$ Grundschülerinnen und -schülern vor, die von der vierten bis zur sechsten Klassenstufe an der Studie teilgenommen haben. In der Sekundarstufe sind es $N = 375$ Schülerinnen und Schüler, die in Klassenstufe sieben, acht und neun bei der Befragung mitgemacht haben.

Die Daten werden mithilfe von hierarchischen Regressionsmodellen unter Berücksichtigung des geschachtelten Stichprobendesigns analysiert. Von Interesse sind hier allerdings nur die Prädiktoren auf Individualebene. Die Einschätzungen der Schülerinnen und Schüler zu Lebenszufriedenheit, subjektivem Wohlbefinden in der Schule und subjektiver Gesundheit bilden die abhängigen Variablen. Als unabhängige Variablen dienen die Angaben zu Geschlecht, Migrationshintergrund und sozialer Herkunft, wobei je abhängige Variable zwei Modelle berichtet werden. Der Migrationshintergrund wird dabei stets im zweiten Modell einbezogen, um zunächst den Effekt der sozialen Herkunft abzuschätzen und anschließend den Einfluss des Migrationshintergrunds über die sozioökonomischen Lebensumstände hinaus zu betrachten. Dieses Vorgehen beruht auf dem bekannten Befund, dass Migrationshintergrund und soziale Herkunft konfundiert sind, da die zugewanderte Population überproportional in den unteren sozialen Schichten vertreten ist. Für den vorliegenden Beitrag werden die Forschungsfragen jeweils für die beiden Schulstufen getrennt bearbeitet, wobei die Jahrgänge innerhalb beider Analysen konstant gehalten werden.

Im Folgenden werden die analysierten Variablen vorgestellt, wobei ein besonderes Augenmerk auf die Skala zum physischen Wohlbefinden gelegt wird (siehe deskriptive Statistiken in Tab. 1). Diese basiert auf vier Items zu unterschiedlichen Gesundheitsproblemen mit Bezug zu Schule und Lernen. Die Reliabilität der Skalen (interne Konsistenz, Cronbachs α) ist über die drei Messzeitpunkte hinweg sehr zufriedenstellend. Bei den beiden Variablen zum subjektiven (psychischen) Wohlbefinden im Leben allgemein bzw. in der Schule handelt es sich um einzelne Items: „In meinem Leben fühle ich mich alles in allem wohl" sowie „In der Schule fühle ich mich meistens wohl" (siehe Tab. 2).

Als unabhängige Variablen dienen sozioökonomischer Status (1 = Dienstklasse/Hochqualifizierte, 2 = Angestellte mit mittlerer Bildung in nicht-manuellen Berufen sowie Facharbeiter, 3 = nicht oder gering qualifizierte Arbeiter) und der Migrationshintergrund (0 = Kind/Jugendlicher sowie mindestens ein Elternteil in Luxemburg geboren; kein Migrationshintergrund, 1 = Kind oder beide Elternteile nicht in Luxemburg geboren; erste und zweite Migrantengeneration). Das Geschlecht wurde – nach einem Screening in den Schulklassen, ob es Schüler/innen gibt, welche sich einem „dritten Geschlecht" oder „divers" zuordnen würden – dichotom erhoben (0 = weiblich, 1 = männlich).

7 Ergebnisse

In diesem Abschnitt stellen wir die Ergebnisse der Regressionsanalysen zur Vorhersage der drei Dimensionen des subjektiven Wohlbefindens von luxemburgischen Kindern und Jugendlichen vor. Für die Grund- und Sekundarschülerinnen und -schüler werden jeweils pro abhängige Variable zwei Modelle präsentiert, einmal mit und einmal ohne Einbezug des Migrationshintergrunds.

7.1 Allgemeine Lebenszufriedenheit

Wie Tab. 3 zu entnehmen ist, lässt sich in der Grundschule kein signifikanter Zusammenhang zwischen dem sozioökonomischen Hintergrund und der allgemeinen Lebenszufriedenheit von Kindern feststellen. Das Modell unter Berücksichtigung des Migrationshintergrunds zeigt jedoch, dass Schülerinnen und Schüler, die selbst oder deren Eltern nicht in Luxemburg geboren sind, eine geringere Lebenszufriedenheit aufweisen als Kinder ohne Migrationshintergrund. In der Sekundarstufe zeigt sich zunächst ein anderes Bild (Modell 1). Jugendliche

Tab. 1 Deskriptive Statistiken der Items zur Erfassung subjektiver Gesundheitsprobleme im Zusammenhang mit der Schule

Item	Grundschule Mittelwert (Standardabweichung)			Sekundarschule Mittelwert (Standardabweichung)		
(Antwortkategorien: 1 ... nie ... 6 sehr oft)	Klasse 4/ Cycle 3.2	Klasse 5/ Cycle 4.1	Klasse 6/ Cycle 4.2	Klasse 7	Klasse 8	Klasse 9
Kam es in den letzten paar Wochen vor, dass du Bauchschmerzen wegen der Schule hattest?	2.03 (1.68)	1.87 (1.47)	2.12 (1.58)	2.20 (1.60)	2.21 (1.63)	2.19 (1.60)
Kam es in den letzten paar Wochen vor, dass du wegen Prüfungsstress keinen Appetit hattest?	2.36 (1.63)	2.31 (1.75)	2.30 (1.71)	2.28 (1.70)	2.40 (1.73)	2.33 (1.73)
Kam es in den letzten paar Wochen vor, dass dir schlecht wurde vor lauter Aufregung?	2.17 (1.75)	2.17 (1.67)	2.08 (1.56)	2.06 (1.54)	2.19 (1.60)	2.21 (1.57)
Kam es in den letzten paar Wochen vor, dass du während des Unterrichts starke Kopfschmerzen hattest?	2.56 (1.77)	2.64 (1.83)	2.60 (1.75)	2.64 (1.75)	2.88 (1.63)	2.79 (1.74)
Gesamtskala Interne Konsistenz	2.28 (1.38) $\alpha = .80$	2.25 (1.25) $\alpha = .73$	2.28 (1.28) $\alpha = .77$	2.30 (1.32) $\alpha = .82$	2.43 (1.40) $\alpha = .83$	2.38 (1.38) $\alpha = .85$

Anmerkungen. Angaben auf Basis der Luxemburger Stichproben (Grund-/Sekundarschule) des Projekts SASAL – Schulentfremdung in der Schweiz und in Luxemburg, Wellen 1–3. (eigene Darstellung).

Tab. 2 Deskriptive Kennwerte der Variablen zum psychischen Wohlbefinden

Schulstufe	Jahrgang	Wohlbefinden im Leben	Wohlbefinden in der Schule
		Mittelwert M (Standardabweichung SD)	
Grundschule	Klasse 4/Cycle 3.2	3.44 (.69)	3.31 (.76)
	Klasse 5/Cycle 4.1	3.34 (.77)	3.24 (.73)
	Klasse 6/Cycle 4.2	3.25 (.77)	3.16 (.77)
Sekundarschule	7. Klasse	3.40 (.85)	3.44 (.82)
	8. Klasse	3.38 (.80)	3.49 (.74)
	9. Klasse	3.28 (.87)	3.37 (.76)

Anmerkungen. Angaben auf Basis der Luxemburger Stichproben (Grundschule: $N = 354$ bis 376, Sekundarschule $= 210$ bis 334 je nach Welle) des Projekts SASAL – Schulentfremdung in der Schweiz und in Luxemburg, Wellen 1–3. (eigene Darstellung).

aus der unteren und mittleren Mittelklasse sowie der Arbeiterklasse fühlen sich im Leben im Allgemeinen weniger wohl als Jugendliche aus der höchsten Statusgruppe. Der um den Migrationsstatus bereinigte Effekt des sozioökonomischen Hintergrunds ist allerdings nicht mehr signifikant (Modell 2). Dies deutet darauf hin, dass die Schülerinnen und Schüler mit Zuwanderungsgeschichte, die zugleich auch gesellschaftlich weniger privilegiert sind, im ersten Modell für den signifikanten Statuseffekt verantwortlich zeichneten. Die signifikanten Kovariaten der höheren Jahrgangsstufen in der Sekundarstufe machen zudem deutlich, dass die Lebenszufriedenheit mit zunehmendem Alter bzw. in höheren Klassenstufen signifikant abnimmt.

7.2 Subjektives Wohlbefinden in der Schule

Die Regressionsmodelle für das subjektive Wohlbefinden in der Schule zeigen mit Blick auf das Grundschulalter ein ähnliches Bild wie die Modelle zur Lebenszufriedenheit (Tab. 4). Die soziale Herkunft hat hier keinen Einfluss darauf, wie wohl sich Kinder in der Schule fühlen. Allerdings tritt hier der erwartete Geschlechtseffekt zutage: Jungen fühlen sich in der Schule signifikant weniger wohl als Mädchen. Der Migrationshintergrund (Modell 2) wiederum hat allenfalls dann einen Effekt auf das Wohlbefinden, wenn man ein Signifikanzniveau von 10 % anlegt und so der eher kleinen Stichprobengröße Rechnung trägt. In der Sekundarstufe zeigen sich erneut deutlichere Effekte und komplexere Zusammen-

Tab. 3 Prädiktion der Lebenszufriedenheit von Kindern und Jugendlichen an Grund- und Sekundarschulen

	Modell 1 Welle, Geschlecht, soziale Herkunft	Modell 2 Welle, Geschlecht, soziale Herkunft, Migrations-hintergrund	Modell 1 Welle, Geschlecht, soziale Herkunft	Modell 2 Welle, Geschlecht, soziale Herkunft, Migrations-hintergrund
	Grundschule		*Sekundarschule*	
Klassenstufe (Welle) (Ref. Klasse 4/C3.2; Klasse 7)				
Klasse 5/C4.1; Klasse 8	–.03	–.03	–.12 **	–.12 **
Klasse 6/C4.2; Klasse 9	–.11	–.10	–.21 ***	–.21 ***
Geschlecht (Ref. Schülerinnen)				
Schüler	.03	.03	.04	.04
Soziale Herkunft (Ref. Obere Mittelklasse)				
Untere und mittlere Mittelklasse	–.07	–.05	–.16 *	–.11
Arbeiterklasse	–.14	–.07	–.19 *	–.09
Migrationshintergrund (Ref. kein Migrationshintergrund oder 2.5-Generation)				
Migrationshintergrund		–.17 *		– 17 **

(Fortsetzung)

Tab. 3 (Fortsetzung)

	Modell 1 Welle, Geschlecht, soziale Herkunft	Modell 2 Welle, Geschlecht, soziale Herkunft, Migrations-hintergrund	Modell 1 Welle, Geschlecht, soziale Herkunft	Modell 2 Welle, Geschlecht, soziale Herkunft, Migrations-hintergrund
Zufallseffekte				
Klassenebene (sd)	.28	.29	.00	.00
Individualebene (sd)	.29	.27	.38	.37
Residual (sd)	.73	.73	.62	.62
N	333	333	374	374
Wald Chi-Square	5.13 (df = 5)	11.05 (df = 6)	27.82 (df = 5)	35.87 (df = 6)
Konstante	3.45 ***	3.53 ***	3.56 ***	3.59***

Anmerkungen. Signifikanz-Niveaus: †.10, *.05, **.01, ***.001.
Datensatz: SASAL – Schulentfremdung in der Schweiz und in Luxemburg, Luxemburger Stichproben (Grund-/Sekundarschule), Wellen 1–3. (eigene Darstellung).

Tab. 4 Prädiktion des schulischen Wohlbefindens von Kindern und Jugendlichen an Grund- und Sekundarschulen

	Grundschule		Sekundarschule	
	Modell 1 Welle, Geschlecht, soziale Herkunft	Modell 2 Welle, Geschlecht, soziale Herkunft, Migrations-hintergrund	Modell 1 Welle, Geschlecht, soziale Herkunft	Modell 2 Welle, Geschlecht, soziale Herkunft, Migrations-hintergrund
Klassenstufe (Welle) (Ref. Klasse 4/C3.2; Klasse 7)				
Klasse 5/C4.1; Klasse 8	.02	.02	−.07 †	−.17 †
Klasse 6/C4.2; Klasse 9	−.09	−.09	−.17 **	−.17 **
Geschlecht (Ref. Schülerinnen) Schüler	−.13 *	−.14 *	−.18 *	−.18 *
Soziale Herkunft (Ref. Obere Mittelklasse)				
Untere und mittlere Mittelklasse	.06	−.01	−.14 *	−.12 †
Arbeiterklasse	−.03	.11	−.17 †	−.13
Migrationshintergrund (Ref. kein Migrationshintergrund oder 2.5-Generation)				
Migrationshintergrund		−.12 †		−.08

(Fortsetzung)

Tab. 4 (Fortsetzung)

	Modell 1 Welle, Geschlecht, soziale Herkunft	Modell 2 Welle, Geschlecht, soziale Herkunft, Migrations-hintergrund	Modell 1 Welle, Geschlecht, soziale Herkunft	Modell 2 Welle, Geschlecht, soziale Herkunft, Migrations-hintergrund
Zufallseffekte				
Klassenebene (sd)	.00	.00	.00	.00
Individualebene (sd)	.32	.32	.42	.42
Residual (sd)	.68	.67	.59	.59
N	333	333	374	374
Wald Chi-Square	10.35 (df = 5)	14.04 * (df = 6)	30.60 ** (df = 5)	32.21 ** (df = 6)
Konstante	3.54	3.60	3.53	3.55

Anmerkungen. Signifikanz-Niveaus: †.10, *.05, **.01, ***.001.
Datensatz: SASAL – Schulentfremdung in der Schweiz und in Luxemburg, Luxemburger Stichproben (Grund-/Sekundarschule), Wellen 1–3. (eigene Darstellung).

hänge. Zum einen schlägt hier der Effekt der sozialen Herkunft stärker durch, insbesondere im Hinblick auf den Unterschied zwischen oberer und unterer/ mittlerer Mittelklasse. Zum anderen ist der Effekt des Geschlechts hier stärker als in der Grundschule und erneut sinkt die Schulfreude in höheren Klassenstufen ab. Der Migrationshintergrund bleibt in der Sekundarstufe anders als bei der Lebenszufriedenheit ohne Einfluss, was auf die Unabhängigkeit von schulischem und allgemeinem Wohlbefinden hindeutet.

7.3   Physisches Wohlbefinden

Zuletzt werden die Modelle zur Prädiktion des physischen Wohlbefindens vorgestellt (Tab. 5). Erstaunlich ist hier auf den ersten Blick sowohl für die Grundschule als auch für die Sekundarschule der deutliche signifikante Effekt der sozialen Herkunft auf die selbst berichteten Gesundheitsprobleme. Kinder und Jugendliche aus der unteren/mittleren Klasse sowie der Arbeiterklasse berichten ein geringeres physisches Wohlbefinden als ihre jeweiligen Altersgenossen aus der gehobenen Mittelklasse. Kinder von Eltern in privilegierten gesellschaftlichen Positionen haben demzufolge weniger häufig Kopfschmerzen und psychosomatische Stresssymptome. Dieser Effekt bleibt auch bei Berücksichtigung des Migrationshintergrunds stabil. Letzterer hat demgegenüber keinen statistisch bedeutsamen Einfluss auf die subjektive Gesundheit. Demgegenüber zeigt sich wieder ein profunder Effekt der Geschlechtszugehörigkeit. Diesmal sind es jedoch die Jungen, die eine um beinahe eine Drittel Standardabweichung besseres Wohlbefinden aufweisen als Mädchen. Somit lässt sich der diametrale Befund festhalten, dass sich Mädchen zwar in der Schule wohler fühlen als Jungen, allerdings in höherem Maße von potenziell schulisch verursachten Gesundheitsproblemen betroffen sind.

8   Diskussion

Insgesamt zeigen die Ergebnisse, dass subjektives Gesundheitsempfinden und die Zufriedenheit mit dem Leben und der Schule in je spezifischer Weise nach sozialer Herkunft, Geschlecht und Migrationshintergrund variieren.

Hinsichtlich der aufgestellten Hypothesen zeigt sich, dass diese nie für alle Wohlbefindensaspekte gleichermaßen gestützt werden konnten, obwohl sich im Forschungsstand tendenziell nur Indizien für differentielle Befunde hinsichtlich der Achse Geschlechtszugehörigkeit fanden. Für die Hypothese 1 zum positiven

Tab. 5 Prädiktion schulischer Gesundheitsprobleme von Kindern und Jugendlichen an Grund- und Sekundarschulen

	Grundschule		Sekundarschule	
	Model 1 Welle, Geschlecht, soziale Herkunft	Model 2 Welle, Geschlecht, soziale Herkunft, Migrations-hintergrund	Model 1 Welle, Geschlecht, soziale Herkunft	Model 2 Welle, Geschlecht, soziale Herkunft, Migrations-hintergrund
Klassenstufe (Welle) (Ref. Klasse 4/C3.2; Klasse 7)				
Klasse 5/C4.1; Klasse 8	.03	.03	−.12 †	−.12 †
Klasse 6/C4.2; Klasse 9	.01	.01	−.07	−.07
Geschlecht (Ref. Schülerinnen)				
Schüler	.28 *	.28 *	.21 †	.21 †
Soziale Herkunft (Ref. Obere Mittelklasse)				
Untere und mittlere Mittelklasse	−.40 *	−.39 *	−.34 *	−.34 *
Arbeiterklasse	−.45 *	−.39 *	−.45 *	−.44 *

(Fortsetzung)

Tab. 5 (Fortsetzung)

	Model 1 Welle, Geschlecht, soziale Herkunft	Model 2 Welle, Geschlecht, soziale Herkunft, Migrations-hintergrund	Model 1 Welle, Geschlecht, soziale Herkunft	Model 2 Welle, Geschlecht, soziale Herkunft, Migrations-hintergrund
Migrationshintergrund (Ref. kein Migrations-hintergrund oder 2.5-Generation) Migrationshintergrund		-.14		-.00
Zufallseffekte				
Klassenebene (sd)	.19	.19	.16	.96
Individualebene (sd)	.80	.79	.96	.16
Residual (sd)	.98	.98	.94	.94
N	338	338	375	375
Wald Chi-Square	19.59 * (df = 5)	21.23 * (df = 6)	14.37 * (df = 5)	14.37 * (df = 6)
Konstante	4.86	4.92	4.83	4.83

Anmerkungen. Signifikanz-Niveaus: †.10, *.05, **.01, ***.001.
Datensatz: SASAL – Schulentfremdung in der Schweiz und in Luxemburg, Luxemburger Stichproben (Grund-/Sekundarschule), Wellen 1–3. (eigene Darstellung).

Einfluss der sozialen Herkunft auf das Wohlbefinden fanden sich nur im Hinblick auf das physische Wohlbefinden (Gesundheitsprobleme) belastbare Belege, sowohl in der Grundschul- als auch in der Sekundarschulstichprobe. Schüler/innen aus privilegierten Sozialschichten berichteten weniger Gesundheitsprobleme. In der Lebenszufriedenheit und im Wohlbefinden in der Schule fanden sich nur punktuelle Hinweise auf ähnliche Trends.

Für die Hypothese 2a zu Geschlechterunterschieden in der Lebenszufriedenheit kann unabhängig von der Schulstufe kein Beleg gefunden werden. Dagegen zeigen sich hypothesenkonforme Effekte für das Wohlbefinden in der Schule (Hypothese 2b), wo sich Jungen weniger wohl fühlen als Mädchen – und zwar sowohl in der Grund- als auch in der Sekundarschule. Im Hinblick auf das physische Wohlbefinden bestätigt sich Hypothese 2c für die Grundschule, während in der Sekundarstufe lediglich in der Tendenz von einem Geschlechtereffekt auszugehen ist: Mädchen berichteten ein geringeres physisches Wohlbefinden und damit mehr Gesundheitsprobleme als Jungen.

Hinsichtlich eines belegenden Befunds zur Hypothese 3 zum Migrationshintergrund ist nur zu konstatieren, dass in der Grund- und Sekundarschule Schüler/innen mit Migrationshintergrund eine geringere allgemeine Lebenszufriedenheit aufweisen als Schüler/innen, die selbst oder zumindest ein Elternteil in Luxemburg geboren wurde.

Generell erweisen sich die drei untersuchten Aspekte des Wohlbefindens – Lebenszufriedenheit, Wohlbefinden in der Schule und physisches Wohlbefinden/Gesundheitsprobleme – in der Grundschule als relativ konstant. In der Sekundarschule erweisen sich die Gesundheitsprobleme als eher stabil, während die Lebenszufriedenheit und das Wohlbefinden in der Schule absinkt. Mechanismen hinter dieser Entwicklung sind neben der zunehmenden Adoleszenz sicher auch die sich mit dem Übergang von der Grund- in die Sekundarschule verändernden Schulumwelten und Lehrstile sowie insbesondere die über die Sekundarbildung zunehmenden Leistungsanforderungen (vgl. Grecu et al. 2019).

Die dargestellten (sparsamen) Modelle sind vor dem Hintergrund einiger Limitationen zu interpretieren. Die Stichprobe ist nicht repräsentativ für Luxemburg. Da der Fokus auf Zusammenhängen zwischen Ungleichheitsachsen soziale Herkunft, Geschlecht und Migrationshintergrund – und nicht auf der Beschreibung des Ausmaßes – lag, geben die Ergebnisse aber durchaus Auskünfte über Trends. Die Abbildung des Migrationshintergrunds entspricht einer eher abstrakten Darstellung, welche der Heterogenität innerhalb der luxemburgischen Migrant/innen nicht Rechnung trägt. Während durch die gleichzeitige Betrachtung des sozioökonomischen Hintergrunds die Heterogenität hinsichtlich dieser Variablen Berücksichtigung fand, blieben ethnische Unterschiede (etwa zwischen Migrant/innen portugiesischer Herkunft und Migrant/innen aus Frankreich) unberücksichtigt. Komplexere Modelle unter Berücksichtigung der Schulnoten und der verschiedenen Sekundarschulzweige (in den Modellen auf Basis der Sekundarschuldaten) ergaben vergleichbare Ergebnisse. Entsprechend sind die dargestellten Trends als robust anzusehen.

Alles in allem zeigt sich, dass bestimmten Risikogruppen hinsichtlich Wohlbefinden im Luxemburgischen Schulsystem besser Rechnung getragen werden sollte. Dies gilt hinsichtlich Schüler/innen mit Migrationshintergrund (insbesondere mit Blick auf die Lebenszufriedenheit), hinsichtlich Jungen mit Blick auf das Wohlbefinden in der Schule, hinsichtlich Mädchen sowie Schülern und Schülerinnen aus benachteiligten sozialen Herkunftsschichten mit Blick auf Gesundheitsprobleme im Sinne eines Mangels an physischem Wohlbefinden.

Literatur

Adamson, Peter. 2010. *The children left behind. A league table of inequality in child well-being in the world's rich countries.* 09. Florence: UNICEF Innocenti Research Centre.

Andresen, S., K. Hurrelmann & U. Schneekloth. 2012. Care and Freedom: Theoretical and Empirical Aspects of Children's Well-Being in Germany. *Child Indicators Research* 5:437–48.

Andresen, S. & U. Schneekloth. 2014. Wohlbefinden und Gerechtigkeit. Konzeptionelle Perspektiven und empirische Befunde der Kindheitsforschung am Beispiel der World Vision Kinderstudie 2013. *Zeitschrift für Pädagogik* 60:535–51.

Axford, N., D. Jodrell & T. Hobbs. 2014. Objective or Subjective Well-Being? In *Handbook of Child Well-Being: Theories, Methods and Policies in Global Perspective,* Hrsg. A. Ben-Arieh, F. Casas, I. Frønes & J. E. Korbin, 2699–2738. Dordrecht: Springer.

Ben-Arieh, Asher. 2005. Where Are the Children? Children s Role in Measuring and Monitoring Their Well-Being. *Social Indicators Research* 74:573–96.

Betz, Tanja. 2008. *Ungleiche Kindheiten: Theoretische und empirische Analysen zur Sozialberichterstattung über Kinder.* Weinheim: Juventa.

Betz, Tanja. 2010. Modern Children and their Well-Being Dismantling an Ideal.In *Children and the Good Life: New Challenges for Research on Children.* Hrsg. S. Andresen, I. Diehm, U. Sander & H. Ziegler, 13–28. Dordrecht: Springer.

Boekaerts, Monique. 2001. Context sensitivity: Activated motivational beliefs, current concerns and emotional arousal. In *Motivation in learning contexts: Theoretical advances and methodological implications. Advances in learning and instruction series.*, Hrsg. von S. Volet & S. Järvelä, 17–32. Elmsford, NY: Pergamon Press.

Boudon, Raymond. 1974. *Education, Opportunity and Social Inequality.* New York: John Wiley & Sons.

Bourdieu, Pierre. 1983. Ökonomisches Kapital, kulturelles Kapital, soziales Kapital. In *Soziale Ungleichheiten.* Sonderband 2. Soziale Welt, Hrsg. R. Kreckel, 183–198. Göttingen: Schwartz.

Bradshaw, J., B. Martorano, L. Natali & C. de Neubourg. 2013. Children's Subjective Well-Being in Rich Countries. *Child Indicators Research* 6: 619–35.

Bradshaw, J., G. Rees, A. Keung & H. Goswami. 2010. The subjective well-being of children. In *Child Well-Being: Understanding Children's Lives. London: Jessica Kingsley Publishers*, Hrsg. C. McAuley & W. Rose, 181–206. London: Jessica Kingsley.

Currie, C., M. Molcho, W. Boyce, B. Holstein, T. Torsheim & M. Richter. 2008. Researching Health Inequalities in Adolescents: The Development of the Health Behaviour in School-Aged Children (HBSC) Family Affluence Scale. *Social Science & Medicine* 66: 1429–36.

Fattore, T., J. Mason & E. Watson. 2007. Children's Conceptualisation(s) of Their Well-Being. *Social Indicators Research* 80: 5–29.

Fend, Helmut. 1997. *Der Umgang mit Schule in der Adoleszenz: Aufbau und Verlust von Lernmotivation, Selbstachtung und Empathie*. Bd. IV. Bern: Huber.

Fend, H. & Sandmeier, A. (2004). Wohlbefinden in der Schule: "Wellness" oder Indiz für gelungene Pädagogik? In *Schule positiv erleben. Ergebnisse und Erkenntnisse zum Wohlbefinden von Schülerinnen und Schülern*, Bd. 10, Hrsg. T. Hascher, 161–183. Bern: Haupt Verlag.

Grecu, A., T. Hascher & A.. 2019. Teachers' images of the ideal student as a marker for school culture and its role in school alienation during the transition from primary to secondary education in Luxembourg. *Studia Paedagogica* 24: 85–108.

Gutman, L. M., J. Brown, R. Akerman & P. Obolenskaya. 2010. *Change in wellbeing from childhood to adolescence: risk and resilience*. 34. London: Institute of Education, University of London.

Gysin, Stefanie. 2017. *Subjektives Wohlbefinden von Schülerinnen und Schülern*. Weinheim: Beltz Juventa.

Hadjar, A., A. Fischbach, R. Martin & S. Backes. 2015. Bildungsungleichheiten im luxemburgischen Bildungssystem. In *Bildungsbericht Luxemburg 2015. Analysen und Befunde*, Hrsg. Ministère de l'Éducation nationale, de l'Enfance et de la Jeunesse, SCRIPT & Université du Luxembourg, FLSHASE, 34–56. Luxembourg: MENEJ/SCRIPT & University of Luxembourg.

Hadjar, A., J. Lupatsch & E. Grünewald-Huber. 2010, Bildungsverlierer/-innen, Schulentfremdung und Schulerfolg. In *Bildungsverlierer. Neue Ungleichheiten*, Hrsg. G. Quenzel & K. Hurrelmann, 223–244. Wiesbaden: VS.

Hadjar, A., J. Scharf & A. Grecu. 2019. Schulische Kontexte, Schulentfremdung und Bildungsarmut. In Handbuch Bildungsarmut, Hrsg. G. Quenzel & K. Hurrelmann, 183–209. Wiesbaden: Springer VS.

Hall-Lande, J. A., M. E. Eisenberg, S. L. Christenson & D. Neumark-Sztainer. 2007. Social Isolation, Psychological Health, and Protective Factors in Adolescence. *Adolescence* 42:265–86.

Harazd, B. & S. Schürer. 2006. Veränderung der Schulfreude von der Grundschule zur weiterführenden Schule. In *Risikofaktoren kindlicher Entwicklung: Migration, Leistungsangst und Schulübergang*, Hrsg. A. Schründer-Lenzen, 208–222. Wiesbaden: VS.

Hascher, Tina. 2003. Well-being in school - why students need social support. In *Learning emotions. The influence of affective factors on classroom learning*, Hrsg. P. Mayring & C. von Rhoeneck. Frankfurt am Main: Peter Lang.

Hascher, Tina. 2004. *Wohlbefinden in der Schule*. Munster: Waxmann.

Hascher, T. & G. Hagenauer. 2010. Alienation from Schoo. *International Journal of Educational Research* 49:220–32.

Hascher, T. & G. Hagenauer. 2011a. Schulisches Wohlbefinden im Jugendalter – Verläufe und Einflussfaktoren. In *Jahrbuch Jugendforschung*. Bd. 10 Hrsg. A. Ittel, H. Merkens & L. Stecher, 14–45. Wiesbaden: VS.

Hascher, T. & G. Hagenauer. 2011b. Wohlbefinden und Emotionen in der Schule als zentrale Elemente des Schulerfolgs unter der Perspektve geschlechtsspezifischer Ungleichheiten. In *Geschlechtsspezifische Bildungsungleichheiten*, Hrsg. A. Hadjar. 285–308. Wiesbaden: VS.

Haubl, Rolf. 2007. Schule als pathogener Ort. *Gruppenpsychotherapie und Gruppendynamik*, 4/2007, 259–276

Jungbauer-Gans, M. & P. Kriwy. 2004. Ungleichheit und Gesundheit von Kindern und Jugendlichen. In *Soziale Benachteiligung und Gesundheit bei Kindern und Jugendlichen*, Hrsg. M. Jungbauer-Gans & P. Kriwy, 9–23. Wiesbaden: VS.

Låftman, S. B. & B. Modin. 2012. School-Performance Indicators and Subjective Health Complaints: Are There Gender Differences?: School-Performance Indicators and Subjective Health Complaints. *Sociology of Health & Illness* 34:608–25.

Lampert, T. & M. Richter. 2006. Gesundheitliche Ungleichheit bei Kindern und Jugendlichen". In *Gesundheitliche Ungleichheit: Grundlagen, Probleme, Konzepte*, Hrsg. M. Richter & K. Hurrelmann, 199–220. Wiesbaden: VS.

Lindenberg, S. 1996 Continuities in the Theory *of* Social Production Functions". In *Verklarende Sociologie*, Hrsg. H. Ganzeboom & S. Lindenberg, 169-184. Amsterdam: Thesis Publishers.

McLeod, J. D. & T. J. Owens. 2004. Psychological Well-Being in the Early Life Course: Variations by Socioeconomic Status, Gender, and Race/Ethnicity. *Social Psychology Quaterly* 67:257–78.

Moor, I., M. Richter, U. Ravens-Sieberer, V. Ottova-Jordan, F. J. Elgar & T.-K. Pförtner. 2015. Trends in Social Inequalities in Adolescent Health Complaints from 1994 to 2010 in Europe, North America and Israel: The HBSC Study. *The European Journal of Public Health* 25(Supplement 2):57–60.

Moreno, E. S. & A. Barrón López de Roda. 2003. Social Psychology of Mental Health: The Social Structure and Personality Perspective. *The Spanish Journal of Psychology* 6:3–11.

Morinaj, J., J. Scharf, A. Grecu, A. Hadjar, T. Hascher & K. Marcin. 2017. School Alienation: A Construct Validation Study. *Frontline Learning Research* 5: 36–59.

Ormel, J., S. Lindenberg, N. Steverink & L. M. Verbrugge. 1999. Subjective Well-Being and Social Production Functions. Social Indicators Research. 46, 61–90.

Pollard, E. & P. D. Lee. 2003. Child well-being: A systematic review of the literature. *Social Indicators Research* 61:59–78.

Proctor, C. L., P. A. Linley & J. Maltby. 2009. Youth Life Satisfaction: A Review of the Literature. *Journal of Happiness Studies* 10:583–630.

Quenzel, G. & Hurrelmann, K. (2011). Entwicklungsaufgaben und Schulerfolg. Stehen geschlechts-spezifische Bewältigungsmuster hinter dem Bildungserfolg von Frauen? In *Ge-schlechtsspezifische Bildungsungleichheiten. Systematischer Überblick zur Frage der Bildungungleichheit zwischen den Geschlechtern*, Hrsg. A. Hadjar, 125–148. Wiesbaden: VS.

Qvortrup, Jens. 2005. Kinder und Kindheit in der Sozialstruktur. In *Kindheit soziologisch*, Hrsg. H. Hengst & H. Zeiher, 27–47. Wiesbaden: VS.

Ravens-Sieberer, U., J. Freeman, G. Kokonyei, C. A. Thomas & M. Erhart. 2009. School as a Determinant for Health Outcomes – a Structural Equation Model Analysis. *Health Education* 109:342–56.

Ravens-Sieberer, U., G Kökönyei & C. Thomas. 2004. School and health. In *Young people's health in context. Health behaviour in school-aged children (HBHC) study: international report from the 2001/2002 survey, Health Policy for Children and Adolescents*, Hrsg. C. Currie, C. Roberts, A. Morgan, R. Smith, W. Settertobulte, O. Samdal & V. B. Rasmussen, 184–196. Kopenhagen: World Health Organization.

Rayce, S. L. B., B. E. Holstein & S. Kreiner. 2008. Aspects of Alienation and Symptom Load among Adolescents. *The European Journal of Public Health* 19:79–84.

Rubin, K. H., K. B. Burgess, A. E. Kennedy & S. L. Stewart. 2003. Social withdrawal in childhood. In *Child psychopathology*, E. J. Mash & R. A. Barkley, 372–406. New York: Guilford Press.

Saab, H. & D. Klinger. 2010. School Differences in Adolescent Health and Wellbeing: Findings from the Canadian Health Behaviour in School-Aged Children Study. *Social Science & Medicine* 70:850–58.

Scharf, J., A. Hadjar & A. Grecu. 2019. Applying social production function theory to benefits of schooling: the concept of values of education. *British Journal of Sociology of Education* 40: 847–867.

Shaw, S. R., P. Gomes, A. Polotskaia & A. M. Jankowska. 2015. The relationship between student health and academic performance: Implications for school psychologists. *School Psychology International* 36:115–134.

Torsheim, T. & B. Wold. 2001. School-Related Stress, Support, and Subjective Health Complaints among Early Adolescents: A Multilevel Approach. *Journal of Adolescence* 24:701–13.

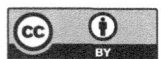

Working Conditions of Young People in Luxembourg – A Health Perspective

Philipp E. Sischka und Georges Steffgen

1 Introduction

1.1 Labor Market Entry and Working Conditions

The transition from youth to adulthood can be described as a sequence of events that includes finishing (school) education, entering labor market, gaining financial independence from the family of origins, setting up a separate household, establishing a long-term relationship with a life partner, becoming a parent (Elfering et al. 2007; Nilsen et al. 2018). Thus, adulthood marks the 'mature individual' and is associated with autonomy and independence from the family of origin (Nilsen et al. 2018). However, recent research showed that structural changes in Western societies during the past decades lead to greater variability and fragmentation in transitions to adulthood, questioning the prototypical sequence of these social markers (Billari et al. 2019; Buchmann and Kriesi 2011; Hellevik and Settersten 2013). In this context, the successful integration in the labor market plays an important role for young people (Buchmann and Kriesi 2011). However, the employment prospects of youths and young people are more dependent on

P. E. Sischka (✉) · G. Steffgen
Department of Behavioural and Cognitive Sciences, University of Luxembourg, Esch-sur-Alzette, Luxembourg
E-Mail: philipp.sischka@uni.lu

G. Steffgen
E-Mail: georges.steffgen@uni.lu

© Der/die Autor(en) 2022
A. Heinen et al. (Hrsg.), *Wohlbefinden und Gesundheit im Jugendalter*,
https://doi.org/10.1007/978-3-658-35744-3_12

macro-economic developments compared to adults.[1] Young people are labor market outsider as they possess only limited exploitable human capital (Lange and Reiter 2018). Thus, they have to prove potential employers that they possess an extraordinary willingness to learn and work. Therefore, many of them try to engage in continuative educational activity and low paid (or unpaid) internships (Lange and Reiter 2018). Thus, with regard to the labor market, young persons are in situations where they are more exploitable. Moreover, there have been many changes in the labor market in recent decades, such as the delocalization of production, the development of non-permanent and part-time work, the introduction of new technologies (digitalization) and, thus, an increased demand of flexible employees with varied skills (Balliester and Elsheikhi 2018). Young people might be more vulnerable to this increase in employment flexibility because many of them had not a chance to gain work experience yet, lack of seniority and professional networks and many employers might use temporary contracts as screening instrument, when dismissal of permanent employees is costly (Bukodi et al. 2008).

The concrete experiences that young people encounter during the transition from school/education into work depend also on their specific working conditions. The working conditions have a strong influence on "whether the transition is experienced as predominantly stressful or as predominantly rewarding and challenging" (Elfering et al. 2007, 98). Thus, the beginning of a job may be a time when a young person's health and well-being is challenged. Indeed, the link between poor psychosocial job quality and health and well-being among young people have been well established (e.g., Milner et al. 2017). What constitutes high job quality is still under debate (Steffgen et al. 2020). However, there is a consensus that it includes positive interactions with others (colleagues, supervisors, clients, etc.), feedback about job performance, working autonomously, skill development and learning, as well as providing benefits such as pay and security (Gallie 2007; Milner et al. 2017).

1.2   Working Conditions and Health and Well-being

Some authors (e.g., Muñoz de Bustillo et al. 2011; Van Aerden et al. 2016) decompose job quality into two broad areas: employment quality and quality of work. Employment quality describe all job characteristics that can be perceived

---

[1] For instance, young people in Europe suffered a disproportionate share of job losses during the global economic crisis (Bell and Blanchflower 2011).

as the framework surrounding the intrinsic activity of work (e.g., career advancement, work-life balance). Employment quality includes income satisfaction, training opportunities, career advancement, job security, difficulty of job change, and work-life-conflict. Income is an important concern for employees. However, what seems to be more important for well-being and job satisfaction than income is satisfaction with income that is affected by the discrepancy of income that employees think they should receive and their actual income (Williams et al. 2006). Indeed, research has shown that high income does not improve emotional well-being (Kahneman and Deaton 2010) and that rank of income, not income per se, affects life satisfaction (Boyce et al. 2010). Therefore, income satisfaction can be seen as key contributor to job satisfaction (Williams et al. 2006). Training opportunities have been linked with job satisfaction (Schmidt, 2007), increased work engagement (Bakker 2011) and reduced turnover intentions (Koster et al. 2011). Career advancement has been linked with higher job satisfaction (Kalleberg 1977), higher affective commitment and higher work engagement (Poon 2013), as well as reduced turnover (Kraimer et al. 2011). Job insecurity has been meta-analytically linked to various negative outcomes such as reduced job satisfaction and mental health (Sverke et al. 2002). Furthermore, employability is also linked to well-being (De Cuyper et al. 2008). Moreover, low work-life-balance (i.e., work-life conflict) has been found to be related with strain and poor psychological health (Lunau et al. 2014; Nohe et al. 2015).

Quality of work refers to the ways and conditions under which the activity of work can affect the well-being of workers, often focusing on job design, work intensity, social and physical conditions. Job design includes participation in decision making, feedback about their job performance and working autonomously. Participation refers to the involvement of employees in decision-making processes. Previous research has shown that this form of participation is linked with less role stress (e.g., role conflict, role ambiguity; Jackson 1983), perceived supervisor and organizational support (Reeves et al. 2012), job satisfaction, skill use and skill enhancement (Gallie 2013). Feedback reflects the degree to which other organizational members (i.e., colleagues, supervisors) provide information about the work output. It has been meta-analytically linked with burnout and engagement (Crawford et al. 2010). Autonomy reflects if an employee has ample opportunities to do his/her work autonomously (i.e., decide when and how to do the work as well as the content and order of tasks). It is one of the most often researched job resources (Nielsen et al. 2017) and has been meta-analytically linked with burnout (Alarcon 2011) and work engagement (Halbesleben 2010). The different dimensions of work intensity are job demands that are also related to employee's well-being. High mental demands can decrease well-being, when no recovery takes place (Meijman and Mulder 1998). It has been linked with psychological ill health (Michélsen and Bildt 2003). Time pressure has been meta-analytically linked to reduced well-being (LePine et al. 2005), also on a day-to-day level (Ilies et al. 2010) and might also lead to a lack of psychological detachment (Sonnentag et al. 2014). Emotional demands have been meta-analytically linked with reduced well-being and job attitudes (Hülsheger and Schewe 2011; Zapf 2002). Additionally, a plethora of studies has shown that social conditions have a strong influence on employee's health, attitude and behavior. One of the most often studied condition is social support (Nielsen et al. 2017). Social support represents a job resource that reflects the degree to which an employee gets advice and assistance from others when needed. Social support has various effects on well-being as it reduces the experienced strain, mitigates perceived stressors and buffers the stressor-strain relationship (Viswesvaran et al. 1999). In contrast, competition and mobbing can be seen as special job stressors. Competition has been linked to workaholism (Keller et al. 2016), and thus, might also have an influence on employee's well-being. Workplace mobbing refers to a situation, where the employee is being subjected to a series of negative and/or hostile acts or other behaviors that are experienced as annoying and/or oppressive at the workplace (Agervold and Mikkelsen 2004). It is a serious phenomenon that has various negative consequences for the targeted employees' health (e.g., depression, burnout), attitudes (e.g., lower job commitment), and work-related behavior (e.g., absence; see Nielsen and Einarsen 2012; Sischka et al. 2020a, 2021). Finally, physical conditions can be seen as job demands that are related to well-being and health. Risk of accidents and physical burden have been linked to well-being and physical health (e.g., Nahrgang et al. 2011; Bailey et al. 2015; Burr et al. 2017). To summarize, there is a vast amount of studies showing that working conditions affect well-being, health, and motivation among others (Bakker and Demerouti 2017; Oldham and Fried 2016; Parker 2014).

1.3   Aims of the Current Study

It is important to research working conditions in a Luxembourgish context to guide possible policy interventions. The Luxembourgish labor market differs in some respect from labor markets in other European countries. For instance, compared to young employees in other European countries, the percentage of young employees in Luxembourg with a permanent contract is quite high, the same applies to full-time employment (Nunez and Livanos 2015; Rokicka et al. 2015). Moreover, regarding working conditions there also exists quite some variation between European countries. Recent research has revealed that Luxembourg has a high mobbing (Sischka and Steffgen 2019a) and risk of depression prevalence (Sischka and Steffgen 2020) at the workplace. Thus, it is important to study how Luxembourg performs in relation to other working conditions and health and well-being dimensions. Furthermore, as younger and older workers differ regarding their needs, attitudes, and skills, it is important to employ a lifespan development perspective on working conditions and job design (Truxillo et al. 2012). Age is associated with personality (Roberts et al. 2006), cognitive functions (Craik and Salthouse 2008), physical ability, work experience, health (Kanfer and Ackerman 2004; Kooij et al. 2008), and family demands (Thrasher et al. 2016) among others, with the possible consequence that working conditions might be perceived differently by employees in different age ranges. Indeed, research has revealed that the association between certain working conditions (e.g., autonomy) and well-being and health (e.g., burnout; Ng and Feldman 2015) as well as between working conditions and job attraction (Zacher et al. 2017) is moderated by age. For instance, a meta-analysis (Ng and Feldman 2015) found that the association between job autonomy and job satisfaction is weaker for older employees. However, the moderation effect of age on the association between many other working conditions (e.g., career advancement) and different well-being dimensions have not been studied so far.

This chapter focuses on the working conditions of young employees in Luxembourg from a health perspective. It sheds light on the development of employment quality, quality of work and well-being dimensions for young employees (between 16 and 29 years) and compares this with the development of these dimensions for older employees. Furthermore, this chapter explores the intercorrelations between different working conditions and different well-being dimensions and investigates if these intercorrelations are different between young employees and older ones. Moreover, with regression analyses it is explored whether certain working conditions are more important for younger employees compared to older ones. By this, the chapter wants to give answers to the following questions: How do young employees perceive their working environment compared to older ones? Does the influence of certain working conditions on well-being and health differ between young employees and older ones? Are certain working conditions more important for young employees than for older ones regarding well-being and health?

Table 1 Quality of Work project description (own illustration)

Dimension	Description
Aim of study	Investigation of the work situation and quality of employees in Luxembourg
Conceptual design, implementation, analysis	University of Luxemburg: INSIDE, Luxembourgish Chamber of Labor, since 2014 Infas Institute, before TNS-ILRES
Survey methodology	Computer-assisted telephone interview (CATI) or computer-assisted web interview (CAWI, since 2018) in Luxembourgish, German, French, Portuguese or English
Sample size for the last waves	2016: 1506, 2017: 1522, 2018: 1689; 2019: 1495

2   Methods

2.1   Data

The Quality of Work project aims to assess the work quality and its effects on well-being among employees working in Luxembourg. It was implemented by the University of Luxembourg in collaboration with the Luxembourg Chamber of Labor (a council that aims to defend the employees' rights with regards to legislation) as an assessment over yearly waves since 2014[2]. Data are entailed via Computer-Assisted Telephone Interviews (CATI) and (since 2018) via computer-assisted web interview (CAWI) and represent a stratified random sample that is also representative in terms of workers' state of residency in Luxembourg (see Table 1 for the project description). The annually survey is conducted according to the Declaration of Helsinki (i.e., voluntary participation, participants were free to withdraw their consent at any time throughout the interviews without negative consequences for them). Data from the most recent 2019 wave was used for the correlation and regression analyses. A weighting variable was used that accounts for unequal sample selection probability and adjusts the sample so that it reflects the socio-demographic structure of the target population[3] (i.e., post-stratification; for a detailed discussion

---

[2] The project started in 2013 with a pilot survey (Steffgen and Kohl 2013).

[3] A different socio-demographic structure between the sample and the population can result from non-response.

of the data collection and weighting procedure see Schütz and Thiele 2019). Finally, the development of employment quality, quality of work and well-being dimensions between 2016 and 2019 was described with data from these waves.[4]

2.2 Measures

The project assesses annually information on employment quality (i.e., income satisfaction, training opportunities, career advancement, job security, difficulty to change job, work life conflict), quality of work (i.e., participation, feedback, autonomy, social support, mobbing, competition, mental demands, time pressure, emotional demands, physical burden, risk of accident) and well-being (i.e., work satisfaction, vigor, burnout, general well-being, subjective health problems) dimensions. These dimensions are measured with 2–7-item scales (see the Table in the Appendix for number of items and internal consistencies). A 5-point Likert response format was used, either with frequency categories (never, seldom, sometimes, often, (almost) always) or with degree of extent (to a very low extent, to a low extent, to a medium extent, to a large extent, to a very large extent). Additionally, work satisfaction, vigor (Schaufeli et al. 2006) burnout, general well-being (Topp et al. 2015; Sischka et al. 2020b), and health problems are assessed. All scales are standardized so that they have a possible range between 0–100 (for a detailed discussion and in-depth psychometric analyses on these scales see Sischka and Steffgen 2019b and Steffgen et al. 2020).[5]

3 Results

3.1 Demographic and Employment Characteristics

Table 2 shows some demographic characteristics and employment conditions across the three age groups. Only 48.8% of the employees between 16 and 29 years are currently in a partnership, compared to 77.8% of employees between 30 and 54 years and 81.8% of employees that are 55 years old or older.

---

[4] Although this project is partially conceptualized as a longitudinal study, the data were treated only in a trend design matter (i.e., each wave as independent from each other).

[5] See Table 3 in the Appendix for the scale reliabilities of the employment quality, quality of work and well-being scales.

Table 2 Demographics and employment characteristics for age groups (in 2019) (own illustration)

Variables	N	16–29 years n (%)	30–54 years n (%)	55 + years n (%)	p (χ^2-test)
Sex – female	1494	145 (42.0)	410 (41.0)	56 (37.8)	.685
Partnership – yes	1494	168 (48.8)	780 (77.8)	121 (81.8)	.000
Children – yes	1495	53 (15.4)	690 (68.9)	87 (58.4)	.000
Supervisor – yes	1495	60 (17.4)	286 (28.6)	47 (31.8)	.000
Permanent contract – yes	1494	308 (89.3)	981 (97.9)	144 (97.3)	.000
Full-time employment – yes	1494	319 (92.5)	797 (79.6)	112 (75.7)	.000
	N	16–29 years M (SD)	30–54 years M (SD)	55 + years M (SD)	p (F-test)
Contractual working hours (per week)	1486	38.8 (4.7)	37.5 (6.0)	36.7 (6.8)	.000
Actual working hours (per week)	1484	42.3 (7.9)	40.2 (8.6)	39.0 (9.3)	.000

Furthermore, only 15.4% of the younger employees live with at least one child in the household compared to 68.9% of employees between 30 and 54 years. Regarding employment characteristics, about 17.4% of the young employees have supervisor responsibilities, compared to 28.6% of the employees in the middle age category and 31.8% in the oldest age category. Moreover, younger employees have less often a permanent contract (89.3% compared to 97.9% and 97.3% in the middle and oldest age group) and more often a full-time employment (92.5% vs. 79.6% and 75.7%). This is also reflected by the contractual and actual working hours per week: On average, employees between 16 and 29 years have longer contractually arranged working hours (38.8 h) and longer actual working hours (42.3 h) per week compared to employees in the middle (37.5 h and 40.2 h) and in the oldest (36.7 h and 39.0 h) age category.

3.2　Mean Differences Across Age Groups

Figure 1 shows the mean-centered employment quality dimensions across the three age groups. A positive value indicates that the group mean is above the total mean, whereas a negative value indicates that the group mean is below the total mean. The younger employees are significantly less satisfied with their income compared to older employees (see the non-overlapping confidence intervals). On the other hand, younger employees perceive more training opportunities and more career advancement than the older age groups. Moreover, they perceive lower levels of job change difficulties. The oldest age group perceives the lowest level of work-life conflict.

Figure 2 shows the Quality of work dimensions. Younger employees get more feedback and more social support, compared to the older age groups. On the other hand, they perceive their work situation as less autonomous. Compared with employees between 30 and 54 years, younger employees report higher levels of physical burden and risk of accident.

Figure 3 shows the different well-being and health dimensions across age groups. There are no significant differences for work satisfaction, burnout and health problems. However, employees with an age of 55 years and more report higher levels of vigor and general well-being compared with employees between 16 and 29 years and employees between 30 and 54 years.

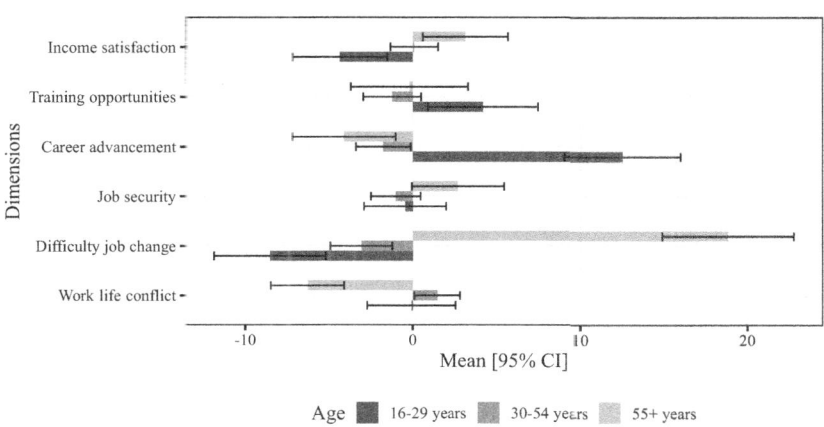

Fig. 1 Means of Employment quality dimensions (mean-centered) across age groups (2019) (own illustration)

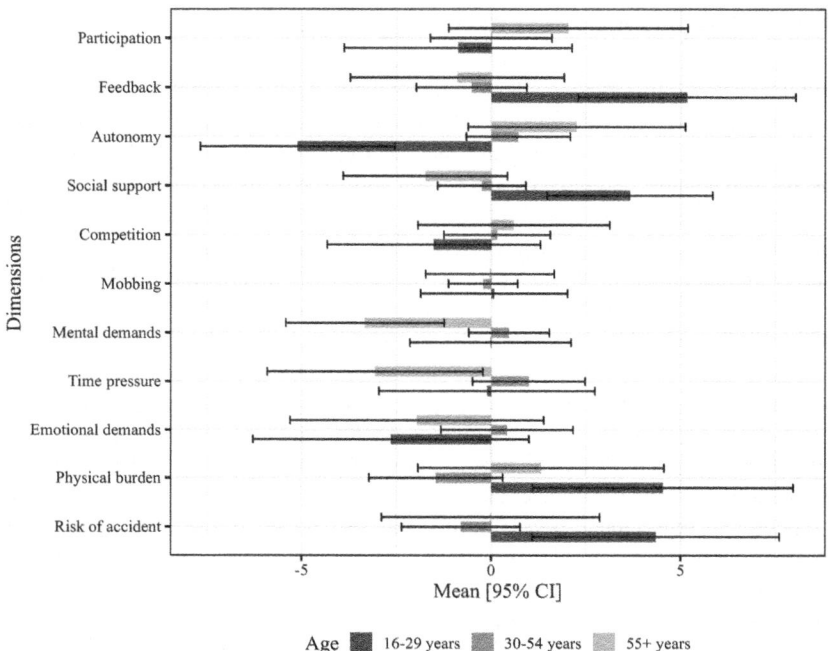

Fig. 2 Means of Quality of work dimensions (mean-centered) across age groups (2019) (own illustration)

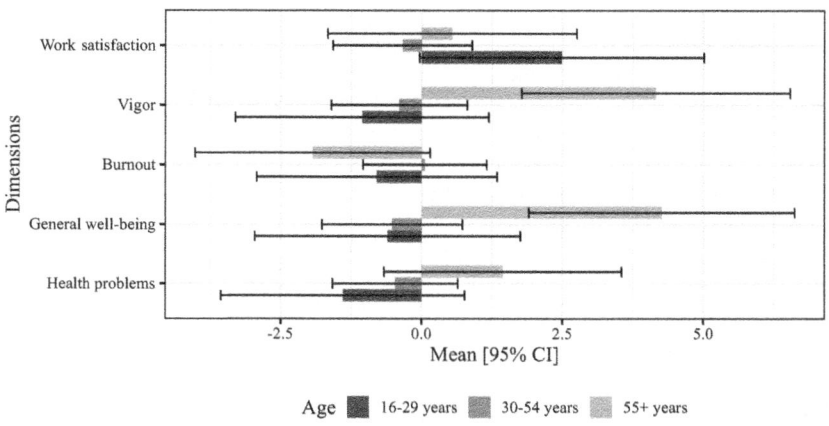

Fig. 3 Means of Well-Being dimensions (mean-centered) across age groups (2019) (own illustration)

3.3   Intercorrelations Between Working Conditions and Well-being Across Age Groups

Figure 4 shows the intercorrelations between the different working conditions and health and well-being measures across the different age groups. Generally, the correlations do not differ much between the age groups. Interestingly, difficulty to change the job is not related to any of the health and well-being measures for the youngest employees, whereas for the older age groups it is associated with less health and well-being. Work satisfaction is strongly positively intercorrelated with participation, feedback, social support and income satisfaction and strongly negatively intercorrelated with mobbing. Vigor is negatively interrelated with mobbing and work-life-conflict. Burnout shows the strongest intercorrelations with mobbing, emotional demands and work life conflict. General well-being is strongly positively associated with income satisfaction and negatively associated with mobbing and work life conflict. Finally, health problems are most strongly correlated with physical burden and work life conflict.

3.4   Regression Analyses with Well-being Measures as Outcomes

Table 3 shows the result of the regression analyses with the different well-being measures as outcome variables and age groups, the different working conditions and the product terms of age groups and working conditions (interaction effects) as predictors. The age group 16–29 years represents the reference group. Thus, the regression coefficients of the working conditions represent those of the youngest employees. The interaction effects represent the change in the main effects for the two other age groups. Regarding work satisfaction, participation, social support, mobbing, time pressure, income satisfaction and training opportunities showed significant effects on the outcome variable. There were two significant interaction effects. The slopes of the variables physical burden and job security changed for one of the two other age groups. Physical burden and job security had stronger effects on work satisfaction for the oldest age group. Higher levels of physical burden and higher level of job security corresponded with higher levels of work satisfaction in the oldest age group. Regarding vigor as outcome variable, feedback, training opportunities, career advancement and job security were significant predictors in the youngest age group. One inter-action term was significant. For employees in the middle age group, difficulties

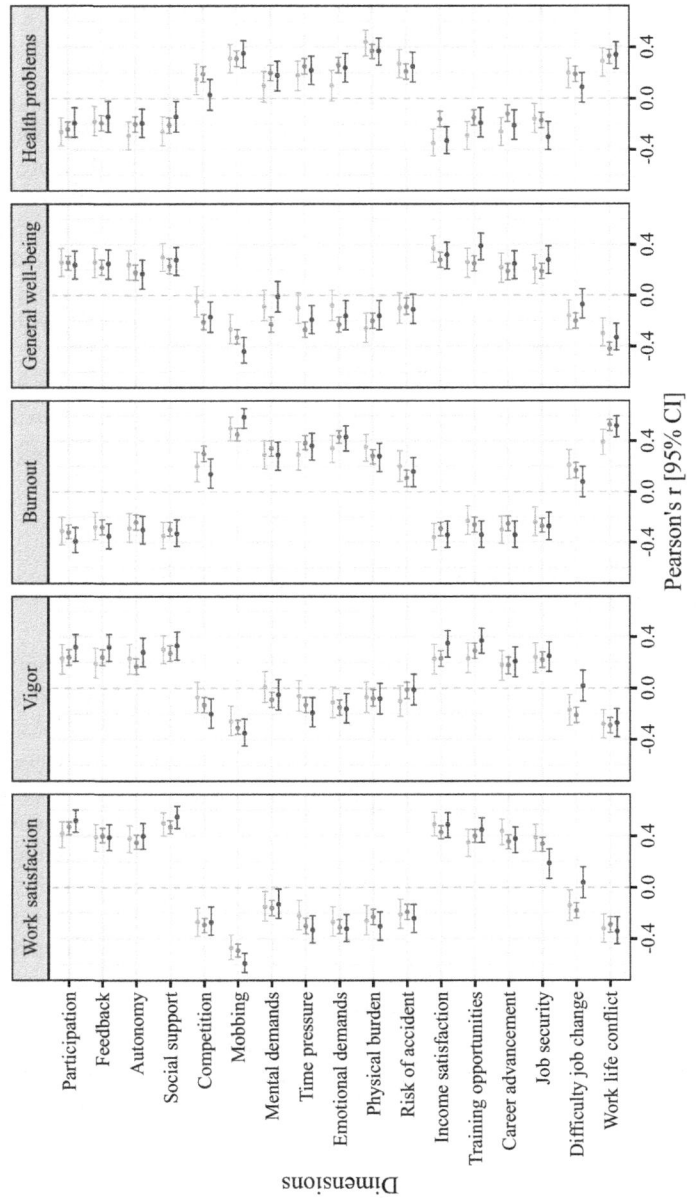

Fig. 4 Intercorrelations between working conditions and well-being dimensions across age groups (2019) (own illustration)

Age ⊹ 16-29 years ⊹ 30-54 years ⊹ 55+ years

Table 3 Regression results using well-being dimensions as criteria

Predictor	Work satisfaction b	95% CI [LL, UL]	Vigor b	95% CI [LL, UL]	Burnout b	95% CI [LL, UL]	General well-being b	95% CI [LL, UL]	Health problems b	95% CI [LL, UL]
Intercept	42.30***	[30.30, 54.30]	22.95***	[9.03, 39.06]	22.08**	[12.05, 33.84]	49.34***	[34.62, 64.06]	21.30**	[7.86, 34.74]
Reference: age group: 16-29 years										
age group: 30-54 years	-4.28	[-18.19, 9.63]	-1.26	[5.25, 40.05]	-0.71	[-13.88, 11.36]	-10.27	[5.02, 39.14]	-0.27	[-25.85, 5.30]
age group: 55+ years	-12.99	[-37.10, 11.00]	-3.33	[19.14, 38.35]	-0.01	[-13.46, 18.54]	-6.72	[-38.97, 27.49]	-0.72	[-32.46, 19.02]
Participation	0.13***	[0.05, 0.20]	0.02	[-0.06, 0.13]	0.02	[-0.05, 0.08]	0.05	[-0.07, 0.12]	0.05	[-0.03, 0.13]
Feedback	0.01	[-0.06, 0.09]	-0.07	[0.02, 0.22]	0.02	[-0.13, 0.00]	0.02	[-0.07, 0.12]	0.02	[-0.07, 0.10]
Autonomy	0.02	[-0.06, 0.11]	-0.02	[-0.01, 0.20]	-0.05	[-0.09, 0.06]	0.03	[-0.15, 0.05]	0.03	[-0.06, 0.13]
Social support	0.28***	[0.18, 0.38]	-0.01	[-0.05, 0.20]	0.01	[-0.10, 0.08]	0.01	[-0.11, 0.14]	0.01	[-0.11, 0.12]
Competition	0.00	[-0.07, 0.07]	-0.09**	[-0.10, 0.08]	0.02	[-0.16, -0.03]	-0.12**	[-0.46, -0.16]	0.20**	[-0.20, -0.05]
Mobbing	-0.21***	[-0.40, -0.17]	0.40***	[-0.21, 0.03]	-0.31***	[1.29, 0.50]	0.20**	[0.02, 0.26]	0.06	[0.06, 0.33]
Mental demands	-0.01	[-0.11, 0.09]	0.06	[-0.08, 0.17]	0.14*	[-0.03, 0.15]	0.06	[-0.19, 0.01]	0.02	[-0.05, 0.17]
Time pressure	-0.09*	[-0.18, -0.01]	0.10***	[-0.20, 0.00]	-0.01	[-0.03, 0.11]	0.06*	[-0.08, 0.05]	0.18***	[-0.07, 0.11]
Emotional demands	-0.03	[-0.09, 0.02]	0.10**	[-0.05, 0.12]	-0.03	[0.03, 0.16]	-0.01	[-0.11, 0.06]	-0.01	[0.00, 0.12]
Physical burden	-0.05	[-0.12, 0.02]	-0.08*	[-0.05, 0.13]	0.00	[-0.14, -0.01]	-0.09	[-0.09, 0.09]	-0.01	[0.10, 0.25]
Risk of accident	-0.04	[-0.11, 0.04]	-0.05	[-0.05, 0.13]	-0.03	[0.12, 0.02]	-0.04	[-0.04, 0.14]	-0.15***	[-0.09, 0.08]
Income satisfaction	0.18***	[0.10, 0.25]	0.09	[-0.18, 0.26]	0.19***	[1.00, 0.01]	-0.15***	[0.10, 0.27]	-0.01	[-0.24, -0.07]
Training opportunities	0.13***	[0.05, 0.21]	0.17***	[-0.22, -0.04]	-0.09*	[-0.08, 0.03]	-0.02	[-0.17, 0.00]	-0.15***	[-0.06, 0.11]
Career advancement	-0.01	[-0.08, 0.06]	0.13**	[-0.05, 0.09]	-0.01	[-0.18, -0.04]	-0.17***	[0.07, 0.26]	0.04	[-0.26, -0.09]
Job security	-0.05	[-0.12, 0.03]	0.02	[-0.13, 0.16]	0.16***	[-0.01, 0.09]	-0.03	[-0.09, 0.04]	-0.02	[-0.02, 0.10]
Difficulty job change	0.03	[-0.03, 0.08]	0.04	[-0.07, 0.39]	-0.03	[-0.32, 0.01]	0.12**	[-0.11, 0.09]	0.04	[0.05, 0.22]
Work life conflict	-0.04	[-0.11, 0.04]	-0.11**	[-0.11, 0.25]	0.05	[-0.08, 0.18]	-0.11*	[-0.11, 0.24]	-0.17***	[-0.20, -0.01]
a.g. 30-54 y. x Participation	-0.04	[-0.12, 0.05]	0.04	[-0.18, 0.01]	0.07	[0.02, 0.17]	-0.04	[-0.26, -0.07]	0.04	[-0.19, 0.11]
a.g. 55+ y. x Participation	-0.11	[-0.25, 0.02]	0.22***	[-0.10, 0.11]	0.17	[0.15, 0.29]	-0.06	[-0.02, 0.19]	0.13**	[0.05, 0.22]
a.g. 30-54 y. x Feedback	0.02	[-0.06, 0.11]	-0.06	[-0.28, 0.30]	0.07	[-0.14, 0.02]	-0.05	[-0.13, 0.20]	-0.11**	[-0.20, -0.01]
a.g. 55+ y. x Feedback	0.09	[-0.05, 0.24]	-0.13	[-0.24, 0.05]	0.19	[-0.15, 0.11]	-0.04	[-0.09, 0.13]	-0.04	[-0.19, 0.11]
a.g. 30-54 y. x Autonomy	0.04	[-0.06, 0.13]	0.03	[-0.27, 0.21]	0.09	[-0.03, 0.32]	0.03	[-0.15, 0.30]	-0.01	[-0.14, 0.06]
a.g. 55+ y. x Autonomy	-0.01	[-0.06, 0.24]	0.04	[-0.07, 0.29]	0.02	[-0.09, 0.08]	0.01	[-0.09, 0.14]	0.03	[-0.13, 0.19]
a.g. 30-54 y. x Social support	-0.08	[-0.06, 0.13]	0.01	[-0.09, 0.04]	0.02	[-0.18, 0.08]	-0.03	[-0.06, 0.29]	-0.05	[-0.14, 0.08]
a.g. 55+ y. x Social support	-0.04	[-0.19, 0.04]	-0.05	[-0.13, 0.16]	0.03	[-0.11, 0.05]	-0.07	[-0.20, 0.06]	-0.07	[-0.20, 0.06]
a.g. 30-54 y. x Competition	-0.07	[-0.22, 0.15]	-0.15	[-0.07, 0.39]	0.17	[-0.32, 0.01]	-0.10	[-0.06, 0.39]	-0.10	[-0.31, 0.10]
a.g. 55+ y. x Competition	0.05	[-0.21, 0.07]	0.10*	[-0.05, 0.16]	-0.01	[0.02, 0.17]	0.12*	[-0.11, 0.09]	0.12*	[0.03, 0.21]
a.g. 30-54 y. x Mobbing	-0.09	[-0.09, 0.19]	0.05	[-0.26, 0.09]	0.07	[-0.08, 0.18]	0.09	[-0.11, 0.24]	0.09	[-0.06, 0.25]
a.g. 55+ y. x Mobbing	0.05	[-0.10, 0.36]	0.01	[-0.28, 0.30]	0.17	[-0.33, 0.08]	-0.06	[0.00, 0.34]	-0.05	[-0.22, 0.09]
a.g. 30-54 y. x Mental demands	0.13	[-0.13, 0.11]	0.07	[-0.24, 0.05]	0.19	[-0.35, 0.08]	-0.05	[-0.09, 0.48]	0.03	[-0.31, 0.21]
a.g. 55+ y. x Mental demands	-0.01	[-0.33, 0.05]	-0.13	[-0.27, 0.21]	-0.29***	[-0.03, 0.18]	0.00	[-0.43, -0.15]	0.01	[-0.10, 0.16]
a.g. 30-54 y. x Time pressure	-0.14	[-0.06, 0.13]	0.07	[-0.24, 0.05]	-0.26*	[-0.03, 0.32]	0.01	[-0.49, -0.03]	0.00	[-0.22, 0.21]
a.g. 55+ y. x Time pressure	0.13	[-0.02, 0.27]	-0.01	[0.01, 0.24]	0.06	[-0.09, 0.08]	0.03	[-0.06, 0.29]	0.03	[-0.09, 0.21]
a.g. 30-54 y. x Emotional demands	-0.01	[-0.09, 0.05]	-0.02	[-0.09, 0.29]	0.03	[-0.16, 0.10]	-0.05	[-0.05, 0.17]	-0.05	[-0.13, 0.19]
a.g. 55+ y. x Emotional demands	-0.03	[-0.19, 0.09]	-0.06	[-0.21, 0.08]	0.04	[-0.08, 0.24]	-0.11	[-0.12, 0.09]	-0.11	[-0.24, 0.02]
a.g. 30-54 y. x Physical burden	0.07	[-0.01, 0.15]	0.01	[-0.07, 0.90]	0.02	[0.17, 0.04]	-0.02	[-0.12, 0.08]	-0.01	[-0.13, 0.16]
a.g. 55+ y. x Physical burden	0.14*	[0.00, 0.27]	0.09	[-0.07, 0.25]	-0.04	[-0.05, 0.10]	0.02	[-0.20, 0.11]	0.02	[-0.08, 0.11]
a.g. 30-54 y. x Risk of accident	0.00	[-0.08, 0.09]	0.00	[-0.11, 0.10]	0.02	[-0.01, 0.24]	0.01	[-0.08, 0.13]	0.01	[-0.08, 0.11]
a.g. 55+ y. x Risk of accident	-0.06	[-0.20, 0.08]	0.12	[-0.28, 0.06]	0.07	[-0.01, 0.04]	0.06	[0.14, 0.19]	0.06	[-0.09, 0.21]
a.g. 30-54 y. x Income satisfaction	0.00	[-0.08, 0.09]	-0.04	[-0.11, 0.10]	-0.04	[-0.18, 0.09]	-0.04	[-0.04, 0.18]	-0.04	[0.06, 0.25]
a.g. 55+ y. x Income satisfaction	0.03	[-0.12, 0.18]	0.12	[0.19, 0.18]	0.15	[-0.08, 0.07]	-0.06	[-0.03, 0.33]	-0.06	[-0.11, 0.22]
a.g. 30-54 y. x Training opportunities	-0.07	[-0.15, 0.02]	-0.04	[-0.15, 0.06]	0.00	[-0.08, 0.07]	-0.04	[-0.22, -0.01]	-0.04	[-0.13, 0.06]
a.g. 55+ y. x Training opportunities	-0.11	[-0.23, 0.02]	-0.05	[-0.26, 0.06]	0.02	[-0.09, 0.14]	-0.06	[-0.30, 0.02]	-0.06	[-0.21, 0.08]
a.g. 30-54 y. x Career advancement	0.08	[0.00, 0.16]	0.08	[-0.03, 0.18]	-0.02	[-0.09, 0.06]	0.05	[-0.04, 0.16]	0.05	[-0.04, 0.14]
a.g. 55+ y. x Career advancement	0.06	[-0.07, 0.20]	0.10	[-0.07, 0.27]	-0.14	[-0.14, 0.11]	-0.05	[-0.13, 0.30]	-0.05	[-0.20, 0.11]
a.g. 30-54 y. x Job security	0.14*	[0.00, 0.17]	-0.10	[-0.21, 0.09]	0.18**	[0.01, 0.16]	-0.18**	[-0.28, -0.07]	0.15**	[0.06, 0.25]
a.g. 55+ y. x Job security	0.09	[-0.09, 0.27]	-0.04	[0.01, 0.99]	-0.04	[-0.06, 0.06]	-0.16	[-0.14, 0.19]	0.25***	[0.01, 0.41]
a.g. 30-54 y. x Difficulty job change	0.00	[-0.08, 0.09]	0.00	[0.11, 0.10]	0.02	[-0.05, 0.10]	0.01	[-0.08, 0.13]	0.05	[-0.13, 0.16]
a.g. 55+ y. x Difficulty job change	-0.04	[-0.18, 0.10]	-0.02	[-0.11, 0.10]	-0.05	[-0.01, 0.24]	0.06	[-0.04, 0.18]	0.06	[-0.04, 0.16]
a.g. 30-54 y. x Work life conflict	-0.02	[-0.11, 0.07]	0.04	[0.19, 0.18]	-0.03	[-0.11, 0.04]	0.02	[-0.03, 0.33]	0.02	[-0.08, 0.12]
a.g. 55+ y. x Work life conflict	-0.07	[-0.23, 0.09]	-0.15	[0.35, 0.04]	0.00	[0.18, 0.11]	0.05	[-0.22, 0.17]	0.05	[-0.13, 0.23]
Fit	$R^2 = .56***$		$R^2 = .26***$		$R^2 = .54***$		$R^2 = .33***$		$R^2 = .32***$	

Note. b represents unstandardized regression weights. *LL* and *UL* indicate the lower and upper limits of a confidence interval, respectively. * indicates $p < .05$. ** indicates $p < .01$. *** indicates $p < .001$. (own illustration)

in changing the job had a negative influence on vigor. For burnout as outcome variable, competition, mobbing, emotional demands, physical burden, risk of accident, job security and work-life-conflict were significant predictors for employees in the youngest age group. Three interaction effects got significant. Compared with employees in the youngest age group competition and job security were more and mobbing was less important for burnout for employees in the middle age group. Regarding general well-being, mobbing, mental demands, training opportunities, career advancement, job security and work-life-conflict were significant predictors for the youngest employees. The lower mobbing and work-life-conflict and the higher mental demands, training opportunities, job security the higher was the general well-being. Compared with the youngest employees, mental demands had a negative and job security and training opportunities no effect on general well-being for employees in the middle age group. For health problems, competition, mobbing emotional demands, physical burden, income satisfaction, job security and work-life-conflict were significant predictors. Compared with the youngest employees, for employees in the middle age group participation was more and competition, income satisfaction and job security were less important for health problems. Again, compared with the youngest employees for employees in the oldest age group job security was less important for health problems.

3.5   Development of the Working Conditions and Well-being Dimensions

Figure 5 shows the development of the employment quality across the three age groups between 2016 and 2019. Most of the dimensions are quite stable over time. Younger employees perceive more training opportunities and stronger career advancement compared to older employees, a stable finding over time. Younger employees also perceive less difficulties in changing the job compared with employees that are 55 years old or older. Regarding income satisfaction, there is a small downturn for the youngest employees and a small upturn for the oldest employees. The oldest employees perceive their job as more secure compared to the employees in the youngest and middle age groups. On the other hand, employees that are 55 years old or older on average perceive less work life conflicts.

Figure 6 shows the development of the Quality of Work dimensions. Employees between 16 and 29 years reported more feedback and social support compared to older employees. However, young employees also report higher levels of physical burden and risk of accident over the years. There seems to be a slight trend downwards in all age groups for these dimensions. There are no clear differences regarding, participation, mobbing, competition, mental demands, time pressure and emotional demands.

Figure 7 shows the development of the different well-being dimensions for the three age groups. Employees between 16 and 29 years report higher levels of work satisfaction and lower levels of subjective health problems; these differences are quite stable over time. However, there are no age remarkable differences with regards to vigor, burnout and general well-being.

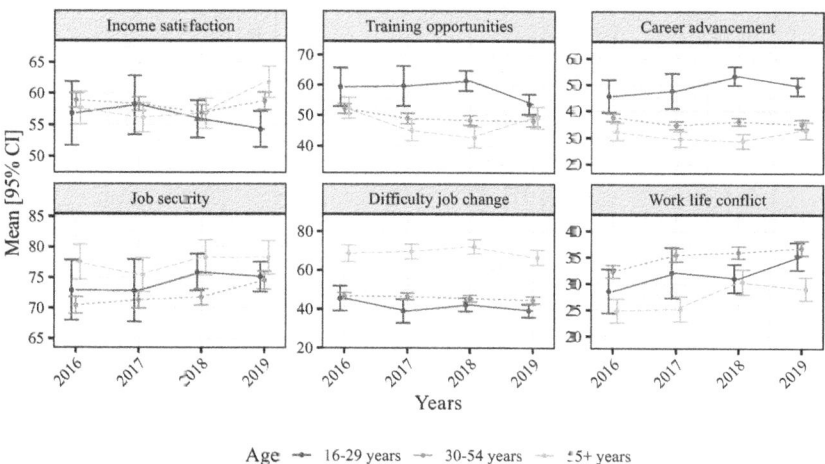

Fig. 5 Development of the Employment Quality dimensions across age groups (own illustration)

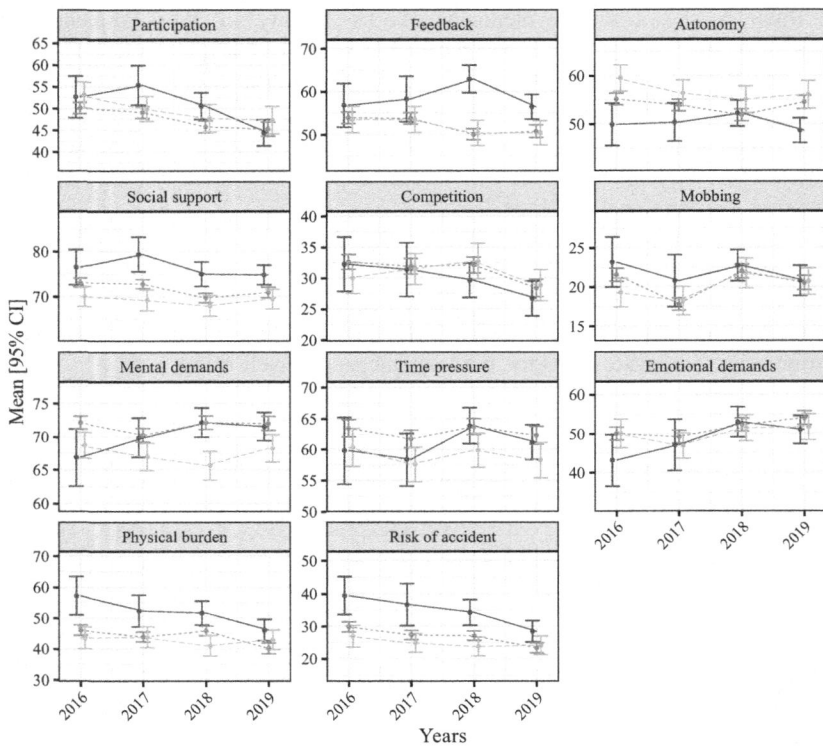

Fig. 6 Development of the Quality of work dimensions across age groups (own illustration)

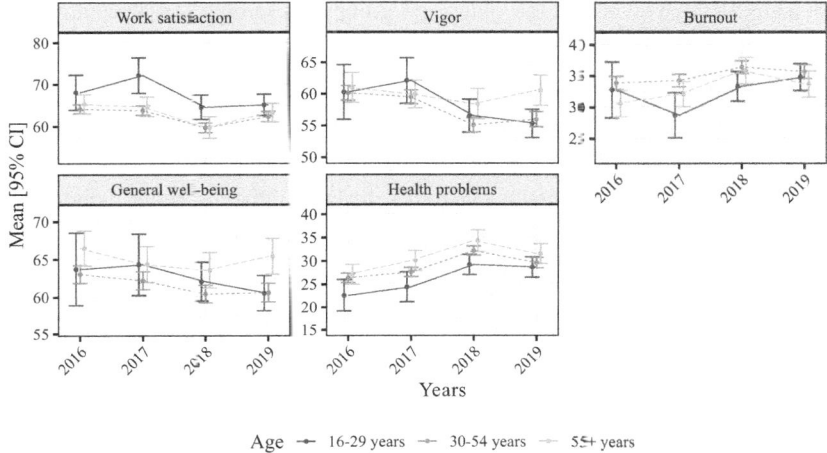

Fig. 7 Development of the Well-Being dimensions across age groups (own illustration)

4   Discussion and Conclusion

In this chapter the working conditions of younger employees (between 16 and 29 years old) compared with older ones were analyzed. Younger employees have less often a permanent contract and more often a full-time employment compared to the older age group. The large percentage of young employees with full-time employment is also reflected by the fact that this group on average works longer compared with employees in the older age group. With regard to employment quality, younger employees perceive more training opportunities and stronger career advancement as well as less difficulties in job change compared to employees in the older age group. Thus, one might conclude that young employees in Luxembourg are not particularly affected by "precarious" (Kretsos and Livanos 2016) or "insecure work" (Heery and Salmon 2000) that can be described as "uncertain, unpredictable and risk from the point of view of the worker" (Kalleberg 2009, p. 2) and that is characterized by fixed-term contracts, involuntary part-time work, and lack of training possibilities (Kretsos & Livanos 2016). On the other hand, the percentage of young employees and new hires with a fixed-term contract increased over the last years in Luxembourg (Eichhorst et al. 2017). With regard to job design, young employees perceive more feedback from their colleagues and their supervisors, but less autonomy at work compared to employees in the older age groups. Regarding social conditions, young employees perceive more social support from their colleagues. There is no difference for perceived competition and mobbing between the age groups. However, young employees report higher levels of physical burden and risk of accident. With regard to the well-being, younger employees report lower levels of vigor and general well-being.

Correlational and regression analyses revealed that working conditions are associated with employee's well-being and health, and that mobbing and work-life conflicts are especially detrimental. Moreover, regression analyses showed that the effects of certain working conditions on different well-being dimensions are not the same for the three age groups. Levels of work satisfaction of young employees seem to be less affected by lower job security compared to employees in the older age group. On the other side, the burnout level of young employees seems to be more affected by mobbing compared to the older age groups. Moreover, for the employees in the youngest age group mental demands is a positive predictor for general well-being, whereas it is a negative predictor for employees in the older age groups. A possible explanation for this finding might be the decline of cognitive functioning with age (Fisher et al. 2017) and the following different appraisal of mental demands. Whereas younger employees might regard mental demands more as a challenge, older employees might frame this work characteristic more as a hindrance[6] (Li et al. 2020). On the other hand, income satisfaction and job security are stronger predictors for health problems in employees in the youngest age group compared with older employees.

4.1   Practical Implications

The present study has shown that working conditions have not the same effects on well-being dimensions for all age groups, a finding that has been supported by previous research (Converso et al. 2018; Ramos et al. 2016; Zaniboni et al. 2013, 2016). Therefore, job design interventions should employ a lifespan development perspective (Truxillo et al. 2012, 2015) as working conditions seem to have different levels of importance for younger employees. If policy makers want to adapt a health perspective on working conditions of younger employees, there

---

[6]Challenges are job demands that appraise employees as potentially promoting their personal growth and achievement, while hindrances are job demands that appraise employees as potentially constraining their personal development and work-related accomplishment (Podsakoff et al. 2007).

exists feasible and effective intervention strategies (LaMontagne et al. 2010). However, the current study showed that they should try to improve the social conditions (i.e., reduction of mobbing incidents, increase of social support) as these are strong predictors of the younger employees health and well-being. Moreover, training opportunities and job security are especially important for younger employees' general well-being. Finally, mental demands seem to have beneficial effects for younger employees as opposed to older employees.

Recent research has indicated that working conditions have indeed changed since the last decades (Holman and Rafferty 2018; Wegman et al. 2018). The present study has also shown that small changes of working conditions can be observed within a short time period. It is important that these changes are monitored, and that negative developments are counteracted.

4.2   Limitations and Outlook

Some limitations of the present study need to be considered that provide directions for future research. First, it is important to note that the present study did not differentiate between educational levels due to sample size restrictions. Several studies showed that low-educated and low-skilled young people are more likely to be in a precarious/insecure working situation (e.g., Berloffa et al. 2019; de Grip and Wolbers 2006). Moreover, previous studies have found that especially young employees with lower educational levels report higher levels of adverse working conditions and lower health and well-being (Akkermans et al. 2013). Thus, future studies might also research education as possible boundary conditions of the present results. Second, the data analysis was only correlational, thus lacking time precedence. Therefore, causal assumptions cannot be drawn. Third, the present study used self-reported measures to assess working conditions. Strictly speaking, these are measures of perception, not objective working conditions (Bonde 2008). Moreover, the mono-method design may have led to an overrating of effects (i.e., common method variance; Podsakoff et al. 2012). Future studies might include additional data sources (e.g., observational studies, third-party reports) to assess the working conditions in a more objective way. Finally, the present study used a variable-oriented approach. Futures studies might employ a person-oriented approach that focus on identifying subpopulations of employees who show different patterns of working conditions (Mäkikangas et al. 2018).

Appendix

Table 4.

Table 4 Reliability of the scales (own illustration)

			Cronbach's α			
Area	Dimension	Number of items	2016	2017	2018	2019
Quality of Work	Participation	2	.73	.72	.75	.76
	Feedback	2	.70	.71	.74	.74
	Autonomy	4	.75	.74	.76	.74
	Social support	4	.79	.80	.82	.83
	Competition	4	.79	.77	.83	.81
	Mobbing	5	.71	.72	.77	.72
	Mental demands	4	.75	.74	.77	.75
	Time pressure	2	.70	.70	.76	.75
	Emotional demands	2	.79	.82	.85	.84
	Physical burden	2	.68	.71	.73	.74
	Risk of accident	2	.75	.78	.79	.79
Employment Quality	Income satisfaction	2	.89	.87	.89	.88
	Training opportunities	2	.87	.87	.85	.82
	Career advancement	2	.84	.84	.86	.87
	Job security	2	.76	.76	.77	.76
	Difficulty job change	2	.81	.83	.82	.84
	Work life conflict	3	.75	.78	.77	.80
Well-Being	Work satisfaction	3	.79	.83	.82	.80
	Vigor	3	.70	.65	.71	.70
	Burnout	6	.81	.80	.83	.82
	General well-being	5	.85	.83	.87	.87
	Health problems	7	.73	.72	.76	.76

References

Agervold, M., & Mikkelsen, E. G. (2004). Relationships between bullying, psychosocial work environment and individual stress reactions. *Work & Stress, 18*, 336-351. doi: https://doi.org/10.1080/02678370412331319794

Akkermans, J., Brenninkmeijer, V., Van Den Bossche, S. N., Blonk, R. W., & Schaufeli, W. B. (2013). Young and going strong? A longitudinal study on occupational health among young employees of different educational levels. *Career Development International, 18*, 416-435. doi: https://doi.org/10.1108/CDI-02-2013-0024

Alarcon, G. M. (2011). A meta-analysis of burnout with job demands, resources, and attitudes. *Journal of Vocational Behavior, 79*, 549-562. doi: https://doi.org/10.1016/j.jvb.2011.03.007

Bailey, T. S., Dollard, M. F., McLinton, S. S., & Richards, P. A. (2015). Psychosocial safety climate, psychosocial and physical factors in the aetiology of musculoskeletal disorder symptoms and workplace injury compensation claims. *Work & Stress, 29*, 190-211. doi: https://doi.org/10.1080/02678373.2015.1031855

Bakker, A. B. (2011). An Evidence-Based Model of Work Engagement. *Current Directions in Psychological Science, 20*, 265–269. doi: https://doi.org/10.1177/0963721411414534

Bakker, A. B., & Demerouti, E. (2017). Job demands–resources theory: taking stock and looking forward. *Journal of Occupational Health Psychology, 22*(3), 273-285. doi: https://doi.org/10.1037/ocp0000056

Balliester, T., & Elsheikhi, A. (2018). *The future of work: A literature review.* ILO, Working Paper, 29. Retrieved from https://www.ilo.org/wcmsp5/groups/public/---dgreports/---inst/documents/publication/wcms_625866.pdf

Bell, D. N. F., & Blanchflower, D. G. (2011). Youth unemployment in Europe and the United States. *Nordic Economic Policy Review, 1(2011)* 11–37. doi: https://doi.org/10.6027/9789289330541-3-en

Berloffa, G., Matteazzi, E., Şandor, A., & Villa, P. (2019). The quality of employment in the early labour market experience of young Europeans. *Cambridge Journal of Economics, 43*, 1549-1575. doi: https://doi.org/10.1093/cje/bez010

Billari, F. C., Hiekel, N., & Liefbroer, A. C. (2019). The social stratification of choice in the transition to adulthood. *European Sociological Review, 35*, 599-615. doi: https://doi.org/10.1093/esr/jcz025

Buchmann, M. C., & Kriesi, I. (2011). Transition to adulthood in Europe. *Annual Review of Sociology, 37*, 481-503. doi: https://doi.org/10.1146/annurev-soc-081309-150212

Bukodi, E., Ebralidze. E., Schmelzer, P., & Blossfeld, H.-P. (2008). Struggling to become an insider: Does increasing flexibility at labor market entry affect early careers? A theoretical framework. In H.-P. Blossfeld, S. Buchholz, E. Bukodi, & K. Kurz (Eds.), *Young workers, globalization and the labor market: Comparing early working life in eleven countries* (pp. 3-28). Northampton, MA: Edward Elgar

Bonde, J. P. E. (2008). Psychosocial factors at work and risk of depression: a systematic review of the epidemiological evidence. *Occupational and Environmental Medicine, 65*, 438-445. doi: https://doi.org/10.1136/oem.2007.038430

Boyce, C. J., Brown, G. D., & Moore, S. C. (2010). Money and happiness: Rank of income, not income, affects life satisfaction. *Psychological Science, 21*, 471-475. doi: https://doi.org/10.1177/0956797610362671

Burr, H., Pohrt, A., Rugulies, R., Holtermann, A., & Hasselhorn, H. M. (2017). Does age modify the association between physical work demands and deterioration of self-rated general health? *Scandinavian Journal of Work, Environment & Health, 43*, 241-249. doi: https://doi.org/10.5271/sjweh.3625

Converso, D., Sottimano, I., Guidetti, G., Loera, B., Cortini, M., & Viotti, S. (2018). Aging and work ability: the moderating role of job and personal resources. *Frontiers in Psychology, 8*, 2262. doi: https://doi.org/10.3389/fpsyg.2017.02262

Craik, F. I. M., Salthouse, T. A. (Eds.). (2008). *The handbook of aging and cognition*. New York: Psychology Press.

Crawford, E. R., LePine, J. A., & Rich, B. L. (2010). Linking job demands and resources to employee engagement and burnout: a theoretical extension and meta-analytic test. *Journal of Applied Psychology, 95*, 834-848. doi: https://doi.org/10.1037/a0019364

De Cuyper, N., Bernhard-Oettel, C., Berntson, E., Witte, H. D., & Alarco, B. (2008). Employability and employees' well-being: Mediation by job insecurity. *Applied Psychology, 57*, 488-509. doi: https://doi.org/10.1111/j.1464-0597.2008.00332.x

De Grip, A., & Wolbers, M. H. (2006). Cross-national differences in job quality among low-skilled young workers in Europe. *International Journal of Manpower, 27*, 420-433. doi: https://doi.org/10.1108/01437720610683930

Eichhorst, W., Marx, P., & Wehner, C. (2017). Labor market reforms in Europe: towards more flexicure labor markets? *Journal for Labour Market Research, 51*, 3. doi: https://doi.org/10.1186/s12651-017-0231-7

Elfering, A., Semmer, N. K., Tschan, F., Kälin, W., & Bucher, A. (2007). First years in job: A three-wave analysis of work experiences. *Journal of Vocational Behavior, 70*, 97-115. doi: https://doi.org/10.1016/j.jvb.2006.07.001

Fisher, G. G., Chaffee, D. S., Tetrick, L. E., Davalos, D. B., & Potter, G. G. (2017). Cognitive functioning, aging, and work: A review and recommendations for research and practice. *Journal of Occupational Health Psychology, 22*, 314-336. doi: https://doi.org/10.1037/ocp0000086

Gallie, D. (2007). Production regimes, employment regimes, and the quality of work. In D. Gallie (ed.), *Employment regimes and the quality of work* (pp. 1–33). Oxford: University Press.

Gallie, D. (2013). Direct participation and the quality of work. *Human Relations, 66*, 453-473. doi: https://doi.org/10.1177/0018726712473035

Halbesleben, J. R. (2010). A meta-analysis of work engagement: Relationships with burnout, demands, resources, and consequences. In A. B. Bakker & M. P. Leiter (Eds.), *Work engagement: A handbook of essential theory and research* (pp. 102-117). Hove: Psychology Press.

Heery, E., & Salmon, J. (2000). The insecurity thesis. In E. Heery, & J. Salmon (Eds.), *The insecure workforce* (pp. 13-36). London: Routledge.

Hellevik, T., & Settersten Jr, R. A. (2013). Life planning among young adults in 23 European countries: The effects of individual and country security. *European Sociological Review, 29*, 923-938. doi: https://doi.org/10.1093/esr/jcs069

Holman, D., & Rafferty, A. (2018). The convergence and divergence of job discretion between occupations and institutional regimes in Europe from 1995 to 2010. *Journal of Management Studies, 55*, 619-647. doi: https://doi.org/10.1111/joms.12265

Hülsheger, U. R., & Schewe, A. F. (2011). On the costs and benefits of emotional labor: a meta-analysis of three decades of research. *Journal of Occupational Health Psychology, 16,* 361-389. doi: https://doi.org/10.1037/a0022876

Ilies, R., Dimotakis, N., & De Pater, I. E. (2010). Psychological and physiological reactions to high workloads: implications for well-being. *Personnel Psychology, 63,* 407-436. doi: https://doi.org/10.1111/j.1744-6570.2010.01175.x

Jackson, S. E. (1983). Participation in decision making as a strategy for reducing job-related strain. *Journal of Applied Psychology, 68,* 3-19. doi: https://doi.org/10.1037//0021-9010.68.1.3

Kahneman, D., & Deaton, A. (2010). High income improves evaluation of life but not emotional well-being. *Proceedings of the National Academy of Sciences, 107,* 16489-16493. doi: https://doi.org/10.1073/pnas.1011492107

Kalleberg, A. L. (1977). Work values and job rewards: A theory of job satisfaction. *American Sociological Review, 42,* 124-143. doi: https://doi.org/10.1111/j.1467-9914.2010.00496.x

Kalleberg, A. L. (2009). Precarious work, insecure workers Employment relations in transition. *American Sociological Review, 74,* 1–22. doi:

Kanfer, R., & Ackerman, P. L. (2004). Aging, adult development, and work motivation. *Academy of Management Review, 29,* 440-458. doi: https://doi.org/10.5465/amr.2004.13670969

Keller, A. C., Spurk, D., Baumeler, F., & Hirschi, A. (2016). Competitive climate and workaholism: Negative sides of future orientation and calling. *Personality and Individual Differences, 96,* 122-126. doi: https://doi.org/10.1016/j.paid.2016.02.061

Kooij, D. T. A. M., de Lange, A. H., Jansen, P. G. W., & Dikkers, J. S. E. (2008). Older workers' motivation to continue to work: Five meanings of age: A conceptual review. *Journal of Managerial Psychology, 23,* 354–394. doi: https://doi.org/10.1108/02683940810869015

Koster, F., De Grip, A., & Fouarge, D. (2011). Does perceived support in employee development affect personnel turnover? *International Journal of Human Resource Management, 22,* 2403-2418. doi: https://doi.org/10.1080/09585192.2011.584404

Kraimer, M. L., Seibert, S. E., Wayne, S. J., Liden, R. C., & Bravo, J. (2011). Antecedents and outcomes of organizational support for development: The critical role of career opportunities. *Journal of Applied Psychology, 96,* 485-500. doi: https://doi.org/10.1037/a0021452

Kretsos, L., & Livanos, I. (2016). The extent and determinants of precarious employment in Europe. *International Journal of Manpower, 37,* 25-43. doi: https://doi.org/10.1108/IJM-12-2014-0243

LaMontagne, A. D., Keegel, T., Louie, A. M., & Ostry, A. (2010). Job stress as a preventable upstream determinant of common mental disorders: A review for practitioners and policy-makers. *Advances in Mental Health, 9,* 17-35. doi: https://doi.org/10.5172/jamh.9.1.17

Lange, A., & Reiter, H. (2018). Gesellschaftsdiagnostische Annäherungen an die Rahmenbedingungen des Aufwachsens in der späten Moderne. In A. Lange, H. Reiter, S. Schutter, & Ch. Steiner (Eds.), Handbuch Kindheits- und Jugendsoziologie, (pp. 13-34). Wiesbaden: Springer.

LePine, J. A., Podsakoff, N. P., & LePine, M. A. (2005). A meta-analytic test of the challenge stressor–hindrance stressor framework: An explanation for inconsistent relationships among stressors and performance. *Academy of Management Journal, 48*, 764-775. doi: https://doi.org/10.5465/amj.2005.18803921

Li, P., Taris, T. W., & Peeters, M. C. (2020). Challenge and hindrance appraisals of job demands: one man's meat, another man's poison?. *Anxiety, Stress, & Coping, 33*, 31-46. doi: https://doi.org/10.1080/10615806.2019.1673133

Lunau, T., Bambra, C., Eikemo, T. A., van Der Wel, K. A., & Dragano, N. (2014). A balancing act? Work–life balance, health and well-being in European welfare states. *European Journal of Public Health, 24*, 422-427. doi: https://doi.org/10.1093/eurpub/cku010

Mäkikangas, A., Tolvanen, A., Aunola, K., Feldt, T., Mauno, S., & Kinnunen, U. (2018). Multilevel latent profile analysis with covariates: Identifying job characteristics profiles in hierarchical data as an example. *Organizational Research Methods, 21*, 931-954. doi: https://doi.org/10.1177/1094428118760690

Meijman, T. F., & Mulder, G. (1998). Psychological aspects of workload. In P. J. D. Drenth, H. Thierry & C.J. d. Wolff (Eds.), *Handbook of Work and Organizational Psychology, Vol. 2, Work psychology* (2nd ed.) (pp. 5–39). Hove, England: Psychology Press.

Michélsen, H., & Bildt, C. (2003). Psychosocial conditions on and off the job and psychological ill health: depressive symptoms, impaired psychological wellbeing, heavy consumption of alcohol. *Occupational and Environmental Medicine, 60*, 489-496. doi: https://doi.org/10.1136/oem.60.7.489

Milner, A., Krnjacki, L., & LaMontagne, A. D. (2017). Psychosocial job quality and mental health among young workers: a fixed-effects regression analysis using 13 waves of annual data. *Scandinavian Journal of Work, Environment & Health, 43*, 50-58. doi: https://doi.org/10.5271/sjweh.3608

Muñoz de Bustillo, R., Fernández-Macías, E., Esteve, F., & Antón, J. I. (2011). E pluribus unum? A critical survey of job quality indicators. *Socio-Economic Review, 9*, 447–475. doi: https://doi.org/10.1093/ser/mwr005

Nahrgang, J. D., Morgeson, F. P., & Hofmann, D. A. (2011). Safety at work: a meta-analytic investigation of the link between job demands, job resources, burnout, engagement, and safety outcomes. *Journal of Applied Psychology, 96*, 71-94. doi: https://doi.org/10.1037/a0021484

Ng, T. W., & Feldman, D. C. (2015). The moderating effects of age in the relationships of job autonomy to work outcomes. *Work, Aging and Retirement, 1*(1), 64-78. doi: https://doi.org/10.1093/workar/wau003

Nielsen, M. B., & Einarsen, S. (2012). Outcomes of exposure to workplace bullying: A meta-analytic review. *Work & Stress, 26*, 309–332. doi: https://doi.org/10.1080/02678373.2012.734709

Nielsen, K., Nielsen, M. B., Ogbonnaya, C., Känsälä, M., Saari, E., & Isaksson, K. (2017). Workplace resources to improve both employee well-being and performance: A systematic review and meta-analysis. *Work & Stress, 31*, 101-120. doi: https://doi.org/10.1080/02678373.2017.1304463

Nilsen, A., Brannen, J., & Vogt, K. C. (2018). Transitions to Adulthood: An Intergenerational Lens. In A. Lange, H. Reiter, S. Schutter, & Ch. Steiner (Eds.), *Handbuch Kindheits- und Jugendsoziologie*, (pp. 83-96). Wiesbaden: Springer.

Nohe, C., Meier, L. L., Sonntag, K., & Michel, A. (2015). The chicken or the egg? A meta-analysis of panel studies of the relationship between work–family conflict and strain. *Journal of Applied Psychology, 100*, 522-536. doi: https://doi.org/10.1037/a0038012

Nunez, I., & Livanos, I. (2015). Temps "by choice"? An investigation of the reasons behind temporary employment among young workers in Europe. *Journal of Labor Research, 36*, 44-66. doi: https://doi.org/10.1007/s12122-014-9195-3

Oldham, G. R., & Fried, Y. (2016). Job design research and theory: Past, present and future. *Organizational Behavior and Human Decision Processes, 136*, 20-35. doi: https://doi.org/10.1016/j.obhdp.2016.05.002

Parker, S. K. (2014). Beyond motivation: Job and work design for development, health, ambidexterity, and more. *Annual Review of Psychology, 65*, 661-691. doi: https://doi.org/10.1146/annurev-psych-010213-115208

Podsakoff, N. P., LePine, J. A., & LePine, M. A. (2007). Differential challenge stressor-hindrance stressor relationships with job attitudes, turnover intentions, turnover, and withdrawal behavior: a meta-analysis. *Journal of Applied Psychology, 92*, 438-454. doi: https://doi.org/10.1037/0021-9010.92.2.438

Podsakoff, P. M., MacKenzie, S. B., & Podsakoff, N. P. (2012). Sources of method biasin social science research and recommendations on how to control it. *Annual Review of Psychology, 63*, 539–569. doi: https://doi.org/10.1146/annurev-psych-120710-100452

Poon, J. M. (2013). Relationships among perceived career support, affective commitment, and work engagement. *International Journal of Psychology, 48*, 1148-1155. doi: https://doi.org/10.1080/00207594.2013.768768

Ramos, R., Jenny, G., & Bauer G. (2016). Age-related effects of job characteristics on burnout and work engagement. *Occupational Medicine, 66*, 230-237. doi: https://doi.org/10.1093/occmed/kqv172

Reeves, D. W., Walsh, B. M., Tuller, M. D., & Magley, V. J. (2012). The positive effects of participative decision making for midlevel correctional management. *Criminal Justice and Behavior, 39*, 1361-1372. doi: https://doi.org/10.1177/0093854812453127

Roberts, B. W., Walton, K. E., & Viechtbauer, W. (2006). Patterns of mean-level change in personality traits across the life course: a meta-analysis of longitudinal studies. *Psychological Bulletin, 132*, 1-25. doi: https://doi.org/10.1037/0033-2909.132.1.1

Rokicka, M. (Ed.), Kłobuszewska, M., Palczyńska, M., Shapova, N., Stasiowski, J. (2015). *Composition and cumulative disadvantage of youth across Europe.* EXCEPT Working Papers, WP No 1. Tallinn University, Tallinn. http://www.except-project.eu/working-papers/

Schaufeli, W. B., Bakker, A. B., & Salanova, M. (2006). The measurement of work engagement with a short questionnaire: A cross-national study. *Educational and Psychological Measurement, 66*, 701-716. doi: https://doi.org/10.1177/0013164405282471

Schmidt, S. W. (2007). The relationship between satisfaction with workplace training and overall job satisfaction. *Human Resource Development Quarterly, 18*, 481-498. doi: https://doi.org/10.1002/hrdq.1216

Schütz, H., & Thiele, N. (2019). *Bericht – Quality of Work Luxembourg, 2019.* Infas, Institut für angewandte Sozialwissenschaft: Bonn.

Sischka, P. E., Schmidt, A. F., & Steffgen, G. (2020a). Further evidence for criterion validity and measurement invariance of the Luxembourg Workplace Mobbing Scale. *European Journal of Psychological Assessment, 36*, 32-43. doi: https://doi.org/10.1027/1015-5759/a000483

Sischka, P. E., Costa, A. P., Steffgen, G., & Schmidt, A. F. (2020b). The WHO-5 well-being index–validation based on item response theory and the analysis of measurement invariance across 35 countries. *Journal ofAffective Disorders Reports, 1,* 100020. doi: https://doi.org/10.1016/j.jadr.2020.100020

Sischka, P. E., Melzer, A., Schmidt, A. F., & Steffgen, G. (2021). Psychological contract violation or basic need frustration? Psychological mechanisms behind the effects of workplace bullying. *Frontiers in Psychology, 12,* 627968. doi: https://doi.org/10.3389/fpsyg.2021.627968

Sischka, P., & Steffgen, G. (2019a). Arbeitsplatzmobbing in Luxemburg – Wie groß ist das Problem? Aktuelles vom „Quality of Work Index" Nr. 14. *Better Work Newsletter, 5/2019,* 1–7. https://www.csl.lu/bibliotheque/newsletters/40173187a9.pdf

Sischka, P., & Steffgen, G. (2019b). *Quality of Work-Index. 5. Forschungsbericht zur Weiterentwicklung des Arbeitsqualitätsindexes in Luxemburg.* Inside Research Report. Luxembourg: University of Luxembourg.

Sischka, P., & Steffgen, G. (2020). Depressionen am Arbeitsplatz in Luxemburg: Ein Handlungsfeld? Aktuelles vom „Quality of Work Index" Nr. 15. *Better Work Newsletter, 1/2020,* 1–7. https://www.csl.lu/bibliotheque/newsletters/da26bb6dfb.pdf

Sonnentag, S., Arbeus, H., Mahn, C., & Fritz, C. (2014). Exhaustion and lack of psychological detachment from work during off-job time: Moderator effects of time pressure and leisure experiences. *Journal of Occupational Health Psychology, 19,* 206-216. doi: https://doi.org/10.1037/a0035760

Steffgen, G.; Kohl, D. (2013): *Rapport final sur le développement d'un indicateur de la qualité du travail au Luxembourg.* Working Paper. Luxembourg: University of Luxembourg.

Steffgen, G., Sischka, P. E., & Fernandez de Henestrosa, M. (2020). The quality of work index and the quality of employment index: a multidimensional approach of job quality and its links to well-being at work. *International Journal of Environmental Research and Public Health, 17,* 7771. doi: https://doi.org/10.3390/ijerph17217771

Sverke, M., Hellgren, J., & Näswall, K. (2002). No security: a meta-analysis and review of job insecurity and its consequences. *Journal of Occupational Health Psychology, 7,* 242-264. doi: https://doi.org/10.1037//1076-8998.7.3.242

Thrasher, G. R., Zabel, K., Wynne, K., & Baltes, B. B. (2016). The importance of workplace motives in understanding work–family issues for older workers. *Work, Aging and Retirement, 2*(1), 1-11. doi: https://doi.org/10.1093/workar/wav021

Topp, C. W., Østergaard, S. D., Søndergaard, S., & Bech, P. (2015). The WHO-5 Well-Being Index: A systematic review of the literature. *Psychotherapy and Psychosomatics, 84,* 167–176. doi: https://doi.org/10.1159/000376585

Truxillo, D. M., Cadiz, D. M., & Hammer, L. B. (2015). Supporting the aging workforce: A review and recommendations for workplace intervention research. *Annual Review of Organizational Psychology and Organizational Behavior, 2,* 351-381. https://doi.org/10.1146/annurev-orgpsych-032414-111435

Truxillo, D. M., Cadiz, D. M., Rineer, J. R., Zaniboni, S., & Fraccaroli, F. (2012). A lifespan perspective on job design: Fitting the job and the worker to promote job satisfaction, engagement, and performance. *Organizational Psychology Review, 2,* 340-360. doi: https://doi.org/10.1177/2041386612454043

Van Aerden, K., Puig-Barrachina, V., Bosmans, K., & Vanroelen, C. (2016). How does employment quality relate to health and job satisfaction in Europe? A typological approach. *Social Science & Medicine, 158*, 132-140. doi: https://doi.org/10.1016/j.socscimed.2016.04.017

Viswesvaran, C., Sanchez, J. I., & Fisher, J. (1999). The role of social support in the process of work stress: A meta-analysis. *Journal of Vocational Behavior, 54*, 314-334. doi: https://doi.org/10.1006/jvbe.1998.1661

Wegman, L. A., Hoffman, B. J., Carter, N. T., Twenge, J. M., & Guenole, N. (2018). Placing job characteristics in context: Cross-temporal meta-analysis of changes in job characteristics since 1975. *Journal of Management, 44*, 352-386. doi: https://doi.org/10.1177/0149206316654545

Williams, M. L., McDaniel, M. A., & Nguyen, N. T. (2006). A meta-analysis of the antecedents and consequences of pay level satisfaction. *Journal of Applied Psychology, 91*, 392-413. doi: https://doi.org/10.1037/0021-9010.91.2.392

Zacher, H., Dirkers, B. T., Korek, S., & Hughes, B. (2017). Age-differential effects of job characteristics on job attraction: a policy-capturing study. *Frontiers in Psychology, 8*, 1124. doi: https://doi.org/10.3389/fpsyg.2017.01124

Zaniboni, S., Truxillo, D. M., & Fraccaroli, F. (2013). Differential effects of task variety and skill variety on burnout and turnover intentions for o der and younger workers. *European Journal of Work and Organizational Psychology 22*, 306-317. doi: https://doi.org/10.1080/1359432X.2013.782288

Zaniboni, S., Truxillo, D. M., Rineer, J. R., Bodner, T. E., Hammer, L. B., & Krainer, M. (2016). Relating age, decision authority, job satisfaction, and mental health: a study of construction workers. *Work, Aging and Retirement, 2*, 428-435. doi: https://doi.org/10.1093/workar/waw006

Zapf, D. (2002). Emotion work and psychological well-being: A review of the literature and some conceptual considerations. *Human Resource Management Review, 12*, 237-268. doi: https://doi.org/10.1016/s1053-4822(02)00048-7

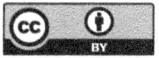

Fremdplatzierte Kinder und Jugendliche in luxemburgischen Institutionen: Befinden und Erleben von Betroffenen

Lisa Clees und Georges Steffgen

1 Einleitung

Zahlreiche Gründe können vorliegen, wenn Kinder und Jugendliche ihr familiäres Umfeld verlassen müssen und vom Jugendgericht in Heimen, in Kinder- und Jugendpsychiatrien oder im Jugendgefängnis platziert werden. Insbesondere wenn eine angemessene psychische Entwicklung des Kindes auf Grund multipler innerfamiliärer Probleme nicht mehr gewährleistet ist, kann das Jugendgericht zum Schutz des Kindes die Platzierung von Säuglingen, Kleinkindern und Schulkindern in Pflegefamilien oder in Institutionen einleiten. Bei älteren Schulkindern und Jugendlichen erfolgt die richterliche Anordnung zur Fremdunterbringung und Trennung vom Elternhaus meist auf Grund ausgeprägter Verhaltensauffälligkeiten der Kinder und Jugendlichen, wie z. B. wiederholtes Schwänzen der Schule, vermehrte verbale oder körperliche Aggressionen, Selbstverletzung, Alkohol- und Drogenkonsum bis hin zu delinquentem Verhalten. Die Herkunftsfamilie sieht sich in diesen Fällen in ihren Erziehungskompetenzen häufig überfordert und steht den Verhaltensauffälligkeiten des Kindes bzw. des Jugendlichen oft hilflos gegenüber.

L. Clees (✉)
Mamer, Luxemburg
E-Mail: lisa.clees@pt.lu

G. Steffgen
Department of Behavioural and Cognitive Sciences,
University of Luxembourg, Esch-sur-Alzette, Luxemburg
E-Mail: georges.steffgen@uni.lu

© Der/die Autor(en) 2022
A. Heinen et al. (Hrsg.), *Wohlbefinden und Gesundheit im Jugendalter,*
https://doi.org/10.1007/978-3-658-35744-3_13

Den Kindern und Jugendlichen ist häufig gemein, dass sie zahlreiche belastende, zum Teil traumatisierende Situationen erlebt haben, ehe es zu einer Fremdunterbringung gekommen ist. Die manchmal unvorbereitete Herausnahme aus dem familiären Milieu wird von den Betroffenen oftmals als zusätzliche emotionale Belastung wahrgenommen. Kinder und Jugendliche sind selten in der Lage, eine Trennung von ihren primären Bezugspersonen als entwicklungsförderlich anzusehen. Die Sehnsucht nach einer Rückkehr ins familiäre Umfeld bleibt meistens über die gesamte Dauer der Fremdplatzierung bestehen. Selbst wenn die Beziehung der Kinder zu den Eltern in der Vergangenheit von Vernachlässigung und Gewalt geprägt war, beeinflusst der Wunsch nach stabilen familiären Beziehungen das psychische Wohlergehen der Kinder und Jugendlichen über Jahre hinweg.

Was benötigen diese Kinder und Jugendlichen, damit sie sich in den Institutionen, die zu ihrem neuen Lebensumfeld geworden sind, wohl fühlen und sich besser entwickeln können, als dies im familiären Umfeld der Fall war? Der folgende Beitrag wird sich mit dieser Fragestellung auseinandersetzen. Dabei werden in einem ersten Schritt theoretische Grundlagen und Befunde bezüglich des Bindungsverhaltens und Beziehungsaufbaus von Neugeborenen und Säuglingen erörtert und deren Bedeutung für eine psychisch gesunde Entwicklung aufgezeigt. Daraufhin folgt die Erläuterung frühkindlicher Traumatisierung sowie die Auswirkungen extremer Belastungssituationen auf die Entwicklung von Kindern. Dieser Teil wird durch eine kurze Beschreibung von resilientem Verhalten bei traumatisierten Kindern ergänzt. Der nachfolgende Abschnitt wird sich mit den Merkmalen und Herausforderungen der Fremdplatzierung von Kindern und Jugendlichen in Institutionen auseinandersetzen und in einem letzten Schritt wird eine derzeit durchgeführte Studie vorgestellt, die zu der erwähnten Fragestellung über das Wohlbefinden fremdplatzierter Kinder und Jugendlicher in luxemburgischen Institutionen relevante Befunde vorlegen wird. In diesem Teil werden Ziele und Methodik der Studie erläutert und erste vorläufige Befunde vorgestellt.

2 Theoretischer Teil

2.1 Bindungstheoretische Grundlagen

Spätestens seit Anfang des 19. Jahrhunderts wird darauf hingewiesen, dass Kinder für ihre gesunde psychische Entwicklung präsente, zuverlässige und wertschätzende Beziehungspersonen benötigen. Bereits 1901 bemängelte der österreichische Kinderarzt Meinhard von Pfaundler die systematische und „widernatürliche" Trennung der Neugeborenen von ihren Müttern. In seinem *„Handbuch der Geburtshilfe"* (1915) brachte er die Entstehung und die Bedingungen des Hospitalismus bei Säuglingen und Kindern mit einer längeren Mutter-Kind-Trennung in Verbindung. Einige Jahre später verglich Eriksson (1925) Anstaltskinder, die aus wohlhabenden Elternhäusern stammten mit Kindern aus einem Armenviertel. Er stellte fest, dass die Kinder aus dem Armenviertel, die bei ihren Familien aufwuchsen, deutlich intelligentere und sozialere Verhaltensmuster aufwiesen als die Anstaltskinder. Bei den Anstaltskindern stand zu diesem Zeitpunkt die strenge Beachtung der Hygienebedingungen im Vordergrund des Wohlergehens, dem emotionalen Wohlbefinden wurde kaum Beachtung geschenkt. Einige Jahrzehnte später befasste sich der Psychoanalytiker René Spitz (1945) mit dem emotionalen Wohlbefinden des Säuglings und rückte dabei die Bedeutsamkeit der Mutter-Kind-Beziehung in den Vordergrund einer gesunden psychischen Entwicklung.

Die Säuglings- und Kleinkindforschung gewann zunehmend an Beachtung. Forscher wie Bowlby (1969) und Ainsworth (1985) haben beobachtet, dass das Neugeborene bereits kurz nach seiner Geburt in der Lage ist, mit seiner Bezugsperson in Beziehung zu treten. Der Säugling sendet mithilfe seiner angeborenen Fähigkeiten Signale an die Umwelt, die bei einer feinfühligen Person intuitiv eine schnelle und angemessene Reaktion auslösen. Durch diese sich ständig wiederholenden Interaktionen zwischen dem Säugling und seiner Bezugsperson baut sich nach und nach eine intensive und anhaltende Beziehung auf. In seinen Arbeiten betont Bowlby (1969, 1973, 1980), dass Säuglinge ab dem dritten Lebensmonat ein spezifisches Bindungsverhalten zu einer bestimmten Person zeigen, die fortan als primäre Bindungsperson bezeichnet werden kann. Das Bindungsverhalten manifestiert sich in der Interaktion zu einigen wenigen Bezugspersonen, wobei es sich im Kontakt mit der primären Bindungsperson am stärksten auszudrücken scheint. Die Forschungsarbeiten von Ainsworth (1985) haben Bowlbys Theorien um das Bindungsverhalten erweitert. Die Bindungsforscherin konnte in einer künstlich hergestellten Situation *("strange situation test")* beobachten, dass ein *sicher gebundenes* Kind sich bei Stress von seiner primären Bindungsperson ohne weiteres trösten und beruhigen lässt, während dies einer dem Kind fremden Pflegeperson eher weniger gelingt. Laut Bowlby (1969, 1973, 1980) sind die primären Bezugspersonen wegen der ausgeprägten Individualität dieser Beziehung nicht ohne weiteres austauschbar. Je weiter der Prozess des Bindungsaufbaus zu der primären Person fortgeschritten ist, umso stärker scheint eine längere Trennung von dieser Person die weitere Entwicklung des Kindes zu beeinträchtigen.

Weitere Studien zum Bindungsverhalten weisen darauf hin, dass Säuglinge und Kleinkinder, die in der Interaktion mit ihren primären Bezugspersonen ein sicheres Bindungsmuster aufbauen, bessere soziale, emotionale, motivationale und kognitive Fähigkeiten entwickeln und ein höheres Selbstwertgefühl aufweisen als Kinder mit unsicheren Bindungsmustern (Bretherton 1985; Decarli 2019; George und Main 1979; Sroufe 1983; Zimmermann 2004). Des Weiteren wurde in zahlreichen Publikationen der Einfluss der Qualität, der aus den frühkindlichen Interaktionen resultierenden Bindung des Säuglings zu seiner primären Bezugsperson auf die Fähigkeit zur affektiven Selbstregulation beschrieben (Ainsworth 1985; Crittenden 1995; Dornes 1993; Papousek et al. 2004). Laut Schore (1994) übernimmt die primäre Bezugsperson die Rolle eines externen psychoneurologischen Regulators. Gerät das Kind in eine Stresssituation, reagiert eine aufmerksame und feinfühlige Bezugsperson unmittelbar auf den emotionalen Zustand ihres Kindes und hilft dem Kind mittels ihres eigenen, ruhigen Gefühlszustandes, sich zu beruhigen. Schore (1994) betont, dass das Kind durch diese sich wiederholenden Eltern-Kind-Interaktionen schon früh lernt, dass negative Gefühlszustände ausgehalten und bewältigt werden können. Von den internen Arbeitsmustern (neurologischen Verbindungen), die sich in Folge dieser Erfahrungen beim Kind bilden, wird das Kind bis ins Erwachsenenalter profitieren. In schwierigen Situationen wird es die erlernten Arbeitsmuster immer öfters aktivieren und sich auf seine Gefühle und Gedanken verlassen, um die in der Situation entstandenen negativen Gefühle eigenständig zu bewältigen. Solche Selbsterfahrungen verstärken beim Kind nach und nach das Gefühl von Kontrolle, Selbstwirksamkeit und eigener Kompetenz. Befindet sich das Kind in einer Situation, in der es ihm nicht gelingt, sich selbst zu regulieren, wird es weiterhin auf die positiven Beziehungserfahrungen zurückgreifen und sich Beruhigung und Unterstützung bei einer ihm vertrauten Person suchen (Schore 2003).

Grossmann und Grossmann (2011) kritisieren an der Bindungstheorie, dass sich Bowlbys Theorie hauptsächlich auf die Beziehung zwischen Mutter und Kind beschränkt. Rezentere Forschungsergebnisse betonen neben der Rolle der Mutter auch die Bedeutung des Vaters, der Großeltern oder die einer Tagesmutter für die Bindung und Entwicklung des Kindes (Chambers et al. 2000; Papoušek et al. 1987). Dornes (1997) sieht als weiteren Kritikpunkt, dass der Rolle des kindlichen Temperamentes in den Bindungstheorien wenig Beachtung geschenkt wird. Zudem betont er, dass der Bindungsstil eines Kindes nicht nur von der durchgehenden Anwesenheit seiner primären Bezugsperson abhängt, sondern vor allem von der Qualität dieser Beziehung. Roth und Strüber (2014) weisen ihrerseits daraufhin, dass unsere Persönlichkeit aus einem Zusammenwirken von

genetisch-epigenetischen Einflüssen sowie vorgeburtliche und früh nachgeburt-
liche Ereignisse bestimmt wird. Sie sehen in der Qualität der Beziehung zwischen
dem Säugling und seiner primären Bezugsperson einen wichtigen Einflussfaktor,
der auf die genetisch angelegten sozialen Fähigkeiten des Kindes einwirken und
diese ausdifferenzieren kann.

Trotz diverser Kritik besteht in der Bindungsforschung weiterhin Konsens,
dass die frühen positiven Bindungserfahrungen eine wesentliche Grundlage
für eine angemessene psychische Entwicklung bilden. Sie sollen dem Kind vor
allem während der ersten Lebensjahre, aber auch später durch einfühlsame und
beständige Bezugspersonen vermittelt werden (Crittenden 1995; Papousek et al.
2004).

2.2 Frühkindliche Traumatisierung und ihre Folgen

Kinder und Jugendliche, die unter Störungen in der Selbst-, Affekt- und Impuls-
regulation leiden, haben in ihrer frühen Kindheit die Fähigkeit zur Selbstregulation und das Sicherheitsgefühl, das ihnen in stabilen und feinfühligen
Beziehungsangeboten vermittelt werden sollte, kaum oder nur unvollständig
erworben (Egle et al. 2005; Papoušek et al. 2004). Die Ursachen hierfür sind
multifaktoriell, wobei diese Kinder und Jugendliche oft frühen Traumatisierungen
und dysfunktionalen Beziehungsmustern ausgesetzt waren. Die schwache Form
der Selbstregulation kann sich in der Kindheit und in der Adoleszenz nicht nur
durch mangelnde Impulskontrolle, sondern auch in destruktiven Handlungen
gegenüber sich selbst und gegenüber anderen manifestieren (van der Kolk und
Fisler 1994; Streeck-Fischer 2004). Hinzu kommen Aufmerksamkeitsstörungen,
Hyperaktivität, aggressives Verhalten sowie zahlreiche andere Verhaltensauffälligkeiten. Ackermann und seine Mitarbeiter (1998) konnten bei einer Gruppe
von Kindern, die sexualisierte und körperliche Gewalt erlebt hatten, als häufigste
Diagnose Trennungsangst, gefolgt von gestörtem Sozialverhalten, Phobien,
Aufmerksamkeitsdefizit-/Hyperaktivitätsstörung   (ADHS),   Posttraumatische
Belastungsstörung (PTBS), Depression, Zwangsstörungen und weitere Auffälligkeiten diagnostizieren. Zahlreiche weitere Studien bestätigen die Annahme,
dass stressreiche und traumatische Erlebnisse in der Kindheit erhebliche Risikofaktoren für die Entstehung von psychischen und körperlichen Erkrankungen
sind. Solche Auffälligkeiten können sich bis ins Erwachsenenalter manifestieren
(Entringer et al. 2016; Entringer und Heim 2016; Heim und Binder 2012).

In einem Beitrag über männliche, aggressive Jugendliche hebt Streeck-Fischer
(2004) hervor, dass sämtliche Jugendliche in einem schwierigen familiären

Umfeld aufgewachsen sind und schweren Traumatisierungen ausgesetzt waren. Ein weiterer Befund dieser Studie zeigt auf, dass die weiblichen Jugendlichen, die unter ähnlichen problematischen Bedingungen aufgewachsen sind, wesentlich resistenter auf chronisch traumatischen Stress reagiert haben. Sie zeigten in der Kindheit ein eher angepasstes Verhalten und fielen gelegentlich durch schlechte Schulleistungen und Symptome wie Einnässen oder Stehlen auf. Streeck-Fischer (2004) erklärt das Verhalten dieser jungen Mädchen dadurch, dass die betroffenen Mädchen oft eine verantwortungsvolle Rolle für die kleineren Geschwister und für die psychisch überforderten Eltern übernahmen. Die unverarbeiteten traumatischen Erlebnisse drücken sich erst im Alter der Adoleszenz vermehrt durch selbstdestruktive Verhaltensweisen wie Essstörungen, Selbstverletzungen, Schulabbruch, massive Regelverletzungen oder Drogenkonsum aus. In dieser schwierigen Zeit der Adoleszenz kommt es bei den traumatisierten Jugendlichen oft zu Re- und Neutraumatisierungen (Bryson et al. 2017; Cromer und Villodas 2017).

Die Auswirkungen belastender, unverarbeiteter Stresssituationen aus der Kindheit auf die Entwicklung des Gehirns in Bezug auf Gefühle und Verhalten können hierbei aufgezeigt werden (Anda et al. 2006; Roth und Strüber 2014). In den ersten 18–24 Monaten nach der Geburt bildet sich der größte Teil der neuronalen Vernetzungen. Die frühen Beziehungserfahrungen werden im Rechtshirn gespeichert, welches mit dem limbischen System – dort werden die Emotionen verarbeitet – verbunden ist. Erlebt das Kind Angst und emotionale Verunsicherungen, wird unter anderem das limbische System aktiviert und es werden vermehrt Botenstoffe und Hormone ausgeschieden. Die Hormone führen ihrerseits zu einer Verfestigung der neuronalen Verschaltungen, die in Stresssituationen Verhaltensmuster einleiten, damit das emotionale Gleichgewicht wiederhergestellt werden kann. Diese im Säuglings- und Kleinkindalter entstandenen neuronalen Verschaltungen im frontalen Kortex beeinflussen unsere Kognitionen, Gefühle und unser Handeln noch im Erwachsenenalter. Sie können bei Stress Verhaltensmuster von funktionaler aber auch von dysfunktionaler Natur einleiten (Schore 2003).

2.3   Trauma und Resilienz

Nicht alle Kinder und Jugendlichen, die in ihrer Kindheit traumatischen Situationen ausgesetzt waren, entwickeln erkennbare Belastungssymptome. Sowohl in psychosozialen Risikofamilien wie auch in stationären Hilfsmaßnahmen finden sich immer wieder Kinder und Jugendliche, die trotz zahlreicher Belastungssituationen ein eher unauffälliges Verhalten zeigen (Clerverley und Kidd 2011; Sattler und Font 2018). Diesen Kindern gelingt es, sich in die Wohngruppen zu integrieren, Beziehungen zu den Gleichaltrigen und den Betreuungspersonen aufzubauen und die Schule regelmäßig und ohne größere Schwierigkeiten zu besuchen. Wissenschaftliche Befunde bestätigen, dass diese Kinder eine erstaunliche Widerstandskraft gegenüber dem erlebten Leid zeigen, während andere Kinder wesentlich verletzbarer sind (Freedman und DeBoer 1979; Gunnar 1993). Die Forscher erklären dieses Verhalten dadurch, dass diese Kinder über eine höhere Resilienz verfügen. Resilienz wird dabei als eine Kompetenz, schwierige und belastende Situationen aufgrund persönlicher Ressourcen, Fähigkeiten und Potenziale angemessen zu bewältigen, definiert (Luthar et al. 2000; Rutter 2000). In rezenten Studien wird der Begriff auch als *„ein dynamischer und damit adaptiver Prozess beim Vorhandensein belastender Ereignisse und Schwierigkeiten"* beschrieben (Lindert et al. 2018). Neueste Erkenntnisse weisen darauf hin, dass Resilienzverläufe über die verschiedenen Altersstufen hin veränderlich sind, die Resilienz nicht als eine anhaltende, stabile Fähigkeit gesehen werden kann, und dass unterschiedliche Faktoren eine Rolle beim Auftreten von resilientem Verhalten spielen (Lindert et al. 2018; Rutter 2000; Scheithauer et al. 2000). So konnten Laucht et al. (2002) nachweisen, dass die Entwicklung von Verhaltensauffälligkeiten bei Kindern nicht allein von den erlebten Situationen abhängt, sondern dass neben der Veranlagung und den persönlichen Ressourcen, die Qualität der frühen Mutter-Kind-Beziehung eine wesentliche Rolle in den langfristigen Auswirkungen von belastenden und traumatisierenden Ereignissen spielt. Die Studie belegt, dass Kinder, die eine Bezugsperson haben, die sich angemessen und einfühlend um ihr Wohl kümmert, eine ausgeprägtere Resilienz aufweisen und demnach bessere Bewältigungsmöglichkeiten zeigen als Kinder, deren primäre Bezugsperson auf einer ungünstigen, dysfunktionalen Beziehungsebene zu ihnen steht. Weitere Faktoren, die das resiliente Verhalten von Kindern begünstigen, konnten in einer Studie von Sattler und Font (2018) dokumentiert werden. Die Autoren beziehen sich auf das Modell von Bronfenbrenner (1994), indem sie Schutzfaktoren auf den unterschiedlichsten Ebenen – die individuelle Ebene, die familiäre Ebene und die gesellschaftliche Ebene – sowie über eine Zeitspanne hinweg identifizierten. Die Studie ergab, dass ein Zusammenhang zwischen den familiären Faktoren und der kindlichen Resilienz auf sozio-emotioneller, kognitiver und allgemeiner Ebene besteht. Die kognitiven Stimulationen und die emotionale Unterstützung durch die Familie konnten dabei als wichtigste Einflussfaktoren bestimmt werden.

Bezüglich der wissenschaftlichen Befundlage über resilientes Verhalten mehrfach traumatisierter Kinder stellt sich Panksepp (2004) die Frage, ob bei den nach

außen hin resilient scheinenden Kindern nicht das Risiko besteht, teilweise dysfunktionale Abwehrmechanismen zu entwickeln, die sie ein Leben lang begleiten.
Um diese Frage angemessen zu beantworten, sind im Bereich der Resilienz-
forschung weitere Längsschnittstudien erforderlich.

2.4 Fremdplatzierung von Kindern und Jugendlichen

Wie bereits aufgeführt, werden zum Teil Kinder, die sich in Heimen oder bei
Pflegeltern befinden, schon im Säuglings- und Kleinkindalter aus dem familiären
Milieu herausgenommen. Andere kommen erst im Schulkindalter oder im Alter
der Adoleszenz in eine außerfamiliäre Betreuung. Bei älteren Kindern und
Jugendlichen sind es vor allem die sich wiederholenden und gravierenden Verhaltensauffälligkeiten, die dazu führen, dass das soziale Umfeld auf diese Kinder
aufmerksam wird. In solchen Fällen wird das Jugendgericht über die Verhaltensauffälligkeiten des Kindes informiert und eine sozialpädagogische Untersuchung des familiären Milieus eingeleitet. Wenn die Eltern in ihrer Fähigkeit
als Erziehungs- und Beziehungspersonen als unfähig oder in ihren Erziehungskompetenzen als überfordert beurteilt werden, erfolgt in den meisten Fällen ein
ambulantes Hilfsangebot. Erst wenn die ambulanten Maßnahmen scheitern, die
familiäre Situation weiterhin angespannt ist und im erweiterten Familiensystem
keine stabilen Familienmitglieder vorhanden sind, welche die Erziehungsauf-
gaben übernehmen können, werden die Kinder aus der Familie herausgenommen
und fremdplatziert.

Je älter die Kinder sind, desto schwieriger erweist es sich, eine geeignete
Pflegefamilie zu finden. Die meisten Kinder und Jugendlichen werden dann in
Kinderwohngruppen und Jugendgruppen untergebracht.

Da viele dieser jungen Menschen jahrelang entwicklungsschädigenden
Erziehungsmethoden und -bedingungen ausgesetzt waren und unter traumatischen
Belastungserfahrungen leiden, stellt dies sowohl die Pflegeltern wie auch
die Betreuer der Kinder- und Jugendwohngruppen vor eine große Herausforderung (Schmid 2013). Auf Grund eines hohen persönlichen Belastungs-
grades sind die leiblichen Eltern der Heimkinder oftmals nicht in der Lage,
ihren Kindern ein sicheres Bindungsmuster zu vermitteln. Bei diesen Kindern
werden häufig unsichere bis hin zu desorganisierte Bindungsmuster beobachtet
(George et al. 1985; Howe und Fearnly 2003; Lionetti et al. 2015; Tizard und
Rees 1975). Zahlreiche Studien belegen, dass dysfunktionale Bindungsmuster
bereits im Säuglings- und Kleinkindalter zu Verhaltensauffälligkeiten wie

Regulationsstörungen und mit fortschreitendem Alter zu exzessivem Trotzen, Impulsivität oder aggressiven Verhaltensweisen führen können (Lyons-Ruth und Jacobvitz 2008; Spangler 2011; Teicher 2011). Die meist unverarbeiteten Erlebnisse wirken bei den Kindern und Jugendlichen jahrelang nach und beeinflussen deren physisches und physisches Wohlergehen, sowie deren Verhalten (Felitti et al. 1998). Internationale Forschungsarbeiten, die sich mit dem psychischen Wohl von Heimkindern befassen, berichten diesbezüglich über eine außergewöhnlich stark belastete Population (Ford et al 2007; Hukkanen et al. 1999; McCann et al. 1996; Schmid 2007). Die Prävalenz psychischer Erkrankung bei Heimkindern und -jugendlichen liegt bei 60–70 % (Ford et al. 2007; Schmid 2007), wobei die Rate psychisch stark belasteter Jugendlicher im Jugendstrafvollzug und in justiziellen Institutionen bis auf 80 % steigt (Fazel et al. 2008; Grisso 2004). In einer epidemiologischen Untersuchung von 592 Jugendlichen und jungen Erwachsenen, die in Schweizer Heimen und im Jugendstrafvollzug untergebracht waren (Durchschnittsalter 16,1 Jahren), berichteten 80 % der Teilnehmer von mindestens einem traumatischen Erlebnis und ein Drittel von mehreren traumatischen Erlebnissen (Schmid et al. 2011). 74 % der Jugendlichen litten gemäß den psychiatrischen Diagnosekriterien (DSM-IV-TR oder ICD-10) an mindestens einer, 44 % an zwei oder mehreren psychischen Erkrankungen. Solche Ergebnisse unterstreichen den hohen Belastungsgrad von Heimkindern und -jugendlichen und machen den Bedarf nach einer intensiven pädagogischen Unterstützung und Betreuung sowie einer psychiatrisch-psychotherapeutischen Hilfe deutlich (Schmid 2013). Kinder und Jugendliche, bei denen zunehmende Selbstverletzungen und Selbstgefährdungen wie z. B. exzessiver Alkohol- oder Drogenkonsum oder Fremdgefährdung (verbale oder körperliche Gewalt, delinquentes Verhalten, usw.) beobachtet wird, erhalten oft vor oder während ihrer Platzierung in einer Kinder- oder Jugendwohngruppe eine stationäre psychiatrische Behandlung. Bei andauernden kriminellen Tätigkeiten (Einbrüche, Überfälle, Drogenhandel usw.) droht den Jugendlichen eine Unterbringung im Jugendgefängnis.

Bei diesen komplex traumatisierten Kindern und Jugendlichen ist das Risiko eines Abbruchs der erfolgten Hilfsmaßnahme stark erhöht und führt häufig zu sich wiederholenden Abbrüchen der stationären Hilfsmaßnahmen (Schmid 2007, 2008, 2010; Tornow und Ziegler 2012). Die reduzierte Bindungsfähigkeit erschwert die Eingliederung in Kinder- und Jugendwohngruppen. Dumais und seine Mitarbeiter (2014) berichten in ihrer Meta-Analyse über Bindungsmuster von Kindern, die in Heimen leben, dass viele dieser Kinder einen unsicheren-desorganisierten Bindungsstil aufweisen. Bei Kindern mit einem unsicher-desorganisierten Bindungsstil steigt das Risiko, Auffälligkeiten auf der kognitiven und auf der sozialen Ebene zu entwickeln. Zudem können bei diesen Kindern vermehrt psychopathologische Verhaltensmuster beobachtet werden (Lyons-Ruth und Jacobvitz 2008). Das pädagogische Betreuungspersonal steht Kindern mit solchen dysfunktionalen Bindungsmustern oft hilflos und überfordert gegenüber (Schmid und Kind 2018). Die aggressiven Verhaltensweisen der Kinder können bei den Erziehern emotionale Reaktionen wie Gefühle der Überforderung, Aggressionen und Ablehnungstendenzen auslösen (Schmid 2010). Nach der *„Replikationshypothese"* wiederholen sich in der sozialpädagogischen Arbeit mit den Kindern und Jugendlichen Beziehungsmuster, welche die Kinder aus ihrem familiären Umfeld übernommen haben (Schmid und Fegert 2012). Der so entstandene Teufelskreis kann in besonders schwerwiegenden Fällen zu einer Aktualisierung traumatischer Erfahrungen führen und das Eingewöhnen in die Wohngruppe massiv erschweren. In Folge kann es zum Abbruch der Hilfsmaßnahmen kommen, was bei den Kindern und Jugendlichen zu erneuten Beziehungsabbrüchen führt. Internationale Studien belegen, dass viele fremdplatzierte Kinder und Jugendliche mehrere Pflegefamilien oder Heimplatzierungen durchlaufen (Jaritz et al. 2008; Schmid und Fegert 2012). Solche Abbrüche verstärken nicht nur die Bindungsproblematik der betroffenen Kinder und Jugendlichen, sondern werden auch von den sozialpädagogischen Fachkräften als erschwerend erlebt. Diese bauen häufig eine emotionale Beziehung zu den Kindern und Jugendlichen auf und erleben dann, dass ihr Beziehungsangebot von den Jugendlichen nicht als solches wahrgenommen und genutzt wird. Grenzüberschreitende Verhaltensweisen der Kinder und Jugendlichen den Fachkräften gegenüber hinterlassen bei den Betroffenen oft Gefühle der Verunsicherung und Überforderung. Vielfach lösen die persönlichen Verletzungen am Arbeitsplatz Scham und Schuldgefühle aus und in Folge ein Verlust der Freude an der Arbeit (Schmid und Kind 2018). Laut Schmid (2013) sollten pädagogische Fachkräfte auf die aus vorausgegangenen traumatischen Erlebnissen entstandenen, dysfunktionalen Verhaltensmuster der Kinder und Jugendlichen vorbereitet und dementsprechend ausgebildet sein.

Wie dargelegt, erweist sich die Arbeit mit fremdplatzierten, meist psychisch belasteten Kindern und Jugendlichen vielfach als schwierig und langwierig. Trotz diesen erschwerenden Bedingungen ist eine Herausnahme aus den psychosozial stark belasteten Familien oftmals eine Chance für das Kind. Durch die Meta-Analyse von Knorth et al. (2008) konnte eine Verbesserung des psychosozialen Verhaltens von fremduntergebrachten Kindern und Jugendlichen belegt werden. Da sich die Ergebnisse dieser Analyse auf kurzzeitige Effekte (drei bis vier Monate nach Beendigung der Maßnahme) beziehen, hat das Forschungsteam um Knorth (Harder et al. 2017) versucht, Faktoren zu identifizieren, die zu einer langzeitigen Verbesserung des Verhaltens der betroffenen Kinder und Jugendlichen beitragen. Die Suche nach diesen Faktoren hat auf mehreren Ebenen stattgefunden. In der von Harder und ihren Mitarbeitern (2017) durchgeführten Studie waren die befragten Jugendlichen und deren Eltern der Ansicht, dass eine Verbesserung des Verhaltens der Jugendlichen während ihres Aufenthaltes in der Institution in erster Linie durch das institutionelle Umfeld bedingt gewesen sei. Da die Institution ein angemessenes Verhalten verlangt habe, sollen die Jugendlichen ihr Verhalten nur während der Dauer ihres Aufenthaltes den institutionellen Anforderungen und Regeln angepasst haben. Diese rein externalisierte Motivation einer Verhaltensveränderung könnte erklären, wieso viele Jugendliche nach ihrer Entlassung aus der Institution wieder ihre alten, dysfunktionalen Verhaltensmuster übernehmen (Ryan und Deci 2000). Für Harder und ihre Mitarbeiter zeigt dieser Befund, dass die persönliche Motivation, am eigenen Verhalten etwas verändern zu wollen – und nicht die durch institutionelle Regeln und Maßnahmen erzwungenen Verhaltensveränderungen – einer der Hauptfaktoren ist, um eine anhaltende positive Veränderungsbereitschaft bei den Jugendlichen zu bewirken. Ein weiterer Befund der Studie von Harder et al. (2017) besteht darin, dass die verschiedenen Fachkräfte, die die Kinder und Jugendlichen betreut haben, unterschiedliche Ansichten und Erklärungen bezüglich der Ursachen, die zu einer erfolgreichen Verhaltensveränderung der Jugendlichen geführt haben, aufweisen. Diese Feststellung bekräftigt die Befunde der Studie von Knorth et al. (2010), die belegt, dass Mitarbeiter aus dem Erziehungsbereich im generellen Kinder und Jugendliche nach ihren eigenen, individuellen Ansichten und mittels ihres persönlichen Stils behandeln und betreuen. Um jedoch in der stationären Kinder- und Jugendhilfe positive Effekte zu bewirken, ist es, laut Knorth et al. (2010), notwendig, dass alle Mitarbeiter einer Institution dieselben Zielsetzungen zeigen und den Kindern und Jugendlichen gegenüber dieselben Erziehungspraktiken und Einstellungen aufweisen.

Aufgrund dieser erschwerenden Bedingungen rund um die stationäre Jugendhilfe wird die Wirksamkeit der Fremdunterbringung von Kindern und Jugendlichen in der Forschung kontrovers diskutiert. Neben Befunden zu kurzeitigen positiven Effekten der Fremdunterbringung in Institutionen (De Swart et al. 2012; Knorth et al. 2008) liegen auch Befunde vor, die diesbezüglich keine oder negative Effekte nachweisen (Dumais und Michel 2014; Strijbosch et al. 2015). Einige Forscher bemängeln zudem das Fehlen von Befundlagen zu den Langzeitwirkungen institutioneller Fremdbetreuung von Kindern und Jugendlichen (De Swart et al. 2012; Knorth et al. 2008).

2.5 Anzahl stationär untergebrachter Kinder und Jugendlicher in Luxemburg

Um einen Einblick in die Anzahl, der in Luxemburg in Institutionen platzierten Kinder und Jugendlichen zu bekommen, wird die Zahl, der im April 2019 in Luxemburg durchs Jugendgericht platzierten Kinder und Jugendlichen tabellarisch dargestellt. Die in Pflegefamilien lebenden Kinder und Jugendlichen werden hierbei nicht berücksichtigt. Bei den Angaben, die aus dem Jahresbericht des *„Office National de l'Enfance"* (vgl. ONE 2019) entnommen wurden, handelt es sich um Kinder und junge Erwachsene, wobei sich der Begriff „Kinder" auf Minderjährige unter 18 Jahren und „junge Erwachsene" auf junge Menschen zwischen 18 und weniger als 27 Jahren bezieht.

Die meisten minderjährigen Kinder und Jugendlichen wurden vom Jugendgericht in die diversen Strukturen platziert, ein kleiner Teil war freiwillig oder auf Wunsch der Eltern in den Institutionen untergebracht. Der Vollständigkeit halber wird in der folgenden Tabelle auch die Anzahl der nicht platzierten Kinder aufgeführt (Tab. 1).

Insgesamt befanden sich im April 2019 *770 Kinder und Jugendliche* in einer stationären Hilfsmaßnahme. 577 (74,94 %) waren vom Jugendgericht platziert, 193 (25,06 %) waren freiwillig in der Maßnahme. Diese Daten belegen, dass auch in Luxemburg eine relevante Zahl vom Jugendgericht platzierter Kinder und Jugendlichen vorliegt. Mit Blick auf die in internationalen Studien aufgeführten 80 % Prozent traumatisierter Kinder und Jugendlichen, die in Institutionen leben (Schmid et al. 2011) wie auch auf die erwähnte Prävalenz von 60 bis 70 % psychischer Erkrankungen dieser Kinder (Ford et al. 2007; Schmid 2007) lässt sich annehmen, dass auch ein vergleichbarer Prozentsatz in luxemburgischen Institutionen zu erwarten ist. Dies legt nahe, dass es sich ebenso bei den in Luxemburg lebenden Heimkindern um eine vulnerable und stark belastete Population handelt, die das luxemburgische psycho-soziale Betreuungssystem in unterschiedlicher Weise fordert.

3 Empirischer Teil

Dieser Teil des Beitrags befasst sich mit einer im August 2018 an der Universität Luxemburg begonnenen Studie, deren Ziel es ist, die Faktoren zu erfassen, die einerseits zum Wohlbefinden und zu einer positiven Entwicklung fremdplatzierter Kinder und Jugendlichen an luxemburgischen Institutionen beitragen sowie

Tab. 1 Überblickstabelle der am 1. April 2019 in luxemburgischen Institutionen unter-gebrachten Kinder und jungen Erwachsenen

	Gesamtanzahl	Davon platziert	Davon freiwillig
Klassische Institutionen[1]	418	340	78
Notaufnahmen[2]	45	34	11
Centre Socio-Educative de l'Etat (CSEE)	50	50	0
Unité de sécurité (Unisec)	8	8	0
Institut Etatique d'Aide à l'Enfance et à la Jeunesse (AITIA)[3]	69	45	24
Spezialisierte Strukturen[4]	40	31	9
Unbegleitete Minderjährige	41		41
Auslandsmaßnahmen	99	69	30
	770	**577** (74,94 %)	**193** (25,06 %)

Erläuterungen: [1]Der Begriff „Klassische Institutionen" bezeichnet vom Staat sub-ventionierte Strukturen wie „*Foyers*", Strukturen, die Kinder unter 3 Jahren empfangen oder Strukturen mit einem „*accueil orthopédagogique*" (eine stationäre Unterbringung mit einer intensiven pädagogischen Betreuung); [2]Der Begriff „Notaufnahmen" bezeichnet Strukturen für psychosoziale Notsituationen; [3]Die „Instituts Etatiques d'Aide à l'Enfance et à la Jeunesse" hießen früher „Maisons d'enfants de l'Etat"; [4]Der Begriff „Spezialisierte Strukturen" bezeichnet spezifische Strukturen, wie zum Beispiel Kinder- und Jugend-psychiatrien

diejenigen, die andererseits zu Belastungen oder Traumatisierungen bei den Betroffenen führen können.

3.1 Studie über das Wohlbefinden von Kindern und Jugendlichen, die in luxemburgischen Institutionen platziert sind

Die aufgeführten wissenschaftlichen Grundlagen zu den Bindungstheorien und zur frühkindlichen Traumatisierung geben einen Einblick in die Komplexität der Betreuung und Förderung fremdplatzierter Kinder und Jugendlicher. Zahlreiche wissenschaftliche Studien belegen, dass die Mehrzahl der platzierten Kinder und Jugendlichen traumatischen Ereignissen ausgesetzt war, bevor sie auf Beschluss des Jugendgerichts aus den Familien herausgenommen wurden (Jackson et al. 2019; Ptacek et al. 2012; Zeanah et al. 2012). Ziel ist es, diesen Kindern und Jugendlichen ein Umfeld zu bieten, in dem sie ihre traumatischen Erlebnisse aufarbeiten können, sich sicher und geborgen fühlen und sich auf psychischer wie auch physischer Ebene angemessen entwickeln können. In den letzten Jahrzehnten sind bedeutende Fortschritte auf dem Gebiet der Heimbetreuung festzustellen (Bryson et al. 2017; Gahleitner 2009; Gahleitner et al. 2018; Schmid 2018) und dennoch kommt es bei dieser sensiblen und belasteten Population weiterhin zu Retraumatisierungen und den daraus resultierenden Verhaltensauffälligkeiten.

Die vorliegende Studie setzt sich mit dieser Thematik auseinander, indem sie die Befindlichkeit betroffener Kinder und Jugendlicher untersucht und die Faktoren, die zu einer Retraumatisierung führen können, identifiziert. Mit Hilfe der Befragung von Jugendlichen sollen Antworten auf folgende Fragen eruiert werden: *„Welche Faktoren erhöhen das Wohlbefinden von Kindern und Jugendlichen, die in luxemburgischen Institutionen fremdplatziert worden sind?"* und *„Welche Faktoren erschweren die Entwicklung dieser Kinder und Jugendlichen?"*. Zusätzlich werden neue Erkenntnisse im Forschungsgebiet der stationären Jugendhilfe erwartet, die es erlauben, Retraumatisierungen in Zukunft zu vermeiden und entwicklungsförderliche Veränderungen in diesem Handlungsfeld zu bewirken. Sämtliche Befunde stützen sich auf die Aussagen der befragten Jugendlichen und geben die von den Studienteilnehmern retrospektiv betrachteten persönlichen Wahrnehmungen und Beschreibungen des Erlebten wieder.

Im Folgenden werden zuerst die Teilnehmer der Befragung sowie der Interviewleitfaden und das Auswertungsverfahren kurz dargestellt, um anschließend erste Befunde der Studie vorzustellen. Die Darstellung der Ergebnislage wird sich dabei auf einzelne Faktoren beschränken, die von den Jugendlichen als entwicklungsförderlich oder entwicklungserschwerend beschrieben wurden. Die gesamte Befundlage der Studie wird voraussichtlich Anfang 2021 vorliegen.

3.1.1 Methode

Um die in der Fragestellung genannten Faktoren zu identifizieren wurden 30 Jugendliche über ihre Erfahrungen, die sie in den unterschiedlichen Institutionen gemacht haben, befragt. Als Einschlusskriterium für die Teilnahme an der Studie galt eine Platzierung durch das Jugendgericht in einer luxemburgischen Institution während der Kindheit oder im Jugendalter (unter 18 Jahren) mit einer Aufenthaltsdauer von mindestens vier Monaten. Als Ausschlusskriterium galt, wenn der Jugendliche sich zum Zeitpunkt der Befragung in einer emotional instabilen Phase befand oder unter einer diagnostizierten schwerwiegenden psychiatrischen Erkrankung litt. An der Studie nahmen 16 minderjährige Jugendliche (zwischen 15 und 17 Jahren) und 14 junge Erwachsene (zwischen 18 und 27 Jahren) teil. Davon waren 16 weibliche und 14 männliche Teilnehmer. Die Teilnahme erfolgte auf freiwilliger Basis, wobei den Jugendlichen absolute Anonymität garantiert wurde. Die Studie wurde im Vorfeld durch die Ethik-Kommission der Universität Luxemburg („*Ethics Review Panel*") bewilligt.

Die Rekrutierung erfolgte durch direktes Ansprechen betroffener Jugendlicher sowie durch das Vorstellen der Studie und die Anwerbung zur Teilnahme in unterschiedlichen Institutionen. Da die Institutionen im Allgemeinen ein großes Interesse an der Studie zeigten, wirkten sie aktiv bei der Suche nach Teilnehmern und unterstützend bei der Durchführung der Interviews mit. Einige Teilnehmer meldeten sich spontan, nachdem sie durch andere Jugendliche von der Studie erfahren hatten. Die Rekrutierung der Teilnehmer erwies sich als unproblematisch, da der Wunsch, sich mitzuteilen und über persönliche Erfahrungen und Erlebnisse zu berichten, bei den betroffenen Jugendlichen sehr ausgeprägt war.

Die Befragung fand anhand eines semi-strukturierten Interviews statt. Neben der Erhebung demographischer Daten wurden die Teilnehmer gebeten, über ihre ersten Lebensjahre zu berichten. Anschließend wurde eine Traumaanamnese über die Zeit vor der ersten Platzierung durch das Jugendgericht erhoben, wobei die Jugendlichen darauf hingewiesen wurden, dass sie keine Einzelheiten zu den erlebten Belastungssituationen erzählen sollten. Nach der Traumaanamnese wurden die Teilnehmer gebeten, den Grund ihrer ersten Platzierung mitzuteilen. Im Folgenden sollten die Jugendlichen ihr eigenes Problemverhalten vor und während der Fremdplatzierung, sowie auch ihre aktuellen Schwierigkeiten, falls vorhanden, beschreiben. Der Schwerpunkt des Interviews lag auf der Befragung über die positiven und entwicklungsförderlichen wie auch belastenden Erfahrungen der Jugendlichen während der Dauer ihrer Platzierung. Hier konnten die Teilnehmer zuerst frei berichten, anschließend wurden sie zu spezifischen Themen befragt. Die durchschnittliche Dauer eines Interviews betrug 57 min.

Die Audioaufnahmen wurden transkribiert und anhand eines Kategoriensystems analysiert. Hierbei wurde sich an der qualitativen Inhaltsanalyse nach Mayring (2015), Schreier (2012) und Kuckartz (2018) orientiert.

3.1.2 Erste Befunde

Da eine umfassende Auswertung der Interviews erst Mitte 2022 vorliegen wird, werden im Folgenden nur erste, eingeschränkte Befunde dargelegt und einige zentrale Themenbereiche der Studie erläutert.

Erstplatzierung: Die Gründe der ersten Platzierung der Interviewteilnehmer in einer Institution variierten je nach Alter der Betroffenen. Dort, wo die erste Fremdbetreuung im Säuglings-, Kleinkind- oder Schulkindalter erfolgte, berichteten alle Jugendlichen von einer Kindeswohlgefährdung. Die Kinder wurden entweder körperlich und psychisch vernachlässigt und/oder sie waren Opfer von körperlicher, sexueller oder psychischer Gewalt. Einige der betroffenen Jugendlichen beschrieben die frühe Herausnahme aus der Familie als eine Chance, den Belastungen und traumatischen Ereignissen, denen sie im familiären Umfeld ausgesetzt waren, zu entkommen. Bei Studienteilnehmern, die bei ihrer ersten Platzierung bereits das Alter der Adoleszenz erreicht hatten, waren die Gründe dieser Platzierung meistens gehäufte und anhaltende Verhaltensauffälligkeiten, wie zum Beispiel Schule schwänzen, Drogenkonsum, Regelmissachtungen bis hin zu delinquentem Verhalten. Manche Jugendlichen klagten, dass sie noch immer nicht nachvollziehen könnten, wieso sie wegen wiederholtem Schulschwänzen oder Regelmissachtungen aus der Familie genommen und in einer Institution untergebracht worden seien *(„Ech hun vill blo gemacht...do ass d'Decisioun vum Gericht einfach komm, dass ech géif placéiert gin")*. Andere wiederum bedauerten, dass sie nicht viel früher aus der Familie herausgenommen wurden. In diesen Fällen lag bei den Eltern meistens eine starke Suchtproblematik oder eine psychiatrische Erkrankung vor.

Traumatisierungen und psychische Belastungen im familiären Umfeld: Bis auf eine Jugendliche berichteten sämtliche Teilnehmer von traumatischen Ereignissen und/oder Trennungssituationen während der Kindheit und/oder Jugend. Die Jugendlichen sprachen über psychische, körperliche oder sexuelle Gewalt, der sie selbst ausgesetzt waren *(„geschloen, Zigaretten u mir ausgedreckt gi sin...")* oder die sie beobachtet haben. Hinzu kamen Vernachlässigung und psychische Erkrankungen der Eltern, wie zum Beispiel Depressionen, Drogen- oder Alkoholabhängigkeit.

Wechsel und Abbrüche: Die Zahl der Wechsel und Abbrüche in den unterschiedlichen Institutionen variierte zwischen einer einzigen Platzierung in einer Institution bis zu 11 Abbrüchel oder Wechsel zwischen unterschiedlichen Institutionen. Die Wechsel kamen gelegentlich auf Anfrage der Jugendlichen zustande, jedoch fand ein Abbruch oder ein Wechsel in den meisten Fällen ohne die Zustimmung des Kindes oder des Jugendlichen statt. In solchen Fällen war die aktuelle Institution meistens nicht mehr in der Lage, den Bedürfnissen des Jugendlichen gerecht zu werden und eine angemessene Entwicklung zu gewährleisten. Die Wechsel waren, nach Aussagen der Jugendlichen, immer mit Beziehungsabbrüchen sowie Eingewöhnungs- und Anpassungsschwierigkeiten verbunden. Die bei dem Wechsel gelegentlich stattgefundene Trennung von Geschwisterkindern wurde von den Jugendlichen als besonders schwierig beschrieben (siehe hierzu weiter unten).

Gruppengröße: Die meisten Jugendlichen zogen kleinere Gruppen von 8–12 Kindern oder Jugendlichen vor. Sie gaben an, dass auftretende Konflikte in kleineren Gruppen eher erkannt und gelöst werden konnten (*„Mir waren ze vill Jugendlécher ob enkem Raum. Dat kann sou net goen"*) und kleinere Gruppen eher einen familiären Charakter hatten. Zudem soll die Beziehung zwischen den Heimbewohnern und dem Betreuungspersonal in kleineren Gruppen intensiver gewesen sein, was den Vorteil hatte, dass sich die Jugendlichen dem Personal eher anvertrauten. Einige wenige der befragten Jugendlichen fühlten sich in größeren Gruppen wohler (*„Am beschten hu mir éischter esou grouss Gruppe wéi ... gefall.... ...t'ass méi cool, du hues méi Leit, du hues méi Ofwiesselung, net ëmmer die Nämmlecht an jo."*). An größeren Gruppen gefiel ihnen, dass sie mehr Auswahl hatten, was Freundschaften betraf. Außerdem wurden größere Gruppen von vereinzelten Teilnehmern als abwechslungsreicher beschrieben.

Beziehungen: Die Beziehung zu den Mitarbeitern der Institutionen wie auch die Beziehung zu den Mitbewohnern spielte für die Studienteilnehmer eine zentrale Rolle für ihr Wohlbefinden. Wertschätzende und stabile Beziehungen steigerten offensichtlich das Wohlbefinden der Kinder und Jugendlichen und trugen zu deren positiven Entwicklung bei. Die Jugendlichen schätzten es, wenn sich ein Betreuer Zeit für sie nahm und ihnen aufmerksam zuhörte (*„...un sech hun ech mech guéd gefillt, well et war een do. Et war een do an déi hun mer ëmmer nogelauschtert. An sie hun mat dir geschwad. An sie hun dech fier eescht geholl"*). Auch scheint die jahrelange Anwesenheit desselben Betreuers für vereinzelte Jugendliche einen großen Stellenwert gehabt zu haben (*„An do war en Erzéier do, den ech vun klengem un kennen also karnt hun, dat heescht, ech hat awer eng gud Bindung zu engem .... dat war eng mega wichteg Persoun."*). Einige Teilnehmer nannten die Köchin oder die Haushälterin als wichtigste Bezugsperson (*„D'Botzfra hat eng mega grouss Roll a mengem Liewen.... sie ass do, sie hëlleft eis, sie kacht eis, sie hëlleft mir"*). Die gute Beziehung zu den Fachkräften wurde als ebenso bedeutend für das allgemeine Wohlbefinden beschrieben wie die freundschaftliche Beziehung zu den anderen Heimbewohnern, wobei der Einfluss dieser Freundschaften auf die eigene Entwicklung im Nachhinein nicht in allen Fällen als entwicklungsförderlich angesehen wurde. Ein weiterer wichtiger Faktor, der von den Jugendlichen als unterstützend beschrieben wurde, war der regelmäßige Kontakt zur eigenen Familie.

Diverse weitere Faktoren: Die Ausstattung der Gemeinschaftsräume, der Schlafzimmer und der sanitären Anlagen schienen einen direkten Einfluss auf das Wohlbefinden der Jugendlichen gehabt zu haben. Die Beschreibungen variierten von wohnlich, großräumig und sauber bis hin zu klein, alt, kaputt und ekelig. In einigen Institutionen wurde kritisiert, dass die Schlafzimmer zu klein waren und noch Spuren von den Vorgängern enthielten *(„et war en plus iwerall gemolt... do war nëmmen fier ze schlofen gudd soss war et net gemittlech an esou...").* So wurden z. B. defektes Mobiliar und unhygienische sanitäre Bedingungen bemängelt. Die institutionsinternen Freizeitaktivitäten wie z. B. gemeinsam das Freibad besuchen oder ins Kino gehen, hatten bei den befragten Jugendlichen einen hohen Stellenwert. Sämtliche Teilnehmer schienen von den angebotenen Freizeitaktivitäten profitiert zu haben und beschrieben diese als einen wichtigen Faktor, der zu ihrem allgemeinen Wohlbefinden beigetragen hat. Sie bedauerten lediglich, dass solche Aktivitäten nicht oft genug stattgefunden hätten. Des Weiteren gaben einige Jugendliche an, dass die therapeutische Arbeit mit einem Psychologen oder Psychiater sie in ihrer persönlichen Entwicklung gestärkt und weitergebracht habe. Andere Jugendliche wiederum hätten sich öfters Gespräche mit ihrem Therapeuten gewünscht oder sie fühlten sich von ihrem Psychologen nicht verstanden *(„also fier mech, mein Psycholog huet et net bruecht...t'ass die eenzeg Persoun, déi mir hätt wierklech kéinten héllefen").* Institutionelle Regeln und Einschränkungen konnten von den Jugendlichen relativ gut angenommen werden und wurden sogar teilweise als hilfreich beschrieben.

Retraumatisierung und entwicklungserschwerende Bedingungen während der Fremdplatzierung: Viele der befragten Jugendlichen berichteten von traumatischen Ereignissen und schwierigen Zeiten während der Fremdplatzierung. Die meisten traumatischen Ereignisse seien von anderen Heimbewohner ausgegangen. Die Jugendlichen sprachen von Drohungen und Erpressungen, körperlicher und verbaler Gewalt, Mobbingsituationen, sexuellen Übergriffen und Vergewaltigung durch andere Bewohner der Institution. Einige der Kinder und Jugendlichen erzählten, dass sie mit niemandem über das Erlebte gesprochen hätten. In den meisten Fällen befürchteten die Kinder und Jugendlichen noch heftigere Reaktionen von Seiten der Täter, wenn sie über die Vorfälle reden würden. Einige wenige Jugendliche berichteten, sie hätten mit Erziehern über die Vorfälle geredet, es sei jedoch von Seiten der Institution keine angemessene Reaktion erfolgt *(„T'ass einfach ënnert den Teppech gekiert gin a fäerdeg").* Als weitere extreme Belastungssituation wurde, wie bereits erwähnt, die Trennung von den Geschwistern beschrieben. Solche Trennungen seien schmerzhaft gewesen und hätten bei den Kindern und Jugendlichen oft zu einer Zunahme ungünstiger Verhaltensmuster geführt. Auch soll die Unterbringung in diversen Institutionen das Unwohlsein gesteigert und demnach zu vermehrten

Verhaltensauffälligkeiten und Drogenkonsum bei den Jugendlichen geführt haben. Einige Jugendliche berichteten, dass sie während der Fremdplatzierung ihren ersten Kontakt mit Drogen hatten. Was die Betreuer betraf, sollen die Kinder und Jugendliche selten körperliche, sondern eher verbale Gewalt wie Demütigungen und Erniedrigungen durch die Betreuer erlebt haben (*„T'es bon à rien"*). Auch sollen verschiedene institutionelle Konsequenzen, die auf Fehlverhalten erfolgt seien, als ziemlich belastend empfunden worden sein und eher eine Verhaltensverschlechterung anstelle einer Verbesserung bewirkt haben. Als besonders belastend wurde die Bestrafung durch mehrtägige Isolation in einem dafür vorgesehenen Bestrafungsraum empfunden (*„...dat mëscht een krank am Kapp"*).

3.1.3 Interpretation der Befunde

Der im theoretischen Teil bereits thematisierte hohe Prozentsatz an traumatisierten fremdplatzierten Kindern und Jugendlichen wird in dieser Studie ebenso belegt. Fast alle Studienteilnehmer waren in ihrer Kindheit und Jugend anhaltend belasteten Situationen ausgesetzt, ehe es zu einer ersten Fremdplatzierung kam. Obwohl die erhaltenen Befunde und Aussagen der Jugendlichen nur eine vorläufige Analyse der Interviews wiederspiegeln, weisen sie deutlich daraufhin dass die Mehrheit der Studienteilnehmer auch während ihrer Fremdplatzierung traumatisierenden Situationen ausgesetzt waren. Die Jugendlichen berichteten unter anderem über vermehrten Drogenkonsum während der Zeit ihrer Fremdplatzierung, über körperliche, sexuelle und psychische Gewalt durch andere Heimbewohner, über körperliche, vor allem psychische Gewalt auf Ebene der Erzieher und anderen Fachkräften, über übertriebene institutionelle Konsequenzen und über einen hohen Belastungsgrad durch die Trennung von ihren Geschwistern. Einige Jugendliche sahen einen Zusammenhang zwischen dem Erlebten und der Entstehung weiterer Verhaltensauffälligkeiten.

Bezüglich der Faktoren, die zum Wohlbefinden der Kinder und Jugendlichen beigetragen haben standen für fast sämtliche Teilnehmer die zwischenmenschlichen Beziehungen an oberster Stelle. Eine vertrauensvolle Beziehung zu einer pädagogischen Fachkraft, einem Angestellten oder einem Therapeuten, enge Freundschaften zu Gleichaltrigen und/oder die Unterstützung durch Familienangehörige wurden hierbei als die wirksamsten Faktoren beschrieben. Hinzu kamen unter anderem gemeinsame Freizeitaktivitäten mit der Wohngruppe, ein angenehmes Wohnumfeld, kleine Gruppen und angemessene institutionelle Verhaltensregeln.

4 Fazit und Ausblick

Die bisherige Befundlage der empirischen Studie zeigt deutlich, dass die Jugendlichen, die an der Studie teilgenommen haben, häufig schwierigen Lebensbedingungen ausgesetzt waren. Dies sowohl vor ihrer ersten Platzierung im familiären Milieu wie auch während der Zeit ihrer Platzierung in den diversen Institutionen. Die vorliegende Analyse der Daten bestätigt, dass es sich bei Kindern und Jugendlichen, die in einem außerfamiliären Umfeld aufwachsen, um eine stark belastete Population handelt. Interviewaussagen weisen darauf hin, dass den Bedürfnissen dieser Populationsgruppe nicht ausreichend Rechnung getragen wird und deren psychische Entwicklung weiterhin erschwert bleibt. Zudem unterstreichen sie die Notwendigkeit einer weiterführenden Analyse der Daten zur Fremdplatzierung. Je mehr Klarheit über die emotionalen Bedürfnisse dieser vulnerablen Kinder und Jugendlichen besteht, umso besser können die Betreuungsstrukturen und -formen angepasst und die Entwicklungschancen dieser jungen Menschen erhöht werden.

Aufgrund zahlreicher Beobachtungen und Forschungsergebnissen konnten auf dem Gebiet der Heimunterbringung in den vergangenen Jahrzehnten bereits eine Reihe von positiven und entwicklungsfördernden Veränderungen erzielt werden (Gahleitner et al. 2018; Harder et al. 2017; Knorth et al. 2008; Schmid 2018). Dennoch bleibt es eine bedeutsame Aufgabe zu prüfen, welche weiteren Veränderungen vorgenommen werden sollten, um den Bedürfnissen der betroffenen Kinder und Jugendlichen gerecht zu werden. Anzunehmen ist, dass nicht nur Veränderungen bezüglich der Handlungsweisen der Fachkräfte notwendig sind, sondern dass auch insbesondere angemessene strukturelle Maßnahmen erforderlich sind.

Literatur

Ackerman, P.T., Newton, J.E., McPherson, W.B., Jones, J.G., & Dykman, R.A. (1998). Prevalence of posttraumatic stress disorder and other psychiatric diagnoses in three groups of abused children (sexual, physical and both). In: *Child Abuse and Neglect, 22* (8), 759–774.

Ainsworth, M.D.S. (1985). Patterns of infant-mother attachment: Antecedents and effects on development. In: *Bulletin of the New York Academy of Medicine*, 61, 771–791.

Anda, R.F., Felitti, V.J., Bremner, J.D., Walker, J.D., Whitfield, C., Perry, B.D., Dube, S.R., & Giles, W.H. (2006). The enduring effects of abuse and related adverse experiences in childhood. A convergence of evidence from neurobiology and epidemiology. *In: European Archives of Psychiatry Clinical Neuroscience, 256* (3), 174–186.

Bowlby, J. (1969). Attachment. *Attachment and Loss, Vol. 1.* New York: Basic Books.
Bowlby, J. (1973). Separation: Anxiety and Anger. *Attachment and Loss, Vol. 2.* New York: Basic Books.
Bowlby, J. (1980). Loss: Sadness and Depression. *Attachment and Loss, Vol. 3.* New York: Basic Books.
Bretherton, I. (1985). Attachment theory: Retrospect and prospect. In: I. Bretherton & E. Waters (Eds.): *Growing Points of Attachment. Theory and Research. Monograph of the Society for Research in Child Development,* 50, 3–35. Chicago: Univ. Chicago Pr.
Bronfenbrenner, U. (1994). Ecological models of human development. In: Husen, T., Postlethwaite, TN. (Eds.), *international encyclopedia of education,* 3, 1643–1647. Oxford, England: Pergamon Press/Elsevier Science.
Bryson, S.A., Gauvin, E., Jameson, A., Rathgeber, M., Fau kner-Gibson, L., Bell, S., Russel, J. & Burke, S. (2017). What are effective strategies for implementing trauma-informed care in youth inpatient psychiatric and residential treatment settings? A realist systematic review. In: *International Journal of Mental Health Systems,* 11.
Chambers, J.A., Power K. G., Loucks N., Swanson V. (2000). Psychometric properties of the Parental Bonding Instrument and its association with psychological distress in a group of incarcerated young offenders in Scotland. In: *Social Psychiatry and Psychiatric* Epidemiology. 35, 318–325. Springer.
Cleverley, K. & Kidd, S.A. (2011). Resilience and suicidality among homeless youth. In: *Journal of Adolescence, 34,* 1049–1054.
Crittenden, P. (1995). Attachment and Psychopathologie. In: S. Goldberg, R. Muir & J. Kerr (Eds.) *Attachment Theory. Social, Developmental and Clinical Perspectives* (376–406). Hilldale, N.Y.: The Analytic Press.
Cromer, K.D. & Villodas M.T. (2017). Post-traumatic stress as a pathway to psychopathology among adolescents at high-risk for victimization. In: *Child Abuse and Neglect,* 67, 182.192.
Decarli, A. (2019). *Mental health and wellbeing in adolescence* The role of child attachment and parents' representation of their children. Dissertation.
De Swart, J.J.W., Van den Broek, H., Stams, G.J.J.M., Asscher, J.J., Van der Laan, G.A., Holsbrink-Engels, G.A. & Van der Helm, G.H.P. (2012). The effectiveness of institutional youth care over the past three decades: A meta-analysis. In: *Children and Youth Services reviews,* 34, 1818–1824.
Dornes, M. (1993). Der kompetente Säugling. Die präverbale Entwicklung des Menschen. Frankfurt am Main: Fischer Verlag.
Dornes, M. (1997). *Die frühe Kindheit. Entwicklungspsychologie der ersten Lebensjahre.* Fischer: Frankfurt am Main.
Dumais, M., Cyr, C. & Michel, G. (2014). L'attachement chez les enfants institutionnalisés: une récension narrative et méta-analytique des études sur les facteurs de risque. In: *Revue européenne de psychologie appliquée, 64,* 181–194.
Egle, U.T., Hoffmann, S.O. & Joraschky, P. (2005). *Sexueller Missbrauch, Misshandlung, Vernachlässigung. Erkennen, Therapie und Prävention der Folgen früher Stresserfahrungen.* Schattauer GmbH: Stuttgart, New York.
Entringer, S., Buss, C. & Heim C. (2016). Frühe Stresserfahrungen und Krankheitsvulnerabilität. In: *Bundesgesundheitsblatt,* 59, 1255–1261. Springer: Berlin, Heidelberg.

Entringer, S, & Heim, C. (2016). BiologischeGrundlagen. In: U. Ehlert (Hrsg), *Verhaltensmedizin*. Springer: Berlin, Heidelberg.

Eriksson, Z. (1925). *Hospitalismus in Kinderheimen: Über Anstaltsschäden der Kinder*. Akad. Abh. aus der Münchener Kinderklinik. M.v. Pfaundler. Akademiska Bokhandeln.

Fazel, S. & Langstrom, N. (2008). Mental disorder among adolescents in juvenile detention and correctional facilities: a systematic review and metaregression analysis of 25 surveys. In: *Journal of the American Academy of Child and Adolescent Psychiatry*, *47* (9), 1010–1019.

Felitti, V.J., Anda, R.F., Nordenberg, D., Williamson, D.F., Spitz, A.M. & Edwards. (1998). The Relationship of adult health status to childhood abuse and household dysfunction. In: *American journal of preventive medicine*, *14*, 245–258.

Ford, T., Vostanos, P., Meltzer, H. & Goodman, R. (2007). Psychiatric disorder among British children looked after by local authorities: comparison with children living in private households. In: *The British Journal of Psychiatry*, *190*, 319–325.

Freedmann, D.G. & DeBoer, M.M. (1979). Biological and cultural differences in early child development. In: *Annual Review of Anthropology*, *8*, 579–600.

Gahleitner, S.B. (2009). *Was hilft ehemaligen Heimkindern bei der Bewältigung ihrer komplexen Traumatisierung?* Expertise im Auftrag des Runden Tisches Heimerziehung.

Gahleitner, S.B., Frank, Ch., Gerlich, K., Hinterwallner, H., Schneider, M. & Radler, H. (2018). „Otherwise I might not have been able to cope at all": A research project on the residential care of children and adolescents. In: *International Journal of Child, Youth and Family Studies, 9 (1), 31–53*.

George, C. & Main, M. (1979). Social interaction of young, abused children: Approach, avoidance and aggression. In: *Child Development*, *50*, 306–318.

George, C., Kaplan, N. & Main, M. (1985). *The Adult Attachment Interview*. Unpublished manuscript, University of Califirnia Berkley.

Grisso, T. (2004). *Double Jeopardy*. New York: Guilford.

Grossmann, K. E., Grossmann, K. (2011). Bindung, innere Arbeitsmodelle und psychologische Anpassung. In: Grossmann, K. E. und Grossmann, K. (Hrsg.): *Bindung und menschliche Entwicklung – John Bowlby, Mary Ainsworth und die Grundlagen der Bindungstheorie*, 307–317, 2. Auflage, Stuttgart: Klett-Cotta, Stuttgart.

Gunnar, M.R. (1998). Quality of early care and buffering of neuroendocrine stress reactions: Potential effects on the developing brain. In: *Preventive Medicine*, *27*, 208–211.

Harder, A.T., Knorth, E.J. & Kalverboer, M.E. (2017). The Inside Out? Views of Young People, Parents and Professionals Regarding Successful Secure Residential Care. In: *Child Adolescent Social Work*, *34*, 431–441.

Heim, C. & Binder, E.B. (2012). Current research trends in early life stress and depression: Review of human studies on sensitive periods, gene-environment interactions, and epigenetics. In: *Experimental Neurology*, 233, 102–111.

Howe, D. & Fearnley, S. (2003). Disorders of Attachment in Adopted and Fostered Children: Recognition and Treatment. In: *Clinical Child Psychology and Psychiatry*, *8* (3). 369–387.

Hukkanen, R., Sourander, A., Bergroth, L. & Piha, J. (1999). Psychosocial factors and adequacy for children in children's home. In: *European Child and Adolescent Psychiatry*, *8* (4), 268–275.

Jackson, A.L., McKenzie, R. & Frederico, M. (2019). Addressing pain and pain-based behaviors for children and young people in child protection and out-of-home care. In: *International Journal of Child, Youth and Family Studies, 10, 103–125.*

Jaritz, C., Wiesinger, D. & Schmid, M. (2008). Traumatische Lebensereignisse bei Kindern und Jugendlichen in der stationären Jugendhilfe. In: *Trauma und Gewalt, 2* (4), 266–277.

Knorth, E.J., Harder, A.T., Zandberg, T. & Kendrick, A.J. (2008). Under one roof: A review and selective analysis on the outcomes of residential child and youth care. In: *Children and Youth Services Review, 30,* 123–140.

Knorth, E.J., Harder, A.T., Huyghen, A.M.N., Kalverboer, M E. & Zandberg, T. (2010). Residential youth care and treatment research: Care workers as key factor in outcomes? In: *International Journal of Child and Family Welfare, 13,* 49–67.

Kolk van der, B.A. & Fisler, R.E. (1994). Childhood abuse and neglect and loss of self-regulation. In: *Bulletin of the Menninger Clinic. 58, 145–168.*

Kuckartz, U. (2018). *Qualitative Inhaltsanalyse. Methoden, Praxis, Computerunterstützung.* Weinheim Basel: Beltz Juventa.

Laucht, M., Schmidt, M. & Esser, G. (2002). Motorische, kognitive und sozial-emotionale Entwicklung von 11jährigen mit frühen Risikobelastungen: späte Folgen? In: *Zeitschrift der Kinder- und Jugendpsychiatrie, 30,* 5–20.

Lindert, L., Schick, A., Reif, A., Kalisch, R. & Tüscher, O. (2018). Verläufe von Resilienz – Beispiele aus Längsschnittstudien. In: *Nervenarzt* 89, 759–756.

Lionetti, F., Pastore, M. & Barone, L. (2015). Attachment in institutionalized children: A review and meta-analysis. In: *Child Abuse and Neglect, 42,* 135–145.

Luthar, S.S., Cicchetti, D. & Becker, B. (2000). The construct of resilience: a critical evaluation and guidelines for future work. In: *Child development,* 71, 543–62.

Lyons-Ruth, K. & Jacobvitz, D. (2008). Attachment disorganization: genetic factors, parenting contexts and developmental transformation from infancy to adulthood. In: J. Cassidy & P.R. Shaver (Eds.), *Handbook of attachment* (2nd ed.), 666–697. New York: Guildford Press.

McCann, J.B., James, A., Wilson, S. & Dunn, G. (1996). Prevalence of psychiatric disorders in young people in the care system. In: *British Medical Journal, 313* (7071), 1529–1530.

Mayring, P. (2015). *Qualitative Inhaltsanalyse. Grundlagen und Techniken.* Weinheim und Basel: Beltz Verlag.

Office national de l'enfance. (2019). Children and young adults in alternative care. Luxembourg: Ministère de l'Education, de l'Enfance et de la Jeunesse.

Panksepp, J. (2004). Die biologischen Langzeitfolgen der emotionalen Umwelten von Kleinkindern für das spätere Gefühlsleben – Forschungsperspektiven für das 21. Jahrhundert. In: A. Streeck-Fischer (Hrsg.), *Adoleszenz – Bindung – Destruktivität.* Stuttgart: Klett-Cotta.

Papoušek, M., Papoušek H. & Haekel M. (1987). Didactic adjustments in fathers' and mothers' speech to their 3-month-old infants. In: *Journal of Psycholinguistic Research.* Springer, 1987.

Papoušek, M., Schieche, M & Wurmser, H. (2004). Regulationsstörungen der frühen Kindheit. Frühe Risiken und Hilfen im Entwicklungskontext der Eltern-Kind-Beziehungen. Bern: Hans-Huber Verlag.

Pfaundler, M.v. (1915). Physiologie des Neugeborenen. In: A. Döderlein (Hrsg.): *Handbuch der Geburtshilfe*. Bd.1, München/Wiesbaden.

Ptacek, R., Kuzelová, H., Celedova, L. & Cevela, R. (2012). Trauma and sings of psychopathology in children in foster and institutional care. In: *European psychiatry, 27, 1.*

Roth, G. & Strüber, M. (2014). Wie das Gehirn die Seele macht. Stuttgart: Klett-Cotta.

Rutter M. (2000). Resilience reconsidered: conceptual considerations,empirical findings, and policy implications. In J.P. Shonkoff & S.J. Meisels (Eds.), *Handbook of early childhood intervention*. 651–82. Cambridge: Cambridge University Press.

Ryan, R.M. & Deci, E.L. (2000). Intrinsic and extrinsic motivations: Classic definitions and new directions. In: *Contemporary Educational Psychology, 25,* 54–67.

Sattler, K.M.P. & Font, S. (2018). Resilience in Young Children with Child Protective Services. In: *Child Abuse and Neglect, 75,* 104–144.

Scheithauer, H., Petermann, F. & Niebank, K. (2000). Frühkindliche Entwicklung und Entwicklungsrisiken. In: F. Petermann, K. Niebank & H. Scheithauer (Hrsg.) *Risiken in der frühkindlichen Entwicklung: Entwicklungspsychopathologie der ersten Lebensjahre.* 15–38. Göttingen: Hogrefe.

Schmid, M. (2007). Psychische Gesundheit von Heimkindern. Eine Studie zur Prävalenz psychischer Störungen in der stationären Jugendhilfe. Weinheim: Juventa.

Schmid, M. (2008). Entwicklungspsychopathologische Grundlagen einer Traumapädagogik. In: *Traum & Gewalt, 2 (4),* 288–309.

Schmid, M. (2010). Umgang mit traumatisierten Kindern und Jugendlichen in der stationären Jugendhilfe: „Traumasensibilität" und „Traumapädagogik". In: Fegert, J.M., Ziegenhain, U. & Goldbeck, L. (Hrsg.). *Traumatisierte Kinder und Jugendliche in Deutschland. Analysen und Empfehlungen zur Versorgung und Betreuung.* Juventa, Weinheim, 36–60.

Schmid, M. (2013). Psychisch belastete Kinder und Jugendliche in der stationären Kinder- und Jugendhilfe – eine kooperative Herausforderung. In: Integras (Ed.), *Leitfaden Fremdplatzierung.* 142–160. Zürich: Integras.

Schmid, M. (2018). Zur Diskussion: Traumapädagogik und geschlossene Unterbringung – ein Widerspruch? In: *Unsere Jugend,* 70, 376–385.

Schmid, M., Fegert, J.M., Kölch, M. & Schmeck, K. (2011). Abschlussbericht des Modellversuchs Abklärung und Zielerreichung in stationären Maßnahmen, MAZ. Bundesamt für Justiz. Bern.

Schmid, M. & Fegert, J.M., (2012). Fremdplatzierte Kinder in Pflegefamilien und stationärer Jugendhilfe. In: J.M. Fegert, Ch. Eggers & F. Resch (Hrsg.), *Psychiatrie und Psychotherapie des Kindes- und Jugendalters,* 63–74. Berlin, Heidelberg: Springer Verlag.

Schmid, M. & Kind, N. (2018). Folgen der Grenzverletzungen an sozialpädagogischen Fachkräften in stationären Settings. In: Birts, V., Kurz-Adam, M., Lippmann, C., Merten, R. & Speck, K. (Hrsg.) *Unsere Jugend, 70,*11–20. München, Basel: Ernst Reinhard Verlag.

Schore, A.N. (1994). Affect Regulation and the Origin of the Self. The Neurobiology of Neuronal Development. Philadelphia: Psychology Press.

Schore, A. N. (2003). *Affect Regulation and the Repair of the Self.* London: W.W. Norton & Company.

Schreier, M. (2012). *Qualitative Content Analysis in Practice.* London: SAGE Publications Ltd.

Spangler, G. (2011). Bindung und Gene: Bio-psycho-soziale Grundlagen emotionaler (Dys-) Regulation und ihre Bedeutung für die Entwicklung von Verhaltensauffälligkeiten. In: K.H. Brisch (Hrsg.), *Bindung und frühe Störung der Entwicklung.* Stuttgart: Klett-Cotta.

Spitz, R. (1945). Hospitalism: An Inquiry into the Genesis of Psychiatric Conditions in Early Childhood. In: *The Psychoanalytic Study of the Child. 1*, 53–74.

Sroufe, A. (1983). Infant-caregiver attachment and patterns of adaption in preschool: The roots of maladaptation and competence. In: M. Perlmutter (Eds.): *The Minnesota Symposia on Child Psychology, 16*, 41–84.

Streeck-Fischer, A. (2004). Selbst- und fremddestruktives Verhalten in der Adoleszenz – Folgen von Traumatisierung in der Entwicklung. In A. Streeck-Fischer (Hrsg.), *Adoleszenz – Bindung – Destruktivität.* Stuttgart: Klett-Cotta.

Strijbosch, E.L.L., Huijs J.A.M., Stams G.J.J., Wissink I.B., van der Helm G.H.P., de Swart J.J.W. & van der Veen Z. (2015). The outcome of institutional care compared to non-institutional youth care for Children of primary school age and early adolescence: A multi-level meta-analysis. In: *Children and Youth Services Review, 58*, 208–218.

Teichler, M. H. (2011). Frühe Misshandlungs- und Missbrauchserfahrungen: Gene, Gehirn, Zeit und Pathologie. In K.H. Brisch (Hrsg.), In: *Bindung und frühe Störung der Entwicklung.* Stuttgart: Klett-Cotta.

Tizard, B. & Rees, J. (1975). The effect of early institutional rearing on the behavior problems and affectional relationship of four-year-old children. In: *Journal of Child Psychology and Psychiatry, 16* (1), 61–73.

Tornow, H. & Ziegler, H. (2012). Ursachen und Begleitumstände von Abbrüchen stationärer Erziehungshilfen (ABiE). In: Tornow, H, Ziegler, H. & Sewenig, J., *Abbrüche in stationären Erziehungshilfen (ABiE). Praxisforschungs- und Praxisentwicklungsprojekt. Analysen und Empfehlungen.* Schriftenreihe 3/2012.

Zeanah, Ch.H., Wallin, R. & Shauffer, C. (2012). Institutional Care for Young Children: Review of Literature and Policy Implications. In: *Social Issues and Policy Review, 6(1),* 1–25.

Zimmermann, P. (2004). Attachment representations and characteristics of friendship relations during adolescence. In: *Journal of Experimental Child Psychology, 88,* 83–101.

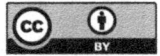

Jugendliches Handeln als Ressource oder Risiko für Wohlbefinden und Gesundheit

Gesundheit, die aus der Bewegung kommt: Wie körperlich aktiv sind Jugendliche in Luxemburg?

Andreas Bund, Georges Steffgen, Melanie Eckelt und Djenna Hutmacher

1 Einführung

Die Bedeutung ausreichender und regelmäßiger Bewegung für die Gesundheit von Jugendlichen ist weitgehend unstrittig und in einer Vielzahl von Studien belegt (z. B. Janssen und LeBlanc 2010; Poitras et al. 2016). Dabei spielen zwei Aspekte eine bedeutsame Rolle:

- Die mit regelmäßiger Bewegung einhergehende erhöhte körperliche Fitness stellt – neben einem intakten sozialen Umfeld und einer ausgewogenen Ernährung – eine Gesundheitsressource dar, die dafür sorgt, dass die Jugendlichen trotz oft hoher Anforderungen in Schule, Familie und Freizeit gesund bleiben.
- Im Jugendalter bilden sich Verhaltensmuster und -gewohnheiten heraus, die u. U. für die gesamte Lebensspanne beibehalten werden. Das heißt: Bewegen

A. Bund (✉) · M. Eckelt
Department of Education and Social Work, University of Luxembourg,
Esch-sur-Alzette, Luxembourg
E-Mail: andreas.bund@uni.lu

M. Eckelt
E-Mail: melanie.eckelt@uni.lu

G. Steffgen · D. Hutmacher
Department of Behavioural and Cognitive Sciences, University of Luxembourg,
Esch-sur-Alzette, Luxembourg
E-Mail: georges.steffgen@uni.lu

D. Hutmacher
E-Mail: djenna.hutmacher.001@student.uni.lu

© Der/die Autor(en) 2022
A. Heinen et al. (Hrsg.), *Wohlbefinden und Gesundheit im Jugendalter,*
https://doi.org/10.1007/978-3-658-35744-3_14

sich Jugendliche zu wenig, tun sie das im Erwachsenenalter in der Regel auch und eine wichtige Gesundheitsressource fällt weg. Bewegung im Jugendalter (und ihre Förderung z. B. durch schulische oder kommunale Programme) hat somit immer auch einen kaum zu überschätzenden präventiven Wert.

Die Frage, wieviel Bewegung Jugendliche für eine gesunde Entwicklung benötigen, beantwortete die WHO schon vor einigen Jahren mit einer Richtlinie, an der sich inzwischen viele Staaten und im Übrigen auch die Forschung orientieren. Demnach sollten sich Kinder und Jugendliche täglich mindestens 60 min *mo-derat bis intensiv* bewegen (WHO 2010); praktisch bedeutet das, dass die Herzfrequenz deutlich erhöht ist und sie zumindest etwas schwitzen.

2   Bisher vorliegende Studien zu Luxemburg

Was ist vor diesem Hintergrund bisher zu Umfang und Intensität der Bewegungsaktivitäten von Jugendlichen in Luxemburg bekannt? Bös et al. befragten 2006 in Kooperation mit dem Ministerium für Bildung und berufliche Ausbildung (heute: Ministerium für Bildung, Kinder und Jugend) 1253 Kinder und Jugendliche der Altersgruppen 9, 14 und 18 Jahre zu ihren körperlich-sportlichen Aktivitäten und ihrer Gesundheit. Dabei zeigte sich, dass nur 26 % der 14- und 18-Jährigen sich gemäß der WHO-Richtlinie ausreichend bewegen; männliche Jugendliche erreichten das 60 min-Limit zu 35 %, weibliche Jugendliche nur zu 18 %. Immerhin war aber knapp die Hälfte aller Jugendlichen Mitglied in einem Sportverein, auch hier deutlich mehr Jungen als Mädchen. Schule und Sportunterricht können das Bewegungsdefizit offenbar nicht ausgleichen; schulische Angebote wie Sport-AGs werden nur von wenigen Jugendlichen genutzt und nur jede/r Fünfte berichtete, dass sie oder er im Sportunterricht sich anstrengt und „ins Schwitzen kommt".

Neuere Ergebnisse sind der „Health Behaviour in School-aged Children"-Studie (HBSC) zu entnehmen, einer im Auftrag der WHO regelmäßig durchgeführten internationalen Erhebung, in der Jugendliche im Alter von 11, 13 und 15 Jahren zu ihrer körperlichen Aktivität und anderen gesundheitsrelevanten Verhaltensweisen befragt werden. Die Daten werden u. a. in länderspezifischen „Factsheets" zusammengefasst (Heinz et al. 2018) und gehen in internationale Übersichtsstudien ein (z. B. Guthold et al. 2019). Demnach sind aktuell nur knapp 21 % der luxemburgischen Jugendlichen mindestens 60 min täglich in

Bewegung, ca. jeder vierte männliche Jugendliche (26 %) und jede siebte weibliche Jugendliche (14 %) erreicht diesen Wert. Mit zunehmenden Alter nimmt die körperliche Aktivität weiter ab. Im Vergleich mit den anderen in die HBSC-Studie einbezogenen europäischen und nordamerikanischen Staaten liegt Luxemburg damit im Mittelfeld (Guthold et al. 2019). Bewegungsmangel im Jugendalter ist – mit den entsprechenden gesundheitlichen Konsequenzen – ein globales Problem.

In beiden Studien gaben die Jugendlichen selbst in einem Fragebogen an, wie oft und wie intensiv sie sich in einer normalen Woche bewegen. Im Projekt „Physical Activity Behavior of Children and Youth in Luxembourg: The Role of Physical Education" (PALUX) haben wir mit der Akzelerometrie zusätzlich ein objektives Verfahren eingesetzt, um die spezifischen Vorzüge subjektiver und objektiver Methoden miteinander zu kombinieren. Im Folgenden werden Methode und ausgewählte Ergebnisse des PALUX-Projekts dargestellt, letzteres v. a. mit Blick auf das Verhältnis von Bewegung und Gesundheit. Zuvor soll aber in einem kurzen Exkurs darauf eingegangen werden, wie körperliche Aktivität gemessen werden kann und welche Vor- und Nachteile die verschiedenen Methoden aufweisen.

3   Methoden zur Messung körperlicher Aktivität

Die Messung körperlicher Aktivität kann prinzipiell auf subjektiver oder objektiver Grundlage erfolgen. Zu den subjektiven Methoden zählen Fragebögen, Interviews sowie Bewegungs- bzw. Aktivitätstagebücher; die UntersuchungsteilnehmerInnen werden zu Umfang, Intensität und eventuell auch den Inhalten ihrer körperlichen Aktivitäten befragt bzw. protokollieren diese. Insbesondere Fragebögen kommen häufig zum Einsatz, zum einen, weil sie es ermöglichen zeit- und kostengünstig viele Personen zu befragen (v. a. wenn sie in digitaler Form vorliegen), zum anderen, weil eine Reihe validierter Instrumente vorliegt (in deutscher Sprache z. B. Schmidt et al. 2016; Fuchs et al. 2015). Die Stärke subjektiver Methoden ist, dass mit ihnen Inhalt, Kontext und ggf. auch der Zweck körperlicher Aktivitäten erfasst werden können und dass sie konsequent die Selbstwahrnehmung der befragten Personen abbilden. Das ist v. a. aus psychologischer Sicht von Bedeutung, da verhaltensrelevante Faktoren wie Einstellungen, Erwartungen und Ziele auf der Selbstwahrnehmung beruhen. Diesen Vorteilen steht jedoch der Nachteil mangelnder Genauigkeit bezüglich der faktischen Bewegungsaktivitäten gegenüber, der darauf zurückgeht, dass Berichte zu den eigenen Aktivitäten durch soziale Erwünschtheit beeinflusst sind und/oder lückenhaft erinnert werden (Arvidsson et al. 2019). Letzteres wird bei Kindern und Jugendlichen vermutlich dadurch verstärkt, dass ihre Aktivitätsmuster im Alltag weniger regelmäßig sind als die Erwachsener (Müller et al. 2010).

Objektive Methoden wie Schrittzähler, Akzelerometer und die Kalorimetrie erfassen die körperliche Aktivität einer Person über physikalische und/oder physiologische Parameter und führen so zu genauen Ergebnissen. Sie sind aber auf eben diese Parameter beschränkt; um welche Aktivitäten es sich handelt, wo und mit welcher Absicht sie stattfinden, kann nur mit Hilfe zusätzlicher Informationsquellen ermittelt werden. Daneben weisen objektive Methoden jeweils spezifische Vor- und Nachteile auf. Schrittzähler sind heute in vielen Activity Trackern und Smartphones integriert und können geh- und laufbasierte Aktivitäten meist zuverlässig messen. Sie sind aber für andere Bewegungsformen wie Fahrradfahren, Schwimmen oder dem Gerätetraining ungeeignet. Die Aufzeichnung der Herzfrequenz über einen längeren Zeitraum gibt ebenfalls Aufschluss darüber, wann, wie lange und wie intensiv jemand körperlich aktiv war. Der Zusammenhang zwischen Herzfrequenz und v. a. leichter körperlicher Betätigung ist jedoch nicht konstant und die Herzfrequenz kann auch durch Stress und Medikationen verändert werden. Die Kalorimetrie sowie das Doubly Labeled Water-Verfahren stellen laborbasierte Methoden dar, die den Energieverbrauch bei körperlicher Aktivität über die CO_2-Produktion sehr genau messen. Sie werden deshalb in Validierungsstudien oft als Referenzmethode verwendet, der mit ihnen verbundene Aufwand und die Kosten stehen aber einer breiten Anwendung, z. B. in epidemiologischen Studien, entgegen.

Die Akzelerometrie bietet derzeit das ausgewogenste Verhältnis von Anwendbarkeit und Validität und ist deshalb in der Forschung die aktuell am häufigsten verwendete objektive Methode (Almeida Mendes et al. 2018). Moderne Akzelerometer sind etwa so groß wie eine Armbanduhr und können bequem und ohne dass sie die betreffende Person einschränken am Handgelenk oder an der Hüfte getragen werden. Sie erfassen direkt, in Echtzeit und bei Bedarf über mehrere Tage die Beschleunigung des Körpers, rechnen sie in „Activity counts" um und ermöglichen so eine hinreichend genaue Messung der körperlichen Aktivität und des Energieverbrauchs. Allerdings fehlen einheitliche Standards bei der Messwertaufnahme und -verarbeitung, z. B. bezüglich der Frequenz und Dauer der Einzelmessung, der Tragezeit oder der Grenzwerte, anhand derer verschiedene Intensitätsstufen körperlicher Aktivität voneinander unterschieden werden. Diese Kriterien müssen angegeben werden, damit die Ergebnisse korrekt bewertet werden können (Thiel et al. 2016).

4   Das PALUX-Projekt

Das Forschungsprojekt „Physical Activity Behaviour of Children and Youth in Luxembourg: The Role of Physical Education" (PALUX) ist auf drei Jahre angelegt und wird zur Zeit von den AutorInnen dieses Beitrags in Zusammenarbeit mit dem Ministerium für Bildung, Kinder und Jugend (Abteilung Script) sowie der Vereinigung der Luxemburgischen Sportlehrer (APEP) durchgeführt. Die Finanzierung erfolgt durch die Universität Luxemburg. Die Ethikkommission der Universität hat das Projekt zudem geprüft und zugelassen.

4.1   Ziele und theoretische Grundlagen

Die Ziele des PALUX-Projekts lassen sich in Kurzfassung wie folgt beschreiben:

* Die Erhebung und Analyse subjektiver und – erstmalig – objektiver Daten zur körperlichen Aktivität von Jugendlichen in Luxemburg. Dabei wird zwischen Schulzeit und Freizeit unterschieden.
* Die Erhebung und Analyse motivationaler Aspekte der körperlichen Aktivität. Hier soll u. a. geklärt werden, ob die Jugendlichen ihre Motivation z. B. vom Sportunterricht auf die Freizeit übertragen.

Während das erstgenannte Ziel eher einen beschreibenden Charakter hat und in den Aufgabenbereich der Sportwissenschaft fällt, hat die Analyse der motivationalen Grundlagen v. a. eine erklärende Funktion und ist fachlich der Psychologie zuzuordnen. Das PALUX-Projekt umfasst also Theorien, Variablen und Methoden beider Disziplinen und ist damit explizit interdisziplinär ausgerichtet.

Der Sportunterricht hat eine einzigartige und vorteilhafte Position, wenn es darum geht, eine erhebliche Anzahl von Kindern und Jugendlichen in Bezug auf deren körperliche Aktivität zu unterstützen. Dies unterstreicht wiederum seine Bedeutung für die Förderung von Kompetenzen in der Schule, die den Jugendlichen auch in ihrem Alltag hilfreich sind. Im Allgemeinen ist eine der Hauptkomponenten, um das Lernen, oder die Absicht zu handeln, zu fördern, die Stärkung der autonomen Motivation (Froiland und Worrell 2016; Krapp 1999). Basierend auf der Selbstbestimmungstheorie (Deci und Ryan 1985), wurde in diesem Zusammenhang die Motivation der Jugendlichen im Sportunterricht untersucht. Um die körperliche Aktivität allerdings auch langfristig außerhalb des schulischen Kontextes zu fördern, wurde gleichermaßen evaluiert, ob die Motivation gegenüber körperlicher Aktivität im Sportunterricht über diesen Kontext hinaus mit der Motivation in der Freizeit zusammenhängt. Dieser kontextübergreifende Transfer der Motivation konnte bereits in der Forschung bestätigt werden (Hagger und Chatzisarantis 2016). Die vorliegende Studie überprüft diese Ergebnisse erstmalig im Längsschnitt, um herauszufinden, ob dieser Motivationstransfer auch tatsächlich über die Zeit gegeben ist.

Die Selbstbestimmungstheorie unterscheidet zwischen intrinsisch motivierten Verhaltensweisen, welche als interessenbestimmte Handlungen ohne extern geleitete Anstöße definiert werden. Die *intrinsische Motivation* geht mit Neugier, Exploration, Spontaneität und Interesse an den unmittelbaren Gegebenheiten des Verhaltens einher. Im Gegenzug beschreibt die extrinsische Motivation Verhaltensweisen, die aufgrund von instrumentellen Absichten ausgeführt werden. Diese Verhaltensweisen treten häufig infolge von Aufforderungen auf, deren Befolgung eine interne oder externe Bekräftigung erwarten lässt. Die Selbstbestimmungstheorie betrachtet die extrinsische Motivation allerdings anhand eines Kontinuums, mit mehreren Motivationstypen. So zählt die *externale Regulation* zur Verhaltensregulation, die lediglich durch fremdbestimmte Einflüsse entsteht. In diesem Sinne sind Handlungen gemeint, die ausgeführt werden, um eine Belohnung zu erhalten oder einer Bestrafung zu entgehen. Der Typus der *introjizierten Regulation* wiederum bezieht sich auf Verhaltensweisen, die internen Anstößen und innerem Druck folgen, welche für die Selbstachtung relevant sind: Man tut etwas, „weil es sich gehört". *Die identifizierte Regulation* hingegen beinhaltet Verhaltensweisen, welche vom Selbst als persönlich wichtig oder wertvoll anerkannt werden. Hierbei tut man etwas, „weil es einem wichtig ist", da man sich mit den zugrundeliegenden Werten und Zielen identifiziert. Schließlich beschreibt die *integrierte Regulation* die Form der extrinsischen Motivation mit dem höchsten Grad an Selbstbestimmung. Sie beinhaltet Verhaltensweisen, welche die Ziele, Normen und Handlungsstrategien beinhaltet, mit denen sich das Individuum identifiziert und in sein/ihr Selbstkonzept integriert hat. Im Gegenzug zur intrinsischen und extrinsischen Motivation steht die „Amotivation", wodurch Verhaltensweisen als nicht motiviert und ohne erkennbares Ziel gekennzeichnet werden. Übergeordnet werden die intrinsische Motivation und identifizierte Regulation als autonome Verhaltensregulation zusammengefasst, wohingegen die externale und introjizierte Regulation kontrollierte Verhaltensregulationsformen darstellen.

4.2   Stichprobe

Die Stichprobe der PALUX-Studie setzt sich aus ca. 2000 Kindern und Jugendlichen im Alter von 10 bis 20 Jahren zusammen, die zum Zeitpunkt der Datenerhebung 9 Grund- und 5 Sekundarschulen in Luxemburg besuchten. Sämtliche Daten wurden zweimal erhoben, das erste Mal von Oktober bis Dezember 2018 und das zweite Mal von Mai bis Juli 2019. Es liegt somit ein echter Längsschnitt vor, der es z. B. ermöglicht, die körperliche Aktivität von Kindern und Jugendlichen in verschiedenen Jahreszeiten miteinander zu vergleichen. Die exakten Zahlen zur Stichprobe, insbesondere die Verteilung auf die beiden Erhebungsmethoden Fragebogen und Akzelerometer, sind Tab. 1 zu entnehmen. Die deutliche geringere Stichprobengröße bei der Akzelerometermessung erklärt sich aus dem höheren Aufwand dieser Methode und der Tatsache, dass bestimmte Tragezeitkriterien für eine valide Messung erfüllt sein müssen.

4.3   Instrumente

Die subjektive körperliche Aktivität wurde mit dem Motorik-Modul Aktivitätsfragebogen (MoMo-AFB) von Schmidt et al. (2016) erfasst. Der Fragebogen kommt regelmäßig im Motorik-Modul der Langzeitstudie des Robert-Koch-Instituts zur gesundheitlichen Lage der Kinder und Jugendlichen in Deutschland (KiGGs) zum Einsatz und erfragt Häufigkeit, Dauer, Intensität und Art der habituellen körperlichen Aktivität in drei Bereichen: 1) Altersspezifisches Setting, bei Kindern und Jugendlichen die Schule (6 Items, Beispielitem: „Wie sehr strengst du dich durchschnittlich im Sportunterricht an?"), 2) Alltag (4 Items, Beispielitem: „Wie groß ist die Entfernung, die du täglich zu Fuß gehst?") und 3) Freizeit, wobei zwischen Aktivitäten im Sportverein (7 Items, Beispielitem: „Welche Sportart(en) betreibst du im Verein?") und außerhalb des Sportvereins (6

Tab. 1 Stichprobe der PALUX-Studie. (Eigene Darstellung)

Erhebungsmethode	TeilnehmerInnen 1. Erhebungswelle	TeilnehmerInnen 2. Erhebungswelle	TeilnehmerInnen 1. u. 2. Erhebungswelle
Fragebogen	1808 (m 918/w 890)	1738 (m 865, w 873)	1681 (m 828, w 853)
Akzelerometer	249 (m 110, w 139)	166 (m 65, w 101)	150 (m 60, w 90)

Items, Beispielitem: „Welche Sportart(en) betreibst du außerhalb des Vereins?") unterschieden wird. Zwei weitere Items beziehen sich auf die allgemeine körperliche Aktivität (Beispielitem: „An wie vielen Tagen einer normalen Woche bist du mindestens 60 min am Tag körperlich aktiv?"). Für die PALUX-Studie wurde der Fragebogen digitalisiert, sodass er von den Jugendlichen am Laptop bzw. Tablet bearbeitet werden konnte.

Die objektive körperliche Aktivität wurde mit dem Akzelerometer GT3X-BT der Firma ActiGraph erhoben. Das an der Hüfte befestigte Gerät zeichnet jede Bewegungsaktivität in Form von „Activity counts" auf, aus denen sich später Dauer und Intensität der Aktivität sowie der damit verbundene Energieverbrauch ermitteln lassen. Mithilfe altersspezifischer Schwellenwerte wird zwischen Ruhe, leichter, moderater und intensiver Aktivität unterschieden. Als maßgebliche Größe für eine gesundheitsförderliche Aktivität hat sich die moderate bis intensive körperliche Aktivität etabliert, dem englischen Ausdruck folgend als „MVPA" abgekürzt. Auf diese Größe bezieht sich auch die eingangs erwähnte Richtlinie der WHO zur körperlichen Aktivität. Im PALUX-Projekt trugen die Jugendlichen den Akzelerometer an sieben aufeinander folgenden Tagen, zum Schlafen wurde er abgelegt.

Zur Erfassung der Motivation im Sportunterricht wurde der „Revised Perceived Locus of Causality in Physical Education" (PLOC-R; Vlachopoulos et al. 2011) Fragebogen genutzt ($\alpha = .78$). Die Amotivation (Beispielitem: „Ich nehme am Sportunterricht teil, aber ich weiß nicht wirklich warum"), die externale Regulation (Beispielitem: „Ich nehme am Sportunterricht teil, weil das die Regel ist"), die introjezierte Regulation (Beispielitem: Ich nehme am Sportunterricht teil, weil ich mich schlecht fühlen würde, wenn der/die Lehrer/-in denkt, dass ich nicht gut im Sportunterricht bin"), die identifizierte Regulation (Beispielitem: „Ich nehme am Sportunterricht teil, weil es mir wichtig ist, die Übungen im Sportunterricht auszuprobieren"), und die intrinsische Motivation (Beispielitem: „Ich nehme am Sportunterricht teil, weil der Sportunterricht Spaß macht"), wurden anhand von jeweils 4 Items erfasst. Antworten aller Items können anhand einer 7-Punkt-Likert-Skala von 1 („trifft überhaupt nicht zu") bis 7 („trifft voll und ganz zu") beantwortet werden. Zur Erfassung der kontrollierten Motivation wurden die Skalen externale und introjezierte Regulation zusammengefasst, wobei die autonome Motivation aus den Skalen intrinsische Motivation und identifizierte Regulation besteht.

Zur Erfassung der Motivation gegenüber körperlicher Aktivität in der Freizeit wurde die überarbeitete Version des Behavioral Regulation in Exercise Questionnaire (BREQ-II; Markland und Tobin 2004) genutzt ($\alpha = .82$). Die Amotivation (Beispielitem: „Ich weiß nicht, warum ich körperlich aktiv sein sollte"), die externale Regulation (Beispielitem: „Ich bin körperlich aktiv, weil andere Personen sagen, dass ich dies tun sollte"), die identifizierte Regulation (Beispielitem: „Ich mag den Nutzen von körperlicher Aktivität"), und die intrinsische Motivation (Beispielitem: Ich bin körperlich aktiv, weil es Spaß macht"), wurden anhand von jeweils 4 Items erfasst. Die introjezierte Regulation wurde anhand von 3 Items erfasst (Beispielitem: „Ich fühle mich schuldig, wenn ich nicht körperlich aktiv bin"). Antworten aller Items können anhand einer 7-Punkt-Likert-Skala von 1 („trifft überhaupt nicht zu") bis 7 („trifft voll und ganz zu") beantwortet werden. Zur Erfassung der kontrollierten Motivation wurden ebenfalls die Skalen externale und introjezierte Regulation genutzt, wobei die autonome Motivation aus den Skalen intrinsische Motivation und identifizierte Regulation gebildet wird.

4.4   Durchführung

In Zusammenarbeit mit dem Ministerium für Bildung, Kinder und Jugend wurden insgesamt 14 Grund- und Sekundarschulen aus allen Landesteilen Luxemburgs zufällig ausgewählt und kontaktiert. Die Teilnahme an der Studie erfolgte im Klassenverband; an den Grundschulen wurden 31 Klassen des Cycle 4 und an den Sekundarschulen 104 Klassen der Stufen 3, 5 und 7 untersucht. Für die Akzelerometermessung wurden aus diesen Klassen – wieder nach dem Zufallsprinzip – 9 Grundschul- und 15 Sekundarschulklassen bestimmt.

Die Direktion der Schulen sowie die Klassen- und Sportlehrkräfte wurden in persönlichen Gesprächen über Ablauf und Zielsetzung der Studie informiert. Des Weiteren wurden die Erhebungstermine vereinbart. Die Schüler und Schülerinnen erhielten ein Informationsblatt sowie eine Einverständniserklärung, die vor dem jeweiligen Termin (ggf. von einem Elternteil) unterschrieben vorliegen musste. Der MoMo-Fragebogen zur Erfassung der subjektiven Aktivität wurde zusammen mit den Motivationsskalen in digitaler Form auf der von der Universität Luxemburg erstellten Plattform OASYS (LUCET 2019) bearbeitet. Damit war sichergestellt, dass die Daten nicht an Dritte weitergeleitet werden können. Das Ausfüllen dauerte ca. 40 min, eine geschulte Testleiterin beantwortete Fragen und half bei Verständnisproblemen. Die Akzelerometer zur Messung der objektiven körperlichen Aktivität wurden in Absprache mit den Lehrkräften während der Unterrichts ausgegeben. Die Schüler und Schülerinnen wurden umfassend mündlich eingewiesen und erhielten zusätzlich ein Informations- und Merkblatt. Anschließend wurden Körpergröße und Körpergewicht gemessen. Während der einwöchigen Messung war das schon erwähnte Trageprotokoll zu führen. Danach wurden die Akzelerometer wieder eingesammelt und die Schüler und Schülerinnen gaben in einem kurzen Fragebogen an, ob sich ihre körperliche Aktivität in der zurückliegenden Woche stark von einer „normalen" Woche unterschieden hatte und falls ja, wie und warum. Von den Sportlehrkräften erhielten wir ebenfalls via Fragebogen einige Informationen zu Dauer und Inhalt des Sportunterrichts in dieser Woche.

4.5   Datenverarbeitung und -analyse

Die aus dem Fragebogen resultierenden Daten wurden in Microsoft Excel eingelesen und auf Plausibilität geprüft. Die Verarbeitung der Akzelerometerdaten erfolgte mit der dafür vorgesehenen Software ActiLife v6.13.3. Die individuellen Tragezeiten wurden ermittelt und Schüler und Schülerinnen, die den Akzelerometer nicht an mindestens 4 Tagen (davon ein Samstag oder Sonntag) für jeweils mindestens 480 min getragen hatten, wurden ausgeschlossen. Für die Abgrenzung der Aktivitätsstufen wurden die von Evenson et al. (2008) und Troiano et al. (2008) speziell für Kinder und Jugendliche entwickelten Schwellenwerte zum Energieverbrauch verwendet; daraus ergab sich auch die wichtige Messgröße der moderat-intensiven Aktivität, also der MVPA. Zuletzt wurden auch diese Werte in einer Excel-Datei zusammengeführt. Die statistischen Analysen erfolgten mit den Programmen SPSS Statistics 25, IBM SPSS Amos 26 und R 3.6.1 (R Core Team 2019).

4.6   Ergebnisse

In den folgenden Abschnitten werden v. a. die Ergebnisse der PALUX-Studie vorgestellt, die einen direkten oder indirekten Bezug zur Gesundheit der Jugendlichen haben. Dazu zählen z. B. Antworten auf die Fragen, wie viel und mit welcher Intensität sich die Jugendlichen bewegen, welche Rolle dabei das Geschlecht und das Alter spielen und ob sie selbst den Umfang ihrer körperlichen Aktivitäten realistisch einschätzen oder nicht. Eine wichtige Richtschnur bei der Bewertung unserer Ergebnisse ist die Empfehlung der WHO, nach der sich Kinder und Jugendliche jeden Tag mindestens 60 min moderat bis intensiv bewegen sollten. Dieser Wert ist deshalb in einige der folgenden Abbildungen eingezeichnet.

Umfang und Intensität der objektiven körperlichen Aktivität

Wie aktiv sind also die Jugendlichen in Luxemburg und wie oft strengen sie sich dabei so sehr an, dass es der Fitness und damit der Gesundheit nützt? Abb. 1 gibt die auf den Tag umgerechneten Ergebnisse der Akzelerometermessung wieder, es geht somit zunächst um die objektive körperliche Aktivität. Auf den ersten Blick wird deutlich, dass die Jugendlichen den weitaus größten Teil des Tages in Ruhe, also sitzend oder liegend, verbringen, nämlich durchschnittlich 594 (Welle 1) bzw. 603 (Welle 2) Minuten. Das sind rund 10 der insgesamt 13 bis 14 h, die der Akzelerometer an einem Tag getragen wurde. Leichte körperliche Aktivitäten, z. B. langsames Gehen oder einfache Haushaltstätigkeiten, sind für 168 (Welle 1) bzw. 170 (Welle 2) Minuten verzeichnet. Gesundheitsrelevante Aktivitäten auf moderatem oder intensivem Niveau, Sport und andere etwas anstrengendere Bewegungsaktivitäten, sind dagegen auf 30 und 17 (Welle 1) bzw. 33 und 19 (Welle 2) Minuten beschränkt. Hier macht sich also durchaus auch die Jahreszeit bemerkbar; im Sommer waren die Jugendlichen täglich 5 min länger moderat oder intensiv in Bewegung als im Winter.

In beiden Erhebungswellen waren männliche Jugendliche aber etwas aktiver als weibliche Jugendliche. So verbrachten die Jungen in Welle 1 durchschnittlich 575 min in Ruhe und 35 bzw. 22 min mit moderater und intensiver körperlichen Aktivität. Die Mädchen waren dagegen 609 min in Ruhe und nur 26 bzw. 13 min moderat und intensiv aktiv.

Diese Zahlen machen deutlich, dass schon Kinder und Jugendliche den Tag hauptsächlich sitzend und mit einem entsprechend niedrigen Energieumsatz verbringen. Für Sport und Bewegung bleiben in der Regel nur wenige Minuten Zeit. Ist das eventuell auf (zu) lange Schulzeiten zurückzuführen oder sind die Jugendlichen auch in ihrer Freizeit (zu) wenig aktiv?

Verteilung der objektiven körperlichen Aktivität auf Freizeit, Schule und Sportunterricht

Im Weiteren konzentrieren wir uns auf den für die Gesundheit wichtigen Aspekt der moderaten und intensiven körperlichen Aktivität, also der MVPA. Abb. 2 zeigt, wie sich die objektiv gemessene MVPA der Jugendlichen auf Freizeit, Schule und Sportunterricht verteilt. Die Darstellung bezieht sich diesmal auf die individuelle Gesamttragezeit des Akzelerometers, da Schule nur an 5 der 7 Tage stattfindet und die in dieser Zeit anfallende MVPA deshalb bei einer Umrechnung auf den Tag zu niedrig angesetzt würde.

Es liegen zur Zeit nur die Ergebnisse für die Erhebungswelle im Winter 2018 vor. Sie zeigen, dass intensivere Bewegungsaktivitäten v. a. in der Freizeit statt-

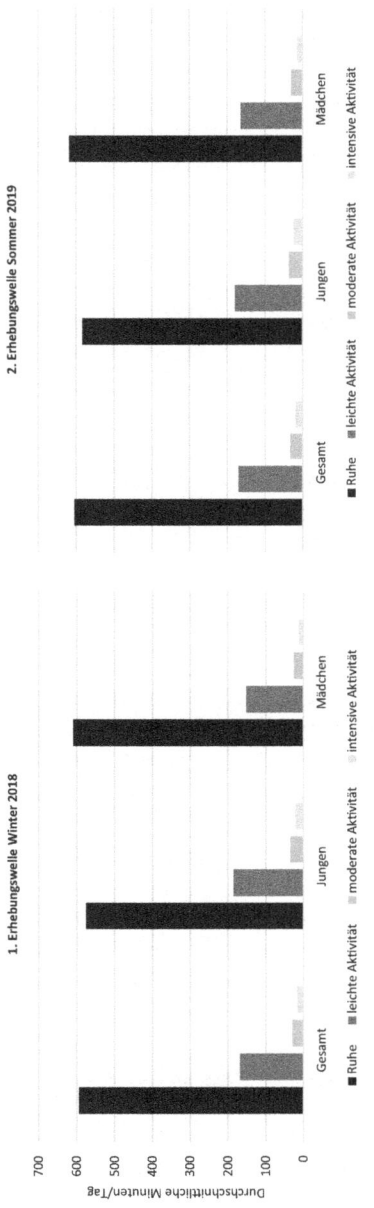

Abb. 1 Umfang und Intensität der objektiven körperlichen Aktivität je Tag. (Eigene Abbildung)

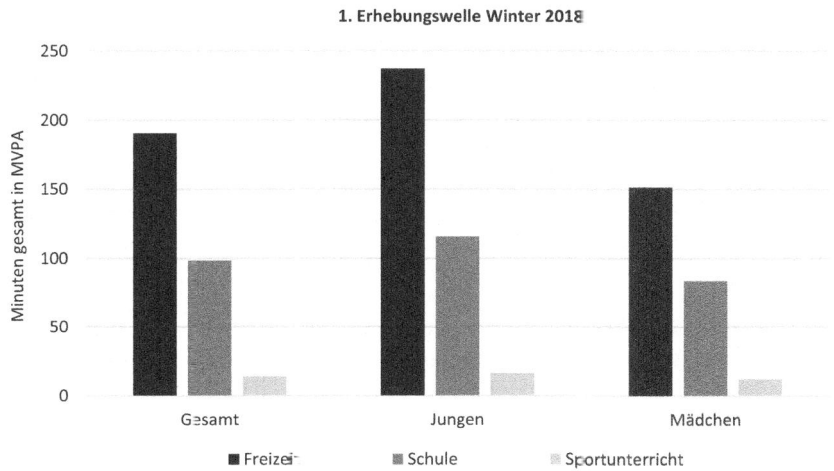

Abb. 2 Verteilung der objektiven moderat-intensiven körperlichen Aktivität (MVPA) auf Freizeit, Schule und Sportunterricht. (Eigene Abbildung)

finden; durchschnittlich 190 der 300 Gesamt-MVPA-Minuten zeichneten die Akzelerometer in dieser Zeit auf. Immerhin 98 min MVPA fielen aber auch in der Schule an, dazu kommen noch knapp 14 min in den zwei bzw. drei Stunden Sportunterricht. Bemerkenswert sind die Unterschiede zwischen männlichen und weiblichen Jugendlichen. Während die Jungen in der Freizeit auf 237 min in MVPA kamen, waren es bei den Mädchen nur 151 min. In der Schule liegt das Verhältnis bei 115 zu 83 min und selbst im Sportunterricht waren die Jungen mit 16 min moderat-intensiver Bewegungszeit deutlich aktiver als die Mädchen mit 12 min.

Insgesamt ergibt sich damit ein Bild, nach dem moderate und intensive Bewegungsaktivitäten v. a. in der Freizeit der Jugendlichen stattfinden. Den Angaben aus dem MoMo-Fragebogen zufolge, sind hier sowohl der selbstorganisierte Sport als auch der Vereinssport gleichermaßen wichtig. Als nicht unerheblich haben sich aber auch die schulischen Bewegungsaktivitäten herausgestellt, die mehr als ein Drittel der gesamten MVPA der Jugendlichen ausmachen. Neben dem Sportunterricht dürften hier die Unterrichtspausen und Sport-AGs eine Rolle spielen.

WHO-Richtlinie und Vergleich von objektiver und subjektiver körperlicher Aktivität

Mit den nun folgenden Analysen nehmen wir zwei weitere Aspekte in den Blick: Genügen die Bewegungsaktivitäten luxemburgischer Jugendlicher der 60 min-Richtlinie der WHO? Und wird der Umfang der eigenen Aktivitäten eigentlich realistisch wahrgenommen? Abb. 3 zeigt für beide Erhebungswellen, wie viele Minuten täglich Jungen und Mädchen moderat oder intensiv aktiv waren – und zwar objektiv in der Akzelerometermessung und subjektiv in der Selbsteinschätzung mittels Fragebogen. Es wird deutlich, dass sich die Jugendlichen objektiv zu wenig auf MVPA-Niveau bewegen, nämlich durchschnittlich nur 47 (Welle 1) bzw. 52 (Welle 2) Minuten. Gerade die Mädchen meiden oft körperlich anstrengende Aktivitäten; für sie wurden im Winter 39 und im Sommer 47 min aufgezeichnet. Aber auch die Jungen erfüllen mit 61 min das WHO-Maß nur in der im Sommer durchgeführten Erhebung. Natürlich handelt es sich hier um statistisch ermittelte Durchschnittswerte. Nimmt man die individuellen MVPA-Zeiten in den Blick, zeigt sich, dass nur etwa 12 % der Mädchen und 41 % der Jungen in Luxemburg der WHO-Empfehlung genügen.

Gleichzeitig belegen die Daten zur subjektiven körperlichen Aktivität, dass die Jugendlichen glauben, sich mehr zu bewegen als dies im Vergleich mit den objektiven Daten der Fall ist. Den objektiv gemessenen 47 (Welle 1) bzw. 52 (Welle 2) MVPA-Minuten stehen im Fragebogen die Angaben von 73 (Welle 1) bzw. 77 (Welle 2) Minuten gegenüber. Das entspricht einer Überschätzung der eigenen Bewegungsaktivitäten um 55 % (Welle 1) bzw. 48 % (Welle 2). Interessanterweise überschätzen v. a. die weiblichen Jugendlichen den Umfang ihrer Aktivitäten; in Welle 1, also im Winter, überschätzen sie sie um 74 %, in Welle 2 um 57 %. Bei den männlichen Jugendlichen beziffert sich die Überschätzung auf 40 % (Welle 1) bzw. 34 % (Welle 2).

Neben dem Geschlecht spielt auch das Alter der Jugendlichen eine wichtige Rolle. In Abb. 4 werden deshalb die täglichen MVPA-Minuten für verschiedene Altersgruppen dargestellt. Im Ergebnis der objektiven Messung erweisen sich die 10- bis 12-Jährigen, also die Grundschüler und -schülerinnen, mit durchschnittlich 53 (Welle 1) bzw. 60 (Welle 2) Minuten als die körperlich aktivste Gruppe. Die älteren Jugendlichen bewegen sich weniger und verfehlen die WHO-Richtlinie demzufolge deutlich. So kommt die Gruppe der 13- bis 16-Jährigen nur auf 39 (Welle 1) bzw. 45 (Welle 2) Minuten in MVPA und die 17- bis 20-Jährigen auf jeweils 43 min. Allerdings ist diese Altersgruppe in unserer Stichprobe unterrepräsentiert; in Welle Welle 2 umfasst sie z. B. nur 18 Jugendliche gegenüber 67 und 81 Jugendlichen in den Gruppen der 13-bis 16- und 10- bis 12-Jährigen. Gemein ist allen Altersgruppen, dass sie subjektiv überschätzen, wie aktiv sie

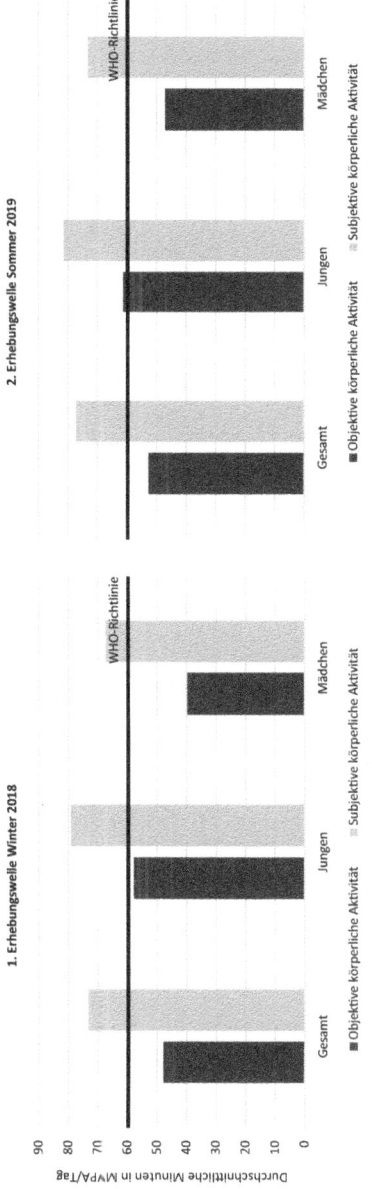

Abb. 3 Die objektive und subjektive moderat-intensive körperlichen Aktivität (MVPA) von Jungen und Mädchen je Tag. (Eigene Abbildung)

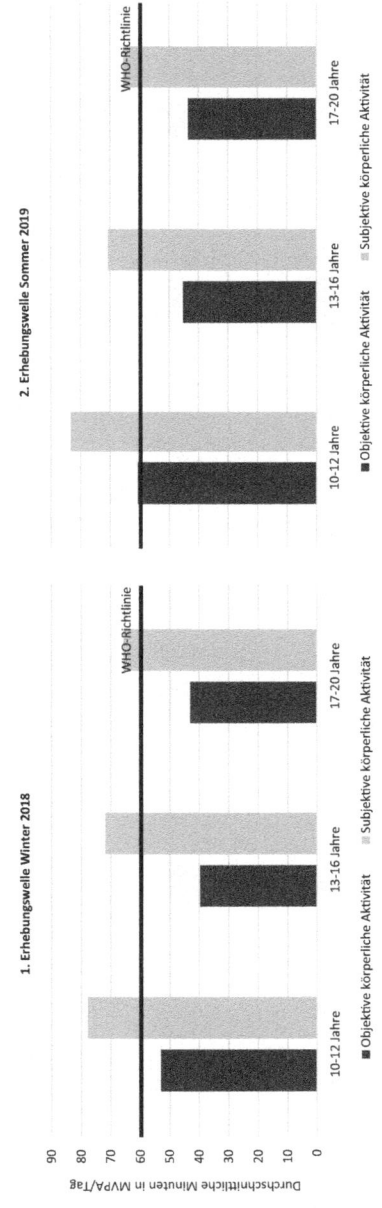

Abb. 4 Die objektive und subjektive moderat-intensive körperlichen Aktivität (MVPA) verschiedener Altersgruppen je Tag. (Eigene Abbildung)

wirklich sind. Die 10- bis 12-Jährigen z. B. gaben im MoMo-Fragebogen eine tägliche Bewegungszeit von 77 (Welle 1) bzw. 84 (Welle 2) Minuten an, was einer Überschätzung von etwa 45 % bzw. 40 % entspricht. In der Gruppe der 13- bis 16-Jährigen sind die Unterschiede zwischen objektiver und subjektiver MVPA-Zeit besonders groß, sie betragen 84 % im Winter und 55 % im Sommer. Die 17- bis 20-Jährigen liegen mit jeweils 51 % daneben.

Zusammenfassend kann damit festgestellt werden: Die Mehrheit der Jugendlichen in Luxemburg erreicht die WHO-Vorgabe nicht, bewegt sich also nicht genug, als dass von einer langfristig gesunden Entwicklung bis in das Erwachsenenalter ausgegangen werden kann. Dies betrifft insbesondere weibliche Jugendliche und die über 16-Jährigen. Darüber hinaus zeigt der Vergleich von objektiv gemessener und subjektiv wahrgenommener körperlicher Aktivität, dass die Jugendlichen ihre Aktivitätszeit in nicht unerheblichem Maße überschätzen; sie geben im Fragebogen an, sich mehr zu bewegen als sie es tatsächlich tun. Dieser Befund tritt in praktisch allen Studien auf, in denen objektive *und* subjektive Methoden zur Messung der Aktivität genutzt werden (z. B. Skender et al. 2016). Insofern wäre eigentlich zu befürchten, dass Studien wie die oben erwähnte HBSC-Studie, in denen die Jugendlichen ausschließlich befragt werden, ein zu positives Bild zeichnen. Tatsächlich liegen aber PALUX- und HBSC-Studie im wichtigsten Ergebnis nicht sehr weit auseinander: Nur jeder vierte bis fünfte Jugendliche in Luxemburg bewegt sich täglich mindestens 60 min und damit genug, um auf lange Sicht gesund zu bleiben.

Körperliche Aktivität im Sportunterricht
Im Lehrplan für das Fach Sport in Luxemburg ist von einem „Doppelauftrag" die Rede: Der Sportunterricht soll erstens den Kindern und Jugendlichen Bewegung, Spiel und Sport erschließen und sie befähigen, daran teilzuhaben und zweitens ihre Entwicklung umfassend fördern. Sportlehrkräfte stehen damit vor der Aufgabe, die sich aus diesem Doppelauftrag ergebenden Lernziele auszubalancieren; es geht eben nicht allein um die Förderung motorischer Kompetenzen, sondern im gleichen Maße um die Entwicklung kognitiver, emotionaler und sozialer Fähigkeiten. Insofern greift die Frage, wie viel sich Jugendliche im Sportunterricht eigentlich bewegen, nur einen Aspekt unter vielen heraus und die Antwort gibt keinesfalls Aufschluss über die Qualität des Sportunterrichts. Sie zu stellen lohnt dennoch, zumal, wenn man bedenkt, dass der Sportunterricht für nicht wenige Jugendliche der einzige regelmäßige Anlass ist, sich sportlich zu bewegen. Fast die Hälfte der am PALUX-Projekt beteiligten Jugendlichen war zum Zeitpunkt der Studie z. B. nicht Mitglied in einem Sportverein.

Von den 24 Klassen, in denen die Akzelerometermessung durchgeführt wurde, hatten 15 Klassen einmal, 8 Klassen zweimal und eine Klasse dreimal pro Woche Sport- bzw. Schwimmunterricht. Da der Unterricht oft in Doppelstunden erfolgte, dauerte eine Sportstunde durchschnittlich 77 min. Abb. 5 zeigt, dass die Jugendlichen davon nur 14 min moderat oder intensiv in Bewegung waren, 63 min verbrachten sie in Ruhe oder mit leichter Aktivität. Für die Jungen wurden 16 min in MVPA aufgezeichnet, für die Mädchen 12 min. Demgegenüber gab immerhin knapp ein Drittel der Jugendlichen im Fragebogen an, im Sportunterricht viel zu schwitzen und weniger als 10 % sprachen davon, überhaupt nicht zu schwitzen. Offenbar zeigt sich auch hier, dass Anstrengung und Aktivität in der Eigenwahrnehmung etwas überschätzt werden.

Insgesamt sind die Jugendlichen im Sportunterricht damit erstaunlich wenig körperlich aktiv. Studien aus anderen Ländern (z. B. Meyer et al. 2013; Nettlefold et al. 2011) kommen aber zu ähnlichen Ergebnissen. Folgt man der vom U.S. Department for Health and Public Services gegebenen Empfehlung, nach der Kinder und Jugendliche mindestens die Hälfte des Sportunterrichts in moderater oder intensiver Bewegung sein sollten, ist das *zu* wenig. Allerdings ist dieser Richtwert weder medizinisch (wie die WHO-Empfehlung) und schon gar nicht pädagogisch-didaktisch begründet; die Bewegungszeit im Sportunterricht hängt natürlich stark von den jeweiligen Inhalten, Methoden und Lernzielen ab. Auch

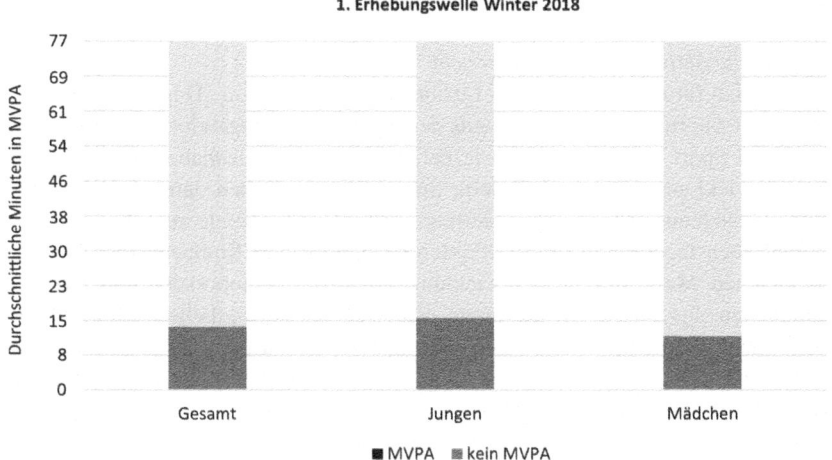

Abb. 5 Die objektive moderat-intensive körperliche Aktivität (MVPA) von Jungen und Mädchen im Sportunterricht. (Eigene Abbildung)

unsere Analyse verkürzt den Sportunterricht auf dieses eine quantitative Merkmal und lässt alles andere außer Acht. Es wird damit aber auch deutlich, dass Bewegung ein substantieller Bestandteil des Sportunterrichts sein muss, nicht (nur) als Ausgleich zum sitzenden Lernen in den anderen Fächern, sondern auch und gerade aus gesundheitlicher Sicht.

In Bezug auf unsere Ausgangsfrage, ob die Motivation zu körperlicher Aktivität über den Schulkontext hinaus auch mit der Motivation im Freizeitsport zusammenhängt, sind wir zu folgenden Ergebnissen gekommen (siehe auch Hutmacher et al. 2020). Jugendliche, die im Sportunterricht autonom motiviert sind, sind auch über die Zeit im Freizeitsport autonom motiviert. Umgekehrt sind autonom motivierte Jugendliche im Freizeitsport aber auch über die Zeit im Sportunterricht stärker autonom motiviert (Abb. 6). Diese Ergebnisse zeigen, dass eine Förderung der autonomen Motivation im Sportunterricht gewinnbringend für den außerschulischen Bereich sein kann. Interventionsprogramme (z. B. Cheon und Reeve 2019) fanden beispielsweise, dass die Förderung von intrinsischen Zielen, das Benutzen einer informellen statt einer kontrollierten Sprache durch den/die Lehrer/in (z. B. „du könntest" anstelle von „du musst"), die Bereitstellung von Erklärungen, Geduld zu zeigen, anstatt Druck auszuüben, und das Akzeptieren von negativen Äußerungen der Jugendlichen, Schlüsselfaktoren darstellen, um deren autonome Motivation zu stärken.

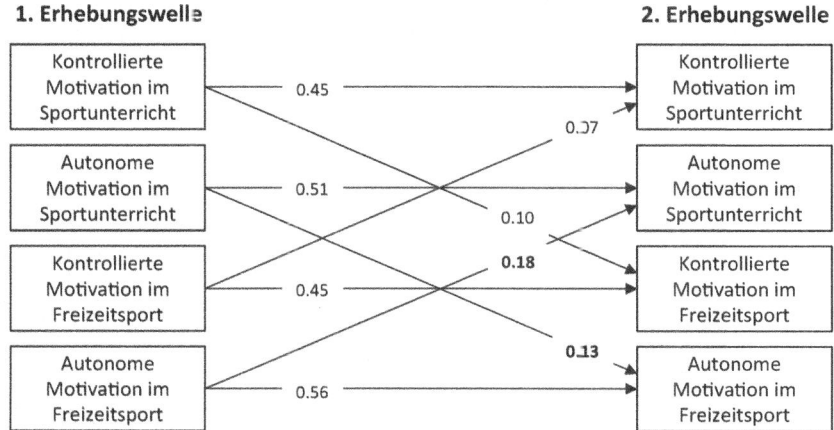

Abb. 6 Zusammenhang der Motivation im Sportunterricht und im Freizeitsport über die Zeit (ein Cross-Lagged-Panel-Design). Alle abgebildeten Pfade sind statistisch signifikant. (Eigene Abbildung)

5 Zusammenfassung und Schlussfolgerungen

Sport und Bewegung sind für die Gesundheit von Jugendlichen in zweifacher Hinsicht wichtig: Kurzfristig als Gesundheitsressource, die den Alltagsanforderungen entgegengestellt werden kann und langfristig als Verhaltensmuster, das im besten Fall über das gesamte Leben beibehalten wird. Einer weithin akzeptierten Richtlinie der WHO zufolge reichen 60 min moderater bis intensiver Bewegung täglich aus.

Zahlreiche Studien (z. B. Guthold et al. 2019) zeigen aber, dass sich Kinder und Jugendliche in praktisch allen Teilen der Welt zu wenig bewegen. Neben der subjektiven Erfassung der körperlichen Aktivität via Fragebogen, werden in den letzten Jahren immer häufiger auch objektive Methoden wie Schrittzähler und v. a. Akzelerometer eingesetzt. In der PALUX-Studie wurde die körperliche Aktivität von ca. 1800 Kindern und Jugendlichen mittels Fragebogen und von ca. 250 Kindern und Jugendlichen zusätzlich mit einem Akzelerometer erhoben. Damit liegen nun für Luxemburg erstmals subjektive *und* objektive Daten darüber vor, wie viel und mit welcher Intensität sich Kinder und Jugendliche in der Schule und in ihrer Freizeit bewegen.

Die Ergebnisse der PALUX-Studie zur körperlichen Aktivität lassen sich wie folgt zusammenfassen:

- Die Jugendlichen verbrachten täglich 12 bis 13 h in Ruhe oder mit körperlich leichten Aktivitäten. Moderate und intensive Aktivitäten, also solche Aktivitäten, die eine positive Wirkung auf Fitness und Gesundheit haben, waren auf täglich 40 bis 50 min beschränkt.
- Etwa zwei Drittel der moderaten und intensiven körperlichen Aktivitäten fanden in der Freizeit der Jugendlichen statt, der Rest in Schule und Sportunterricht.
- Nur 12 % der weiblichen Jugendlichen und 41 % der männlichen Jugendlichen erreichten die WHO-Richtlinie von mindestens 60 min moderat-intensiver körperlicher Aktivität täglich.
- Die Jugendlichen überschätzten den Umfang ihrer moderat-intensiven Aktivitäten erheblich. Den objektiv gemessenen ca. 50 min täglich standen im Fragebogen Angaben von ca. 75 min gegenüber.
- Die männlichen Jugendlichen waren körperlich aktiver als die weiblichen Jugendlichen und die 10- bis 12-Jährigen waren körperlich aktiver als die 13- bis 16- und 17- bis 20-Jährigen.

- Im Sportunterricht verbrachten die Jugendlichen durchschnittlich 14 von 77 min in moderat-intensiver körperlicher Aktivität.

Die Konsequenzen und v. a. praktischen Implikationen, die sich aus diesen Befunden ergeben, liegen auf der Hand: Sport und Bewegung im Kindes- und Jugendalter müssen systematisch und zielorientiert gefördert werden, und zwar stärker als das bisher geschieht. Dabei ist aus unserer Sicht ein ebenso umfassender wie spezifischer Ansatz angezeigt. „Umfassend" meint, dass die kommunalen Akteure – Schulen, Maison Relais, Sportvereine und Gemeindeverwaltungen – in enger Zusammenarbeit vielfältige Bewegungsangebote und -gelegenheiten entwickeln, die Kinder und Jugendliche sowohl in der Schule als auch in der Freizeit nutzen können. Das seit 2017 an immer mehr Schulen implementierte „Clever Move"-Projekt ist dafür ein gutes, wenngleich noch isoliert dastehendes Beispiel. Basierend auf dem in der Schweiz entwickelten Konzept der Bewegten Schule wird hier den Schülerinnen und Schülern während des Unterrichts immer wieder die Gelegenheit gegeben, körperlich aktiv zu werden. Das geschieht z. B. durch Bewegungspausen oder dem so genannten Bewegten Lernen bei dem Bewegung in den Lern- und Arbeitsprozess der Schüler und Schülerinnen eingebunden wird. Eine Evaluation des Projekts durch die Universität Luxemburg (Bund & Scheuer 2017) erbrachte durchweg positive Ergebnisse. So gaben die Schüler und Schülerinnen z. B. an, mehr Spaß am Unterricht zu haben und die Eltern stellten eine bessere Bewegungskoordination fest.

„Spezifisch" sollte der Ansatz in dem Sinn sein, dass neben eher breit und auch durchaus integrativ-inklusiv angelegten Bewegungsangeboten auch solche Programme etabliert werden, die sich gezielt an bestimmte Gruppen richten, indem sie deren Bedürfnisse und Motivationslager berücksichtigen. Hier kann es natürlich um Programme gehen, die nur Jungen oder Mädchen offenstehen oder die sich in ihren Zielsetzungen und Leistungsanforderungen voneinander abgrenzen. Darüber hinaus wären aber auch Angebote denkbar (und wünschenswert) für Kinder und Jugendliche aus sozial benachteiligten Familien, solchen mit Migrationshintergrund oder sogar für Kinder und Jugendliche, die als unbegleitete Flüchtlinge nach Luxemburg gekommen sind und sich hier nun integrieren müssen.

Was setzt eine Bewegungsförderung der hier skizzierten Art voraus? Zum einen sicher eine administrative Struktur, etwa in Form einer Koordinierungsstelle, die z. B. die Zusammenarbeit der verschiedenen Akteure koordiniert, die Durchführung der Projekte und Programme verwaltet und ihre Qualität sicherstellt. Zum anderen müssen Fachkräfte ausgebildet werden, die die Bewegungsprogramme kompetent anleiten und durchführen können. Hier ist auch die Universität Luxemburg gefordert und bietet deshalb mit Beginn des Wintersemesters 2019 eine berufsbegleitende akademische Weiterbildung zur „Bewegungsförderung und -erziehung in formalen und non-formalen Bildungssettings" an, die u. a. Erziehern und Grundschullehrern und -lehrerinnen offensteht und mit einem Zertifikat abschließt.

Literatur

Almeida Mendes, M., da Silva, I.C.M., Ramires, V.V., Reichert, F.F., Martins, R.C., & Tomasi, E. (2018). Cali-bration of raw accelerometer data to measure physical activity: A systematic review. *Gait Posture, 61,* 98–110.

Arvidsson, D., Fridolfsson, & Börjesson, M. (2019). Measurement of physical activity in clinical practice using accelerometers. *Journal of Internal Medicine, 286* (2), 137–153.

Bös, K., Brochmann, C., Eschette, H., Lämmle, L., Lanners, M., Oberger, J., Opper, E., Romahn, N., Schorn, A., Wagener, Y., Wagner, M. & Worth, A. (2006). *Gesundheit, motorische Leistungsfähigkeit und kör-perlich-sportliche Aktivität von Kindern und Jugendlichen in Luxemburg.* Ministère de l'Èducation et de la Formation professionelle: Luxemburg.

Bund, A. & Scheuer, C. (2017). *Abschlussbericht zum Forschungsprojekt „Bewegter Unterricht in Luxemburg".* Universität Luxemburg: Esch sur Alzette.

Cheon, S.H., Reeve, J., Song, Y.-G. (2019). Recommending goals and supporting needs: An intervention to help physical education teachers communicate their expectations while supporting students' psychological needs. *Psychology of Sport & Exercise, 41,* 107–118.

Deci, E. L., & Ryan, R. M. (1985). Cognitive evaluation theory. In *Intrinsic motivation and self-determination in human behavior* (pp. 43–85). Springer: Boston, MA.

Evenson, K.R., Catellier, D.J., Gill, K., Ondrak, K.S., & McMurray, R.G. (2008). Calibration oft wo objective measures of physical activty for children. *Journal of Sport Science, 26* (14), 1557–1565.

Froiland, J. M., & Worrell, F. C. (2016). Intrinsic motivation, learning goals, engagement, and achievement in a diverse high school. *Psychology in the Schools, 53*(3), 321–336.

Fuchs, R., Klaperski, S., Gerber, M. & Seelig, H. (2015). Messung der Sport- und Bewegungsaktivität mit dem BSA-Fragebogen. *Zeitschrift für Gesundheitspsychologie, 23* (2), 60–76.

Guthold, R., Stevens, G.A., Riley, L.M., & Bull, F.C. (2019). Global trends in insufficient physical activity among adolescents: A pooled analysis of 298 population-based surveys with 1.6 million participants. The *Lancet Child & Adolescent Health, 4* (1), 23–35.

Hagger, M. S., & Chatzisarantis, N. L. (2016). The trans-contextual model of autonomous motivation in education: Conceptual and empirical issues and meta-analysis. *Review of Educational Research, 86*(2), 360–407.

Heinz, A., Kern, M R., Residori, C., Catunda, C., van Duin, C. & Willems, H. (2018). *Körperliche Aktivität von Schülern in ihrer Freizeit.* HBSC-Factsheet Nr. 15. Luxemburg.

Hutmacher, D., Eckelt, M., Bund, A., & Steffgen, G. (2020). Does motivation in physical education have an impact on out of school physical activity? A longitudinal approach. *International Journal of Environmental Research and Public Health, 17*(19), 7258.

Janssen I., & LeBlanc, A.G. (2010). Systematic review of the health benefits of physical activity and fitness in school-aged children and youth *International Journal of Behavioral Nutrition and Physical Activity, 7*: https://doi.org/10.1186/1479-5868-7-40.

Krapp, A. (1999). Interest, motivation and learning: An educational-psychological perspective. *European Journal of Psychology of Education, 14*(1), 23–40.

LUCET (2019). *Online assessment system OASYS (version 2).* Esch-sur-Alzette: University of Luxembourg.

Markland, D., & Tobin, V. (2004). A modification to the behavioral regulation in exercise questionnaire to include an assessment of amotivation. *Journal of Sport and Exercise Psychology, 26*(2), 191–196.

Meyer, U., Roth, R., Gerber, M., Puder, J.J., Hebestreit, H., & Kriemler, S. (2013). Contribution of physical education to overall physical activity. *Scandinavian Journal of Medicine & Science in Sports, 23,* 600–606.

Müller, C., Winter, C. & Rosenbaum, D. (2010). Aktuelle objektive Messverfahren zur Erfassung körperlicher Aktivität im Vergleich zu subjektiven Erhebungsmethoden. *Deutsche Zeitschrift für Sportmedizin, 61* (1), 11–18.

Nettlefold, L., McKay, H.A., Warburton, D.E., McGuire, K.A., Bredin, S.S., & Naylor, P.J. (2011). The challenge of low physical activity during the school day: At recess, lunch and in physical education. *British Journal of Sports Medicine, 45,* 813–819.

Poitras, V.J., Gray, C.E., Borghese, M.M., Carson, V., Chaput, J-P., Janssen, I., Katzmarzyk, P.T., Pate, R.R., Gorber, S.C., Kho, M.E., Sampson, M., & Tremblay, M.S. (2016). Systematic review of the relationships between objectively measured physical activity and health indicators in school-aged children and youth. *Applied Physiology, Nutrition, and Metabolism, 41,* 197–239.

R Core Team (2019). *R: A language and environment for statistical computing.* Foundation for Statistical Computing: Vienna, Austria.

Schmidt, S., Will, N., Henn, A., Reimers, A. & Woll, A. (2016). *Der Motorik-Modul Aktivitätsfragebogen MoMo-AFB.* Karlsruher Institut für Technologie (KIT): Karlsruhe.

Skender, S., Ose, J., Chang-Claude, J., Paskow, M., Brühmann, B., Siegel, E. M., Steindorf, K. & Ulrich C. M. (2016). Accelerometry and physical activity questionnaires. A systematic review *BMC Public Health, 16* (1), p. 515.

Thiel, C., Gabrys, L. & Vgt, L. (2016). Registrierung körperlicher Aktivität mit tragbaren Akzelerometern. *Deutsche Zeitschrift für Sportmedizin, 67* (2), 44–48.

Troiano, R.P., Berrigan, D., Dodd, K.W., Mâsse, L.C., Tilert, T., & McDowell, M. (2008). Physical activity in the United States measured by accelerometer. *Medicine & Science in Sport & Exercise, 40* (1), 181–188.

Vlachopoulos, S. P., Katartzi, E. S., Kontou, M. G., Moustaka, F. C., & Goudas, M. (2011). The revised perceived locus of causality in physical education scale: Psychometric evaluation among youth. *Psychology of Sport and Exercise, 12*(6), 583–592.

WHO (2010). *Global recommendations on physical activity for health.* World Health Organization: Geneva.

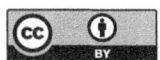

On the Relationship Between Body Perception and Eating Disorders in Adolescents and Young Adults

Zoé van Dyck und Annika P. C. Lutz

1   Eating Disorders

During the last decades, eating disorders have been a frequent topic in the media. Images of emaciated models and Hollywood stars have made the news and the fashion industry has been criticised for its encouragement of extreme dieting behaviours. Western societies' ideals for female and male bodies have become increasingly slender and toned over the second half of the last century (Pope et al. 1999; Spitzer et al. 1999). The media's portrayal of these ideals has often been blamed as the culprit for body dissatisfaction, extreme dieting, and disordered eating behaviour (Levine and Murnen 2009). The introduction of Western television in Fiji in the 1990s was accompanied by the appearance of eating disorder symptoms in adolescent girls (Becker 2004). Yet, the picture is more complex. Not everyone exposed to Western media develops an eating disorder; therefore, additional factors must come into play. In addition, the relentless pursuit of thinness is not the only type of disordered eating behaviour.

The Diagnostic and Statistical Manual of Mental Disorders, fifth edition (American Psychiatric Association 2013), lists three major eating disorders: anorexia nervosa (AN), bulimia nervosa (BN), and binge eating disorder (BED). Anorexia nervosa is characterised by extreme weight-reduction behaviours, leading to underweight, as well as a disturbance in the way in which one's

Z. van Dyck (✉) · A. P. C. Lutz
Department of Behavioural and Cognitive Sciences, University of Luxembourg,
Esch-sur-Alzette, Luxembourg
E-Mail: zoe.vandyck@uni.lu

A. P. C. Lutz
E-Mail: annika.lutz@uni.lu

© Der/die Autor(en) 2022
A. Heinen et al. (Hrsg.), *Wohlbefinden und Gesundheit im Jugendalter,*
https://doi.org/10.1007/978-3-658-35744-3_15

own body is perceived. Individuals with BN engage in recurrent binge eating and compensatory behaviours, e.g. self-induced vomiting. Binge eating is defined as the consumption of large amounts of food in a discrete period of time, accompanied by a perceived loss of control over eating. It is the main characteristic of BED.

Recent prevalence data show that eating disorders are relatively common among women in Europe, with AN affecting <1–4%, BN <1–2%, BED <1–4%, and 2–3% being affected by subthreshold eating disorders (Keski-Rahkonen and Mustelin 2016). Prevalence rates in men are below 1% (Keski-Rahkonen and Mustelin 2016), resulting in a scarcity of research on eating disorders in men, which poses a particular challenge for treatment. Compared to AN and BN, however, BED is more equally distributed between the sexes, with lifetime prevalence rates of 2% for men and 3.5% for women (Hudson et al. 2007). Adolescence is a critical period, as most eating disorders develop during this time of life (Smink et al. 2012). The exact prevalence of eating disorders in Luxembourg is unknown. The only source of information are the statistics on hospitalisations in Luxembourg, which include neither outpatient treatment nor treatment in specialised hospitals abroad, therefore considerably underestimating prevalence rates. The Luxembourg Ministry of Health reported a total of 42 hospitalisations for eating disorders in 2015, with 9 hospitalisations in the age range 0–14 years and 17 hospitalisations in the age range 15–19 years (Ministère de la Santé 2018).

Eating disorders are potentially life threatening. Frequent medical complications include gastrointestinal complications, cardiovascular and pulmonary complications, hormonal disturbance, and effects on the skeletal system (Mitchell and Crow 2006). As a consequence, eating disorders have some of the highest mortality rates of all mental disorders (Harris and Barraclough 1998). Compared to the general population, mortality is almost 6 times higher in individuals with AN and almost 2 times higher in individuals with BN (Smink et al. 2012). Despite the availability of effective treatment approaches, such as cognitive behaviour therapy, outcome for eating disorders remains poor, especially for AN. In a large longitudinal study in Germany, only 40% of patients with AN showed full remission 20 years after inpatient treatment (Fichter et al. 2017). Therefore, research into the mechanisms underlying these debilitating disorders is essential, to define targets for novel approaches to intervention, and eventually improve treatment outcome.

2   Body Perception

When asked about the image of our body, which we have in our mind, most of us will think about a visual image of their body. This body image has four components: cognitive, emotional, perceptual and behavioural (Cash and Green 1986; Vocks et al. 2006). The cognitive and emotional components describe how we think and feel about our own body. Negative feelings about the body and thoughts of being too fat are hallmarks of body dissatisfaction, which is a well-established risk factor for dieting and eating disorders (Jacobi et al. 2004; Stice 2002). The perceptual component encompasses the frequently replicated phenomenon that individuals with eating disorders overestimate their body size, even in an emaciated state (Cash and Deagle 1997; Sepúlveda et al. 2002; Smeets 1997). Body size overestimation, and feelings and thoughts of being too fat may lead to extreme weight-loss behaviours, such as strict fasting, excessive exercising, self-induced vomiting, or misuse of laxatives and diuretics. These in turn may facilitate the development of binge eating. Thus, body image is at the heart of cognitive-behavioural models of eating disorders (Fairburn et al. 2003).

Yet, visual information is not the only type of information, which is integrated in the brain to form the body image. The brain constantly receives information from the body's interior, a process called *interoception*. This includes information on the position of the body and its limbs in space, and the condition of muscles, tendons, and joints, (proprioception) on the one hand, and information about the state of inner organs (visceroception) on the other hand (Birbaumer and Schmidt 2006; Schandry 2003; Vaitl 1996). In eating disorders, body perception is fundamentally altered, including distortions in the visual, as well as the interoceptive components of body image.

Adolescence is a critical developmental period. The body changes from the outside, with increasing sex characteristics, as well as from the inside, with profound changes in hormonal and central-nervous functioning. In addition, pressure to conform to societal ideals increases. Researchers have hypothesized that it might be the interaction of these combined changes in adolescence, which, together with predisposing factors such as perfectionism, lead to the development of eating disorders, especially AN (Kaye et al. 2013). Therefore, it is during adolescence that alterations in the perception of the body's shape and its internal signals play a crucial role.

In the present book chapter, a model is proposed which considers interoception as a multilevel process originating in the visceral organ, where a stimulus, for example, food in the stomach, is registered by receptors, for example, mechanoceptors in the stomach wall (Vaitl 1996). The receptor generates a signal, which is transmitted to the central nervous system. There, the signal is registered and made available for further processing. The intensity with which the visceral signal is processed in the brain can be assessed with electroencephalography (Schandry et al. 1986). Neuroimaging studies have identified several brain regions implicated in interoceptive processing. In this context, the insular cortex plays a major role (Craig 2002; Critchley et al. 2004; Pollatos et al. 2005).

Further processing of the visceral signal includes homeostatic processes occurring outside of conscious awareness, as well as conscious processes. For example, the sensation of stomach fullness triggers the release of hormones (outside of conscious awareness), and generates a sensation of satiety, which is accessible to conscious perception. The ultimate purpose of interoception is to maintain homeostatic balance, that is, to respond to internal and external stimuli in a way that maintains optimal physiological conditions. Therefore, after processing of the interoceptive signal, processes of homeostatic regulation are initiated in the brain, if required. These include non-conscious physiological processes, but also behavioural responses. For example, during meal consumption, the stretching of the stomach walls and the secretion of certain hormones is registered and eventually leads to meal termination. The motivational state generating this behaviour may be consciously perceived as satiety, but this is not necessary for the behaviour to be performed. Disordered eating behaviours may be seen as an attempt at homeostatic regulation in the short term, but which causes disruptions in interoceptive processing in the long term. For example, repeated binge eating may distend stomach walls, and alternating binge eating and vomiting causes cardio-vascular abnormalities due to electrolyte imbalance (Mitchell and Crow 2006). Thereby, the input into the interoceptive system is altered over the course of the disorder.

In summary, we construe interoceptive processing in eating disorders as a circular multilevel model, in which the visceral signal is processed in the brain (with or without conscious perception), and causes behaviours intended to maintain homeostatic balance, but causing visceral alterations and thereby disrupting interoceptive processing. For example, in an individual with BN, an elevated heartrate may be interpreted in terms of an unbearable emotion, such as anxiety. This emotion is downregulated through binge eating. Binge eating leads to uncomfortable sensations of stomach fullness and feelings of guilt. These are downregulated through self-induced vomiting. In the long term, the dysfunctional emotion regulation behaviours "binge eating and vomiting" lead to gastric and cardiac abnormalities, which cause abnormal sensations, which, in turn, maintain disordered eating behaviour. As an example, distended stomach walls lead to a delayed perception of satiety and thereby facilitate the ingestion of large amounts of food during binge eating.

In consequence, it is necessary to assess interoceptive processing at various levels in eating disorders, that is, the viscera organ, central nervous system representation, conscious perception, motivational interpretation, and dysfunctional regulatory behaviours. In addition, different organ systems, such as the heart and the stomach, need to be taken into account. Our model calls for a more complex investigation of interoception in eating disorders and challenges the assumption of a general interoceptive deficit (Bruch 1962; Klabunde et al. 2017). In the following, we will review the extant literature on body perception, including (visual) body image and interoception, in AN, BN, and BED, while adopting a multilevel perspective.

3   Anorexia Nervosa—Body Image, Interoception, and Multi-sensory Integration

Anorexia nervosa (AN) is an eating disorder characterised by extreme weight-reduction behaviours, leading to underweight, as well as a disturbance in the way in which one's own body is perceived (American Psychiatric Association 2013). Recent epidemiological data show that 0.8% of adolescents and young adults in Germany have suffered from AN at some point (Nagl et al. 2016). Despite these low numbers, AN is associated with severe medical complications, e.g. cardiovascular problems, osteoporosis, alterations in linear growth, and structural and functional brain abnormalities (Katzman 2005). There is still insufficient evidence as to how medical complications during the critical developmental period of adolescence affect health and well-being later in life (Katzman 2005). Moreover, a recent study assessing outcome of AN 20 years after inpatient treatment reported that mortality was increased more than fivefold compared to people of similar age and sex from the general population (Fichter and Quadflieg 2016).

Cognitive behavioural models of AN describe a vicious cycle, in which dietary restriction is maintained through an enhanced experience of control over eating, weight and shape (Fairburn et al. 1999). Experimental research has shown that already in pre-adolescent girls (aged 11–12 years) watching thin-ideal focused television shows (e.g. shows about fashion models) increases the body dissatisfaction and makes them desire a thinner body (Anschutz et al. 2011). Indeed, thin-ideal media images have often been blamed as being responsible for body image dissatisfaction and AN, but the relationship is not as direct as one might be tempted to think (Levine and Murnen 2009). Thin-ideal media exposure only leads to body dissatisfaction, if the media ideal is adopted as one's personal ideal and if a discrepancy between the actual and the ideal body shape is detected (Dittmar et al. 2009). Body dissatisfaction, in turn, is only one of many established risk factors for AN. Additional factors take effect throughout the life span, including genetic factors, pregnancy and birth problems, feeding and gastro-intestinal problems in early childhood, adverse life events, and perfectionism, to name only a few examples, culminating in the development of eating disorder symptoms during adolescence (Jacobi et al. 2004). In the light of these findings, recent numbers of body dissatisfaction in Luxembourgish adolescents give rise to concern. The 2013/2014 Health Behaviour in School-Aged Children survey (World Health Organization 2016) reported that among 15-year-old girls, 56% perceived themselves as being too fat and 29% engaged in weight-reduction behaviours. Only 15% were actually overweight or obese. Although these girls are by no means predetermined to develop AN, they are certainly at risk.

Body dissatisfaction reflects the cognitive-affective level of body image disturbance in AN (Gleaves et al. 1995). On the behavioural level, excessive weight-loss behaviours, such as strict fasting, are prominent. Another aspect, which has drawn a lot of attention in the literature, is that individuals with AN, who are underweight by definition, significantly overestimate their body dimensions (Cash and Deagle 1997). This is a striking symptom and accompanied by alterations in other aspects of body perception, namely interoception (Lutz et al. 2019). The presence of body image disturbance is a negative prognostic factor for treatment outcome (Garfinkel et al. 1977; Slade and Russell 1973), which is why research on this aspect of AN is especially important.

In our own research (Lutz et al. 2019), we were able to show that body perception is not necessarily reduced on all levels, as suggested by early theories of AN (Bruch 1962). Previous studies confirming interoceptive deficits focused mainly on the conscious perception of cardiac signals (Pollatos et al. 2008, 2016). We investigated interoception of cardiac signals in young women (mean age 25 years) from Luxembourg and inpatients with AN, based on our multilevel model of interoception in eating disorders. On a first level, we found no group differences regarding heart rate and its variability, suggesting the signals arriving in the brain were similar in both groups. On a second level, we investigated how this information from the heart is processed in the brain. To this end, we analysed brain potentials, which occur around 500 ms after the heartbeat (as indexed by the R-peak of the electrocardiogram). These heartbeat-evoked potentials reflect brain processing of cardiac information on a pre-conscious level, i.e. they are visible even when the individual is not actively directing their attention to the heartbeat (Schandry et al. 1986). On this level, we found enhanced processing of heartbeats in the brain. When looking at conscious perception of heartbeats (third level), we found no difference between individuals with or without AN in how well they were able to count their own heartbeats or how they judged their own heartbeat-counting performance. Moving to the fourth level of interpretation of body sensations, individuals with AN reported increased problems with the perception of emotions and other body sensations, as assessed via questionnaire. This clearly shows that prominent symptoms of AN, such as difficulties perceiving and interpreting emotions, are not necessarily based on reduced interoception. Instead, our study showed that some aspects of interoception may be unaltered or even enhanced in AN. This supports our notion that different levels need to be distinguished when assessing interoception in eating disorders.

Other studies showed increased interoceptive processing in AN during meal and food stimulus anticipation (Khalsa et al. 2015; Oberndorfer et al. 2013). Meals are inherently aversive events for individuals with AN and this aversiveness could be, at least partially, maintained by increased interoception, that is, a stronger experience of the uncomfortable sensations around eating. This would explain why fasting, rather than eating, would have a positive connotation and serve as a reward in individuals with AN (Kaye et al. 2013). In conclusion, increased interoceptive processing, rather than interoceptive deficits, may be present in AN at least at some levels (central nervous system representation). The strict fasting behaviour, which is characteristic of the disorder, might help to reduce aversive body sensations which are amplified by distorted interoceptive processing (Kaye et al. 2013). These alterations might play a particularly important role during adolescence, as during this developmental period the balance between prefrontal and limbic brain structures changes. This makes adolescents sensitive to disruptions in the balance between controlled and intuitively motivated behaviours (Kaye et al. 2013). In that sense, altered interoceptive processing might contribute to the need for cognitive control over eating behaviour, to compensate for distorted intuitive processes.

4   Interoceptive Processes in Bulimia Nervosa and Binge-Eating Disorder

As mentioned above, BN and BED are both characterised by recurrent episodes of binge eating, referring to the consumption of large amounts of food in a short period of time, accompanied by a sense of loss of control over eating (American Psychiatric Association 2013). These episodes have been termed objective bulimic episodes (Fairburn and Cooper 1993). While BN is marked by the oscillation between objective bulimic episodes and compensatory behavior to prevent weight gain (e.g., vomiting), along with an undue influence of shape on self-evaluation, BED entails recurrent binge eating in the absence of such compensatory behaviors (American Psychiatric Association 2013). Hence, it is little surprising that BED is strongly related to obesity (Dingemans et al. 2002), and that the prevalence of BED is high among individuals who seek weight control treatment (up to 30%; de Zwaan 2001). Furthermore, obese individuals with regular binge eating episodes seem to be especially at risk for further weight gain (Yanovski 2002). With 26% of the adult population in Luxembourg being obese (World Health Organization 2018), and a recent increase in the proportion of overweight or obese adolescents (Heinz et al. 2020), a better understanding of the factors underlying binge eating is important when aiming to tackle the obesity epidemic.

Binge eating behaviours are not solely found in clinical populations, but are also very common in the general population. Recent prevalence rates suggest that worldwide more than 20% of adolescents report binge eating episodes, with even higher rates among overweight and obese youth (He et al. 2017; Van Malderen et al. 2019). Similarly, Goossens et al. (2009) found that nearly 17% of adolescents from a community sample had experienced at least one episode of loss of control over eating during the past month. Loss of control over eating, referring to an inability to stop eating once eating has started, irrespective of the amount of food consumed, can be considered the hallmark feature of binge eating (e.g., Colles et al. 2008). Research has shown that loss of control over eating is common among youth in the general population and can be a precursor to eating disorders and other psychiatric disorders (e.g., addiction, depression) (Herpertz-Dahlmann et al. 2015).

Several lines of research have suggested that interoceptive processes play an important role in the development and maintenance of binge eating behaviours (Simmons and DeVille 2017). Altered interoception has been repeatedly associated with overeating, especially with respect to the perception of hunger and satiety and emotion processing. To date, interoceptive processes in eating disorders have primarily been investigated in relation to the awareness of emotional states. Using self-report questionnaires, a substantial body of research has provided evidence that interoceptive sensibility is reduced in individuals engaging in uncontrollable overeating and that these impairments persist even after recovery (for a meta-analysis, see Jenkinson et al. 2018).

Besides self-report measures, behavioural measures have been used to investigate conscious interoceptive accuracy, most of which have focused on people's ability to perceive their own heartbeats (Brener and Kluvitse 1988; Critchley et al. 2004; Schandry 1981; Whitehead et al. 1977). The predominant focus on cardiac interoceptive accuracy is largely due to pragmatic reasons: Heartbeats are distinct and frequent internal events that can be easily discriminated and measured (Garfinkel et al. 2015). These so-called heartbeat perception tasks are well-validated measures, as evidenced by relationships between cardiac interoceptive accuracy and activation in brain structures responsible for the mapping of internal bodily responses, in particular the right anterior insula, and the somatomotor and cingulate cortices (Critchley et al. 2004). While research on cardiac interoceptive accuracy n BED remains scarce, studies on participants with BN show either attenuated interoceptive abilities compared to healthy controls (Klabunde et al. 2013) or no differences (Eshkevari et al. 2014; Pollatos and Georgiou 2016).

This inconsistent evidence raises doubts about the use of measures of cardiac interoception as a proxy for interoception in general, which do not directly address a core aspect of interoceptive deficits in eating disorders, i.e. impaired perception of hunger and satiety cues. A major objective of our working group in recent years has therefore been the development and validation of adequate measures to assess interoceptive processes in eating disorders at multiple levels, based on our model introduced earlier. To do so, we focus on the processing of interoceptive information from two organ systems that are particularly relevant to eating behaviours, that is, the heart and the stomach. Altered processing of cardiovascular activity, as measured by heartbeat perception tasks, has frequently been linked to disturbances in cognitive and emotional processes (e.g., Craig 2009). Difficulties in the processing and regulation of emotions have also been documented in BN and BED (e.g., Harrison et al. 2010), suggesting that interoceptive deficits are indirectly linked to eating disorder symptomatology. Another organ system of relevance for eating behaviours is the gastric system, which might contribute to eating disorder symptoms via altered processing of hunger and satiety cues (Klabunde et al. 2017).

In the self-report domain, our research group has developed a multi-dimensional questionnaire to assess eating disorder-specific interoceptive processes in terms of the ability to perceive emotions, hunger and satiety, and to discriminate between those signals (van Dyck et al. 2017). First results using the eating disorder-specific interoceptive processes-questionnaire (EDIP-Q) are promising and show alterations on all four dimensions in individuals with an eating disorder diagnosis (van Dyck et al. 2017). More importantly, the EDIP-Q subscales were affected to a varying extent and in different directions among eating disorder types, suggesting that the processing of emotions, hunger, and satiety might be of differential relevance in different eating disorder diagnoses. More precisely, participants with BN or BED reported more difficulties perceiving satiety cues and differentiating between hunger and emotional states compared to AN and healthy controls. This finding is in line with the idea that individuals with BN or BED use binge eating as a (dysfunctional) emotion regulation strategy.

With the aim of developing a behavioural measure of interoceptive processing in the gastric system, we developed a water load test as a provocative test of gastric distention (van Dyck et al. 2016). Gastric distention during intake activates vagal and spinal mechanosensitive afferents, which transmit signals from the stomach to the brain and lead to the perception of satiation and fullness (Hellström et al. 2004). Reduced sensitivity to these signals may result in excessive food intake (Wang et al. 2008), a core feature of binge eating. Laboratory studies have shown that patients with BN or BED eat larger meals compared to controls, even under controlled circumstances (Kissileff et al. 1996). Furthermore, patients require much larger amounts of food than healthy control participants to reach similar levels of fullness (Walsh et al. 2003). These findings suggest that individuals with BN or BED process the information on gastric distention differently, which may contribute to altered sensations and physiological and behavioral responses.

Water load test protocols were initially developed to assess gastric sensation and accommodation in patients with functional digestive disorders and, therefore, needed some adaptations to measure sensitivity for eating-related sensations. We developed the water load test-II as a two-step drink test measuring the perception of eating-related satiation, in addition to the experience of maximum stomach fullness. Initial results in a non-clinical sample in Luxembourg suggest that the water load test-II is a simple, reliable test that distinguishes well between sensations of comfortable satiation and unpleasant fullness (van Dyck et al. 2016). Importantly, water volume ingested until satiation was related to bulimic symptoms, suggesting that the development of satiation is altered in individuals who engage in binge eating. Using the water load test-II in combination with psychophysiological methods, we further found that individuals with BN or BED show a delayed response to satiation, together with abnormal gastric motility, as assessed via electrogastrography (van Dyck et al. 2020). Applying the multilevel model of interoception, gastric motility corresponds to the most basic level of gastric interoception, which refers to the rate of stomach contractions and is a central mediator of hunger and satiety (Janssen et al. 2011). Furthermore, we were able to show that the degree of normal gastric activity decreased with the number of binge eating episodes per week in the patient group, suggesting that there is a systematic relationship between the severity of the eating disorder and the extent of disturbances to gastric motor function (van Dyck et al. 2020).

5   Treatment of Interoceptive Deficits

Several implications for the treatment of eating disorders might follow from findings on interoceptive abnormalities, and interventions can occur at each level of our model. One of the best-validated treatment approaches for eating disorders is cognitive behaviour therapy (Linardon et al. 2017). This type of psychotherapy typically focuses on the normalisation of eating behaviour and the treatment of body image disturbance. Interventions targeting eating behaviour usually address maladaptive dieting patterns, such as limiting calorie intake, leaving excessive time between meals, and avoiding "forbidden foods" (Fairburn et al. 1993; Hilbert and Tuschen-Caffier 2010). A pattern of regular eating is established, which patients are required to follow until their hunger and satiety signals are re-established. This pattern of eating also aims at preventing binge eating (Latner and Wilson 2000).

When treating young patients who are living with their family of origin, it is essential to include parents or guardians in the therapeutic process and to build up a solid therapeutic relationship with both the child/adolescent and the parents (Herpertz et al. 2011). Parents can help the young patients to realize the need for treatment and ensure that the treatment is arranged and carried out. For this reason, they should be provided comprehensive information about the eating disorder and the required treatment. Furthermore, it is important to support the emotional functioning of parents in order to strengthen their ability to support their child most effectively during treatment.

Another line of interventions is derived from awareness and mindfulness-based trainings, trying to improve the patients' ability to regulate eating through heightened responsivity to internal hunger and satiety cues. However, although mindfulness-based interventions have become increasingly popular in the treatment of eating disorders (e.g., Dunne 2018), they only target some aspects of interoceptive processing (Khalsa et al. 2008).

Using biofeedback of electrogastrographic activity, Stern and colleagues showed that normal gastric myoelectrical activity can be increased in healthy individuals (Stern et al. 2004). Normal gastric myoelectrical activity corresponds to three cycles per minute and is associated with normal gastric function (Koch and Stern 2004). Hence, electrogastrographic biofeedback constitutes a promising and noninvasive intervention to improve individuals' awareness of their stomach activity and enhance gastric interoceptive processing at the most basic level (the visceral organ).

The visual aspect of body image can be altered, as well (Farrell et al. 2006), and its improvement constitutes a key factor for remission (Key et al. 2002; Vall and Wade 2015). Yet, visual information on the body's state is not processed in isolation, but integrated with interoceptive information. This is termed multisensory integration (Badoud and Tsakiris 2017). Interventions based on multisensory integration are still in the experimental phase, but show promising results. One technique, for example, uses virtual reality to integrate visual information (showing the exterior of the body) and tactile information (a sensation of touch). This technique reduces body size overestimation in AN (Keizer et al. 2016). A current project at the University of Luxembourg expands this line of research, by investigating how the addition of interoceptive (heartbeat-related) information may help to improve body image. This work is essential to improve the poor long-term outcome of AN (Fichter et al. 2017) and support clinicians and patients in Luxembourg and worldwide. As these interventions are performed in virtual reality environments, they might appear particularly appealing to adolescents. Yet, it is important to keep in mind that evidence exists that interoceptive deficits persist even after recovery from an eating disorder (Jenkinson et al. 2018; Klabunde et al. 2013). This raises the question to what extent interoceptive processes are traits that cannot be changed. Further research is needed to investigate whether alterations on interoceptive levels in the cardiac or gastric system can be modified in eating disordered patients. Moreover, we are unaware of any research investigating the long-term consequences of disruptions in interoceptive functioning during the developmentally critical period of adolescence.

6 Summary and Conclusion

In this book chapter, we presented a selective review of the role of body perception in eating disorders, with a special focus on research performed in Luxembourg. We conclude that the visual aspect of the body is perceived in a distorted and negative way in all eating disorders. The picture is much more complex when looking at the perception of signals from within the body. Therefore, we adopted a multilevel perspective on interoception, taking into account different organ systems (e.g. heart, stomach), different levels of processing (visceral organ, central nervous system representation, conscious processing, interpretation, behaviour), and their interactions. Regarding AN, we found that processing on the different levels diverges, and that processing on some levels may even be enhanced (central nervous system representation). Enhanced processing of interoceptive signals in the central nervous system, especially around meals, may directly promote fasting behaviour, as it increases the discomfort associated with eating in these individuals.

Concerning eating disorders in which binge eating is a central feature (BN and BED), we showed that interoceptive deficits exist on different levels (visceral organ, conscious processing, and behaviour) and in both the cardiac and the gastric domains. Studies investigating different levels of interoceptive processing concomitantly within the same sample of eating disordered patients are scarce, which is a gap we are currently attempting to fill in our research at the University of Luxembourg. Furthermore, additional studies are needed to examine the unique associations of binge eating, purging, and prolonged episodes of dietary restriction with interoceptive processes at multiple levels and in different organ systems.

Research on interoception has gained popularity only recently and we are just beginning to understand the complexity of interoceptive alterations in eating disorders. Yet, this area of research opens up several avenues for potential interventions, which are expected to improve current treatment programmes for eating disorders in the future. Regarding adolescents and young adults, research on the relationship between eating disorder symptoms and interoceptive processes is scarce. Few studies have investigated the development of interoceptive ability during youth and throughout the lifespan, and available evidence suggests that interoceptive perception changes with development (Failla et al. 2020). It is, however, not yet known how these age-related interoceptive changes may contribute to the development of healthy or disordered eating behaviours. Yet, it seems likely that they constitute one of the bio-psycho-social changes associated with adolescence, which play a crucial role in the development of eating disorders (Kaye et al. 2013). Eating-disorder research is especially important in Luxembourg, where little is known about the prevalence of eating disorders or about factors contributing to their development.

References

American Psychiatric Association. (2013). *Diagnostic and Statistical Manual of Mental Disorders* (5th ed.). American Psychiatric Publishing.

Anschutz, D. J., Spruijt-Metz, D., Van Strien, T., & Engels, R. C. M. E. (2011). The direct effect of thin ideal focused adult television on young girls' ideal body figure. *Body Image, 8*(1), 26–33. https://doi.org/10.1016/j.bodyim.2010.11.003

Badoud, D., & Tsakiris, M. (2017). From the body's viscera to the body's image: Is there a link between interoception and body image concerns? *Neuroscience and Biobehavioral Reviews, 77*(April), 237–246. https://doi.org/10.1016/j.neubiorev.2017.03.017

Becker, A. E. (2004). Television, Disordered Eating, and Young Women in Fiji: Negotiating Body Image and Identity during Rapid Social Change. *Culture, Medicine and Psychiatry, 28*(4), 533–559. https://doi.org/10.1007/s11013-004-1067-5

Birbaumer, N., & Schmidt, R. F. (2006). *Biologische Psychologie* (6th ed.). Springer Medizin Verlag.

Brener, J., & Kluvitse, C. (1988). Heartbeat detection: Judgments of the simultaneity of external stimuli and heartbeats. *Psychophysiology, 25*(5), 554–561.

Bruch, H. (1962). Perceptual and conceptual disturbances in anorexia nervosa. *Psychosomatic Medicine, 24*(2), 187–194.

Cash, T. F., & Deagle, E. A. (1997). The nature and extent of body-image disturbances in anorexia nervosa and bulimia nervosa: A meta-analysis. *International Journal of Eating Disorders, 22*, 107–125.

Cash, T. F., & Green, G. K. (1986). Body weight and body image among college women: Perception, cognition, and affect. *Journal of Personality Assessment, 50*(2), 290–301.

Colles, S. L., Dixon, J. B., & O'Brien, P. E. (2008). Loss of control is central to psychological disturbance associated with binge eating disorder. *Obesity, 16*(3), 608–614. https://doi.org/10.1038/oby.2007.99

Craig, A. D. (2002). How do you feel? Interoception: The sense of the physiological condition of the body. *Nature Reviews. Neuroscience, 3*(8), 655–666. https://doi.org/10.1038/nrn894

Craig, A. D. (2009). How do you feel — now? The anterior insula and human awareness. *Nature Reviews Neuroscience, 10*(1), 59–70. https://doi.org/10.1038/nrn2555

Critchley, H. D., Wiens, S., Rotshtein, P., Ohman, A., & Dolan, R. J. (2004). Neural systems supporting interoceptive awareness. *Nature Neuroscience, 7*(2), 189–195. https://doi.org/10.1038/nn1176

de Zwaan, M. (2001). Binge eating disorder and obesity. *International Journal of Obesity and Related Metabolic Disorders: Journal of the International Association for the Study of Obesity, 25*(1), 51–55. https://doi.org/10.1038/sj.ijo.0801699

Dingemans, A. E., Bruna, M. J., & Van Furth, E. F. (2002). Binge eating disorder: A review. *Internation Journal of Obesity, 26*(3), 299–307.

Dittmar, H., Halliwell, E., & Stirling, E. (2009). Understanding the impact of thin media models on women's body-focused affect: the roles of thin-ideal internalization and weight-related self-discrepancy activation in experimental exposure effects. *Journal of Social and Clinical Psychology, 28*(1), 43–72. https://doi.org/10.1521/jscp.2009.28.1.43

Dunne, J. (2018). Mindfulness in Anorexia Nervosa: An Integrated Review of the Literature. *Journal of the American Psychiatric Nurses Association, 24*(2), 109–117. https://doi.org/10.1177/1078390317711250

Eshkevari, E., Rieger, E., Musiat, P., & Treasure, J. (2014). An investigation of interoceptive sensitivity in eating disorders using a heartbeat detection task and a self-report measure. *European Eating Disorders Review, 22*(5), 383–388. https://doi.org/10.1002/erv.2305

Failla, M. D., Bryant, L. K., Heflin, B. H., Mash, L. E., Schauder, K., Davis, S., Gerdes, M. B., Weitlauf, A., Rogers, B. P., & Cascio, C. J. (2020). Neural Correlates of Cardiac Interoceptive Focus Across Development: Implications for Social Symptoms in Autism Spectrum Disorder. *Autism Research, 13*(6), 908–920. https://doi.org/10.1002/aur.2289

Fairburn, C. G., & Cooper, Z. (1993). The eating disorder examination. In C. G. Fairburn & G. T. Wilson (Eds.), *Binge eating: Nature, assessment, and treatment* (12th ed., pp. 317–360). Guilford Press.

Fairburn, C. G., Cooper, Z., & Shafran, R. (2003). Cognitive behaviour therapy for eating disorders: a "transdiagnostic" theory and treatment. *Behaviour Research and Therapy, 41*(5), 509–528. https://doi.org/10.1016/S0005-7967(02)00088-8

Fairburn, C. G., Marcus, M. D., & Wilson, G. T. (1993). Cognitive-behavioral therapy for binge eating and bulimia nervosa: A comprehensive treatment manual. In C. G. Fairburn & G. T. Wilson (Eds.), *Binge eating. Nature, assessment, and treatment* (pp. 361–404). Guilford Press.

Fairburn, C. G., Shafran, R., & Cooper, Z. (1999). A cognitive behavioural theory of anorexia nervosa. *Behaviour Research and Therapy, 37*, 1–13.

Farrell, C., Shafran, R., & Lee, M. (2006). Empirically evaluated treatments for body image disturbance: A review. *European Eating Disorders Review, 14*(5), 289–300. https://doi.org/10.1002/erv.693

Fichter, M. M., & Quadflieg, N. (2016). Mortality in eating disorders – Results of a large prospective clinical longitudinal study. *International Journal of Eating Disorders, 49*(4), 391–401. https://doi.org/10.1002/eat.22501

Fichter, M. M., Quadflieg, N., Crosby, R. D., & Koch, S. (2017). Long-term outcome of anorexia nervosa: Results from a large clinical longitudinal study. *International Journal of Eating Disorders, 50*(9), 1018–1030. https://doi.org/10.1002/eat.22736

Garfinkel, P. E., Moldofsky, H. & Garner, D. M. (1977). Prognosis in anorexia nervosa as influenced by clinical features, treatment and self-perception. *Canadian Medical Association Journal, 117*(9), 1041–1045. http://www.ncbi.nlm.nih.gov/pubmed/912628

Garfinkel, S. N., Seth, A. K., Barrett, A. B., Suzuki, K., & Critchley, H. D. (2015). Knowing your own heart: Distinguishing interoceptive accuracy from interoceptive awareness. *Biological Psychology, 104*, 65–74. https://doi.org/10.1016/j.biopsycho.2014.11.004

Gleaves, D., Williamson, D., Eberenz, K., Sebastian, S., & Barker, S. (1995). Clarifying body-image disturbance: Analysis of a multidimensional model using structural modeling. *Journal of Personality Assessment, 64*(3), 478–493.

Goossens, L., Soenens, B., & Braet, C. (2009). Prevalence and characteristics of binge eating in an adolescent community sample. *Journal of Clinical Child and Adolescent Psychology*, *38*(3), 342–353. https://doi.org/10.1080/15374410902851697

Harris, E., & Barraclough, B. (1998). Excess mortality of mental disorder. *British Journal of Psychiatry*, *173*, 11–53.

Harrison, A., Sullivan, S., Tchanturia, K., & Treasure, J. (2010). Emotional functioning in eating disorders: attentional bias, emotion recognition and emotion regulation. *Psychological Medicine*, *40*(11), 1887–1897. https://doi.org/10.1017/S0033291710000036

He, J., Cai, Z., & Fan, X. (2017). Prevalence of binge and loss of control eating among children and adolescents with overweight and obesity: An exploratory meta-analysis. *International Journal of Eating Disorders*, *50*(2), 91–103. https://doi.org/10.1002/eat.22661

Heinz, A., van Duin, C., Kern, M. R., Catunda, C., & Willems, H. (2020). *Trends from 2006–2018 in Health Behaviour, Health Outcomes and Social Context of Adolescents in Luxembourg*. University of Luxembourg.

Hellström, P. M., Geliebter, A., Näslund, E., Schmidt, P. T., Yahav, E. K., Hashim, S. A., & Yeomans, M. R. (2004). Peripheral and central signals in the control of eating in normal, obese and binge-eating human subjects. *British Journal of Nutrition*, *92*(S1), 47–57. https://doi.org/10.1079/BJN20041142

Herpertz-Dahlmann, B., Dempfle, A., Konrad, K., Klasen, F., & Ravens-Sieberer, U. (2015). Eating disorder symptoms do not just disappear: the implications of adolescent eating-disordered behaviour for body weight and mental health in young adulthood. *European Child and Adolescent Psychiatry*, *24*(6), 675–684. https://doi.org/10.1007/s00787-014-0610-3

Herpertz, S., Hagenah, U., Vocks, S., Wietersheim, J. von, Cuntz, U., & Zeeck, A. (2011). The Diagnosis and Treatment of Eating Disorders. *Deutsches Aerzteblatt Online*, *108*(40), 678–685. https://doi.org/10.3238/arztebl.2011.0678

Hilbert, A., & Tuschen-Caffier, B. (2010). *Essanfälle und Adipositas*. Hogrefe.

Hudson, J. I., Hiripi, E., Pope, H. G., & Kessler, R. C. (2007). The prevalence and correlates of eating disorders in the National Comorbidity Survey Replication. *Biological Psychiatry*, *61*(3), 348–358. https://doi.org/10.1016/j.biopsych.2006.03.040

Jacobi, C., Hayward, C., de Zwaan, M., Kraemer, H. C., & Agras, W. S. (2004). Coming to Terms With Risk Factors for Eating Disorders: Application of Risk Terminology and Suggestions for a General Taxonomy. *Psychological Bulletin*, *130*(1), 19–65. https://doi.org/10.1037/0033-2909.130.1.19

Janssen, P., Vanden Berghe, P., Verschueren, S., Lehmann, A., Depoortere, I., & Tack, J. (2011). Review article: The role of gastric motility in the control of food intake. *Alimentary Pharmacology & Therapeutics*, *33*(8), 880–894. https://doi.org/10.1111/j.1365-2036.2011.04609.x

Jenkinson, P. M., Taylor, L., & Laws, K. R. (2018). Self-reported interoceptive deficits in eating disorders: A meta-analysis of studies using the eating disorder inventory. *Journal of Psychosomatic Research*, *110*(November 2017), 38–45. https://doi.org/10.1016/j.jpsychores.2018.04.005

Katzman, D. K. (2005). Medical complications in adolescents with anorexia nervosa: A review of the literature. *International Journal of Eating Disorders*, *37*, S52–S59. https://doi.org/10.1002/eat.20118

Kaye, W. H., Wierenga, C. E., Bailer, U. F., Simmons, A. N., & Bischoff-Grethe, A. (2013). Nothing tastes as good as skinny feels: The neurobiology of anorexia nervosa. *Trends in Neurosciences*, *36*(2), 110–120. https://doi.org/10.1016/j.tins.2013.01.003

Keizer, A., Van Elburg, A., Helms, R., & Dijkerman, H. C. (2016). A virtual reality full body illusion improves body image disturbance in anorexia nervosa. *PLoS ONE*, *11*(10), 1–21. https://doi.org/10.1371/journal.pone.0163921

Keski-Rahkonen, A., & Mustelin, L. (2016). Epidemiology of eating disorders in Europe. *Current Opinion in Psychiatry*, *29*(6), 340–345. https://doi.org/10.1097/YCO.0000000000000278

Key, A., George, C. L., Beattie, D., Stammers, K., Lacey, H., & Waller, G. (2002). Body image treatment within an inpatient program for anorexia nervosa: The role of mirror exposure in the desensitization process. *International Journal of Eating Disorders*, *31*(2), 185–190.

Khalsa, S. S., Craske, M. G., Li, W., Vangala, S., Strober, M., & Feusner, J. D. (2015). Altered interoceptive awareness in anorexia nervosa: Effects of meal anticipation, consumption and bodily arousal. *International Journal of Eating Disorders*, *1 mL*, n/a-n/a. https://doi.org/10.1002/eat.22387

Khalsa, S. S., Rudrauf, D., Damasio, A. R., Davidson, R. J., Lutz, A., & Tranel, D. (2008). Interoceptive awareness in experienced meditators. *Psychophysiology*, *45*(4), 671–677. https://doi.org/10.1111/j.1469-8986.2008.00666.x

Kissileff, H. R., Wentzlaff, T. H., Guss, J. L., Walsh, B. T., Devlin, M. J., & Thornton, J. C. (1996). A direct measure of satiety disturbance in patients with bulimia nervosa. *Physiology and Behavior*, *60*(4), 1077–1085. https://doi.org/10.1016/0031-9384(96)00086-8

Klabunde, M., Acheson, D. T., Boutelle, K. N., Matthews, S. C., & Kaye, W. H. (2013). Interoceptive sensitivity deficits in women recovered from bulimia nervosa. *Eating Behaviors*, *14*(4), 488–492. https://doi.org/10.1016/j.eatbeh.2013.08.002

Klabunde, M., Collado, D., & Bohon, C. (2017). An interoceptive model of bulimia nervosa: A neurobiological systematic review. *Journal of Psychiatric Research*, *94*, 36–46. https://doi.org/10.1016/j.jpsychires.2017.06.009

Koch, K. L., & Stern, R. M. (2004). *Handbook of electrogastrography*. Oxford University Press.

Latner, J. D., & Wilson, G. T. (2000). Cognitive-behavioral therapy and nutritional counseling in the treatment of bulimia nervosa and binge eating. *Eating Behaviors*, *1*(1), 3–21. https://doi.org/10.1016/S1471-0153(00)00008-8

Levine, M. P., & Murnen, S. K. (2009). "Everybody knows that mass media are/are not [pick one] a cause of eating disorders": A critical review of evidence for a causal link between media, negative body image, and disordered eating in females. *Journal of Social and Clinical Psychology*, *28*(1), 9–42. https://doi.org/10.1521/jscp.2009.28.1.9

Linardon, J., Wade, T. D., De La Piedad Garcia, X., & Brennan, L. (2017). The efficacy of cognitive-behavioral therapy for eating disorders: A systematic review and meta-analysis. *Journal of Consulting and Clinical Psychology*, *85*(11), 1080–1094. https://doi.org/10.1037/ccp0000245

Lutz, A. P. C., Schulz, A., Voderholzer, U., Koch, S., van Dyck, Z., & Vögele, C. (2019). Enhanced cortical processing of cardio-afferent signals in anorexia nervosa. *Clinical Neurophysiology*, *130*(9), 1620–1627. https://doi.org/10.1016/j.clinph.2019.06.009

Ministère de la Santé, . (2018). *Carte sanitaire – mise a jour 2017. Grand-Duché de Luxembourg. Fascicule 2: Motifs de recours à l'hospitalisation selon la classification internationale des maladies (ICD 10)*.

Mitchell, J. E., & Crow, S. (2006). Medical complications of anorexia nervosa and bulimia nervosa. *Current Opinion in Psychiatry, 19*(4), 438–443. https://doi.org/10.1097/01. yco.0000228768.79097.3e

Nagl, M., Jacobi, C., Paul, M., Beesdo-Baum, K., Höfler, M., Lieb, R., & Wittchen, H. U. (2016). Prevalence, incidence, and natural course of anorexia and bulimia nervosa among adolescents and young adults. *European Child and Adolescent Psychiatry, 25*(8), 903–918. https://doi.org/10.1007/s00787-015-0808-z

Oberndorfer, T., Simmons, A., McCurdy, D., Strigo, I., Matthews, S., Yang, T., Irvine, Z., & Kaye, W. (2013). Greater anterior insula activation during anticipation of food images in women recovered from anorexia nervosa versus controls. *Psychiatry Research, 214*(2), 132–141. https://doi.org/10.1016/j.pscychresns.2013.06.010

Pollatos, O., & Georgiou, E. (2016). Normal interoceptive accuracy in women with bulimia nervosa. *Psychiatry Research, 240*, 328–332. https://doi.org/10.1016/j. psychres.2016.04.072

Pollatos, O., Herbert, B. M., Berberich, G., Zaudig, M., Krauseneck, T., & Tsakiris, M. (2016). Atypical self-focus effect on interoceptive accuracy in anorexia nervosa. *Frontiers in Human Neuroscience, 10*(484). https://doi.org/10.3389/fnhum.2016.00484

Pollatos, O., Kirsch, W., & Schandry, R. (2005). Brain structures involved in interoceptive awareness and cardioafferent signal processing: A dipole source localization study. *Human Brain Mapping, 26*(1), 54–64. https://doi.org/10.1002/hbm.20121

Pollatos, O., Kurz, A.-L., Albrecht, J., Schreder, T., Kleemann, A. M., Schöpf, V., Kopietz, R., Wiesmann, M., & Schandry, R. (2008). Reduced perception of bodily signals in anorexia nervosa. *Eating Behaviors, 9*(4), 381–388. https://doi.org/10.1016/j. eatbeh.2008.02.001

Pope, H. G., Olivardia, R., Gruber, A., & Borowiecki, J. (1999). Evolving ideals of male body image as seen through action toys. *The International Journal of Eating Disorders, 26*(1), 65–72.

Schandry, R. (1981). Heart beat perception and emotional experience. *Psychophysiology, 18*(4), 483–488. http://www.ncbi.nlm.nih.gov/pubmed/7267933

Schandry, R. (2003). *Biologische Psychologie* (1st ed.). Beltz Verlage.

Schandry, R., Sparrer, B., & Weitkunat, R. (1986). From the heart to the brain: Study of heartbeat contingent scalp potentials. *International Journal of Neuroscience, 30*, 261–275. https://doi.org/10.3109/00207458608985677

Sepúlveda, A. R., Botella, J., & León, J. A. (2002). Body-image disturbance in eating disorders: A meta-analysis. *Psychology in Spain, 6*(1), 83–95.

Simmons, W. K., & DeVille, D. C. (2017). Interoceptive contributions to healthy eating and obesity. *Current Opinion in Psychology, 17*, 106–112. https://doi.org/10.1016/j. copsyc.2017.07.001

Slade, P. D., & Russell, G. F. M. (1973). Awareness of body dimensions in anorexia nervosa: Cross-sectional and longitudinal studies. *Psychological Medicine, 3*(2), 188–199. https://doi.org/10.1017/S0033291700048510

Smeets, M. A. M. (1997). The rise and fall of size estimation research in anorexia nervosa: A review and reconceptualization. *European Eating Disorders Review, 5*(2), 75–95.

Smink, F. R. E., van Hoeken, D., & Hoek, H. W. (2012). Epidemiology of eating disorders: Incidence, prevalence and mortality rates. *Current Psychiatry Reports, 14*(4), 406–414. https://doi.org/10.1007/s11920-012-0282-y

Spitzer, B. L., Henderson, K. A., & Zivian, M. T. (1999). Gender differences in population versus media body sizes: A comparison over four decades. *Sex Roles, 40*(7/8), 545–565.

Stern, R. M., Vitellaro, K., Thomas, M., Higgins, S. C., & Koch, K. L. (2004). Electrogastrographic biofeedback: a technique for enhancing normal gastric activity. *Neurogastroenterology and Motility, 16*(6), 753–757. https://doi.org/10.1111/j.1365-2982.2004.00543.x

Stice, E. (2002). Risk and maintenance factors for eating pathology: A meta-analytic review. *Psychological Bulletin, 128*(5), 825–848. https://doi.org/10.1037/0033-2909.128.5.825

Vaitl, D. (1996). Interoception. *Biological Psychology, 42*(1–2), 1–27. https://doi.org/10.1016/0301-0511(95)05144-9

Vall, E., & Wade, T. D. (2015). Predictors of treatment outcome in individuals with eating disorders: A systematic review and meta-analysis. *International Journal of Eating Disorders, 48*(7), 946–971. https://doi.org/10.1002/eat.22411

van Dyck, Z., Ortmann, J., Lutz, A. P. C., Rose, G., & Vögele, C. (2017). Development and validation of a multidimensional instrument to assess eating disorder-specific interoceptive processes. In A. Schorr (Ed.), *13. Kongress der Fachgruppe Gesundheitspsychologie der DGPs* (pp. 45–47).

van Dyck, Z., Schulz, A., Blechert, J., Herbert, B. M., Lutz, A. P. C., & Vögele, C. (2020). Gastric interoception and gastric myoelectrical activity in bulimia nervosa and binge-eating disorder. *International Journal of Eating Disorders, 18*(S), eat.23291. https://doi.org/10.1002/eat.23291

van Dyck, Z., Vögele, C., Blechert, J., Lutz, A. P. C., Schulz, A., & Herbert, B. M. (2016). The Water Load Test As a Measure of Gastric Interoception: Development of a Two-Stage Protocol and Application to a Healthy Female Population. *PLOS ONE, 11*(9), e0163574. https://doi.org/10.1371/journal.pone.0163574

Van Malderen, E., Goossens, L., Verbeken, S., Boelens, E., & Kemps, E. (2019). The interplay between self-regulation and affectivity in binge eating among adolescents. *European Child and Adolescent Psychiatry, 28*(11), 1447–1460. https://doi.org/10.1007/s00787-019-01306-8

Vocks, S., Legenbauer, T., Troje, N., & Schulte, D. (2006). Körperbildtherapie bei Essstörungen. *Zeitschrift Für Klinische Psychologie Und Psychotherapie, 35*(4), 286–295. https://doi.org/10.1026/1616-3443.35.4.286

Walsh, B. T., Zimmerli, E., Devlin, M. J., Guss, J., & Kissileff, H. R. (2003). A disturbance of gastric function in bulimia nervosa. *Biological Psychiatry, 54*(9), 929–933. https://doi.org/10.1016/S0006-3223(03)00176-8

Wang, G. J., Tomasi, D., Backus, W., Wang, R., Telang, F., Geliebter, A., Korner, J., Bauman, A., Fowler, J. S., Thanos, P. K., & Volkow, N. D. (2008). Gastric distention activates satiety circuitry in the human brain. *NeuroImage, 39*(4), 1824–1831. https://doi.org/10.1016/j.neuroimage.2007.11.008

Whitehead, W. E., Drescher, V. M., Heiman, P., & Blackwell, B. (1977). Relation of heart rate control to heartbeat perception. *Biofeedback and Self-Regulation, 2*(4), 371–392. https://doi.org/10.1007/BF00998623

World Health Organization. (2016). *Growing up unequal: gender and socioeconomic differences in young people's health and well-being* (J. C. Inchley, D. B. Currie, T. Young, O. Samdal, T. Torsheim, L. Augustson, F. Mathison, A. Y. Aleman-Diaz, M. Molcho, M. Weber, & V. Barnekow (Eds.); Issue 7).

World Health Organization. (2018). *Fact sheet on obesity and overweight*. https://www. who.int/en/news-room/fact-sheets/detail/obesity-and-overweight

Yanovski, S. Z. (2002). Binge eating in obese persons. In *Eating disorders and obesity: A comprehensive handbook* (2nd ed., pp. 403–407). Guilford Press.

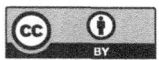

Controlled Drugs, Use, Abuse and Youth: A Meaningful, Yet Evolving Relationship

Alain Origer

1 Drug Use Prevalence in the General and Target Populations

Various indicators allow assessing drug use and its correlates in youngsters, such as the prevalence of lifetime or recent use of different substances in the general population, regular, problem drug use, high-risk drug use, frequency of use, age of substances' use initiation as well as the perception of potential risks and benefits of drugs by young people. However, these indicators merely provide a fragmented picture of the complex and changing bond between psychoactive substances and their users or potential users in a given era and socio-cultural environment. Moreover, national data might not be available, not representative or not comparable to previous data or to data from other countries, due for instance to divergent methodologies or data formatting.

This said, data from representative general population surveys provide a sound framework to discuss patterns of drug use in the general population. Although national data from a series of selective surveys on various target groups at regional or national levels are available, the latter are either outdated or too specific to provide meaningful input to the present analysis.

To date, the sole representative national data on drug use in the general population of Luxembourg stems from the 2014 wave of the *European Health Interview Survey* (EHIS). Prevalence rates of substance use in age group 15–34 years are presented in Fig. 1. Cocaine and ecstasy-type substances appear to be the most used controlled substances (cannabis excluded) in residents aged

A. Origer (✉)
Ministère de la Santé, Direction de la santé, Luxembourg, Luxembourg
E-Mail: alain.origer@ms.etat.lu

© Der/die Autor(en) 2022
A. Heinen et al. (Hrsg.), *Wohlbefinden und Gesundheit im Jugendalter*,
https://doi.org/10.1007/978-3-658-35744-3_16

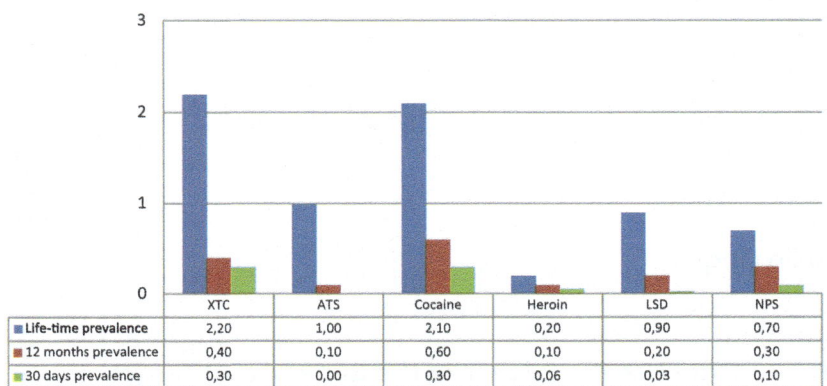

Fig. 1 Life-time, last 12 months and last 30 days prevalence of various psychoactive substances' use (cannabis excluded) according to age 15–34 years (2014) (valid %). *Source* EHIS (2014)—Origer (2018)

15–34 years. Drug prevalence rates applied to age group 15–18 years are not included in Fig. 1 as the latter equal to 0.0% for retained substances (except for LSD: 0.6%).

Cannabis is the most used controlled psychoactive substance at the national level, and thus deserves special attention, notably because of its use prevalence in youngsters. Figure 2 provides an overall picture of national cannabis use prevalence in the general population according to age groups 15–18 years and 15–34 years, based on EHIS data.

To put these results in a European perspective, a comparison with comparable prevalence data from other EU member states has been performed. According to available 2014/2015 data (EMCDDA 2015), national last 12 months prevalence and last 30 days prevalence of cannabis use situate below the EU average and below respective rates in border countries of Luxembourg.

Table 1 shows that first substance use most frequently occurs in age group 15–19 years, with the exceptions of heroin and cocaine, for which first use typically occurs between 20 and 24 years. Virtually, half of youngsters use cannabis for the first time while being still minor of age.

A longitudinal analysis of prevalence trends in the general population cannot be performed since serial data on drug use at the national level are unavailable to date. In contrast, data from school survey allow, to a certain extent, a more in-depth analysis of the evolution of drug use in youngsters over the last decades.

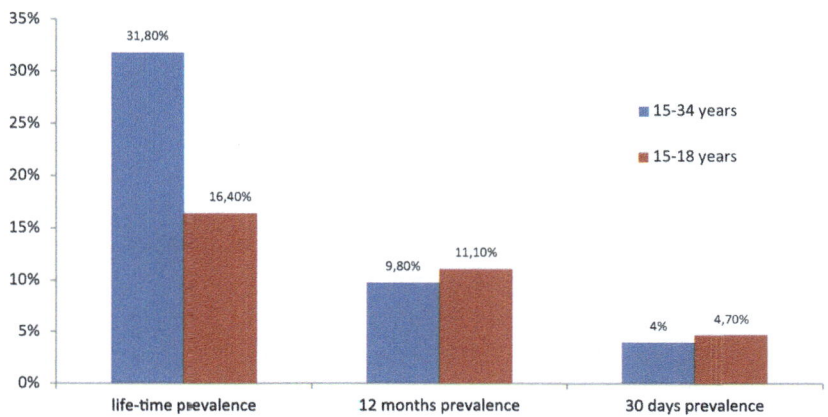

Fig. 2 National life-time (LTF), last 12 months (LYP) and last 30 days (LMP) prevalence of cannabis use according to different age groups (valid %). *Source* EHIS (2014)—Origer (2018)

Table 1 Age distribution of first substance use. *Source* EHIS (2014)—Origer (2018)

	Cannabis	XTC	ATS	Cocaine	Heroin	LSD	NPS
Mean age at first use	18.89 y	21.13 y	20.83 y	24.55 y	22.89 y	18.69 y	22.45 y
Median age at first use	18 y	20 y	20y	22 y	21 y	18 y	19 y
Age<18	47.40%	23.30%	19.20%	7.70%	5.30%	31.10%	18.20%
Min. age	12 y	12 y	13 y	13 y	13 y	10 y	11 y
Max. age	55 y	42 y	45 y	45 y	48 y	27 y	40 y
12–14	6.10%	5.00%	3.80%	1.30%	5.30%	4.40%	9.10%
15–19	**62.40%**	**38.30%**	**42.40%**	25.60%	31.50%	**64.50%**	**45.40%**
20–24	22.30%	**38.40%**	34.60%	**35.90%**	**36.90%**	24.40%	9.10%

First representative school surveys including national data on drug use have been conducted as early as 1992 (Matheis et al. 1995). However, only the first national wave of the *Health Behavior in School Children* (HBSC) survey in 1999

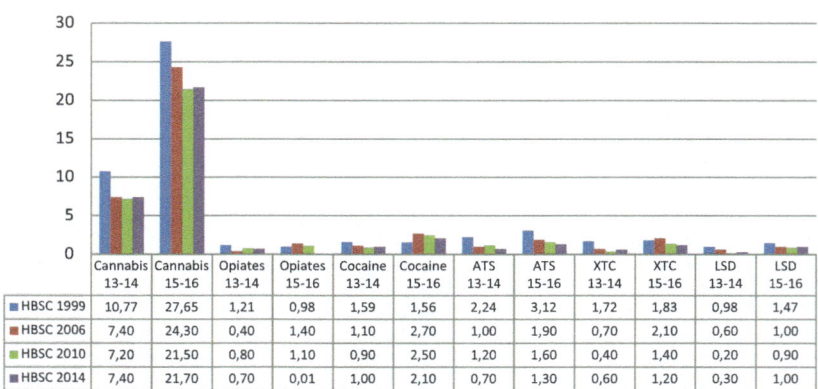

Fig. 3 Life-time prevalence of psychoactive substances' use according to age groups 13–14 years and 15–16 years (1999–2014) (valid %). *Source* HBSC 1999–2014, Université du Luxembourg, Ministère de l'Education Nationale, de l'Enfance et de la Jeunesse, Ministère de la Santé (2002, 2018)

and subsequent serial surveys allowed to validly compare national prevalence data in a longitudinal perspective.

When looking specifically into younger age groups, data from the HBSC study suggest that, among 15–16 years-old, lifetime consumption of illicit drugs has been generally decreasing since 1999, with the notable exception of cocaine use (Fig. 3). As to the age group 13–14 years, similar trends can be observed with the exceptions of cocaine, showing a decreasing use prevalence, and cannabis use, which has been remarkably stable between 2006 and 2014, following a marked decrease compared to 1999 data.

Between 1999 and 2006, last 12 months consumption of cannabis in 15 and 16 years old schoolchildren has been decreasing. Moreover, last 12 months cannabis use prevalence shows a discontinuous decrease for 15 years old and a fair stability for 16 years old between 2006 and 2014 (Fig. 4). As for other controlled substances, cocaine use has been showing a slight increase and ATS and LSD use have been witnessing a decrease in both 15 and 16 old students between 1999 and 2010. No serial last 12 months prevalence data for substances other than cannabis are available for 2014.

Figure 5 shows trends in lifetime, last 12 months and last 30 days prevalence of cannabis use in students aged 13 to 18 years between 2006 and 2014.

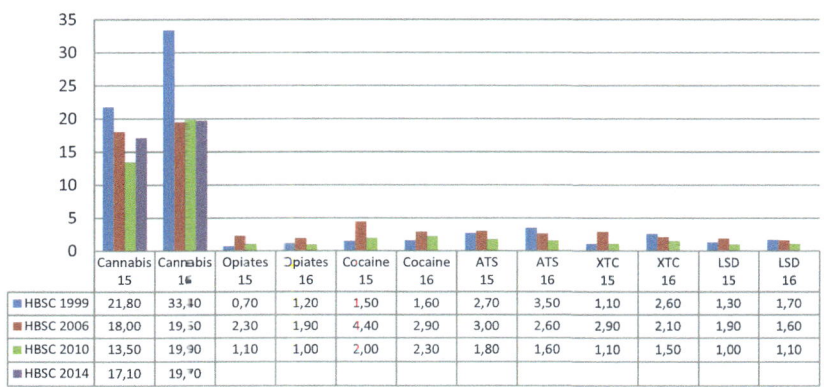

	Cannabis 15	Cannabis 16	Opiates 15	Opiates 16	Cocaine 15	Cocaine 16	ATS 15	ATS 16	XTC 15	XTC 16	LSD 15	LSD 16
■ HBSC 1999	21,80	33,40	0,70	1,20	1,50	1,60	2,70	3,50	1,10	2,60	1,30	1,70
■ HBSC 2006	18,00	19,50	2,30	1,90	4,40	2,90	3,00	2,60	2,90	2,10	1,90	1,60
■ HBSC 2010	13,50	19,90	1,10	1,00	2,00	2,30	1,80	1,60	1,10	1,50	1,00	1,10
■ HBSC 2014	17,10	19,70										

Fig. 4 Last 12 months prevalence of psychoactive substances' use according to age groups 15 years and 16 years (1999–2014) (valid %). *Source* HBSC 1999–2014, Université du Luxembourg, Ministère de l'Education Nationale, de l'Enfance et de la Jeunesse, Ministère de la Santé (2002, 2018)

Last 30 days cannabis use prevalence rates in schoolchildren aged 15 to 18 years, provided by serial HBSC data, have been witnessing an overall increase between 2006 and 2018 (see Fig. 6). A more in-depth analysis has revealed that the increase is statistically significant overall and for girls and that according to specific age groups, cannabis use appears to have been decreasing in younger adolescents (i.e. 15 years) whereas increasing in higher age groups (i.e. 16/17/18 years) since 2006.

In summary, data from general population and school surveys suggest that national drug use prevalence in younger residents (i.e 15–34) situates below the EU average and that drug use in youngsters aged between 13 and 16 years has been generally decreasing since the beginning of the 21st century, except for cocaine in the age group 15–16 years. More detailed national data are available for cannabis use in youngsters between 2006 and 2018. Whereas lifetime and last 12 months use of cannabis in students aged 13–18 years have been stable as a whole during the referred period, recent cannabis use (last 30 days) has been witnessing an overall increase between 2006 and 2018. In terms of international comparison, HBSC data (Inchley et al. 2016) have shown that 15 years old girls and boys in Luxembourg report both a lifetime prevalence of cannabis use of 18%, which appears to be higher than the HBSC average of 13% for girls and 17% for boys.

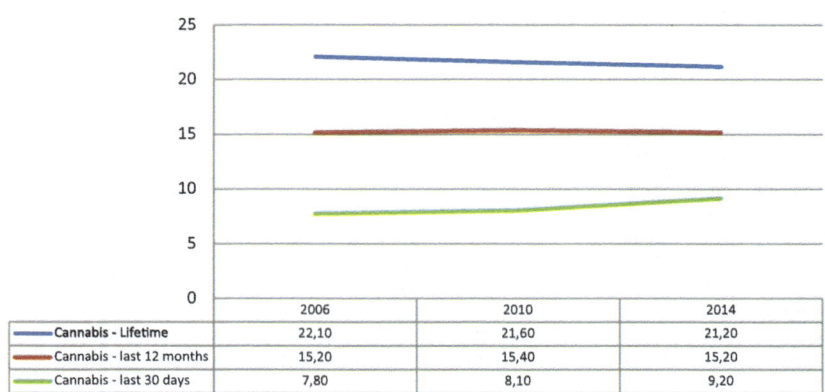

Fig. 5 Lifetime, last 12 months and last 30 days prevalence of cannabis use according to age group 13–18 years (2006–2014) (valid %). *Source* HBSC 1999–2014, Université du Luxembourg, Ministère de l'Education Nationale, de l'Enfance et de la Jeunesse, Ministère de la Santé (2002, 2018)

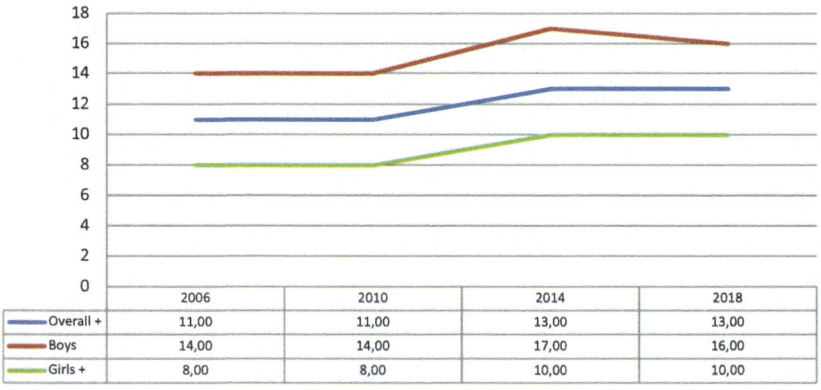

Fig. 6 Last 30 days prevalence of cannabis use according to age group 15–18 years (2006–2018) (valid %). *Source* HBSC 2018, Heinz et al. (2019)

2   High-risk Drug Use

Problem drug use (PDU) or high-risk drug use (HRDU)[1] are further indicators to measure drug use prevalence and drug use patterns in a given population or target group. The number of high-risk drug users has been estimated at 2250 persons based on 2015 national data (Origer et al. 2018) at the national level, which equals to a national prevalence rate of 5.79 high risk drug users in 1000 inhabitants aged 15–64 years. A more recent study on 2018 data, (Berndt et al. 2021) tends to confirm the general downward trend of national HRDU prevalence observed since 2003 (2018: 5.02 HRD users in 1000 inhabitants aged 15-64 years).

According to national drug monitoring data (RELIS), the average age of HRDU has been increasing from 28 years and 4 months in 1995 to 38 years and 6 months in 2017. After a closer look at age distributions over time, it appears that the obvious aging of the national HRDU population is primarily due to a marked increase in the proportion of users aged 40 years and more and to a decreasing proportion of users aged 20 to 29 years and not to any genuine trend in younger users aged 15–19 years. Moreover, the average age of first illicit drugs' use by current HRD users has been increasing from 15 years in 2008 to 16 years in 2017. This observation contrasts with markedly higher average ages of first dug use in the general population (see Table 1).

3   Drug Supply, Quality and Price

On the supply side, special attention is due to cannabis when it comes to drug use in youngsters. Average Δ^9-tetrahydrocannabinol (THC) concentration in cannabis products available on the national illicit market has been increasing over the last decade and is continuing to do so. Maximum concentrations of THC in national samples of cannabis show the same trend as can be seen in Fig. 7, knowing, however, that these very high concentrations are currently exceptional and mostly related to specific extraction methods (e.g. butane hash oil, dab,

---

[1] 'Problem drug use' (PDU) is defined by the EMCDDA as *'injecting drug use or long duration/regular use of opioids, cocaine and/or amphetamines*'. The indicator is currently referred to as '*High risk drug use*' due to the changing drug situation, and focuses on '*recurrent drug use that is causing actual harms (negative consequences) to the person (including dependence, but also other health, psychological or social problems), or is placing the person at a high probability/risk of suffering such harms*'.

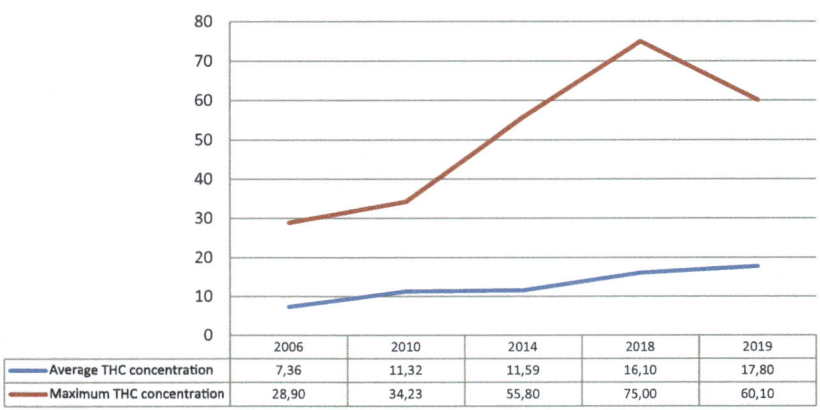

Fig. 7 Average and maximum THC concentrations in cannabis (resin and herbal) in Luxembourg from 2006–2019 (%). *Source* LNS (2020)

shatter). Similar evolutions have been observed in the EU, where cannabis resin and herb potencies have been increasing by 122% and 82% respectively between 2008 and 2020, whereas prices of cannabis resin and herb at retail level have known an increase of 12% over the same period (EMCDDA 2018, 2020). In other words, cannabis users tend to getting more THC for less money over recent years (Fig. 8).

Moreover, new varieties of cannabis have been appearing on the illicit market with high levels of THC and low levels of cannabidiol (CBD[2]). Knowing that emerging evidence suggest that CBD may have the capacity to reduce the psycho-active potential of THC (Wall 2019), these newer varieties are more '*potent*' than varieties with similar THC levels but higher CBD concentrations. These emerging cannabis products as well as the average increase of THC concentrations in cannabis not only bear greater risks in terms of immediate psychological and behavioral effects but also in terms of cerebral maturation and the development of cognitive functions such as working memory, decision-making, impulsivity control, motivation and of mental health in general, according to the frequency of use.

---

[2] CBD is a non-intoxicating cannabinoid found in cannabis.

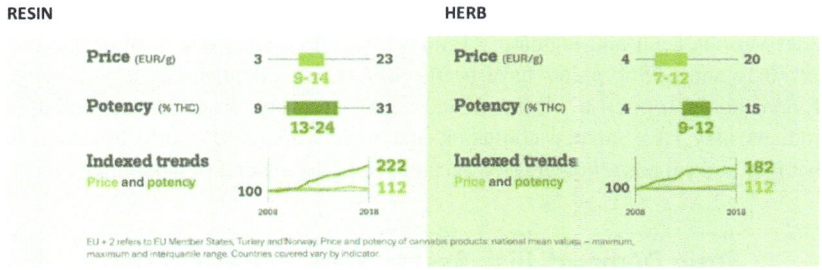

Fig. 8 Cannabis price and potency in Europe 2008–2018. *Source* EMCDDA (2020)

Purity is one aspect of quality; impurity is another one. Drugs sold on the illicit market are knowingly of diverse and changing quality. They may contain cutting agents[3] and other adulterants (Solomini et al. 2017). As far as cannabis is concerned, a considerable variety of impurities has been found in samples worldwide over recent years, including sand, soil, shoe wax, hairspray, henna, glass beads, lead, talcum, etc. Moreover, street cannabis and its derivatives may be contaminated for instance with pesticides, heavy metals, bacteria, fungi and mycotoxins (Buchicchio et al. 2022). A more recent emerging trend that is bearing increased risks appears to be the adulteration of cannabis products with synthetic cannabinoid receptor agonists (Oomen et al. 2022).

As the very characteristics of cannabis and cannabis products have been changing markedly over recent years, the 'image' of cannabis has equally known substantial re-adjustments. Research on the nature and components of cannabis and its potential applications for health related matters, and the fact that an increasing number of countries or jurisdictions throughout the world have put or plan to put legislations in place allowing the use of cannabis and its derivatives for medical and non-medical purposes, supposedly had an impact on how people perceive cannabis and its potential risks and benefits.

Moreover, in recent years, new markets have been developing. One of these relates to cannabidiol (CBD) products, reaching from dried flowering tops of hemp containing less than 0.2% or 0.3% THC and CBD oils and extracts,

---

[3] Regarding impurities, the same applies to heroin and cocaine which according to latest national figures reach average purity levels of 12% and 48% respectively in 2017. (Origer et al. 2018) and 13.4% and 52.7% in 2018 (Berndt et al. 2019)

to infusions and cosmetics containing CBD. Although these products do fall under various legal and regulatory frameworks, the market has been developing nervously and selling points have been proliferating, commending a wide range of beneficial proprieties of hemp and CBD. Notably via CBD, hemp-based products may have created confusion and more importantly curiosity, interest, visibility and supposedly increased acceptance in the general population.

4   Drug Demand, Risk Assessment, Pattern of Use and Trends

This having been said, cannabis and related products sold on the illicit market bear increasing risks, while cannabis as such tends to be perceived as more beneficial, useful and potentially less harmful than half a century ago when cannabis was put in the very same and most restrictive schedules of relevant UN conventions as heroin or desormorphine for instance. These evolutions in somehow opposite directions need to be addressed also because of their likely impact on the perceptions, risk assessment, choices and behaviors of young people, users and potential users. As a matter of fact, the risk perception of cannabis use seems to have changed in EU youngsters aged 15 to 24 years between 2001 and 2014. In 2011, 67% of responding youngsters in a EURO-BAROMETER survey (European Commission 2014) considered regular cannabis use to bearing high risks while in 2014, this rate only reached 63%. The same downward trend has been observed regarding risk assessment of occasional use.

Knowing that numerous studies have found an inverse relationship between risk perception related to cannabis and the prevalence of its use (Bachman et al. 1998; Volkow et al. 2014; Compton et al. 2016; Lynskey and Hall 2016; Parker and Anthony 2018), it seems obvious that these factors and changes have to be addressed in sound prevention strategies, bearing in mind, however, that other factors such as changes in tobacco and cigarettes' use also interfere with cannabis use prevalence (Miech et al. 2017).

As addressed earlier, drug supply and accessibility are relevant factors in the analysis of drug use patterns. Nonetheless, they do evolve according to an equally dynamic demand for psychoactive substances in the course of time.

Why do people start (or do not start) using drugs and what kind of psychoactive substances do they use for which reasons in a given era, in a given environment, during a given time of their life? These questions should be asked when investigating the bond between individuals and psychoactive substances. There seems to be evidence that the decision to use drugs by youngsters tends to be based on a 'rational appraisal process', rather than a passive reaction to the context in which a substance is available' (Boys et al. 1999, 2001; Wibberley and Price 2000). Notwithstanding the potential impact of the interactions between individual genetics and life and social environments on human behaviour, one may categorise the motivation to use psychoactive substances overall in terms of pleasure, relief, and individual functions. (Allen 2003; Boys et al. 1997, 1999, 2001; Kreek et al. 2005; Parks and Kennedy 2004; Van der Poel et al. 2009).

Reasons to start using or to using psychoactive substances commonly cited in literature (Brunelle et al. 2003; McInstosh et al. 2005; Palmqvist et al. 2003; Titus et al. 2007) such as enjoyment, relaxation, curiosity and experimentation, rebellion, non-conformity, escape from reality, defense mechanisms, abuse and trauma, self-medication, boredom, solitude, grief, end of relationship, peer/social-pressure, emotional stress, professional burden, performance enhancing do all fit in one or more of these broad categories.

Moreover, as new drugs have been developed and already existing psycho-active substances have found their ways to recreational drug use over the last decades, their use has been going along with innovation in drug development and societal changes. Since 1971, the Substance Abuse and Mental Health Services Administration, an agency of the U.S. Department of Health and Human Services, coordinates the National Survey on Drug Use and Health (NSDUH), collecting data from a representative sample of U.S. households on their drinking, smoking, and illicit drug use habits. Data were analysed according to 10 different classes of substances throughout several generations of Americans: the Baby Boomers (1943–1962), Generation X (1963–1982), and Millennials (1983–2002). The data allowed to assess the prevalence of past months, past year and lifetime substances' use according to different age groups[4].

Detailed data analysis has been performed, but in the present context, the mere general conclusion of the surveys is at stake; namely: every generation has its trends in psychoactive substance use. Summarily, according to the authors of the analysis, alcohol is the most commonly used substance by all generations, although Baby Boomers show a higher prevalence and have started drinking earlier than other generations. Cannabis is the second most used substance in all generations, with the Baby Boomers, having lived through the 60s, once again showing highest prevalence rates. What characterises Baby Boomers most,

---

[4] https://drugabuse.com/featured/drug-and-alcohol-abuse-across-generations/, accessed 25/07/2020.

however, is their highest use of stimulants and sedatives, which might be linked to the fact that they have lived through a post-World War II period when amphetamines were frequently prescribed as a treatment for depression before they were eventually regulated more strictly due to their widespread abuse. Moreover, in the 60s, new barbiturates were frequently prescribed for insomnia and anxiety but these drugs were progressively replaced by a broader class of medications known as benzodiazepines.

Alcohol and cannabis use of Generation X is lower than the one of the Baby Boomers but higher than the prevalence in Millennials. This said, psychotropic medications (commonly prescribed in case of mental disorders) use is highest in Generation X. This use peaked around the age of 20 years, with about 10% of Generation Xers using these drugs.

After alcohol and cannabis use, Millennials, for their part, seem to be more attracted to painkillers than any previous generation. Their peak shows over 12% painkiller use in age categories 19–20, compared to fewer than eight percent of Baby Boomers and Generation Xers. In the 70s, the prescription of opioid painkillers expanded in the US and by 2013, more than 207 million prescriptions of these medications were registered, compared to 76 million in 1991.[5] Facing the growing problem of opioid painkiller addiction and the increase of accidental opioid overdose deaths between 1999 and 2010, the US government has been undertaking a series of measures to reduce opiate painkiller use and abuse as for instance abuse-deterrent formulation of these medications. This contributed to reduce supply at street level, increase their price and lead numerous users to heroin, a less expensive and more accessible alternative to opioid prescription drugs. (Slevin and Ashburn 2011). As it stands, this is another sound example of how regulations, pharmacological developments and economic aspects may affect drug supply and demand as well as drug use and abuse patterns.

Although these data should not be generalised and applied without restriction to other countries or populations as the survey exclusively includes US citizens, they clearly show differences between generations which were exposed to different social and political contexts and innovations in drug supply/accessibility and pharmacological developments over the past 70 years.

Anther relevant example of contemporary changes might be seen in the emergence of New Psychoactive Substances (NPS). In a commercial perspective,

---

[5] America's Addiction to Opioids: Heroin and Prescription Drug Abuse. (2014, May 14). https://archives.drugabuse.gov/testimonies/2014/americas-addiction-to-opioids-heroin-prescription-drug-abuse accessed 24/07/2020.

NPS are drugs, which were designed or recovered to replicate or mimic the effects of illegal substances while not being controlled by international drug conventions by the time of their appearance on the market. They may, however, pose a public health threat comparable to that posed by substances listed in these conventions[6].

Most of these substances have appeared in Europe in the 1990s and in the beginning of the 2000s. From 2004 onwards, synthetic cannabinoids became available on the market, followed by synthetic cathinones and others. (UNODC 2013).

Precursors and additives used in the manufacturing of NPS are often easily available because they serve other, commercial or industrial legitimate purposes and the production process generally requests reasonable means in terms of investments and knowhow. The prime 'advantages' of NPS compared to substances stemming from naturally grown plants are indeed multifold. Small and inconspicuous production units can be set up conveniently near consumer markets; short distances between producers and user markets, online selling with crypto currencies, small quantities but high potency of products jointly contribute to reducing 'commercial' risks and increasing potential benefits. These parameters together with low initial investments and modest running costs of production units are regrettably making NPS traffic an outstanding '*business model*'.

This to say that illicit drugs, their origin, their very characteristics, their price and purity and finally their targeted user groups are largely conditioned by benefits' optimization and market rules, difficult to influence in a preventive and harm reduction perspective.

In addition, the genuine, praised or supposed legality of these substances and the multitude of expected or hoped for effects make them remarkably attractive especially to young users who may consider that if a substance is not (or said to be not) illegal, it should not be that dangerous. Unfortunately, the contrary is mostly the case. Indeed, the legal status of NPS are often blurry and rapidly changing and many of these man-made substances are potentially more dangerous than plant based drugs or long known psychoactive substances; some of which have been used and studied for decades.

---

[6] For the purposes of this document, NPS are defined as "substances of abuse, either in a pure form or a preparation, that are not controlled by the 1961 Convention on Narcotic Drugs or the 1971 Convention on Psychotropic Substances, but which may pose a public health threat". In this context, the term 'new' does not necessarily refer to new inventions but to substances that have recently become available'. (UNODC 2013)

5   New Information and Communication Technologies and Access to Psychoactive Substances

Availability of and access to an increasing variety of psychoactive substances have become greater. Online selling sites offer a vast range of psychoactive products, providing home delivery and customer reviews, fora and quality ratings. A large variety of psychoactive substances are accessible on the street or online. Access to drugs has probably never been that easy for younger and older regular or first users. Notably NPS and cannabis are increasingly accessible to youngsters, while potentially more harmful on the one hand, whereas various factors, addressed previously, may contribute to lower their risk assessment, on the other hand.

6   Responses

It thus appears essential that information and prevention strategies take into account the dynamic nature of the relationship between drugs, demand and supply, markets and end users.

Drugs are only one of many temptations young people are exposed to. New information and communication technologies, smart communication devices, social media, gaming and online gaming[7], etc. represent as many options and choices to make by youngsters and the risks of excessive and dysfunctional use of the latter have become more and more apparent. Information and prevention strategies should consider these evolutions and constantly adapt to emerging facts and evidence; but ideally in a holistic perspective in which drug use is only one element among others to consider. Consume behavior and wellbeing in general are at stake here. Especially young people should be supported in acquiring overall life competences and resilience based on objective and sound information as well as on skill and capacity building, notably in terms of risk and benefits assessments allowing them to make informed and responsible individual choices, regardless of the object of desire or choice.

---

[7] In 2018 'Gaming disorder' was included in the 11th Revision of the International Classification of Diseases (ICD-11) as a pattern of gaming behavior ("digital-gaming" or "video-gaming") characterized by impaired control over gaming, increasing priority given to gaming over other activities to the extent that gaming takes precedence over other interests and daily activities, and continuation or escalation of gaming despite the occurrence of negative consequences.

7   Conclusions

Drugs and drug use patterns are of changing nature. There is thus no reason why responses to risks, damage and other problems related to drug use should be set in stone. The very nature of drugs are changing as are their access, their attractiveness and the perceptions of their benefits and harm potential. Numerous underlying factors such as market rules, technological innovations and societal changes are difficult to influence. Drug demand, and drug supply in the long term, may, however, be reduced if the underlying mechanisms are understood and duly taken into account.

Moreover, country specific parameters need to be addressed. Social and economic factors are potential determinants of drug use and misuse (Galea 2004; Patrick 2012). Evidence has emerged suggesting that drug abuse tends to be highest in wealthier nations (Degenhardt and Hall 2012). Knowing that Luxembourg ranks among the countries with the highest GDP per capita worldwide, these findings are of particular relevance in a national perspective. More research is needed in this regard, especially on the possible relationship between the power of purchase of youngsters, money at their disposal and drug use patterns and prevalence (Johnston et al. 1980, 1982, 1984, 1986, 2019; McCristal et al. 2007). One should also bear in mind that, more recently, the Covid-19 crises will show how drug use prevalence and patterns might have changed in youngsters also in the aftermath of a pandemic unprecedented for the current generation.

Young people start and continue to use drugs for different reasons and individual factors are clearly at stake as well when it comes to better understand why and how a behavior has become excessive and dysfunctional or addictive whether substance use is involved or any other behaviors with addictive potential. It is essential to closely monitor market evolutions in drugs' supply as well as emerging drug use patterns and addictive behavior in general and to promote early intervention measures especially in young generations in order to timely adapt prevention and response strategies.

Additionally, although sound and objective information is needed, the means and channels by which to reach youngsters, to trigger their curiosity and to maintain their attention are equally important and require a great deal of insight in and understanding of youth culture, values, and communication forms. Combining these transient knowledge and skills in the interaction and communication with young people may be a valuable means to impact beneficially on their perceptions and reflections on their way to self-determination and informed decision making in a world of increasing possibilities, temptations, incertainty and challenges.

References

Allen, D. (2003). Treating the cause not the problem: Vulnerable young people and substance misuse. *Journal of Substance Use*, 8, 47–54.

Bachman, J.G., Johnson, L.D., & O'Malley, P.M. (1998). Explaining recent increases in students' marijuana use: impacts of perceived risks and disapproval, 1976 through 1996. *American journal of public health*. 88(6):887–892.

Berndt, N., Seixas, R., & Origer, A. (2019). National Drug Report 2019. National EMCDDA Focal point. Luxembourg.

Berndt, N., Seixas, R., & Origer, A. (2021). National Drug Report 2020. National EMCDDA Focal point. Luxembourg.

Boys, A., Lenton, S., & Norcross, K. (1997). Polydrug use at raves by a Western Australian sample. *Drug and Alcohol Review*, 16, 227–234.

Boys, A., Marsden, J., Fountain, J., Griffiths, P., Stillwell, G., & Strang, J. (1999). What influences young people's use of drugs? A qualitative study of decision-making. *Drugs: Education, Prevention and Policy*, 6, 373–389.

Boys, A., Marsden, J., & Strang, J. (2001). Understanding reasons for drug use amongst young people: A functional perspective. *Health Education Research*, 16(4), 457–469.

Brunelle, N., Brochu, S., & Cousineau, M. -M. (2003). Points de vue d'adolescents quant aux liens entre leur usage de drogues et leur délinquance. *L'intervenant, revue sur l'alcoolisme et la toxicomanie*, 19(3). (pp. 19–22).

Buchicchio, L., Asselborn, L., Schneider, S., et al. (2022). Investigation of aflatoxin and ochratoxin A contamination of seized cannabis and cannabis resin samples. *Mycotoxin Research, 38,* 71–78. doi: https://doi.org/10.1007/s12550-022-00449-z

Compton, W.M., Han, B., Jones, C.M., Blanco, C., & Hughes, A. (2016).Marijuana use and use disorders in adults in the USA, 2002–14: analysis of annual cross-sectional surveys. *Lancet Psychiatry*. 3(10):954–964. doi: https://doi.org/10.1016/S2215-0366(16)30208-5.

Degenhardt, L., & Hall, W. (2012). Extent of illicit drug use and dependence, and their contribution to the global burden of disease. *Lancet*, 379, 55–70. doi:https://doi.org/10.1016/S0140-6736(11)61138-0.

European Monitoring Centre for Drugs and Drug Addiction. (2018) http://www.emcdda.europa.eu/data/stats2018/ppp_fr. Accessed 25/09/2019.

European Monitoring Centre for Drugs and Drug Addiction. (2019), European Drug Report 2019: Trends and Developments, Publications Office of the European Union, Luxembourg.

European Monitoring Centre for Drugs and Drug Addiction. (2020), European Drug Report 2020: Trends and Developments, Publications Office of the European Union, Luxembourg.

European Commission. 2014. Young people and drugs. Flash Eurobarometer 401. Brussels: Directorate-General Communication – European Commission. https://ec.europa.eu/commfrontoffice/publicopinion/index.cfm/Survey/getSurveyDetail/instruments/FLASH/surveyKy/2029. Accessed 23/09/2019.

Galea, S., Nandi, A., & Vlahov, D. (2004) The Social Epidemiology of Substance Use. *Epidemiologic Reviews*, Volume 26, Issue 1, July 2004, Pages 36–52, https://doi.org/10.1093/epirev/mxh007

Heinz, A., van Duin, C., Kern, MR., Catunda, C., & Willems, H. (2019). Trends from 2006–2018 in Health Behaviour, Health Outcomes and Social Context of Adolescents in Luxembourg. University of Luxembourg. Esch-sur-Alzette.

Inchley, J. et al. (2016). Growing up unequal: gender and socioeconomic differences in young people's health and well-being. Health behaviour in School-aged Children (HBSC) study: International report from 2013/2014 survey. Health policy for Children and Adolescents, N°7. Copenhagen, Denmark: WHO Regional Office for Europe.

Johnston, L.D., Bachmann, J.G., & O'Mally, P.M. (1980, 1982, 1984, 1986): Monitoring the Future: Questionnaire Responses from the Nation's High School Seniors. Volumes for Odd-numbered years 1976 to 1986. Ann Arbor, Michigan.

Johnston, L. D., Miech, R. A., O'Malley, P. M., Bachman, J. G., Schulenberg, J. E., & Patrick, M. E. (2019). Monitoring the Future national survey results on drug use, 1975–2018: Overview, key findings on adolescent drug use. Ann Arbor: Institute for Social Research, The University of Michigan.

Kreek et al. (2005). Influences on impulsivity, risk taking, stress responsivity and vulnerability to drug abuse and addiction. Nat. Neurosci., 8(11). Pp. 1450–1457.

Lynskey, M., & Hall, W. (2016). Cannabis use and cannabis use disorders. Lancet Psychiatry. 3(10):911–912. doi: https://doi.org/10.1016/S2215-0366(16)30270-X.

Matheis,J., Prussen, P.,& Reuter, P. (1995). Schüler und Drogen: Eine repräsentative Untersuchung bei Schülern der 5. Klasse des allgemeinen und technischen Sekundarunterrichts in Luxemburg. Ausmaße, Zusammenhänge, Vergleiche, Präventionsmaßnahmen, Fentage:IEES.

McCrystal, P., Percy, A., & Higgins, K.(2007).The Cost of Drug Use in Adolescence: Young People, Money and Substance Abuse. Drugs: Education, Prevention & Policy, v14 n1 pp19–28.

McInstosh, J., MacDonald, F., & Mckeganey, N. (2005). Pre-teenage children's experiences of drug use. Journal of Drug Policy, 16(1), 37–45.

Miech, R., Johnston, L., & O'Malley, P. M. (2017). Prevalence and Attitudes Regarding Marijuana Use Among Adolescents Over the Past Decade. Pediatrics, 140(6), e20170982. doi:https://doi.org/10.1542/peds.2017-0982.

Ministère de la Santé (2002), Das Wohlbefinden der Jugend – HBSC Studie, Direction de la Santé, Luxembourg.

Oomen, P.E., Schori, D., Tögel-Lins, K., Acreman, D., Chenorhokian, S., Luf, A., Karden. A., Paulos, C., Fornero, E., Gerace. E., Koning, RPJ., Galindo, L., Smit-Rigter, L.A., Measham, F., Ventura, M. (2022). Cannabis adulterated with the synthetic cannabinoid receptor agonist MDMB-4en-PINACA and the role of European drug checking services. International Journal of Drug Policy, 100, 103493. doi: 10.1016/j.drugpo.2021.103493. Epub 2021 Oct 20. PMID: 34687992.

Origer, A. et al. (2018). National Drug Report 2018. National EMCDDA Focal point. Luxembourg.

Palmqvist, R. K., Martikainen, L. K., & VonWright, M. R. (2003). Reasons given for adolescentsfor alcohol and narcotics use, 1984–1999. Journal of Youth and Adolescence, 32(3), 195–203.

Parker, M.A., & Anthony, J.C. (2018). Population-level predictions from cannabis risk perceptions to active cannabis use prevalence in the United States, 1991–2014. Addictive behaviors. 82:101–104. doi: https://doi.org/10.1016/j.addbeh.2018.02.030.

Parks, K. A., & Kennedy, C. L. (2004). Club drugs: reasons for and consequences of use. Journal of Psychoactive Drugs, 36(3), 295–302.

Patrick, M. E., Wightman, P., Schoeni, R. F., & Schulenberg, J. E. (2012). Socioeconomic status and substance use among young adults: a comparison across constructs and drugs. Journal of studies on alcohol and drugs, 73(5), 772–782. doi:https://doi.org/10.15288/jsad.2012.73.772

Slevin, K.A. & Ashburn, M.A., 2011. Primary care physician opinion survey on FDA opioid risk evaluation and mitigation strategies. Journal of opioid management, 7(2), 109–115.

Solimini, R., Rotolo M.C., Pellegrini, M., Minutillo, A., Pacifici, R., Busardo, F.P., Zaami, S. (2017). Adulteration practices of psychoactive illicit drugs: An updated Review. Current Pharmaceutical Biotechnology, 18(7), 524–530. doi: 10.2174/1389201018666170710184531. PMID: 28699480

Titus, J. C., Godley, S. H., & White, M. K. (2007). A post-treatment examination of adolescents' reasons for starting, quitting, and continuing the use of drugs and alcohol. Journal of Child & Adolescent Substance Abuse, 16(2), 31–34.

United Nations Office on Drugs and Crime. (2013), 'The challenge of new psychoactive substances', Vienna: United nations Publications.

Université du Luxembourg, Ministère de l'Education National, de l'Enfance et de la Jeunesse & Ministère de la Santé. (2018). Health Behaviour in School-aged Children – Luxembourg – enquête 2006. Luxembourg, Esch-sur-Alzette: HBSC Data Archive Luxembourg.

Université du Luxembourg, Ministère de l'Education National, de l'Enfance et de la Jeunesse & Ministère de la Santé. (2018). Health Behaviour in School-aged Children – Luxembourg – enquête 2010. Luxembourg, Esch-sur-Alzette: HBSC Data Archive Luxembourg.

Université du Luxembourg, Ministère de l'Education National, de l'Enfance et de la Jeunesse & Ministère de la Santé. (2018). Health Behaviour in School-aged Children – Luxembourg – enquête 2014. Luxembourg, Esch-sur-Alzette: HBSC Data Archive Luxembourg.

Van der Poel, A., Rodenburg, G., Dijkstra, M., Stoele, M., & Mheen, D. (2009). Trends, motivations and settings of recreational cocaine use by adolescents and young adults in the Netherlands. International Journal of Drug Policy, 20, 143–151.

Volkow, N. D., Baler, R. D., Compton, W. M., & Weiss, S. R. (2014). Adverse health effects of marijuana use. The New England journal of medicine, 370(23), 2219–2227. doi:https://doi.org/10.1056/NEJMra1402309

Wall, M.B. et al. (2019). Dissociable effects of cannabis with and without cannabidiol on the human brain's resting-state functional connectivity. Journal of Psychopharmacology. 2019 Jul;33(7):822–830. doi: https://doi.org/10.1177/0269881119841568.

Wibberley, C., & Price, J. (2000). Young People's Drug Use: Facts and Feelings – Implications for the Normalization Debate. Drugs: Education, Prevention and Policy, 7 (2), 147–162.

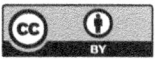

The Evolving Landscape of Sports Betting: A Risk for Young People?

Damien Brevers, Claus Vögele und Joël Billieux

Which Team Will Win The Game? What Will Be The Winning Margin? Which Player Will Score?
While sport fans might differ in their confidence with which they respond to such questions, they will certainly have an answer. Sport events are numerous, easily accessible, and associated with a large number of betting options. Despite being banned for minors, this sort of gambling activity is extensively advertised on television and on social media platforms. Accordingly, there is a legitimate concern on whether this increasing popularization and immediate availability of sport betting has the potential to harm children and adolescents. Assuming that the current landscape of sport betting constitutes an emerging public health issue, the present chapter provides a comprehensive synthesis of the available evidence and to describe the potential impact and consequences of sports betting in young people.

C. Vögele
Department of Behavioural and Cognitive Sciences, University of Luxembourg, Esch-sur-Alzette, Luxembourg
E-Mail: Claus.voegele@uni.lu

D. Brevers (✉)
Psychological Sciences Research Institute, UCLouvain, Louvain-la-Neuve, Belgium
E-Mail: damien.brevers@uclouvain.be

J. Billieux
Institute of Psychology, University of Lausanne, Lausanne, Switzerland
E-Mail: Joel.Billieux@unil.ch

© Der/die Autor(en) 2022
A. Heinen et al. (Hrsg.), *Wohlbefinden und Gesundheit im Jugendalter,*
https://doi.org/10.1007/978-3-658-35744-3_17

363

1   Gambling-related Harm in Young People

Sports betting has become increasingly prevalent among young people, as evidenced by recent cross-sectional studies. For instance, in a recent study undertaken in a convenience sample of 735 young adults (aged 18-25) in Spain (recruited in person at various university faculties and vocational training centres in Madrid, $n = 603$; or through online surveys on social network sites, $n = 132$), 43% (comprising 80% of men) reported to have bet on a sports event at least once (Labrador and Vallejo-Achón 2019). This study also showed that most bets were made online, target football (soccer), and constitute obvious outcomes (e.g., betting on the winning team). With regard to underage youth (< 18-year-old), in a study involving a convenience sample of 1330 male Croatian high-school students, the majority of boys acknowledged to have been involved in sports betting, even though they do not have the legal age to gamble (Ricijas et al. 2011, 2016). Of particular concern is that 24% of male high-school students had already developed severe psychosocial consequences related to gambling (Ricijas et al. 2016). These patterns occurred particularly in sports betting, video lottery terminals, and virtual betting (Ricijas et al. 2016).

An increase in gambling-related harm has also been described for adolescents (see also **BOX 1** for a brief account of hazardous gambling practices in adolescents). For instance, a survey of 12- to 15-year adolescents in Finland (a convenience sample of 988 first-year junior high-school students) found that 3% had a probable gambling disorder and a further 4.9% can be considered at-risk gamblers (Castrén et al. 2015). Hazardous gambling involvement of adolescents has also been found in Australia (Miller 2017; Purdie et al. 2011), Canada (Elton-Marshall et al. 2016), Croatia (Ricijas et al. 2011, 2016), New Zeeland (Volberg et al. 2010), Sweden (Fröberg et al. 2015), the United Kingdom (Gambling Commission UK 2016, 2017), and the United States (Marchica et al. 2017).

With regard to sports betting, recent research has shown that patterns of live betting are very common in young, male, single, educated, full-time employed workers or students (Hing et al. 2016; see also Russel et al. 2018, 2019), with a shorter experience of sports betting (Hing et al. 2018a, b). Other studies have shown that problematic sports bettors are predominantly male adolescents and young adults (Hing et al. 2017a; Humphreys and Pérez 2012; Russel et al. 2018; Wood and Williams 2009).

Importantly, the increase in online sports betting behaviors has also been shown in recent population-based sampling reports. For instance, in France, sports betting represents the type of gambling that has expanded the most in

2019, with 11% of the French population reporting to have bet on sports (three times more than in 2014; Costes et al. 2020). This reports also shows that sports betting is the second most popular type of gambling (second only to playing the lottery), with a 2.8 increase of betting stakes in five years (4.6 increase for online sports betting, which represent 56% of sports betting stakes; Costes et al. 2020). Sports betting is also linked to the type of gambling that is the most regularly played (26.9% of weekly sports bettors; 37.1% of weekly sports bettors for horses racing bets; 26.9% for other types of sports; Costes et al. 2020). Moreover, and in line with the above-mentioned convenience sample studies, Costes and colleagues (2020) observed that sports bettors are most commonly men (89.7%), of a young age 72.2% < 35 years), with a high level of education, and with higher incomes than the other types of gamblers. Critically, among the different types of gambling, sports betting is the most strongly associated with gambling-related issues (3 times more moderate problem gamblers, and 6 six times more high problem gamblers than lottery players), with a quarter of the individuals developing Gambling Disorder being specifically involved in sports betting (Costes et al. 2020).

Another key point is that amongst young people, the loss of control over gambling and related adverse outcomes can occur rapidly, in just a few months (Spritzer et al. 2011; see also *BOX 1*). Specifically, adolescent gambling has been related to poor school performance, isolation, depression, disrupted relationship with family and friends, deleterious financial loss, and problematic substance use (Derevensky 2007, 2012; Miller 2017). Individuals who reported having gambled before the age of fifteen are also at higher risk to experience substance abuse, psychological disorders, and suicidal ideation, compared to late-onset gamblers (Burge et al. 2004, 2006; Hare 2009). Nevertheless, these results are based on cross-sectional studies, which impedes any conclusions about causality. Moreover, longitudinal studies have shown that young people's gambling behavior fluctuates over time and may not necessary lead to continued (problem) gambling in adulthood (Delfabbro et al. 2009, 2014; Edgerton et al. 2015).

Overall, current findings from the literature suggest that, among sports bettors, young male adults are at increased risk for developing gambling problems. Nevertheless, additional research is needed to distinguish temporary maladaptive gambling habits in young adulthood from those that could lead to functionally impairing gambling patterns.

BOX 1. Why Adolescents are More at Risk of Developing Problematic Gambling Habits?

Adolescence represents a distinct developmental period in terms of experimentation and engagement in risky behaviors (e.g., Derevensky 2012). At the neural level, an immature prefrontal cortex is generally considered as the neurobiological correlate of poor decision making and risky behaviors in teenagers (e.g., Casey and Jones 2010).

The prefrontal cortex is one of the last regions of the brain to reach maturation (Arain et al. 2013). This region acquires information from all of the senses and orchestrates thoughts and actions to achieve specific goals (Arain et al. 2013). The prefrontal cortex is thus a key region for cognitive analysis, abstract thought, and the moderation of correct behavior in social situations (e.g., Goldstein and Volkow 2002). Accordingly, adolescents cannot fully access executive and inhibitory control functions due to the immaturity of the prefrontal cortex (Arain et al. 2013).

These processes are not detrimental *per se*, and may also promote a learning drive for optimal adaptation to adult roles (Chambers and Potenza 2003). Nevertheless, this dynamic may also confer an increased vulnerability to addictive behaviors, such as problem gambling. Gambling can be viewed as involving repeated participation in ritualized "impulsive" decision-making, featuring instant monetary rewards (Burge et al. 2004).

Adolescence is a developmental period associated with increased responsibility, autonomy and freedom, thereby facilitating the involvement in problematic and risky activities (e.g., substance use, drinking and driving, unprotected sexual behavior and gambling). All these behaviors represent primary markers for risk taking, and in certain cases are viewed as a *rite of passage* (e.g., MacDonald 1987).

2   Convergence Between Sport, Gaming, and Gambling

Does playing online games influence and shape young people's attitudes and engagement toward (sports) gambling? This question is currently examined by research on Daily Fantasy Sports (DFS). DFS allows players to create their own teams of real-life players and to assume the role of team manager/owner and to potentially win cash prizes, derived from entry fees. The primary aim of

DFS leagues is to accrue the most points on contests that can span an entire sport season. DFS are worldwide popular (especially in North America; e.g., Marchica et al. 2017). Skill-based processes and sports knowledge (e.g., statistics, injury, player drafts, trades) play a critical role in fantasy game participation (e.g., Davis and Duncan 2006). As these games are considered as skill-based games (i.e., unlike traditional gambling involving mainly games of chance), adolescents can legally be involved in these gambling-related activities (Billings et al. 2016).

Some concerns have been expressed regarding the accelerated nature of fees and other DFS features that might promote excessive play and related harm in young people (e.g., Nelson et al. 2019). Indeed, the daily or hourly DFS use mimics online sports betting, as it offers availability and opportunities on the short-term. Accordingly, there is evidence that participating in fantasy sports leagues is associated with sports betting problems (i.e., loss of control over gambling, lying about one's gambling, being preoccupied about one's gambling) in adults (Nower et al. 2018), college students (Marchica and Derevensky 2016; Martin and Nelson 2014; Martin et al. 2016), and adolescents (Marchica et al. 2017).

In addition to DFS, other games may offer a pathway to gambling. For instance, social media sites such as Facebook offer social casino games, e.g. slot games and card games (blackjack). These games are not classified as gambling activities as they are not associated with monetary gains (although monetary expense can result from playing or subscribing). Hence, similar to DFS, these games can be legally provided to adolescents and are very popular among this population (Derevensky and Gainsbury 2016; Gainsbury et al. 2015, 2017; Kim et al. 2017; Teichert et al. 2017; Wohl et al. 2017). Crucially, longitudinal studies have shown that the involvement in simulated gambling via social network sites facilitates the transition to gambling with real money in adolescents (Dussault et al. 2017; Hayer et al. 2018). These findings raise concerns as it suggests that simulated online gambling activities can render gambling as a socially acceptable, enjoyable and risk-free activity.

An increasing convergence of gambling and video gaming has been observed over the last years, facilitated by the advent of incentivized in-game purchasing systems (i.e., micro-transactions), such as the repeat purchase of randomly determined items via "loot box" mechanics (i.e., items in video games that may be bought for real-world money, but which contain randomized contents; Zendle et al. 2020). The basic design and implementation of in-game purchasing options simulates the dynamic and intermittent reward ratios that are typically observed in slot machines (King and Delfabbro 2018), as it features rapid pace, repeatability, and randomness of rewards (e.g., monetized cosmetic in-game items; Hardenstein 2017; Holden and Ehrlich 2017; Macey and Hamari 2018a, b; Gambling Commission UK 2017). These monetized in-game purchasing systems use sophisticated behavioral tracking and machine learning-based algorithms to alter in-game conditions to incentivize continuous spending and persistent playing (King et al. 2019a, b).

The convergence of sport, gaming and gambling is even more pronounced with the unprecedented development of E-sport (Lopez-Gonzalez and Griffiths 2018). This increasingly popular form of sport encompasses video gaming competitions organized into leagues and tournaments, along with streaming practices, which has brought professionalization, regulation, fan communities, and has also resulted in a wide range of new sport betting options (Hamari and Sjoblom 2017).

Overall, the contemporary technological and cultural environment encapsulates gaming and gambling as easy access leisure activities, along with the continuous development of E-sport. The tremendous popularity of video games (and now E-sport) and the implementation of gambling-like in-game purchasing systems in video games (e.g., loot boxes) result in most young people being exposed to gambling situations at a stage of being under age (including situations likely to promote sports betting), which raises important public health issues. In the next section, we will detail on how young people's attitudes and engagement toward gambling is also shaped by the sports betting advertising and its powerful alignment with professional sports sponsorship.

3 Hyper Exposure and Easy Access to Sports Betting

In most European countries, sports betting is legal and highly advertised (see *BOX 2* for an overview of the landscape of sports betting in Luxembourg). As a result, sports fans are directly (e.g., through television advertisements, smartphone notifications) or incidentally exposed to gambling messages while watching sport match-day programs (e.g., team shirt sponsored by gambling companies, pitch side advertising boards, half time entertainment; Sharman et al. 2019). For example, a comprehensive analysis of three full episodes of a popular soccer-related show ("*Match of the Day*", which is broadcasted on a non-commercial British television channel, BBC1) emphasizes an average of over 250 gambling logo exposures per episode (Cassidy and Ovenden 2017). Studies conducted in Australia observed that spectators watch between 10 and 15 minutes of gambling promotions during every single game (Lindsay et al.

2013), and are exposed on average to 107 gambling advertisement per game (Gordon and Chapman 2014). In the English Premier League, the number of teams with gambling shirt sponsors increased from four teams in 2008 to half of all teams in 2017 (Lopez-Gonzalez and Griffiths 2018). Live commentary and half-time studio break also promote gambling-related cues exposure via betting odds discussions (e.g., between match-day programs hosts, featuring celebrities and football experts; Deans et al 2017; Hing et al. 2015). Sports betting is thus becoming increasingly embedded into the sports culture and advertised in prime-time popular TV programs.

Another key aspect of sports betting advertising is that its content features minute-by-minute information (e.g., betting odds dynamically changing according to ongoing games and events), as well as direct incentives to bet (e.g., emails, smartphone notifications on bonus bets, happy hours, multi-bet offers, improved odds, cash out offers, refunds; for a review, see Newall et al. 2019). Hence, since a large range of macro and micro events are available to bet on, merely viewing such advertisements and the related sport events are likely to increase the motivational salience of sports betting-related cues.

These assumptions have recently been investigated in a functional magnetic resonance imaging (fMRI) study on sports betting cue exposure (Brevers et al. 2018). The results show a differential pattern of sport cues information processing, depending on whether sport fans think about a sporting event with the intention of gambling on the outcome or thinking about it with the intention of merely watching it (Brevers et al. 2018). The neural networks mediating these responses to sports betting cues were identified in the orbitofrontal cortex, anterior insula, caudate nucleus, and the hippocampus. These regions represent important brain pathways underlying memory, cognition and emotion as triggered by addiction-related cue reactivity (for a review, see Brevers et al. 2019).

One recent study found evidence for implicit associations between gambling and sport (i.e., spontaneous and fast associations between sports betting brand logos and sport names) in adolescents (Li et al. 2018). This result is important as it illustrates the considerable strength of an associative pathway between sport and gambling in young people. Specifically, the repeated pairing of environmental gambling advertisement with sports might lead these stimuli to acquire increased motivational salience and to take up more attention capacity. These patterns are consistent with those observed in adult samples of frequent gamblers (Brevers et al. 2013a; Flòrez et al. 2016; Yi and Kanetkar 2010; Zack et al. 2005).

The convenient and easy access to sports betting is not only likely to trigger gambling saliency among the population of sports fans but might also increase non-planned betting (e.g., in-play live betting on in-match contingencies). For instance, Hing and colleagues (2016, 2018a, b; see also Browne et al. 2019) showed that live betting is common among sports bettors, and is positively associated with gambling disorder symptoms. This line of research also has shown that patterns of live betting are very common in young men characterized by general trait impulsivity (Hing et al. 2018a, b) and sensation seeking (Martinez-Loredo et al. 2019).

Overall, these findings echo current neurocognitive approaches to gambling disorder (e.g., Brevers and Noël 2013b; Brevers et al. 2020) in that the confrontation with sports-related stimuli in individuals with problematic sports betting habits might lead to the activation of the "sports betting cluster", which would in turn automatically trigger a corresponding impulse, consisting of a positive, fast and intense incentive attributed to gambling and a corresponding behavioral approach schema (see also Hofmann et al. 2009; Stacy and Wiers 2010).

BOX 2. An Overview of the Landscape of Sports Betting in Luxembourg
Gambling has become widely viewed as a socially acceptable and increasingly popular form of recreational activity (e.g., Calado and Griffiths 2016). This also applies to Luxembourg, which has been listed as one of the countries with the highest prevalence rates of gambling, as suggested by gross gambling revenues (Griffiths 2009), and high popularity of gambling among young adults (Duscherer and Paulos 2014).

Sports betting has been legal in Luxembourg since 1987. The minimum age for betting is 18 and **players' winnings are not taxable.** Currently, sports betting is placed under the auspices of the Loterie Nationale (since 2016). Nevertheless, as of February 2017, no foreign-based online sports betting website has been blocked in Luxembourg. Moreover, a high-frequency of sports betting advertisement can be viewed through the media from neighbouring countries (Belgium, Germany and France). Hence, there is a wide variety of options for sports bettors in Luxembourg, just as in many other European countries.

4 Narrative Content of Sports Betting Advertisement

Gambling brand exposure is ubiquitous in most industrialized countries. This section aims to demonstrate how young people are increasingly targeted by the gambling industry through the symbolic content of sports-betting advertising.

A growing body of literature targets the content and impact of the advertising and promotion on sports betting across the world (Deans et al. 2017; Gordon et al. 2014; Lopez-Gonzalez et al. 2018a, b). These studies have disentangled the tactics used by the sport betting industry to promote gambling behavior through online marketing and gambling-related websites, which consist of only 10 ten major strategies These include features such as sports fan rituals and behaviors (e.g., pictures or videos of fans cheering for their teams, waving banners, and wearing team uniforms, jerseys, or scarves), mate ship and peer bonding (e.g., young men watching sport together, socializing at the pub, or at social gatherings such as parties or barbeques), social bonding characterized by an individual betting dynamic (e.g., the bettor is surrounded by people but isolated in their betting), gender stereotypes (e.g., sexual objectification of women, with advertisements often portraying male dominance or power over women), presentation of betting outcomes as predictable and skill-based (e.g., using themes of sports knowledge, calculations, active choice, the bettor identity, masculinity, control over the way in which individual gamble, and when and where they could gamble), social superiority (e.g., financial success from wagering would lead to affluent lifestyles, and control over life choices), in-play live betting, adventure, thrill, and risk (e.g., gamblers need to take risks to reap higher rewards, staking small amounts of money with large potential returns), cash winning emotion and celebration (e.g., themes of personal and group triumph and the social success resulting from monetary gains), and co-consumption with other risky behaviors (e.g., alcohol, junk food; see also Sartori et al. 2018). Humor and celebrity endorsement were also observed. These later two elements have been suggested to normalize gambling behaviors and increase its social acceptance (Derevensky et al. 2010; Hing et al. 2015; Lamont et al. 2016; McMullan and Miller 2008, 2009; Fitt et al. 2017a, b).

Taken together, sports betting advertising relies on narratives themes that exaggerate social acceptance and perceived control over betting (see *BOX 3* for a discussion on illusory active control in sports betting). Previous research also supports the notion that positive attitudes towards sports betting advertisement (e.g. "good/bad"; "like/dislike"; "harmless/harmful"), but not actual frequency of exposure, is associated with problem gambling symptoms (Hing et al. 2017b). Importantly, positive attitudes to sports betting advertisement are also linked to increased levels of awareness of, attention to, and recall of the sponsor's name and their promotions (e.g., through logos on team uniforms), as well as with greater betting intention in young people (Glozah et al. 2019; Hing et al. 2017b; Newall et al. 2019). On the whole, it can be concluded that favorable attitudes and salient recall of sports betting marketing constitute risk factors for problem gambling in young sports bettors.

The rise of betting marketing has also prompted sport fans to describe the betting market as "saturated" (Thomas et al. 2012), and seeing themselves as "desensitized" by the continuous exposure to sports betting related cues (Deans et al. 2017). This is a further signal that gambling becomes increasingly embedded within sport. The next section aims to detail how the onset of sports betting content alongside sports news and events is susceptible to shape positive attitudes toward sport gambling among young people.

BOX 3. Can Sports Knowledge Impact Sports Betting Earnings?

Cantinotti and colleagues (2004) observed that experienced sports bettors achieved higher accuracy rates when picking the results of games, as compared to a random bet selection. The monetary outcomes won by the sports bettors, however, were not significantly higher than the random selection condition. Similar results have been observed in the context of horse-race betting (Ladouceur et al. 1998).

Two studies showed that the level of football expertise did not impact the accuracy of football match prognoses (e.g., to predict the scores of the first 10 matches of the 2008 UEFA European Football Championship; Huberfeld et al. 2013; Khazaal et al. 2012). Hence, results of these studies suggest that sports related knowledge is useless when considering long term monetary gains, and that the so-called "skills" inflate the bettor's confidence. This process is frequently referred to as the "illusion of control" (Langer 1975).

In addition to sports related knowledge, the illusion of control in sports betting could also be fueled by the following factors (Lopez-Gonzalez et al. 2018a):

- A high engagement of attention and decision-making processes, with bettors required to perform composite complex actions and calculations. Hence, as bettors adopt a more active role, betting outcomes (i.e., bet won or lost) are more likely to be misinterpreted as a direct consequence of their strategic thinking.
- Near-miss situations (i.e., a loss that looks almost the same as a win) lead bettors to overestimate bets with low winning probability (Vaughan Williams 1999). For instance, in horse racing, "close finishes" usually describe the features of a good race. Hence, bookmakers have been using this characteristic feature of racing to generate betting odds (Reis 1986).
- The current positive connotations of sports betting in the society reduces the perception of risk pertaining to this type of gambling (e.g., by focusing on its entertainment value; Lopez-Gonzalez et al. 2018a, b).
- With the increasing convergence between sport, gaming, and gambling, sports bettors are increasingly identified as players and not gamblers. The juxtaposition and confusion of skill-based and chance-based roles could thus foster the illusion of control in sports betting.

5 Impact of Sports Betting Advertisement on Children and Adolescents

An important public health concern is that a large number of children and adolescents are currently exposed to sports betting cues during family TV viewing time. For instance, 17% of all advertising displayed around TV's coverage of the 2018 Football World Cup targeted gambling (Duncan et al. 2018; Newall et al. 2019). Moreover, even taking into account advertising restrictions (e.g., in Australia a restriction on advertising in live sport takes place until 8:30 pm), young people report seeing gambling advertisements on social media or on Youtube (e.g., before being able to watch the sport or gaming video they aim to watch; Thomas et al. 2018; see also Houghton et al. 2020; Killick and Griffiths 2019).

Several studies conducted in the recent years have examined the impact of sports betting advertising on gambling attitudes and consumption intentions of children and adolescents. These studies can be clustered around four complementary findings. A first observation is that young people are able to recall the names of sports betting brands, and associate sports betting sponsors with specific sport teams (Bestman et al. 2015; Djohari et al. 2019; Hanss et al.

2015; Nyemcsok et al. 2018; Pitt et al. 2016, 2017a; Thomas et al. 2016, 2018). Moreover, young people seem particularly sensitive to music, voiceovers and catchy slogans featured in advertisements for sports betting or gambling games on social platforms (Abarbanel et al. 2017; Pitt et al. 2017b).

A second important finding is that seeing parents and friends gambling is associated with gambling frequency and gambling disorder symptoms (e.g., Wickwire et al. 2007a, b; Pitt et al. 2017a, b). Social learning theorists have long pointed to the important role of observation and imitation in the acquisition and maintenance of both socially desirable and socially undesirable behaviors (Bandura 1977). Social learning takes place within a specific reference group, and observation of gambling in significant individuals could unsurprisingly affect young people's participation in gambling activities. Studies using focus group designs found that young people involved in betting generally consider this activity as non-risky and as a socially accepted form of gambling (Deans et al. 2017; Gavriel-Fried et al. 2010; Thomas et al. 2015). Furthermore, sports betting is also perceived as an activity that helps to fit in and to share topics of conversation with friends (Deans et al. 2017). These qualitative observations are consistent with the advertisement strategies of the betting industry, which portray sports betting as an activity facilitating social cohesion, mate ship, and social opportunities (e.g., Deans et al. 2017; Lopez-Gonzalez et al. 2018a, b). An increasing number of children also learn about the excitement of gambling by watching the reactions (e.g., emotional state) of their parents during sports watching (Pitt et al. 2017a, b). Betting parents also frequently include their children in their sports betting activities while watching sports (e.g., by asking their advice, by providing an active role in the actual betting activity; Pitt et al. 2017a, b). In this context, children with betting parents are likely to be at increased risk of developing illusory patterns of self-efficacy by observing (i.e., vicarious learning) and gambling with (i.e., verbal persuasion and mastery experiences) significant others.

A third important observation is that young people take promotions at face value and cannot fully grasp the persuasive and cynical aspects of appeal strategies in sports betting advertisements. For instance, young people are attracted by the skill elements depicted in sports betting advertisement, and interpret these messages as relevant information (Pitt et al. 2016, 2017b). Other studies emphasize that the alignment of gambling with culturally valued events (i.e., sport), celebrity endorsement, perceived expert knowledge and understanding of sport, cash back offers, and the positive attitude of parents and peers towards gambling increase perceptions of trust in sports betting in children and adolescents (e.g., "sports betting is a part of the sports fan's identity"; Pitt et al. 2016, 2017a, b).

Fourth, the abiding sports betting marketing has been shown to successfully increase gambling intention and motivation in young people. For instance, over 40% of young people reported that they wanted to gamble after having been exposed to gambling advertisement (Derevensky et al. 2010). A high number of young sports fans also reported that they would like to try sports betting (currently or when being legally authorized to bet on sports; Hing et al. 2014; Pitt et al. 2017b). Besides, sport-related gambling is not necessarily perceived as true gambling, and is associated with a lower degree of stigma (Lopez-Gonzalez et al. 2019; Sproston et al. 2015). Results from recent focus group-based studies support the notion that the positive attitudes and connotations surrounding sports betting might negatively impact upon self-perception of problem gambling (Johansen et al. 2019; Lopez-Gonzalez et al. 2019).

6   Sport Betting in Young Athletes

Throughout the present chapter, we have described how the sports betting industry contributes progressively to the creation of new subcultures (e.g., sports betting is becoming a sports fan ritual) and identities (i.e., bettors are now referred to as "players") associated with their product. This section focuses on young athletes. Specifically, we investigated how young athletes perceive sports betting, and whether the high accessibility, aggressive advertising, and social acceptability of sports betting impact on their gambling behaviors, as well as on their sport performance.

Some of these questions were addressed by Richard et al. (2019) over the course of four study iterations (2004, 2008, 2012 and 2016) in student-athletes from the North American National Collegiate Athletic Association (NCAA). These studies examined gambling behaviors in more than 84.000 student-athletes (22.388 in the 2016 study) across all three NCAA divisions. The participants were surveyed regarding their attitudes toward and engagement in various gambling activities, including sports betting. The results show that, in contrast to the decrease of poker or online casino use over the years, online sports betting, and especially in-game betting, remains popular with student-athletes. Despite NCAA prohibition, 9% of athletes reported betting on sports at least once per month, and 2% met diagnostic criteria for gambling disorder (see also *BOX 4* for a discussion on why athletes could be more at risk to develop problem gambling). Although playing cards for money was the most common first experience with gambling, sports betting was increasingly cited by NCAA men as the preferred and most frequently practiced gambling activity (with 90% of men and 82% of women placing their first bet before entering college). Of particular concern is that 11% percent of Division I football players and 5% of men's basketball players reported betting on a game from their championship (but not involving their team).

A recent qualitative study specifically focused on the betting practices among professional football, handball and basketball players (Moriconi and Cima 2019). This study capitalized on semi-structured interviews to explore why athletes bet on their own competitions and sometimes even on their own games (see also Grall-Bronnec et al. 2016). One striking finding from this study is that, even mindful of the regulations and prohibitions, gambling is described by the athletes as a well-known and recurring practice in their milieu. Sports betting is mostly perceived as a recreational behavior for seeking excitement/stimulation or prestige within the group (e.g., internal rivalry between teammates who bet on opposed results to compete and define who eventually "knows more about sport"). Sport athletes also describe specific strategies that they frequently display to avoid being identified by regulators, such as asking a friend to bet for (and sometimes on) themselves, or betting with low amounts. Interestingly, for some individuals, betting in one's own games can even be a sign of sport integrity and a source of collective motivation (e.g., similar to an official monetary prize or cash bonus). In the players' opinion, problem gambling and financial insecurity were seen as conditions that could lead to match fixing. According to the players, if athletes become indebted, they can be tempted to altering their play on the field to affect the outcome of a game. According to the informants, betting-related behaviors are involved at different levels and conducted by different actors to finance various kinds of activities, from salaries to travel expenses (Moriconi and Cima 2019).

Attitudes towards sports betting were also examined by Richard, Paskus and Derevensky (2019) in a sample of NCAA student-athletes. Around 25% of athletes reported being uncomfortable with the idea of betting on college sports and 50% were against gambling advertising related to college sporting events. Nevertheless, 44% percent of men and 31% of women viewed sports betting as a harmless pastime. This view was more pronounced (76% and 61%) among student-athletes who were involved in sports betting. Moreover, around 50% of men and 25% of women who bet on sports thought that sport betting is a convenient way of winning money. The student-athletes involved in sports betting also reported that a lot of players violate NCAA betting bylaws and 25% think that coaches did not consider these rules seriously.

These findings suggest that online sports betting is already firmly rooted within the sport culture, i.e. not only in sport fans but also in athletes. This high-acceptance of gambling might also change the way young people consider sports (e.g., Thomas et al. 2018; Pitt et al. 2017b). This aspect is especially relevant when tackling the issue of sports betting by adopting a sport psychology perspective. The development that a young elite performer is likely to progress through is completely at odds with the achievement goals conveyed by sports betting. Specifically, young athletes need to develop self-efficacy and self-determined motivation through the experimentation and the observation of task-oriented mastery goals (e.g., Baker et al. 2003; Côté 1999; Kitsantas et al. 2000). These patterns fundamentally contrast with sports betting in which the main motivation is oriented toward an external reward (i.e., money) that is obtained through quantitative indices of performances. Hence, it might be that the sports betting culture increases the normative aspect of performance-oriented goals in young athletes (commonly associated with sport dropout in this population; e.g., Conroy et al. 2003; Duda 2001; Elliot and McGregort 2001), and hamper the development of task-oriented goals (commonly associated with feelings of pleasure and self-efficacy in young athletes; e.g., Smith et al. 2009). Further studies are thus needed to examine whether and how the normalization and acceptance of sports betting impacts on young athletes' motivation and achievement goals toward their sport practice.

BOX 4. Are Athletes More at Risk to Develop Problem Gambling than Non-athletes?

The most frequent motives to gamble among elite athletes tend to be related to their competitive attitude and interest in sport (Curry and Jiobu 1995). More specifically, gambling corresponds well to athletes' desire for competition and challenges, and sometimes their heightened needs to experience sensation and risk-taking (St-Pierre et al. 2014; Håkansson et al. 2018). In addition, athletes tend to think that they know more about their particular sport and, therefore, may view sports betting as an easy opportunity to win money (Curry and Jiobu 1995; Grall-Bronnec et al. 2016). Furthermore, most professional athletes have a lot of free time, which could lead them to bet on sport as an occupational activity of for sharing their knowledge and interest in sport (Nowak and Aloe 2014). Lastly, having a considerable income at a young age has also been linked to gambling behaviors (Hayatbakhsh et al. 2012).

Of particular public health concerns is the reported significant number of athletes who are starting gambling in group and at a young age (e.g., Sullivan-Kerber 2005; Huang et al. 2007). Based on a nationally representative sample of 20.739 student-athletes in the United States, a study reported that 62.4% of males and 42.8% of females were involved in some sort of gambling (Huang et al. 2007). In a sample of European professional athletes, Grall-Bronnec et al. (2016) found that 56.6% of the sample had gambled at least once during the previous year. This rate of gambling frequency is higher than the percentage generally found in the general population in European countries (with variations ranging from 25% in Belgium to 56.2% in France; Costes et al. 2015; Goudriaan et al. 2013; Ekholm et al. 2014).

With regards to problem gambling, recent studies reported lifetime prevalence rates of 7% (in a Swedish sample of university student athletes, $N = 352$; Håkansson et al. 2018) and 8.2% (in a sample of European professional athletes from Grall-Bronnec et al. 2016). These rates are at the upper end of the range reported in the general population, with lifetime rates of problem gambling ranging from 0.7 to 6.5% (Calado and Griffiths 2016). Gambling frequency and problem gambling were also positively linked to participation in competitive sports in high school, in samples of adolescent athletes (Gavriel-Fried et al. 2010; Moore and Ohtsuka 2000).

7   Regulatory Responses and Educational Programmes

Policymakers and legislators are becoming increasingly aware of the potential adverse effects of sports betting in young people. In the last years, various regulatory responses have targeted sports betting advertising, such as discussing with sports clubs strategies to prevent their team and stadium from exposure to gambling sponsorship, or banning all gambling advertising across public spaces and television during a sports event (Thomas et al. 2018). Nevertheless, these regulation strategies contain a number of exemptions which have important implications for young people's continued exposure to sports betting advertising (Thomas et al. 2018). In Belgium, for instance, gambling advertisement is now banned during live sport events, but can still be visualized through stadium and team sponsorships. Moreover, sports betting marketing is still allowed during the other types of sport television programs occurring shortly prior or after the live event. Besides, cut-off time strategies (e.g., no betting ads prior 8:30 pm) are generally inefficient since young people watch media content well beyond e.g. 8:30 pm, or are engaged in media viewing via online digital platforms and social media which are exempted from these regulations, such as Youtube (Thomas et al. 2018).

When asking young people to share their opinions on what could be done for addressing public health concerns on sports betting, they tend to report that sport institutions and government bodies should do more to protect young people from gambling advertisement exposure (Richard et al. 2019; Thomas et al. 2016, 2018). This includes the need to remove all gambling advertising from sport (without exemption rules) and to create educational programs on sport integrity. In other words, regulatory actions need to go beyond the gamble ban message.

It is important to disentangle excitement and knowledge resulting from sports passion from those oriented toward sports betting (e.g., Miller 2017). This aspect is crucial for allowing young people to build a sports fans and/or athletes identity centered around the passion for sports, despite being highly exposed to sports betting advertisement. This view echoes qualitative works on gambling abstinence (Reith and Dobbie 2011, 2012, 2013; Reith 2018). These studies emphasized that the maintenance gambling abstinence revolves around shifting from a gambling self-identity (i.e., a "gambling self", with many becoming unable to fulfill roles associated with their "non-addict selves"; Reith and Dobbie 2012) to a self-identity that is reshaped in harmonious and appropriate ways (e.g., through a renewed interest in activities in line with the individual's life values, which allows him/her to recover a sense of agency and meaning in life). In this context, building a sport fan's or athlete's identity separated from gambling activities is a key feature of young people regulated betting habits. Indeed, a challenge for sport fans who try to diminish or stop betting is to watch sport events without betting on them (e.g., Johansen et al. 2019). In this vein, educational programs promoting harmonious sports passion should help to restore an interest in sports *per se*, that is, without betting on it (i.e. shifting back to a "sport-fan" or "athlete identity").

Interestingly, these initiatives depart from prototypical gambling industry "responsible gambling" practices, which are framed in terms of the individual's responsibility to avoid harm and to act responsibly (Hancock 2011, 2018; Hancock and Smith 2017). Specifically, this "responsible gambling" approach might reinforce individual choice, and shape public policy in ways favorable to the gambling industry (e.g., by avoiding more government regulation through corporate political activity; Baysinger 1984). This dynamic is also likely to divert attention away from banning sports betting advertising during broadcasts by focusing on voluntary self-regulation. It is thus crucial to develop and fund innovative educational programs aiming to protect young people, and to spread these actions to parents, young adults' peers or siblings, teachers and sporting coaches.

8   Conclusion and Perspectives

Given the constantly growing popularity of sports betting, it is important to better characterize young adults' involvement in this new digitalized form of gambling. Little is known about the specific factors that distinguish safe from harmful involvement in sports betting. It will also be important to distinguish excitement and knowledge resulting from sports from those oriented toward the gambling-related reward (e.g., Miller 2017). This aspect is crucial for allowing young people to build a sports fans and/or athletes identity centered around the passion for sports, despite being highly exposed to sports betting advertisement.

This view echoes qualitative works on gambling abstinence (Reith and Dobbie 2011, 2012, 2013; Reith 2018), as well as recent theoretical accounts on addictive behaviors (Miller et al. 2020). These authors emphasize that the maintenance of gambling abstinence revolves around shifting from a gambling self-identity (i.e., a "gambling self", with many becoming unable to fulfill roles associated with their "non-addict selves"; Reith and Dobbie 2012) to a self-identity that is reshaped in harmonious and appropriate ways (e.g., through a renewed interest in activities in line with the individuals' life values, which allows them to recover a sense of agency and optimal engagement with the world; Reith and Dobbie 2012; Miller et al. 2020).

In this context, building a sport fan's or athlete's identity separated from gambling activities is a key process for young people regulating betting habits. A challenge for sport fans who try to reduce or stop betting is to watch sport events without betting on them (e.g., Johansen et al. 2019), which—in a clinical context—would be akin to exposure with response prevention in the cognitive-behavioral treatment of behaviors with a strong compulsion. Another issue is that sports betting is often undertaken in groups (e.g., friends, relatives; Johansen et al. 2019), as a form of rituals as members of a community (Miller et al. 2020). Hence, young adults' identity might be associated with a sense of membership in a gambling community with which the individual identifies (Miller et al. 2020). In this context, educational programs promoting harmonious sports passion should help to restore an interest in sports *per se*, that is, without betting on it (i.e. shifting back to a "sport-fan" or "athlete identity").

This research direction should also be relevant when adopting a longitudinal approach in the investigation of the long-term (mental) health effects of young adults' exposure to sports betting cues, as well as in studying trajectories of problematic gambling habits (initiation, maintenance, disengagement) in the light of other behaviors that might or might not be detrimental to young people (e.g., substance use, videogaming, Internet use).

To conclude, while the long-term effects of early exposure to sports betting cues are still unknown, there is a need to fuel the discussion on how the increasing popularization and ubiquity of sports betting impact young people's mental health. These concerns should address gambling related risks at a global level, and challenge stakeholders' views on the status of gambling in sports.

References

Abarbanel, B., Gainsbury, S. M., King, D., Hing, N., & Delfabbro, P. H. (2017). Gambling games on social platforms: How do advertisements for social casino games target young adults? Policy & Internet, 9(2), 184–209.

Arain, M., Haque, M., Johal, L., Mathur, P., Nel, W., Rais, A., Sandhu, R., & Sharma, S. (2013). Maturation of the adolescent brain. *Neuropsychiatric Disease and Treatment, 9*, 449–461. https://doi.org/10.2147/NDT.S39776

Baker, J. (2003). Early specialization in youth sport: A requirement for adult expertise? *High Ability Studies, 14*(1), 85–94. https://doi.org/10.1080/13598130304091

Bandura, A. (1977). Self-efficacy: Toward a unifying theory of behavioral change. *Psychological Review, 84*(2), 191–215. https://doi.org/10.1037/0033-295X.84.2.191

Baysinger, B. D. (1984). Domain maintenance as an objective of business political activity: an expanded typology. *Academic Managment Review, 9*, 248–258.

Bestman, A., Thomas, S. L., Randle, M., & Thomas, S. D. M. (2015). Children's implicit recall of junk food, alcohol and gambling sponsorship in Australian sport. *BMC Public Health, 15*, 1022. https://doi.org/10.1186/s12889-015-2348-3

Billings, A. B., Ruihley, J., & Yang, Y. (2016). Fantasy gaming on steroids? Contrasting fantasy sport participation by daily fantasy sport participation *Communication & Sport*. https://doi.org/10.1177/21674 79516644445.

Brevers, D., Cleeremans, A., Hermant, C., Tibboel, H., Kornreich, C., Verbanck, P., & Noël, X. (2013a). Implicit gambling attitudes in problem gamblers: Positive but not negative implicit associations. *Journal of Behavior Therapy and Experimental Psychiatry, 44*(1), 94–97. https://doi.org/10.1016/j.jbtep.2012.07.008

Brevers, D., Herremans, S. C., He, Q., Vanderhasselt, M.-A., Petieau, M., Verdonck, D., Poppa, T., De Witte, S., Kornreich, C., Bechara, A., & Baeken, C. (2018). Facing temptation: The neural correlates of gambling availability during sports picture expo-

sure. *Cognitive, Affective & Behavioral Neuroscience*, *18*(4), 718–729. https://doi.
org/10.3758/s13415-018-0599-z

Brevers, D., & Noël, X. (2013b). Pathological gambling and the loss of willpower: A
neurocognitive perspective. *Socioaffective Neuroscience & Psychology*, *3*, 21592.
https://doi.org/10.3402/snp.v3i0.21592

Brevers, D., Sescousse, G., Maurage, P., & Billieux, J. (2019). Examining neural reactivity
to gambling cues in the age of online betting. *Current Behavioral Neuroscience
Reports*, *6*(3), 59–71. https://doi.org/10.1007/s40473-019-00177-2

Brevers D., Vögele, C. & Billieux J. (2020). Cognitive processes underlying impaired
decision-making in gambling disorder. In T. Zaleskiewicz (ed.). Psychological
Perspectives on Financial Decision Making. Springer International Publishing.

Browne, M., Hing, N., Russell, A. M. T., Thomas, A., & Jenkinson, R. (2019). The impact
of exposure to wagering advertisements and inducements on intended and actual
betting expenditure: An ecological momentary assessment study. *Journal of Behavioral
Addictions*, *8*(1), 146–156. https://doi.org/10.1556/2006.8.2019.10

Burge, A. N., Pietrzak, R. H., Molina, C. A., & Petry, N. M. (2004). Age of gambling
initiation and severity of gambling and health problems among older adult problem
gamblers. *Psychiatric Services (Washington, D.C.)*, *55*(12), 1437–1439. https://doi.
org/10.1176/appi.ps.55.12.1437

Burge, A. N., Pietrzak, R. H., & Petry, N. M. (2006). Pre/early adolescent onset of
gambling and psychosocial problems in treatment-seeking pathological gamblers.
Journal of Gambling Studies, *22*(3), 263–274. https://doi.org/10.1007/s10899-006-
9015-7

Calado, F., & Griffiths, M. D. (2016). Problem gambling worldwide: An update and
systematic review of empirical research (2000–2015). *Journal of Behavioral
Addictions*, *5*(4), 592–613. https://doi.org/10.1556/2006.5.2016.073

Cantinotti, M., Ladouceur, R., & Jacques, C. (2004). Sports betting: Can gamblers
beat randomness? *Psychology of Addictive Behaviors: Journal of the Society of
Psychologists in Addictive Behaviors*, *18*(2), 143–147. https://doi.org/10.1037/0893-
164X.18.2.143

Casey, B. J., & Jones, R. M. (2010). Neurobiology of the adolescent brain and behavior:
Implications for substance use disorders. *Journal of the American Academy of Child
and Adolescent Psychiatry*, *49*(12), 1189–1201; quiz 1285. https://doi.org/10.1016/j.
jaac.2010.08.017

Cassidy, R., & Ovenden, N. (2017). Frequency, duration and medium of advertisements
for gambling and other risky products in commercial and public service broadcasts of
English Premier League football. https://doi.org/10.31235/osf.io/f6bu8

Castrén, S., Grainger, M., Lahti, T., Alho, H., & Salonen, A. H. (2015). At-risk and problem
gambling among adolescents: A convenience sample of first-year junior high school
students in Finland. *Substance Abuse Treatment, Prevention, and Policy*, *10*, 9. https://
doi.org/10.1186/s13011-015-0003-8

Chambers, R. A., & Potenza, M. N. (2003). Neurodevelopment, impulsivity, and
adolescent gambling. *Journal of Gambling Studies*, *19*(1), 53–84. https://doi.org/10.10
23/a:1021275130071

Conroy, D. E., Elliot, A. J., & Hofer, S. M. (2003). A 2 × 2 Achievement Goals
Questionnaire for Sport: Evidence for Factorial Invariance, Temporal Stability, and

External Validity. *Journal of Sport and Exercise Psychology*, *25*(4), 456–476. https://doi.org/10.1123/jsep.25.4.456

Costes, J.M., et al. (2015). *Les jeux d'argent et de hasard en France en 2014*. Les notes de l'Observatoire Des Jeux. 4: p. 9.

Costes, J.M., Richard, J.B., Eroukmanoff, V., Philippon, A.. (2020). *Les Français et les jeux d'argent et de hasard: Résultats du Baromètee de Santé publique France 2019*. p. 6.

Côté, J. (1999). The influence of the family in the development of talent in sports. *The Sport Psychologist*, *13*, 395–417.

Curry, T. J. & Jiobu, R. M. (1995). Do motives matter? Modelling gambling on sports among athletes. *Sociology of Sport Journal*, *12*, 21–35.

Davis, N.W. and Duncan, M.C. (2006) Sports knowledge is power: reinforcing masculine privilege though fantasy sport league participation. Journal of Sport and Social Issues 30, 244–264.

Deans, E. G., Thomas, S. L., Derevensky, J., & Daube, M. (2017). The influence of marketing on the sports betting attitudes and consumption behaviours of young men: Implications for harm reduction and prevention strategies. *Harm Reduction Journal*, *14*(1), 5. https://doi.org/10.1186/s12954-017-0131-8

Delfabbro, P., King, D., & Griffiths, M. D. (2014). From adolescent to adult gambling: An analysis of longitudinal gambling patterns in South Australia. *Journal of Gambling Studies*, *30*(3), 547–563. https://doi.org/10.1007/s10899-013-9384-7

Delfabbro, P., Lambos, C., King, D., & Puglies, S. (2009). Knowledge and beliefs about gambling in Australian secondary school students and their implications for education strategies. *Journal of Gambling Studies*, *25*(4), 523–539. https://doi.org/10.1007/s10899-009-9141-0

Derevensky, J. L. (2012). Youth gambling: An important social policy and public health issue. In *Current issues and controversies in school and community health, sport and physical education* (pp. 115–130). Nova Science Publishers.

Derevensky, J. L., & Gainsbury, S. M. (2016). Social casino gaming and adolescents: Should we be concerned and is regulation in sight? *International Journal of Law and Psychiatry*, *44*, 1–6. https://doi.org/10.1016/j.ijlp.2015.08.025

Derevensky, J. L., Pratt, L. M., Hardoon, K. K., & Gupta, R. (2007). Gambling problems and features of attention deficit hyperactivity disorder among children and adolescents. *Journal of Addiction Medicine*, *1*(3), 165–172. https://doi.org/10.1097/ADM.0b013e318142d081

Di, M. (1987). Patterns of alcohol and drug use among adolescents. *Pediatric Clinics of North America*, *34*(2), 275–288. https://doi.org/10.1016/s0031-3955(16)36214-9

Djohari, N., Weston, G., Cassidy, R., Wemyss, M., & Thomas, S. (2019). Recall and awareness of gambling advertising and sponsorship in sport in the UK: A study of young people and adults. *Harm Reduction Journal*, *16*(1), 24. https://doi.org/10.1186/s12954-019-0291-9

Duscherer, K., & Paulos, C. (2014). *Enquête sur la pratique des jeux de hasard auprès des élèves des écoles secondaires luxembourgeoises*. Luxembourg: Centre des Prevention de Toxicomanie.

Edgerton, J. D., Melnyk, T. S., & Roberts, L. W. (2015). Problem Gambling and the Youth-to-Adulthood Transition: Assessing Problem Gambling Severity Trajectories in a

Sample of Young Adults. *Journal of Gambling Studies*, *31*(4), 1463–1485. https://doi. org/10.1007/s10899-014-9501-2

Derevensky, J., Sklar, A., Gupta, R. et al. (2010). An Empirical Study Examining the Impact of Gambling Advertisements on Adolescent Gambling Attitudes and Behaviors. *International Journal of Mental Health and Addiction*, *8*, 21–34. https://doi. org/10.1007/s11469-009-9211-7

Duda, J. L. (2001). Achievement Goal Research in Sport: Pushing the Boundaries and Clarifying Some Misunderstandings. In G. C. Roberts (Ed.), Advances in Motivation in Sport and Exercise (pp. 129–182). Leeds: Human Kinetics.

Duncan, P., Davies, R. & Sweney, M. (2018). Children 'bombarded' with betting adverts during world cup. Retrieved from https://www.theguardian.com/media/2018/jul/15/children-bombarded-with-bettingadverts-during-world-cup

Dussault, F., Brunelle, N., Kairouz, S., Rousseau, M., Leclerc, D., Tremblay, J., ... Dufour, M. (2017). Transition from playing with simulated gambling games to gambling with real money: A longitudinal study in adolescence. *International Gambling Studies*, *17*, 386–400.

Ekholm, O., Eiberg, S., Davidsen, M., Holst, M., Larsen, C. V. L., & Juel, K. (2014). The prevalence of problem gambling in Denmark in 2005 and 2010: A sociodemographic and socioeconomic characterization. *Journal of Gambling Studies*, *30*(1), 1–10. https://doi.org/10.1007/s10899-012-9347-4

Elliot, A. J., & McGregor, H. A. (2001). A 2 X 2 achievement goal framework. *Journal of Personality and Social Psychology*, *80*(3), 501–519. https://doi.org/10.1037/0022-3514.80.3.501

Elton-Marshall, T., Leatherdale, S. T., & Turner, N. E. (2016). An examination of internet and land-based gambling among adolescents in three Canadian provinces: Results from the youth gambling survey (YGS). *BMC Public Health*, *16*, 277. https://doi. org/10.1186/s12889-016-2933-0

Flórez, G., Saiz, P. A., Santamaría, E. M., Álvarez, S., Nogueiras, L., & Arrojo, M. (2016). Impulsivity, implicit attitudes and explicit cognitions, and alcohol dependence as predictors of pathological gambling. *Psychiatry Research*, *245*, 392–397. https://doi. org/10.1016/j.psychres.2016.08.039

Fröberg, F., Modin, B., Rosendahl, I. K., Tengström, A., & Hallqvist, J. (2015). The association between compulsory school achievement and problem gambling among Swedish young people. *The Journal of Adolescent Health: Official Publication of the Society for Adolescent Medicine*, *56*(4), 420–428. https://doi.org/10.1016/j. jadohealth.2014.12.007

Gainsbury, S. M., King, D. L., Russell, A. M. T., Delfabbro, P., & Hing, N. (2017). Virtual addictions: An examination of problematic social casino game use among at-risk gamblers. *Addictive Behaviors*, *64*, 334–339. https://doi.org/10.1016/j. addbeh.2015.12.007

Gainsbury, S. M., Russell, A., Blaszczynski, A., & Hing, N. (2015). The interaction between gambling activities and modes of access: A comparison of Internet-only, land-based only, and mixed-mode gamblers. *Addictive Behaviors*, *41*, 34–40. https://doi. org/10.1016/j.addbeh.2014.09.023

Gambling Commission. Young people and gambling (2017). A research study among 11–16 year olds in Great Britain. Gambling Commission. Available from: http://www.

gamblingcommission.gov.uk/PDF/survey-data/   Young-People-and-Gambling-2017-
Report.pdf
Gambling Commission. Gambling participation in 2016 (2016): behaviour, awareness
    and attitudes. Gambling Commission: Birmingham, England. Available from: http://
    www.gamblingcommission.gov.uk/PDF/survey-data/Gambling-participation-in-2016-
    behaviour-awareness-and-attitudes.pdf
Gavriel-Fried, B., Teichman, M., & Rahav, G. (2010) Adolescent gambling: Temperament,
    sense of coherence and exposure to advertising. Addiction Research & Theory, 18(5),
    586–598. doi:https://doi.org/.0.3109/16066350903428945.
Glozah, F. N., Tolchard, B., & Pevalin, D. J. (2019). Participation and attitudes towards
    gambling in Ghanaian youth: An exploratory analysis of risk and protective factors.
    International Journal of Adolescent Medicine and Health. https://doi.org/10.1515/
    ijamh-2018-0175
Goldstein, R. Z., & Volkow, N. D. (2002). Drug addiction and its underlying neurobio-
    logical basis: Neuroimaging evidence for the involvement of the frontal cortex. The
    American Journal of Psychiatry, 159(10), 1642–1652. https://doi.org/10.1176/appi.
    ajp.159.10.1642
Gordon, R., & Chapman, M. (2014). Brand community and sports betting in Australia.
    https://researchers.mq.edu.au/en/publications/brand-community-and-sports-betting-in-
    australia
Goudriaan, A.E. (2013). Gambling and problem gambling in the Netherlands. Addiction.
Grall-Bronnec, M., Caillon, J., Humeau, E., Perrot, B., Remaud M., Guilleux, A., Rocher,
    B., Sauvaget, A., & Bouju, G. (2016). Gambling among European professional athletes.
    Prevalence and associated factors. Journal of Addictive Diseases, 35(4), 278–290.
    https://doi.org/10._080/10550887.2016.1177807
Håkansson, A., Kenttä, G., & Åkesdotter, C. (2018). Problem gambling and gaming
    in elite athletes. Addictive Behaviors Reports, 8, 79–84. https://doi.org/10.1016/j.
    abrep.2018.08.003
Hancock L. (2011). Regulatory failure: The case of Crown Casino. Melbourne: Australian
    Scholarly Publishing.
Hancock L, & Smith G. (2017). Critiquing the Reno Model I–IV international influence
    on regulators and governments (2004–2015)—the distorted reality of responsible
    gambling. International Journal of Mental Health and Addiction. https://doi.
    org/10.1007/s11469-017-9745-y
Hancock, L., Ralph, N., & Martino, F. P. (2018). Applying Corporate Political Activity
    (CPA) analysis to Australian gambling industry submissions against regulation of tele-
    vision sports betting advertising. PloS One, 13(10), e0205654. https://doi.org/10.1371/
    journal.pone.0205654
Hamari, J., & Sjöblom, M. (2017). What is eSports and why do people watch it? Internet
    research, 27(2). DOI: https://doi.org/10.1108/IntR-04-2016-0085.
Hanss, D., Mentzoni, R. A., Griffiths, M. D., & Pallesen, S. (2015). The impact of
    gambling advertising: Problem gamblers report stronger impacts on involvement,
    knowledge, and awareness than recreational gamblers. Psychology of Addictive
    Behaviors: Journal of the Society of Psychologists in Addictive Behaviors, 29(2), 483–
    491. https://doi.org/10.1037/adb0000062

Hardenstein, T. S. (2017). Skins in the game: Counter-strike, esports, and the shady world of online gambling. *UNLV Gaming LJ, 7*, 117. Retrieved from: http://heinonline.org/hol-cgi-bin/get_pdf.cgi?handle=hein.journals/unlvgalj7&section=14.

Hare, Sarah (2009). A Study of Gambling in Victoria – Problem Gambling from a Public Health Perspective. Available at: http://www.responsiblegambling.vic.gov.au/__data/assets/pdf_file/0013/407/Gambling-in-victoria-problem-gambling-from-a-public-healthperspective.pdf

Hayatbakhsh, M. R., Clavarino, A., Williams, G. M., Bor, W., & Najman, J. M. (2012). Young adults' gambling and its association with mental health and substance use problems. *Australian and New Zealand Journal of Public Health, 36*(2), 160–166. https://doi.org/10.1111/j.1753-6405.2011.00815.x

Hayer, T., Kalke, J., Meyer, G., & Brosowski, T. (2018). Do simulated gambling activities predict gambling with real money during adolescence? Empirical findings from a longitudinal study. *Journal of Gambling Studies, 34*, 929–947.

Hing, N., Breen, H., Gordon, A., & Russell, A. (2014). Risk factors for problem gambling among indigenous Australians: An empirical study. *Journal of Gambling Studies, 30*(2), 387–402. https://doi.org/10.1007/s10899-013-9364-y

Hing, N., Li, E., Vitartas, P., & Russell, A. M. T. (2018a). On the Spur of the Moment: Intrinsic Predictors of Impulse Sports Betting. *Journal of Gambling Studies, 34*(2), 413–428. https://doi.org/10.1007/s10899-017-9719-x

Hing, N., Russell, A., Blaszczynski, A., & Gainsbury, S. M. (2015). What's in a Name? Assessing the Accuracy of Self-identifying as a Professional or Semi-Professional Gambler. *Journal of Gambling Studies, 31*(4), 1799–1818. https://doi.org/10.1007/s10899-014-9507-9

Hing, N., Russell, A. M., & Browne, M. (2017a). Risk Factors for Gambling Problems on Online Electronic Gaming Machines, Race Betting and Sports Betting. *Frontiers in Psychology, 8*, 779. https://doi.org/10.3389/fpsyg.2017.00779

Hing, N., Russell, A. M. T., Lamont, M., & Vitartas, P. (2017b). Bet Anywhere, Anytime: An Analysis of Internet Sports Bettors' Responses to Gambling Promotions During Sports Broadcasts by Problem Gambling Severity. *Journal of Gambling Studies, 33*(4), 1051–1065. https://doi.org/10.1007/s10899-017-9671-9

Hing, N., Russell, A. M. T., Li, E., & Vitartas, P. (2018b). Does the uptake of wagering inducements predict impulse betting on sport? *Journal of Behavioral Addictions, 7*(1), 146–157. https://doi.org/10.1556/2006.7.2018.17

Hing, N., Russell, A. M. T., Vitartas, P., & Lamont, M. (2016). Demographic, Behavioural and Normative Risk Factors for Gambling Problems Amongst Sports Bettors. *Journal of Gambling Studies, 32*(2), 625–641. https://doi.org/10.1007/s10899-015-9571-9

Hofmann, W., Friese, M., & Strack, F. (2009). Impulse and Self-Control From a Dual-Systems Perspective. *Perspectives on Psychological Science: A Journal of the Association for Psychological Science, 4*(2), 162–176. https://doi.org/10.1111/j.1745-6924.2009.01116.x

Holden, J. T., & Ehrlich, S. C. (2017). Esports, skins betting, and wire fraud vulnerability. *Gaming Law Review, 21*, 566–574.

Houghton, S., Moss, M., & Casey, E. (2020). Affiliate marketing of sports betting – a cause for concern? *International Gambling Studies, 0*(0), 1–6. https://doi.org/10.1080/14459795.2020.1718737

Huberfeld, R., Gersner, R., Rosenberg, O., Kotler, M., & Dannon, P. N. (2013). Football gambling three arm-controlled study: Gamblers, amateurs and laypersons. *Psychopathology. 46*(1), 28–33. https://doi.org/10.1159/000338614

Humphreys, B. R., & Perez, L. (2012). Who bets on sports? Characteristics of sports bettors and the consequences of expanding sports betting opportunities. *Estudios de Economía Aplicada, 30(2)*, 579–598.

Jiun-Hau Huang SM S., PhD, D. F. J., PhD, J. L. D., PhD, R. G., & PhD, T. S. P. (2007). A National Study on Gambling Among US College Student-Athletes. *Journal of American College Health, 56*(2), 93–99. https://doi.org/10.3200/JACH.56.2.93-100

Johansen, A. B., Helland, P. F., Wennesland, D. K., Henden, E., & Brendryen, H. (2019). Exploring online problem gamblers' motivation to change. *Addictive Behaviors Reports, 10*, 100187. https://doi.org/10.1016/j.abrep.2019.100187

Khazaal, Y., Chatton A., Billieux, J., Bizzini, L., Monney, G., Fresard, E., Thorens, G., Bondolfi, G., El-Guebaly, N., Zullino, D., & Khan, R. (2012). Effects of expertise on football betting. *Substance Abuse Treatment, Prevention, and Policy, 7*, 18. https://doi.org/10.1186/1747-597X-7-13

Killick, A. E., & Griffiths, M. D. (2019). A Content Analysis of Gambling Operators' Twitter Accounts at the Start of the English Premier League Football Season. *Journal of Gambling Studies.* https://doi.org/10.1007/s10899-019-09879-4

Kim, H. S., Hollingshead, S., & Wohl, M. J. (2017b). Who spends money to play for free? Identifying who makes micro-transactions on social casino games (and why). *Journal of Gambling Studies, 33*, 525–538.

King, D. L., & Delfabbro, P. H. (2018). Predatory monetization schemes in video games (e.g. 'loot boxes') and internet gaming disorder. *Addiction (Abingdon, England), 113*(11), 1967–1969. https://doi.org/10.1111/add.14286

King, D.L., Koster, E., & Billieux, J. (2019a). Study what makes games addictive. Nature, 573 (7774), 346.

King, D.L., Delfabbro, P.H., Gainsbury, S.M., Dreier, M., Greer, N., & Billieux, J. (2019b). Unfair play? Video games as exploitative monetized services: An examination of game patents from a consumer protection perspective. Computers in Human Behaviors, 101, 131–143.

Kitsantas, A., Zimmerman, B. J., & Cleary, T. (2000). The role of observation and emulationin the development of athletic self-regulation. Journal of Educational Psychology, 92, 811–817.

Labrador, F. J., & Vallejo-Achón, M. (2019). Prevalence and Characteristics of Sports Betting in a Population of Young Students in Madrid. *Journal of Gambling Studies.* https://doi.org/10.1007/s10899-019-09863-y

Ladouceur, R., Sylvain, C., Letarte, H., Giroux, I., & Jacques, C. (1998). Cognitive treatment of pathological gamblers. *Behaviour Research and Therapy, 36*(12), 1111–1119. https://doi.org/10.1016/s0005-7967(98)00086-2

Lamont, M., Hing, N., & Vitartas, P. (2016). Affective response to gambling promotions during televised sport: A qualitative analysis. *Sport Management Review, 19*, 319–331.

Langer, E. J. (1975). The illusion of control. *Journal of Personality and Social Psychology, 32*(2), 311–328. https://doi.org/10.1037/0022-3514.32.2.311

Li, E., Langham, E., Browne, M., Rockloff, M., & Thorne, H. (2018). Gambling and Sport: Implicit Association and Explicit Intention Among Underage Youth. *Journal of Gambling Studies, 34*(3), 739–756. https://doi.org/10.1007/s10899-018-9756-0

Lindsay, S., Thomas, S., Lewis, S., Westberg, K., Moodie, R., & Jones, S. (2013). Eat, drink and gamble: Marketing messages about 'risky' products in an Australian major sporting series. *BMC Public Health, 13*(1), 719. https://doi.org/10.1186/1471-2458-13-719

Lopez-Gonzalez, H., & Griffiths, M. D. (2018). Betting, Forex Trading, and Fantasy Gaming Sponsorships-a Responsible Marketing Inquiry into the "Gamblification" of English Football. *International Journal of Mental Health and Addiction, 16*(2), 404–419. https://doi.org/10.1007/s11469-017-9788-1

Lopez-Gonzalez, H., Estévez, A., & Griffiths, M. D. (2018a). Controlling the illusion of control: A grounded theory of sports betting advertising in the UK. *International Gambling Studies, 18*(1), 39–55. https://doi.org/10.1080/14459795.2017.1377747

Lopez-Gonzalez, H., Estévez, A., & Griffiths, M. D. (2019). Can Positive Social Perception and Reduced Stigma be a Problem in Sports Betting? A Qualitative Focus Group Study with Spanish Sports Bettors Undergoing Treatment for Gambling Disorder. *Journal of Gambling Studies, 35*(2), 571–585. https://doi.org/10.1007/s10899-018-9799-2

Lopez-Gonzalez, H., Guerrero-Solé, F., Estévez, A., & Griffiths, M. (2018b). Betting is Loving and Bettors are Predators: A Conceptual Metaphor Approach to Online Sports Betting Advertising. *Journal of Gambling Studies, 34*(3), 709–726. https://doi.org/10.1007/s10899-017-9727-x

Macey, J., & Hamari, J. (2018a). *eSports, skins and loot boxes: Participants, practices, and problematic behaviour associated with emergent forms of gambling. 21*, New Media and Society20–41.

Macey, J., & Hamari, J. (2018b). Investigating relationships between video gaming, spectating esports, and gambling. *Computers in Human Behavior, 80*, 344–353.

Marchica, L., & Derevensky, J. L. (2016). Examining personalized feedback interventions for gambling disorders: A systematic review. *Journal of Behavioral Addictions, 5*(1), 1–10. https://doi.org/10.1556/2006.5.2016.006

Marchica, L., Zhao, Y., Derevensky, J., & Ivoska, W. (2017). Understanding the Relationship Between Sports-Relevant Gambling and Being At-Risk for a Gambling Problem Among American Adolescents. *Journal of Gambling Studies, 33*(2), 437–448. https://doi.org/10.1007/s10899-016-9653-3

Martin, R. J., & Nelson, S. (2014). Fantasy sports, real money: Exploration of the relationship between fantasy sports participation and gambling-related problems. *Addictive Behaviors, 39*(10), 1377–1382. https://doi.org/10.1016/j.addbeh.2014.05.017

Martin, R. J., Nelson, S. E., & Gallucci, A. R. (2016). Game On: Past Year Gambling, Gambling-Related Problems, and Fantasy Sports Gambling Among College Athletes and Non-athletes. *Journal of Gambling Studies, 32*(2), 567–579. https://doi.org/10.1007/s10899-015-9561-y

Martínez-Loredo, V., Grande-Gosende, A., Fernández-Artamendi, S., Secades-Villa, R., & Fernández-Hermida, J. R. (2019). Substance Use and Gambling Patterns Among Adolescents: Differences According to Gender and Impulsivity. *Journal of Gambling Studies, 35*(1), 63–78. https://doi.org/10.1007/s10899-018-09824-x

McMullan, J. L., & Miller, D. (2008). All in! The commercial advertising of offshore gambling on television. *Journal of Gambling Issues, 22*, 230–251.

McMullan, J. L., & Miller, D. (2009). Wins, winning and winners: The commercial advertising of lottery gambling. *Journal of Gambling Studies, 25*, 273–295.

Miller, H. (2017). *Gen Bet: Has gambling gatecrashed our teens?* Victoria. Australia: Victorian Responsible Gambling Foundation.

Miller, M., Kiverstein, J., & Rietveld, E. (2020). Embodying addiction: A predictive processing account. *Brain and cognition, 138*, 105495. https://doi.org/10.1016/j.bandc.2019.105495

Moore, S., & Ohtsuka, K. (2000). The Structure of Young People's Leisure and Their Gambling Behaviour. *Behaviour Change, 17*(3), 167–177. https://doi.org/10.1375/bech.17.3.167

Moriconi, M., & de Cima, C. (2019). Betting Practices Among Players in Portuguese Championships: From Cultural to Illegal Behaviours. *Journal of Gambling Studies*. https://doi.org/10.1007/s10899-019-09880-x

Nelson, S. E., Edson, T. C., Singh, P., Tom, M., Martin, R. J., LaPlante, D. A., Gray, H. M., & Shaffer, H. J. (2019). Patterns of Daily Fantasy Sport Play: Tackling the Issues. *Journal of Gambling Studies, 35*(1), 181–204. https://doi.org/10.1007/s10899-018-09817-w

Newall, P. W. S., Thobhani, A., Walasek, L., & Meyer, C. (2019). Live-odds gambling advertising and consumer protection. *PloS One, 14*(6), e0216876. https://doi.org/10.1371/journal.pone.0216876

Nowak, D. E., & Aloe, A. M. (2014). The prevalence of pathological gambling among college students: A meta-analytic synthesis, 2005–2013. *Journal of Gambling Studies, 30*(4), 819–843. https://doi.org/10.1007/s10899-013-9399-0

Nower, L., Caler, K. R., Pickering, D., & Blaszczynski, A. (2018). Daily Fantasy Sports Players: Gambling, Addiction, and Mental Health Problems. *Journal of Gambling Studies, 34*(3), 727–737. https://doi.org/10.1007/s10899-018-9744-4

Nyemcsok, C., Thomas, S. L., Bestman, A., Pitt, H., Daube, M., & Cassidy, R. (2018). Young people's recall and perceptions of gambling advertising and intentions to gamble on sport. *Journal of Behavioral Addictions, 7*(4), 1068–1078. https://doi.org/10.1556/2006.7.2018.128

Pitt, H., Thomas, S. L., Bestman, A., Daube, M., & Derevensky, J. (2017a). Factors that influence children's gambling attitudes and consumption intentions: Lessons for gambling harm prevention research, policies and advocacy strategies. *Harm Reduction Journal, 14*(1), 11. https://doi.org/10.1186/s12954-017-0136-3

Pitt, H., Thomas, S. L., Bestman, A., Daube, M., & Derevensky, J. (2017b). What do children observe and learn from televised sports betting advertisements? A qualitative study among Australian children. *Australian and New Zealand Journal of Public Health, 41*(6), 604–610. https://doi.org/10.1111/1753-6405.12728

Pitt, H., Thomas, S. L., Bestman, A., Stoneham, M., & Daube, M. (2016). "It's just everywhere!" Children and parents discuss the marketing of sports wagering in Australia. *Australian and New Zealand Journal of Public Health, 40*(5), 480–486. https://doi.org/10.1111/1753-6405.12564

Purdie N, Matters G, Hillman K, Murphy M, Ozolins C, Millwood P. (2011). Gambling and young people in Australia. In: Victoria (AUST): Gambling Research Australia.

Reid, R. L. (1986). The psychology of the near miss. *Journal of Gambling Behavior, 2*(1), 32– 39.

Reith, G. (2018). *Addictive Consumption: Capitalism, Modernity and Excess.* London: Routledge.

Reith, G., & Dobbie F. (2011). Beginning gambling: the role of social networks and environment. *Addiction Research and Theory, 19,* 483–93.

Reith G, & Dobbie F. (2012). Lost in the game: narratives of addiction and identity in recovery from problem gambling. *Addiction Research and Theory, 20,* 511–21.

Reith G, & Dobbie F. (2013). Gambling careers: a longitudinal, qualitative study of gambling behaviour. *Addiction Research and Theory, 21,* 376–90.

Richard, J., Paskus, T. S., & Derevensky, J. L. (2019). Trends in gambling behavior among college student-athletes: A comparison of 2004, 2008, 2012 and 2016 NCAA survey data. *Journal of Gambling Issues, 41,* 73–100.

Ricijas, N., Dodig, D., Huić, A., & Kranzelic, V. (2011). Habits and characteristics of adolescent gambling in urban areas — Research report. Downloaded from: https://bib.irb.hr/datoteka/654654.IZVJESTAJ_-_KOCKANJE_ADOLESCENATA.pdf

Ricijas, N., Dodig D., & Huic, A. (2016). Predictors of adverse gambling related consequences among adolescent boys. *Children and Youth Services Review, 67,* 168–176. https://doi.org/10.1016/j.childyouth.2016.06.008

Russell, A. M. T., Hing, N., Browne, M., Li, E., & Vitartas, P. (2019). Who Bets on Micro Events (Microbets) in Sports? *Journal of Gambling Studies, 35*(1), 205–223. https://doi.org/10.1007/s10899-018-9810-y

Russell, A. M. T., Hing, N., Browne, M., & Rawat, V. (2018). Are direct messages (texts and emails) from wagering operators associated with betting intention and behavior? An ecological momentary assessment study. *Journal of Behavioral Addictions, 7*(4), 1079–1090. https://doi.org/10.1556/2006.7.2018.99

Sartori, A., Stoneham, M., & Edmunds, M. (2018). Unhealthy sponsorship in sport: a case study of the AFL. *Australian and New Zealand journal of public health, 42*(5), 474–479. https://doi.org/10.1111/1753-6405.12820

Sharman, S., Ferreira, C. A., & Newall, P. W. S. (2019). Exposure to Gambling and Alcohol Marketing in Soccer Matchday Programmes. *Journal of Gambling Studies.* https://doi.org/10.1007/s10899-019-09912-6

Smith, R. E., Smoll, F. L., & Cumming, S. P. (2009). Motivational climate and changes in young athletes' achievement goal orientations. *Motivation and Emotion, 33*(2), 173–183. https://doi.org/10.1007/s11031-009-9126-4

Spritzer, D. T., Rohde, L. A., Benzano, D. B., Laranjeira, R. R., Pinsky, I., Zaleski, M., Caetano, R., & Tavares, H. (2011). Prevalence and correlates of gambling problems among a nationally representative sample of Brazilian adolescents. *Journal of Gambling Studies, 27*(4), 649–661. https://doi.org/10.1007/s10899-010-9236-7

Sproston, K., Hanley, C., Brook, K., Hing, N., & Gainsbury, S. (2015). *Marketing of sports betting and racing.* Melbourne: Gambling Research Australia.

Stacy, A. W., & Wiers, R. W. (2010). Implicit cognition and addiction: A tool for explaining paradoxical behavior. *Annual Review of Clinical Psychology, 6,* 551–575. https://doi.org/10.1146/annurev.clinpsy.121208.131444

St-Pierre, R. A., Tencheff, C. E., Gupta, R., Derevensky, J., & Paskus, T. S. (2014). Predicting gambling problems from gambling outcome expectancies in college student-athletes. *Journal of Gambling Studies*, *30*(1), 47–60. https://doi.org/10.1007/s10899-012-9355-4

Sullivan-Kerber, C. (2005). Problem and pathological gambling among college athletes. Annals of Clinical Psychiatry, 17(4), 243–247.

Teichert, T., Gainsbury, S. M., & Mühlbach, C. (2017). Positioning of online gambling and gaming products from a consumer perspective: A blurring of perceived boundaries. *Computers in Human Behavior, 75*, 757–765.

Thomas, S. L., Lewis, S., Duong, J. & McLeod, C. (2012). Sports betting marketing during sporting events: a stadium and broadcast census of Australian Football League matches. Australian and New Zealand Journal of Public Health, 36 (2), 145–152.

Thomas, S. L., Bestman A., Pitt H., Cassidy R., McCarthy S., Nyemcsok C., Cowlishaw S., Daube M. (2018). Young people's awareness of the timing and placement of gambling advertising on traditional and social media platforms: A study of 11–16 years olds in Australia. Harm Reduction Journal, 15(1), 51.

Thomas SL, Bestman A, Pitt H, Deans E, Randle M, Stoneham M, Daube M. (2015). The marketing of wagering on social media: An analysis of promotional content on YouTube, Twitter and Facebook. North Melbourne, V C: Victorian Responsible Gambling Foundation.

Thomas, S. L., David, J., Randle, M., Daube, M., & Senior, K. (2016). Gambling advocacy: Lessons from tobacco, alcohol and junk food. *Australian and New Zealand Journal of Public Health, 40*(3), 211–217. https://doi.org/10.1111/1753-5405.12410

Vaughan Williams, L. (1999). Information efficiency in betting markets: a survey. *Bulletin of Economic Research, 51*(1), 1–39.

Volberg, R. A., Gupta, R., Griffiths, M. D., Olason, D. T., & Delfabbro, P. (2010). An international perspective on youth gambling prevalence studies *International Journal of Adolescent Medicine and Health, 22*(1), 3–38.

Wickwire, E. M., Whelan, J. P., Meyers, A. W., & Murray, D. M. (2007). Environmental correlates of gambling behavior in urban adolescents. *Journal of Abnormal Child Psychology, 35*(2), 179–190. https://doi.org/10.1007/s10802-006-9065-4

Wickwire, E. M., Whelan, J. P., West, R., Meyers, A., McCausland, C., & Leullen, J. (2007). Perceived availability, risks, and benefits of gambling among college students. *Journal of Gambling Studies, 23*(4), 395–408. https://doi.org/10.1007/s10899-007-9057-5

Wohl, M. J., Salmon, M. M., Hollingshead, S. J., & Kim, H. S. (2017). An examination of the relationship between social casino gaming and gambling: The bad, the ugly, and the good. *Journal of Gambling Issues, 35*, 1–23 article 1.

Wood, R. T., & Williams, R. J. (2009). Internet gambling: prevalence, patterns, problems, and policy options. Final report prepared for the Ontario Problem Gambling Research Centre. Guelph, Canada: Ontario Problem Gambling Research Centre

Yi, S., & Kanetkar, V. (2010). Implicit measures of attitudes toward gambling: An exploratory study. Journal of Gambling Issues, 24, 140163.

Zack, M., Stewart, S. H., Klein, R. M., Loba, P., & Fragopoulos, F. (2005). Contingent gambling-drinking patterns and problem drinking severity moderate implicit gambling-alcohol associations in problem gamblers. *Journal of Gambling Studies, 21*(3), 325–354. https://doi.org/10.1007/s10899-005-3102-z

Zendle, D., Meyer, R., Cairns, P., Waters, S., & Ballou, N. (2020). The prevalence of loot boxes in mobile and desktop games. *Addiction, 115*(9), 1768–1772. https://doi.org/10.1111/add.14973

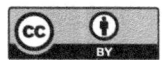

Spielsucht als Herausforderung für Gesundheit und Wohlbefinden von Jugendlichen

Andreas König

1   Einleitung

Die zunehmende Digitalisierung der Gesellschaft hat schon seit langem auch das Freizeitverhalten von Kindern und Jugendlichen durchdrungen. Internet- und Computerspielnutzung sind seit vielen Jahren, unabhängig von Zeit und Ort, über verschiedene Endgeräte möglich und weichen die Abgrenzung zwischen digitaler und physischer Lebenswelt auf, beide Aktionsräume verschmelzen im Alltag. Auch zeitlich intensives Computerspielen ist längst kein Nischenphänomen mehr, sondern betrifft weite Teile insbesondere der männlichen Jugendlichen. Dass während des „Fortnite-Hypes" 2018 auch auf Schulhöfen in Luxemburg beobachtbar reihenweise Siegestänze nachahmende Kinder und Jugendliche zu sehen waren – selbst solche, die diese nur über soziale Medien kannten und das Spiel z. B. aufgrund von Altersrestriktionen nicht selbst spielten – unterstreicht den Bestandteil und die Bedeutung von Computerspielen in der Jugendkultur. Während Social Media und Videospiele zweifelsohne positive Erfahrungen erlauben, die auch soziale und kognitive Vorteile mit sich bringen (Bell et al. 2015), zeigen umfangreiche Studien seit fast drei Jahrzehnten, dass die Nutzung für eine signifikante Minderheit der Nutzer mit sozialen, psychischen und körperlichen Problemen verbunden ist. Der folgende Artikel beleuchtet die Computerspielnutzung Jugendlicher mit Blick auf mögliche positive und negative Folgen, sowie die Häufigkeit, Merkmale und Entstehung problematischen und süchtigen Computerspielens. Abschließend werden Implikationen für die Prävention im Jugendbereich diskutiert.

A. König (✉)
ZEV – Zenter fir exzessiivt Verhalen a Verhalenssucht, route d'Esch, Luxembourg
E-Mail: akoenig@zev.lu

© Der/die Autor(en) 2022
A. Heinen et al. (Hrsg.), *Wohlbefinden und Gesundheit im Jugendalter,*
https://doi.org/10.1007/978-3-658-35744-3_18

2   Wie oft und lange spielen Jugendliche?

Nach Ergebnissen der aktuellen JIM-Studie spielen 80 % der Jungen und 44 % der Mädchen zwischen 12 und 19 Jahren täglich oder mehrmals pro Woche digitale Spiele. Im Alter von 14–15 Jahren zeichnet sich zwar ein leichter Höhepunkt ab, aber die Begeisterung geht mit zunehmendem Alter bei beiden Geschlechtern nur leicht zurück. Dank mobiler und internetfähiger Geräte, sowie einer Vielzahl von Spielformaten, sind Computerspiele längst nicht mehr auf Spielekonsolen und eigens dafür aufgerüstete heimische Computer beschränkt, sondern lassen sich auch zwischendurch im Freizeitalltag, auf dem Schulweg oder in Schulpausen nutzen. So verwundert wenig, dass 45 % der Jugendlichen täglich bzw. mehrmals pro Woche vor allem auf dem Smartphone spielen, gefolgt von 26 % auf Spielekonsolen, 24 % am Computer/Laptop und 7 % auf dem Tablet. Während Mädchen mit 63 % eindeutig das Smartphone als häufigstes Spielgerät nutzen (Jungen 23 %), stellen für Jungen stationäre Spielkonsolen (36 %, Mädchen: 12 %) bzw. Computer (34 %, Mädchen: 13 %) die häufigsten Plattformen für digitale Spiele dar (Feierabend et al. 2020).

Insgesamt nehmen Computerspiele im Jugendalter einen nicht unerheblichen Teil der Freizeit ein: Französische Jugendliche spielen unter Einbezug des Wochenendes durchschnittlich zwei Stunden täglich (Bonnaire und Phan 2017). Deutsche Jugendliche spielen unter der Woche durchschnittlich 81 min (Jungen 116 min, Mädchen 43 min) auf Computer, Smartphone, Tablet und Konsole (Feierabend et al. 2020), in „Corona-Zeiten" sogar 139 min pro Tag (DAK 2020). In Luxemburg erfassten König und Steffgen (2015) die Spielzeiten Jugendlicher getrennt nach schul- und schulfreien Tagen: An Schultagen verbachten 38 % (Jungen: 49 %, Mädchen: 22 %) im Durchschnitt mehr als eine Stunde, 17 % (Jungen: 24 %, Mädchen: 8 %) mehr als zwei Stunden täglich mit Computerspielen. An schulfreien Tagen spielten bereits 56 % (Jungen: 71 %, Mädchen: 35 %) durchschnittlich mehr als eine und 36 % (Jungen: 50 %, Mädchen: 18 %) mehr als zwei Stunden pro Tag. Unter männlichen Jugendlichen von 14 bis 17 Jahren verbrachte fast jeder fünfte an schulfreien Tagen im Schnitt mehr als 4 h mit Computerspielen.

Innerhalb eines Jahrzehnts stieg bei deutschen Jugendlichen zwischen 12 und 17 Jahren 7 % nicht nur die Gesamtzeit der Internetnutzung kontinuierlich, sondern darunter auch der für Computerspiele (26 %) und Unterhaltungsangebote (30 %) aufgebrachte Anteil zulasten des Anteils für Online-Kommunikation und Informationssuche (Feierabend et al. 2020). Dass unter den Unterhaltungsangeboten YouTube dominiert und 52 % der männlichen Jugendliche dort am häufigsten „Let's Play"-Videos konsumieren, lässt vermuten, dass die gedanklich-inhaltliche Beschäftigung mit Computerspielen zumindest bei einigen die reine Spielzeit signifikant übersteigt.

3 Spaßfaktor mit Nutzwert – nicht nur für das Wohlbefinden

Neben Motiven wie Spaß, Unterhaltung und Ablenkung spielen Jugendliche aus Neugierde, Faszination für die Storyline, zur Verbesserung der Fähigkeiten ihres Avatars, zur Stimulation der Imagination, zur Verbesserung von Real-Life-Fähigkeiten, um soziale Beziehungen in der virtuellen Welt zu schließen und zu pflegen, oder um etwas zum Darüber-Reden zu haben (Demetrovics 2011; von der Heiden et al. 2019). Mit am häufigsten nennen Jugendliche als Spielmotiv das Management der eigenen Stimmungslage und die Verbesserung des eigenen emotionalen Zustandes. Für intermittierend nutzbare Spiele, die nur ein kurzzeitiges Commitment erfordern, eine minimalistische Oberfläche aufweisen und leicht zugänglich sind (Candy Crush, Angry Birds, etc.), ist eine kurzfristige stimmungsverbessernde, entspannungsinduzierende und stress-reduzierende Wirkung belegt (z. B. Russoniello et al. 2009). Dass Computer-spielen eine deutliche Wirkung auf Nutzer ausüben kann, zeigt sich auch auf physiologischer Ebene, z. B. über Parameter wie der Hautleitfähigkeit als zuver-lässiges Maß des psychologischen Erregungsniveaus (z. B. Drachen et al. 2010) oder signifikanten Veränderung der Dopaminausschüttung (Koepp et al. 1998), die mitunter mit der Einnahme von Amphetamin vergleichbaren Effekten ein-hergehen (Müller und Wölfling 2017b). Allahverdipour et al. (2010) fanden bei wohlbefindensrelevanten Maßen psychischer Gesundheit einen Vorteil moderat computerspielender gegenüber spielabstinenten Jugendlichen.

Auch die Online-Kommunikation mit existierenden Freunden scheint sich positiv auf das psychologische und soziale Wohlbefinden auszuwirken, während „einzelgängerische" Nutzungsformen keinen Effekt haben (Huang 2010; Wang et al. 2014). Als wichtige mediierende Faktoren sind hier die Selbstoffenbarung und die Qualität der Freundschaft zu nennen (Valkenburg und Peter 2009; Wang et al. 2011). Computerspiele „ziehen" Jugendliche in virtuelle Umgebungen und lassen sie dort auf für sie bedeutsame Ziele hinarbeiten, Beharrlichkeit angesichts mehrfacher Misserfolge zeigen, und die raren Momente des Triumphes nach erfolgreicher Aufgabenbewältigung feiern. Dies könnte einen durch Persistenz und kontinuierliche Bemühung geprägten Motivationsstil fördern (Granic et al. 2014). Das unmittelbare und konkrete Feedback in Computerspielen dient nicht nur als Verstärkung für kontinuierliche Bemühungen, sondern hält Gamer auch in einem motivationalen „Sweet Spot", in dem das Niveau von Herausforderung und Frustration optimal mit Erfahrungen von Erfolg und eigener Leistung ausbalanciert werden. Dies geschieht aufgrund der dynamischen kontinuierlichen Anpassung des Schwierigkeitslevels an die Fähigkeiten des Spielers besonders effektiv, so dass von diesem zunehmend mehr Durchhaltevermögen, bessere Reaktionszeiten und komplexere Lösungen etc. gefordert sind, was das Erleben von „Flow" begünstigt (Granic et al. 2014; Sweetser und Wyeth 2005).

Auch diverse positive Effekte auf kognitive Fähigkeiten sowohl von kurzer, als auch extensiver Nutzung von Computerspielen sind gut belegt. Vor allem hinsichtlich Auge-Hand-Koordination, Reaktionszeit, räumlichem Vorstellungsvermögen, sowie der Aufmerksamkeit, Wahrnehmung und Verarbeitung visueller Reize wird angenommen, dass sich die Effekte auch auf Kontexte außerhalb des Computerspiels generalisieren lassen (Latham et al. 2013). Die Komplexität von Spielen scheint außerdem den Fähigkeiten der Problemlösung und des vernetzten Denkens zu trainieren (Fritz et al. 2011). Aktuelle Längsschnittstudien kommen allerdings zum Schluss, dass kommerzielle Videospiele zumindest keinerlei Vorteil bei der Entwicklung solcher kognitiven Fähigkeiten bieten, von denen auch akademische Leistungen profitieren (z. B. Gnambs et al. 2020).

4 Computerspielen: „exzessiv", „problematisch", „süchtig"?

Bereits 2013 wurde mit Erscheinen des DSM-5 die *Internet Gaming Disorder* in einer Sektion für Störungsbilder berücksichtigt, zu denen weitere Forschung als notwendig erachtet wird. 2019 wurde die *Gaming Disorder (online* und *offline)* schließlich von der WHO, neben der Glücksspielsucht, als zweite eigenständige, nicht-stoffgebundene Abhängigkeit in die ICD-11 aufgenommen und den Suchtstörungen zugeordnet. Als diagnostische Merkmale einer solchen pathologischen Nutzung gelten darin eine verminderte Kontrolle über die Spielaktivität, der eine erhöhte und zunehmende Priorität bis zu einem Ausmaß gegeben wird, dass diese Vorrang vor anderen Lebensinteressen und Alltagsaktivitäten erhält bzw. diese verdrängt. Die Spielaktivität wird ferner trotz des Auftretens negativer Konsequenzen fortgeführt oder sogar gesteigert. Dieses Verhaltensmuster muss zur Diagnosestellung zu einer anhaltenden Beeinträchtigung des psychosozialen Funktionsniveaus in persönlichen, familiären, sozialen, leistungsbezogenen oder anderen wichtigen Funktionsbereichen des Lebens führen und über einen Zeitraum von 12 Monaten persistieren oder wiederkehrend auftreten, wobei der diagnoserelevante Zeitraum bei besonders stark ausgeprägter Symptomatik auch kürzer angesetzt werden darf. Unter klinischen Stichproben erweist sich, dass die Berücksichtigung von Craving (psychisches Verlangen nach dem Suchtmittel) als weiteres Kriterium die diagnostische Genauigkeit erhöht (Müller et al. 2019).

Für die Praxis der Jugendarbeit scheint eine solch dichotom-kategoriale Sichtweise ("krank" vs. "[noch] gesund") wenig sinnvoll. Vielmehr bietet sich eine dimensionale Sichtwiese an, wie sie im DSM-5 mit der Einteilung in verschiedene Schweregrade und der damit einhergehenden funktionalen Beeinträchtigung im Alltag zumindest teilweise umgesetzt ist. Auch die Arbeitsgruppe zweier einschlägiger Fachverbände empfiehlt, die *Gaming Disorder* (GD) als Krankheitsbild und Steigerung sowohl von *exzessivem Spielen* (als zeitlich ausgedehntes Nutzungsverhalten, das phasenweise und temporär die hauptsächliche Freizeitgestaltung ausmacht und mit typischen Adoleszenzkonflikten als Teil der normalen Entwicklung verbunden sein kann), als auch *problematischem Spielen* abzugrenzen, das bereits mit typischen Folgen wie der Vernachlässigung anderer Interessen und (z. B. schulischen) Verpflichtungen, sozialem Rückzug oder fortgesetztem Spielen trotz z. B. sozialer Kritik von Nahestehenden verbunden ist (Deutsche Hauptstelle für Suchtfragen 2020). Insbesondere bei letzterem ist noch nicht vollständig geklärt, inwieweit die Folgen durch das Computerspielen selbst oder durch anders gelagerte Probleme oder Konflikte herbeigeführt werden, die dann mit problematischem Spielen als eine weitere Form des Umgangs damit beantwortet werden. Dass bei Van Rooij et al. (2011) circa ein Drittel der zeitlich auffälligen jugendlichen Nutzer keine erhöhten psychosozialen Symptome aufweist und auch nach einem Jahr signifikant häufiger wieder vom Nutzungsverhalten Abstand nahm, spricht zusätzlich für eine konzeptionelle Differenzierung zwischen suchtartigen Spielern und Intensivspielern.

Im deutschsprachigen Raum etabliert sich der Begriff der "Internetbezogenen Störungen" (IbS), der einen breiteren Betrachtungswinkel eröffnet. Neben der Möglichkeit, dass nicht immer alle diagnoserelevanten Kriterien einer Sucht voll erfüllt sind, obwohl das entsprechende Verhalten für die Betroffenen bereits subjektiv stark beeinträchtigende Folgen hat (z. B. massive Konflikte in der Familie, drastischer Abfall der Schulleistungen), besteht seit geraumer Zeit Konsens unter Forschern und Praktikern, dass auch andere suchtartige Nutzungsformen des Internets (z. B. Pornokonsum oder exzessives Sammeln von Informationen und Musik- und Videodateien) ein klinisch relevantes und behandlungsbedürftiges Ausmaß annehmen können (Eichenberg 2014; Müller und Wöfling 2017). Im Jahr 2018 wurde mit der Erarbeitung einer entsprechenden Behandlungsleitlinie für IbS auf den Niveau S. 1 (Expertenkonsens) begonnen (Thomasius 2018).

Brand et al. (2020) weisen auf die Wichtigkeit der Unterscheidung zwischen einerseits den Symptomen einer Gaming Disorder, und andererseits den beteiligten Mechanismen hin. So müssen spezifische Mechanismen nicht für alle Betroffenen gleichermaßen ein Hauptmerkmal ihres süchtigen Verhaltens darstellen. Zum Beispiel mag die Bewältigung negativer Stimmungslagen für manche die Hauptmotivation für zeitintensives Gaming darstellen, während bei anderen das Verlangen und die Antizipation von Gratifikation (im Sinne eines „Cravings" nach Belohnung) im Vordergrund steht. Beides kann schwer kontrollierbar sein und letztlich zu Symptomen der GD führen, aber beide Phänomene können auch bei nicht-problematischen, leidenschaftlichen Freizeitspielern auftreten. Forschung ist insbesondere hinsichtlich der komplexen Feinheiten in der Beziehung zwischen der mit Spielen verbrachten Zeit und der Symptombildung während der Entwicklung einer GD nötig, da der klinischen und der Praxis der Jugendarbeit keine robuste Datenlage zur Verfügung steht, anhand derer eine eindeutige Linie zwischen gestörtem und nicht-gestörtem Spielverhalten zu ziehen ist (Montag et al. 2019).

Für die Jugendarbeit könnte sich zur Umsetzung einer differenzierteren, stärker dimensionalen Betrachtungsweise eine Orientierung eher an den im DSM-5 genannten Kriterien anbieten. Neben einer mehr oder weniger großen Zahl an infrage kommenden Kriterien kann davon jedes für sich mehr oder weniger stark ausgeprägt sein, wobei das DSM-5 eine Diagnosestellung bei Vorliegen von fünf von neun genannten Symptomen vorsieht (Griffiths et al. 2016): 1) Die betroffene Person ist gedanklich (z. B. durch Nachdenken über vergangene oder Antizipieren der nächsten Spielaktivität) bzw. auf Verhaltensebene (Spielen wird zur dominanten Tätigkeit) stark durch das Spielen eingenommen, 2) bei Konsumverhinderung treten Entzugssymptome auf (typischerweise erhöhte Reizbarkeit, Nervosität oder Traurigkeit, d. h. ohne die physischen Anzeichen eines pharmakologischen Entzugs), 3) Toleranzentwicklung, d. h. das Bedürfnis, zunehmend mehr Zeit mit dem Spielen zu verbringen, 4) der Verlust des früher bestehenden Interesses an anderen Hobbies oder Unterhaltungsformen außer Computerspielen, 5) erfolglose Versuche der Reduktion der Spieleaktivität (Kontrollverlust), 6) Fortführung der Spieleaktivität trotz Wissens um daraus resultierende psychosoziale Probleme, 7) Vertuschen, Verheimlichen über Lügen über das Ausmaß des Spielens gegenüber wichtigen Bezugspersonen, 8) Emotionsregulation durch die Computerspielnutzung (v. a. Eskapismus und Erleichterung von negativen Gefühlen wie z. B. Hilflosigkeit, Schuld oder Angst), sowie 9) die Gefährdung bedeutsamer zwischenmenschlicher Beziehungen oder des Arbeitsplatzes bzw. der schulischen oder beruflichen Ausbildung durch das Computerspielen.

Eine sich an einer solchen Bandbreite von Kriterien orientierende, aber dimensional verstandene Betrachtungsweise vereinfacht nicht nur, kritische Entwicklungen eher entdecken und differenzierter benennen, sondern auch Erfolge und Verbesserungen graduell abbilden zu können, wahrzunehmen und zu würdigen. Sie hilft zudem, eine inflationäre Verwendung des Suchtbegriffes und eine Stigmatisierung als „süchtig" zu vermeiden, bzw. die dadurch bei Jugendlichen oft provozierte Reaktanz und Verteidigungshaltung zu reduzieren.

5   Prävalenz süchtigen und problematischen Spielens

In einer Metaanalyse identifizierten Cheng und Li (2014) eine globale Prävalenz der alle Formen abhängiger Internetnutzung mit einschließenden internetbezogener Störungen (IbS) von 6 % in der Altersspanne von 12 bis 41 Jahren, wobei sich die Prävalenz im Jugendalter stets am höchsten erwies. Unter deutschen Jugendlichen wird die Prävalenz der IbS zwischen 3,2 % (Wartberg et al. 2015) und 6,1 % (Lindenberg et al. 2018) geschätzt. In Luxemburg identifizierten König und Steffgen (2015) bei 3,4 % ein süchtiges, sowie bei weiteren 6,7 % ein problematisches Nutzungsverhalten. Unter der IbS stellt die süchtige Nutzung von Computerspielen den eindeutig größten Anteil. Eine aktuelle Metaanalyse beziffert die internationale Prävalenz der Gaming Disorder mit 4,6 % im Jugendalter, wobei männliche Jugendliche stärker betroffen sind (Fam 2018). In Deutschland variieren die Prävalenzschätzungen im Jugendalter zwischen 1,2 % (Rehbein et al. 2015) und 5,7 % (Wartberg et al. 2017). Eine französische Studie kommt auf eine Schätzung von 8,8 % Problemspielern, ohne den enthaltenen Anteil süchtiger Computerspieler separat auszuweisen (Bonnaire und Phan 2017). In Luxemburg fanden König und Steffgen (2015) eine Prävalenz von 2,2 % für süchtiges, und zusätzliche 4,8 % für problematisches Computerspielen. Die Heterogenität in den Prävalenzangaben ist in erster Linie auf methodische Abweichungen zurückzuführen, wie z. B. uneinheitliche Definitionskriterien und unterschiedliche Operationalisierungen.

Bei allen substanzgebundenen und -ungebundenen Süchten übersteigen die in der Bevölkerung gefundenen Prävalenzraten stets bei weitem die Anzahl der Hilfesuchenden, was auf spezifische motivationale Korrelate der Störungen und auf strukturelle Merkmale des Gesundheitssystems zurückzuführen ist (Müller und Wölfling 2017a). Eine Verdreifachung der Anfragen im Bereich exzessiver

Mediennutzung im Zeitraum von 2017 bis 2019 in unserer Einrichtung[1] spiegelt exemplarisch wider, dass das Phänomen auch in Luxemburg in der Bevölkerung zunehmend als professioneller Unterstützung bedürftiges Problem angesehen wird. Ein Anstieg des öffentlichen Bewusstseins darf allerdings nicht mit steigender Prävalenz gleichgesetzt werden: Wenngleich selektive Befunde dies naheliegen, zeigt eine Analyse internationaler Prävalenzdaten zwischen 1998 und 2017, dass die durchschnittliche berichtete Prävalenz für Computerspielsucht konstant bei ca. 4,7 % lag (Feng et al. 2017).

Hinsichtlich der zeitlichen Stabilität des Störungsbildes im Jugendalter schwankt die Studienlage zwischen 27 % und 66 % der Betroffenen, die nach einem Jahr noch die diagnostischen Kriterien erfüllten, bis zu einer Stabilität von 84 % der Betroffenen über den Verlauf von drei Jahren (Chang et al. 2014; Gentile et al. 2011; Rothmund et al. 2018). Je besser die Haltequote in den Studien war, desto höher fiel auch die Stabilität des Störungsbildes aus. Eine erste umfassendere Langzeitstudie mit jährlicher Erhebung der Symptomatik über einen Zeitraum von sechs Jahren deutet darauf hin, dass unter Jugendlichen mit einer moderat ausgeprägten Symptomatik sich diese bei etwa einem Drittel verschlimmert und bei zwei Dritteln auf stabilem Niveau bleibt. Bei Jugendlichen mit eingangs schwach ausgeprägter Symptomatik stellten sich über den Erhebungszeitraum kaum Veränderungen ein (Coyne et al. 2020).

6   Risikofaktoren für problematisches und süchtiges Spielen

Der relevanteste *soziodemographische Risikofaktor* scheint das Geschlecht zu sein: Während das Risiko problematischer Nutzung für Computerspiele bei Jungen deutlich höher ist, ist es für Social Media bei Mädchen höher (Anderson et al. 2016; Bonnaire und Phan 2017; Mérelle et al. 2017; Paulus et al. 2018). Erklären lässt sich die höhere Vulnerabilität männlicher Jugendlicher u. a. durch Merkmale des Inhalts und Designs von Games, wie z. B. gewalthaltige Spieleaktionen, stereotypische Rollenbilder, die kompetitive Struktur der Spiele und nur eingeschränkte bedeutsame soziale Interaktionen (Hartmann und Klimmt 2006),

---

[1] Die vom Verein Anonym Glécksspiller ASBL getragenen Einrichtungen „Game Over"/ „Ausgespillt" (ab Juni 2022: „Zenter fir exzessiivt Verhalen a Verhalenssucht") bieten Prävention und Beratung für Jugendliche, Eltern und Familien im Bereich exzessiver Mediennutzung bzw. ambulante Psychotherapie und Vor- und Nachsorge stationärer Aufenthalte im Bereich Verhaltenssüchte.

was für Mädchen weniger attraktiv zu sein scheint. Hinsichtlich des Alters zeigt sich ein Anstieg der Prävalenz der Gaming Disorder im frühen Jugendalter mit einem Höhepunkt bei 15 bis 16 Jahren, gefolgt von einem Absinken bis zum Alter von 18 Jahren, sowie einem zweiten Höhepunkt in der Spätadoleszenz (Szász-Janocha et al. 2019). In Europa scheint das Risiko problematischen Computerspielens für aus einer nicht-westlichen Kultur stammende Jugendliche höher zu sein (Kuss et al. 2014; Mérelle et al. 2017). Zum Verständnis von Migrationshintergründen als demografischem Risikofaktor liegt allerdings noch wenig systematische Forschung vor.

Als *individuelle Risikofaktoren* konnten in Längsschnittstudien soziale Kompetenzdefizite, eine dysfunktionale Emotionsregulation, sowie andere psychische Störungen wie depressive oder Angststörungen, sowie Aufmerksamkeits-Defizit-Hyperaktivitätsstörungen als individuelle Risikofaktoren identifiziert werden (z. B. Cho et al. 2013; Gentile et al. 2011; Ko et al. 2009; Lemmens et al. 2011). Zudem scheinen prädisponierende Variablen in der Genetik zu bestehen (Jeong et al. 2017; Park et al. 2018). Traumatische Erfahrungen in der Kindheit erhöhen ebenfalls das Risiko problematischer Computerspielenutzung (Shi et al. 2020). Mehrere Studien belegen konsistent eine hohe Impulsivität als Risikofaktor (vgl. Şalvarlı und Griffiths 2019). Unter den Persönlichkeitsmerkmalen wurden ferner Sensation Seeking (z. B. Hu et al. 2017), Neurotizismus (z. B. Mehroof und Griffiths 2010) und Feindseligkeit (z. B. Ko et al. 2009) als Risikofaktoren identifiziert. Insbesondere die Kombination verschiedener Persönlichkeitsmerkmale könnte eine Schlüsselrolle bei der Entwicklung und der Aufrechterhaltung des Störungsbildes spielen, daher ist weitere Forschung, insbesondere zu prädisponierenden Mustern, erforderlich (Gervasi et al. 2017). Problematische Nutzung von Computerspielen könnte auch mit frühen Bindungsstörungen (Lampert-Imkamp und te Wildt 2009) und dem Bindungsstil zusammenhängen, insbesondere dem durch verminderte Öffnungsbereitschaft charakterisierten, ambivalent-verschlossenen Bindungssti. bzw. einem diffus-vermeidender Persönlichkeitsstil (Eichenberg 2014; Grescher et al. 2013; Monacis et al. 2017).

Hinsichtlich *familiärer Kontextfaktoren* zeigen verschiedene Studien einen Zusammenhang zwischen einer schlechten Beziehung zu den Eltern bzw. dysfunktionalen familiären Mustern und dem Schweregrad problematischen Spielens, so z. B. für innerfamiliäres Vertrauen und familiäre Entfremdung (Lei und Wu 2007), Konflikte mit und zwischen den Eltern (Yen et al. 2007) und ein negatives Familienklima (König und Steffgen 2015), habituell konsumierende Geschwister und Eltern, die dem Substanzkonsum gegenüber als positiv-gewährend wahrgenommen werden (Yen et al. 2007). Renbein und Baier (2013)

fanden ein erhöhtes Risiko für IbS bei Jugendlichen, die bei nur einem Eltern-
teil aufwachsen oder sozial schlechter integriert sind. Eine gute Beziehung zum
Vater scheint hingegen ein möglicher protektiver Faktor zu sein (Schneider et al.
2017). Insgesamt kann davon ausgegangen werden, dass Probleme in der Eltern-
Kind-Beziehung einen Risikofaktor darstellen (Sugaya et al. 2019). Zusammen-
hänge mit Lebensereignissen wie finanziellen Problemen der Eltern oder
Scheidung lassen sich entweder nicht identifizieren oder werden im multivariaten
Kontext nicht signifikant (Mérelle et al. 2017; Tang et al. 2014). Dies könnte
dafür sprechen, dass weniger einzelne kritische Lebensereignisse, sondern eher
Situationen mit „milderen", aber dafür chronisch wirkenden Stressoren, wie z. B.
Schulprobleme und ein angespanntes Familienklima, als Risikofaktoren Relevanz
entfalten.

Hinsichtlich *schulischer Kontextfaktoren* gehen IbS mit schlechterer Schulleistung und gehäuften Fehlzeiten einher (Müller et al. 2015; Tsitsika et al. 2011).
Ein früher angenommener Zusammenhang mit dem Niveau der schulischen Lauf-
bahn verschwindet, sobald das Alter als konfundierte Variable kontrolliert wird
(Mérelle et al. 2017; Lindenberg et al. 2018).

Unter den *spiel- und nutzungsbezogenen Risikofaktoren* werden häufig eine
lange Spieldauer (z. B. Gentile et al. 2011) sowie die Nutzung von Onlinerollen-
spielen und etwas eingeschränkter auch Shooter- und Strategiespielen berichtet
(Bonnaire und Phan 2017; van Rooij et al. 2011). Unterschiede im Suchtpotenzial
bestimmter Spielgenres bzw. einzelner Spiele innerhalb eines Genres lassen
sich durch strukturelle Merkmale der Spiele, vor allem die Systematisierung
der Belohnungsvergabe im Sinne bestimmter lernpsychologischer Verstärker-
pläne erklären (Batthyány et al. 2009). Man kann zudem davon ausgehen, dass
die Zunahme an Monetarisierungsstrategien in Onlinespielen über eine Erhöhung
des Commitments auch die Bindung an das entsprechende Computerspiel erhöht
(Müller und Wöfling 2017b). Problemspieler verfügen eher über einen eigenen
Computer (Allahverdipour et al. 2010) und haben signifikant mehr Bildschirm-
geräte zuhause (Bonnaire und Phan 2017) bzw. nutzen insgesamt mehr Geräte für
den Internetzugang (König und Steffgen 2015).

7   Folgen problematischen und süchtigen Spielens

Da die meisten Erkenntnisse zu mit Gaming Disorder assoziierten Problemen
auf Querschnittsdaten beruhen, können Aussagen über die Wirkrichtung oder
den Einfluss bislang nicht untersuchter Drittvariablen derzeit nur eingeschränkt
getroffen werden. Am ehesten weisen Längsschnittstudien auf schädliche Folgen

süchtigen Computerspielens hin. So fanden z. B. Lemmens et al. (2011), dass Computerspielsucht bei männlichen Jugendlichen nach sechs Monaten zu einer erhöhten Aggressivität führte, und zwar auch dann, wenn gewaltfreie Spiele genutzt wurden. Gentile et al. (2011) konnten nachweisen, dass Depressionen, (insbesondere soziale) Angststörungen und schlechtere Schulleistungen über einen Zeitraum von zwei Jahren sowohl als Antezedent, als auch als Konsequenz von GD im Jugendalter auftreten können.

Insgesamt verdeutlicht das breite Spektrum häufig berichteter Komorbiditäten, das ferner Zwangsstörungen, Störungen des Sozialverhaltens, Aufmerksamkeits-Defizit-Hyperaktivitätssörungen, substanzgebundene Abhängigkeiten und externalisierenden Störungen umfasst, Bedeutung und Ausmaß der Folgen einer Gaming Disorder (Anderson et al. 2016; Carli et al. 2013; Ho et al. 2014; Ko et al. 2012; Linderberg et al 2017; Ra et al. 2018). Auch für nicht süchtiges, problematisches Computerspielen finden sich bei Jugendlichen Zusammenhänge mit somatischen Beschwerden wie Kopfschmerzen und trockenen Augen, mit einer allgemeinen psychopathologischen Symptomatik (SCL-90-R), Verhaltensproblemen und Suizidgedanken (Mérelle et al. 2017; Schulte-Markwort et al. 2002; Von der Heiden et al. 2019). Wenngleich die kausalen Wirkmechanismen noch nicht eindeutig geklärt sind, scheint eine reziproke Beziehung zwischen den verschiedenen Störungen am wahrscheinlichsten (Anderson et al. 2016). Die nachstehenden Befunde beschränken sich auf solche, die aus empirischen oder logisch-konzeptuellen Gründen als Folger problematischen Spielens, oder zumindest damit in reziproker Beziehung stehend angesehen werden können.

Hinsichtlich der *sozialen Folgen* ist Computerspielen bereits für problematische Nutzer häufig mit familiären Konflikten über die Nutzungszeiten verbunden. In klinischen Stichproben berichten 80 % der Jugendlichen von stark negative Konsequenzen auf das Familienleben. Eine suchtartige Nutzung führt häufig, meist mit schleichendem Verlauf, zu sozialer Isolation mit Verlust realen sozialen Rückhalts (Müller und Wölfling 2017b). Neben dem Risiko für einen bis zur Vereinsamung reichenden allgemeinen Mangel an sozialen Kontakten, ist dieses auch speziell für romantische Kontakte erhöht (Allison et al. 2006; Porter et al. 2010), bis hin zur dauerhaften Beziehungslosigkeit (Rho et al. 2016) Obwohl das Jugendalter diesbezüglich ein bedeutsames „Übungsfeld" darstellt, erhielten mittel- und langfristig negative Konsequenzen exzessiven Computerspielens Jugendlicher für romantische Beziehungen in der Forschung bislang wenig Aufmerksamkeit.

In der Literatur wurden wiederholt negative *Beeinträchtigungen des Leistungsniveaus* und der Konzentrations- und Aufmerksamkeitsfähigkeit von Jugendlichen durch zeitintensives Computerspielen berichtet und jüngst auch in

Längsschnittstudien belegt (Gnambs et al. 2020; Müller et al. 2015; Wright 2011; Von der Heiden et al. 2019). Eine plausible Erklärung dafür bieten die zwangsläufige Verdrängung anderer Aktivitäten wie Lernen oder Schlafen aufgrund der hohen Zeitintensität des Spielens, sowie die Störung des Aufbaus von Gedächtnisspuren insbesondere in der Konsolidierungsphase im Arbeitsgedächtnis zwischengespeicherter Lerninhalte aufgrund der mit dem Spielen verbundenen psychologischen und physiologischen Erregungszustände (Müller und Wölfling 2017b). Von einer Leistungsbeeinträchtigung scheinen allerdings Basiskompetenzen in Mathematik und Lesen selbst durch exzessives Spielen kaum betroffen zu sein (Drummond und Sauer 2014; Gnambs et al. 2020).

Bei Jugendlichen finden sich signifikante Zusammenhänge zwischen problematischem Computerspielen und vermehrtem *Zigaretten- und Cannabiskonsum* (z. B. Van Rooij et al. 2014; Mérelle 2017). Ein missbräuchlicher Cannabiskonsum zeigt sich in unserer Erfahrung biografisch meist nach der Entwicklung exzessiver Spielgewohnheiten und scheint bei mangelnder Entwicklung bzw. Verlernen anderer Copingstrategien als zusätzliche Strategie zur Stimmungsregulation eingesetzt zu werden. Verhaltenssüchte könnten sich untereinander bzw. mit substanzgebundenen Abhängigkeiten gegenseitig aufschaukeln (Burleigh et al. 2019).

Hinsichtlich der *physischen Gesundheit* sind vor allem Einflüsse auf Schlafdauer und -qualität bedeutsam. Die durchschnittliche tägliche Schlafdauer von Teenagern hat sich in den letzten 30 Jahren um kritische 2 h verringert (Hysing et al. 2015). Hale und Guan (2015) fanden in einem umfangreichen Review in 90 % der gesichteten Studien einen Zusammenhang zwischen Bildschirmzeit Jugendlicher und verringerter Schlafdauer oder späteren Bettzeiten. In einem rezenten Review finden Sugaya et al. (2019) in allen gesichteten Studien bei Vorliegen einer Gaming Disorder negative Effekte auf den Schlaf von Jugendlichen. Jugendliche mit weniger Schlaf haben schlechtere Noten, ein geringeres Selbstwertgefühl, eine schlechtere Emotionsregulation, depressive Symptome, höhere Feindseligkeit und Aggression, eine allgemein schlechtere Stimmung und emotionale Probleme bis hin zu vermehrten Suizidgedanken (Dahl 2006; Fredriksen et al. 2004; Sarchiapone et al. 2014). Physische Auswirkungen von Schlafmangel betreffen vor allem das Risiko für Übergewicht, Fettleibigkeit und Insulinresistenz (Cappuccio et al. 2008; Nightingale et al. 2017). Langfristiger Schlafmangel erhöht, teils vermittelt über ungünstigeres gesundheitsrelevantes Verhalten schlafdeprivierter Jugendlicher (Chen et al. 2006), das allgemeine Krankheitsrisiko, insbesondere für spätere Herz-Kreislauf-Erkrankungen (Figueiro et al. 2011; Fountas et al. 2018). Problematisches Computerspielen geht mit einem sedentären Lebensstil und einem geringeren Ausmaß körperlicher Aktivität einher (Fotheringham et al. 2000; Mérelle et al. 2017). In einer Längsschnittstudie belegen Altenburg et al. (2012) die Kausalitätsrichtung des Zusammenhangs zwischen Bildschirmzeit und Übergewicht von Jugendlichen. Allerdings scheinen die Effekte eher durch die Verlagerung von Aktivitäten ins Digitale verursacht zu werden, als durch die Aktivität des Computerspielens selbst (Bell et al. 2015).

8   Wie wird man computerspielsüchtig?

In einem frühen kognitiv-behavioralen Modell unterscheidet Davis (2001) eine generalisierte (viele bzw. alle Anwendungen umfassend) von einer spezifischen Form pathologischer Internetnutzung (nur spezieller Inhalte, z. B. Online-spiel). Die *generalisierte Form* wird als eigenständige Entität nicht über einen Suchtcharakter definiert, sondern stellt das Vorliegen typischer dysfunktionaler Kognitionen über die Beziehung des Nutzers mit seinem realen und virtuellen sozialen Umfeld in den Vordergrund (z. B. „offline bin ich wertlos, aber online bin ich jemand" oder „online behandeln mich andere Menschen besser als off-line"). Die exzessive Internetnutzung dient dabei zum Ausgleich bestimmter Defizite wie z. B. soziale Isolation oder unzureichende soziale Unterstützung. Die *spezifische Form* wird als Folge bereits zuvor bestehender psychischer Störungen angesehen. Trotz der teilweisen Überholtheit des Dachkonstrukts „Internetsucht", das wichtige Unterschiede zwischen verschiedenen suchtartigen Nutzungs-formen vernachlässigt (Starcevic und Billieux 2017), bleibt Davis' Idee der kompensatorischen Nutzung ein wichtiger Erklärungsansatz.

Ein aktuelles Erklärungsmodell (Scerri et al. 2019) für die Motivation zum zeitintensiven Computerspielen verknüpft Davis' (2001) Ansatz mit Annahmen der Self-Determination-Theory (Ryan und Deci 2000). Der SDT zufolge ist Selbstbestimmung derjenige Mechanismus, über den sich Menschen in Tätig-keiten engagieren, die für die Entwicklung und Erfüllung des eigenen Potenzials für sie von Interesse sind. Die Stärke und Qualität der Motivation dieses Engagements hängt vom Ausmaß ab, in dem die Tätigkeit die Befriedigung von drei nach der SDT permanent und kulturübergreifend existierenden psycho-logischen Grundbedürfnissen ermöglicht: *Kompetenz* (effektiv auf die subjektiv bedeutsamen Dinge einwirken können und die gewünschten Resultate zu erzielen), *Autonomie* (Gefühl der Freiwilligkeit der Ausführung des Verhaltens) und *soziale Eingebundenheit* (gekennzeichnet durch gegenseitig zugemessene Bedeutung einer Person für die Gruppe, und umgekehrt). Die Befriedigung dieser psychologischen Grundbedürfnisse ist sowohl für psychische Gesundheit und Wohlbefinden, als auch für die langfristige Internalisierung und Integration von Verhaltensweisen von zentraler Bedeutung (Deci und Ryan 2000). Aufgrund unzureichender Möglichkeiten zur Bedürfnisbefriedigung oder deren aktiver Frustration durch externe Faktoren der Umwelt können Defizite in den Grundbedürfnissen entstehen. Computerspiele stellen dann ein leicht zugängliches und schnell verfügbares Mittel dar, um diese zu befriedigen: Sie werden freiwillig als Freizeitausgleich zu erlebten Verpflichtungen gewählt *(Autonomieerleben)*, können durch ihre ausgeklügelte Verstärkerstruktur und fortwährend erfasste Daten den Spielverlauf individuell anpassen und sind daher vor allem in der Anfangsphase von vielen kleinen Erfolgen und hohem Selbstwirksamkeitserleben geprägt, führen mithin zu hohem *Kompetenzerleben*. Insbesondere in teambasierten Spielen mit verteilten, durch spezifische Eigenschaften oder Fähigkeiten versehenen Rollen (z. B. Magier, Heiler, etc.), besteht im Team eine hohe gegenseitige Abhängigkeit für den Spieleerfolg (z. B. Erfüllung einer Mission) und eine affektive Aufwertung der Gruppe durch die gemeinsamen positiven Erlebnisse *(soziale Eingebundenheit)*. Insofern kann Computerspielen einerseits grundsätzlich einen positiven Beitrag zum Wohlbefinden leisten. Andererseits kann es der Internalisierung problematischer Strategien Vorschub leisten, wenn Jugendliche sich in einem exzessiven Maß dem Spielen zuwenden, und aufgrund der damit verbundenen Folgen in eine Spirale geraten, in der eine Bedürfnisbefriedigung außerhalb des Spielens immer schwieriger wird. Erste empirische Befunde bestätigen, dass Gamer mit erlebten Defiziten in der Bedürfnisbefriedigung im Sinne der SDT ein geringeres Selbstwertgefühl aufweisen, mit höherer Wahrscheinlichkeit eine depressive Symptomatik und infolge ein suchtartiges Spielverhalten als Emotionsregulationsstrategie entwickeln (Scerri et al. 2019). Die psychologischen Grundbedürfnisse bzw. diesbezügliche Defizite könnten somit als auslösende (bei mangelnder Erfüllung im realen Leben) als auch aufrechterhaltende (wenn das Gaming die Bedürfnisse befriedigt) Faktoren fungieren.

Andere Ansätze zum Verständnis der Manifestation süchtigen Computerspielens sind eher typologischer Natur. Rho et al. (2016) identifizieren bei jungen Computerspielsüchtigen ab 20 Jahren sechs zentrale Prädiktoren: Durchschnittliche tägliche Spielzeit, durchschnittliche Spielzeit an arbeits- bzw. unterrichtsfreien Tagen, Teilnahme an Offline-Treffen mit der Gaming Community, Spielkosten, Beziehungsstatus, sowie ein selbst als süchtig wahrgenommenes Spielverhalten. Deren jeweilige Ausprägungen dienen als Indikatoren, mit denen anhand eines Entscheidungsbaums eine Klassifizierung nach drei verschiedenen Suchtmustern bzw. Typologien vorgenommen wird: „cost consuming" (investiert regelmäßig und in Summe größere Geldbeträge ins Computerspielen), „socializing" (investiert sowohl Zeit als auch Geld und hat physisch Kontakt zur Spielecommunity[2]) und „solidary" (charakterisiert als Single ohne jegliche längerfristige Beziehungserfahrung).

Einem integrativen biopsychosozialen Ansatz folgt das Modell der Interaction of Person-Affect-Cognition-Execution („I-PACE"; Brand et al. 2016 2019), das basierend auf der aktuellen Empirie potenzielle Mechanismen integrierend zusammenfasst, die zur Entwicklung und Aufrechterhaltung von Computerspielsucht beitragen, und sich damit vorbehaltlich der weiteren Validierung des Gesamtmodells gut für eine detailliertere Beschreibung des Prozesscharakters der Suchtentwicklung eignet. Im Zentrum des Modells steht namensgebend die Interaktion zwischen prädisponierenden Merkmalen einer Person (psychologische und neurobiologische Faktoren wie frühe Kindheitserfahrungen, genetische Faktoren), affektiven und kognitiven Prozessen (z. B. Reizreaktivität, Craving und Inhibitionskontrolle), sowie Umweltvariablen bzw. digitalen Medien. Ferner berücksichtigt das Modell verschiedene Mediatoren und Moderatoren (z. B. habituelle Coping-Strategien, subjektive Wirkungserwartungen an die Effekte der Internetnutzung, bestimmte kognitive Verzerrungen).

Je nach persönlichen Eigenschaften und nutzungsspezifischen Bedürfnissen, Motiven und Werten reagiert eine Person mit einer spezifischen Wahrnehmung auf die äußeren und inneren Stimuli, die mit dem Computerspielen verbunden sind. Die jeweilige Wahrnehmung löst eine entsprechende individuelle affektive und kognitive Reaktion aus. Die Summe der Reaktionen des Organismus auf solche Hinweisreize auf physiologischer, behavioraler und subjektiver Ebene wird als Reizreaktivität bezeichnet. Zu Beginn einer Suchtentwicklung folgt noch eine bewusste Entscheidung für das Aufnehmen der Spieltätigkeit, d. h. selbst bei auftretenden starken Spieleimpulsen ist im Zweifelsfall noch eine inhibitorische Kontrolle möglich. Auch wenn durch das Spielen bereits negative Konsequenzen im täglichen Leben auftreten (z. B. Konflikte mit den Eltern), überwiegt anfangs noch der belohnende Charakter (positive Verstärkung). Dies begünstigt sowohl die Herausbildung computerspielassoziierter Belohnungserwartungen, als auch eines bestimmten Coping-Stils im Umgang mit internen Triggern. Belohnungserwartungen und Coping-Stil verändern über die Zeit in einer ständigen Rückkopplungsschleife wiederum die Wahrnehmung der Hinweisreize selbst und die Reaktion auf diese. Im weiteren Verlauf erhöht sich zunehmend die Reizreaktivität im Sinne einer verstärkten Reaktionsbereitschaft auf Stimuli, die das belohnende Verhalten ankündigen, sowie das Verlangen nach

---

[2] gemeint sind die in Korea typischen „Computercafés".

dem Spiel („craving"), was wiederum sukzessive die spezifische inhibitorische Kontrolle über das Nutzungsverhalten beeinträchtig. Mit dem Computerspielen verbundene äußere (z. B. Bildschirm, Tastatur) und innere Reize (z. B. Gefühls-zustände) werden salienter wahrgenommen (Prinzip der Anreizhervorhebung) und teilweise automatisiert durch Ausführen des entsprechenden Nutzungs-verhaltens beantwortet. Die anfangs bewusste Entscheidung zum Spielen wird somit sukzessive durch spezifische habituelle Verhaltensweisen abgelöst, so dass in einem Kontext verminderter exekutiver Kontrolle wiederholt exzessive Konsumsituationen auftreten können, die durch Konditionierungsprozesse immer weiter konsolidiert werden. Daraufhin nehmen die negativen Konsequenzen im täglichen Leben zu (z. B. schulische Leistung, Beziehungsabbrüche), die schließlich die positiven Konsequenzen überwiegen. Dass Betroffene eine akzentuierte emotionale Verarbeitung suchtassoziierter Reize aufweisen, weist, analog zu Substanzabhängigkeiten, auf eine Sensibilisierung des mesolimbischen dopaminergen Belohnungssystems hin (Kuss und Griffiths 2012). Im Extremfall und bei Vorliegen weiterer Risikofaktoren „spezialisiert" sich das Belohnungs-system also bei wiederholter Nutzung aufgrund belohnungsassoziierter Lern-prozesse auf einen schmalen Bereich spielebezogener Reize, was die Aufnahme ursprünglich attraktiver alternativer Verhaltensweisen bzw. Tätigkeiten subjektiv weniger belohnend macht, und Veränderungen mithin erschwert. In späteren Phasen stehen dann bei der Aufrechterhaltung der suchtartigen Nutzung weniger die angenehmen Folgen des Spielens, als vielmehr die Vermeidung unan-genehmer Gefühlszustände, Konflikte und belastender Situationen im Vorder-grund (negative Verstärkung).

9   EXKURS: Problematisches Glückspielen bei Jugendlichen

Wenngleich „Spielsucht"[3] im Jugendkontext eher die Assoziation zu Computer-spielen weckt, sollen überblicksartig auch die mit dem Drängen klassischer Glücksspielangebote verbundenen Risiken in die Welt von Jugendlichen adressiert werden, die sich der massiven Werbung über TV, Webseiten, In-App-Werbung auf dem Smartphone etc. kaum entziehen können. Pathologisches

---

[3]Anders als im Deutschen und Französischen („jeu de hasard") kann Glücksspielen im angelsächsischen Raum mit „Gambling" zurecht auch sprachlich von anderen Formen des Spielens („Games") abgegrenzt werden.

Glücksspielen ist seit über zwei Jahrzehnten als Störungsbild in den Diagnose-systemen DSM und ICD zu finden, und wurde in deren letzten Ausgaben unter der Bezeichnung „Glücksspielstörung" den Abhängigkeitserkrankungen zugeordnet. Dass trotz Altersbeschränkungen und unabhängig vom sozio-kulturellen Kontext mehr als die Hälfte aller Heranwachsenden Erfahrungen mit Glücksspielen unterschiedlicher Art machen, wird in internationalen Studien konsistent belegt (Delfabbro et al. 2016). Eine signifikante Minderheit Jugend-licher erlebt im Zusammenhang mit diesen deutlichen Belastungen: So reichen die Angaben zur Prävalenz glücksspielbezogener Probleme in europäischen Ländern von 0,2 % bis 12,3 % (vgl. Calado et al. 2016). Grundsätzlich gelten Jugendliche und junge Erwachsene als besonders gefährdet, zumindest temporär glücksspielbezogene Probleme und Belastungen zu entwickeln (Fiedler und Hayer 2016). Vor allem Geldspielautomaten, Sportwetten und Poker üben für Jugendliche einen relativ hohen Spielanreiz aus (Hayer 2012).

Erste Kontakte mit *klassischem Glücksspiel* erfolgen zunehmend im „virtuellen Raum". Die aktuelle Expansion des Glücksspielmarktes ist besonders eng mit der Kommerzialisierung des *Sportwettens* verknüpft, für das ein kaum überschaubares Onlineangebot privater Wettanbieter besteht[4]. Die Teilnahme daran fußt im Wesentlichen auf einer generellen Begeisterung für Sport, einem selbstzugeschriebenen Fachwissen und dem damit einhergehenden Irrglauben, diese Expertise in einfacher Weise monetarisieren zu können. Gerade im Jugend-alter dürften kognitive Verzerrungsmuster wie die Überschätzung der eigenen Einflussnahme auf den Spielausgang problematischen Entwicklungen Vorschub leisten (Fiedler und Hayer 2016). Neue Produktformate an der Schnittstelle von Wetten und Geschicklichkeitsspielen richten sich vor allem an junge Menschen. So kann beim *eSports Betting* auf den Ausgang von Computerspielen gewettet werden, während bei *Fantasy Sports* in einer Art Managerspiel eine imaginäre Mannschaft aus tatsächlich existierenden Spielern zusammengestellt wird. Die Umsätze allein aus dem eSports haben sich zwischen 2012 und 2019 um durch-schnittlich 30 % jährlich (in Summe fast 750 %) erhöht. Für 2020 wurde ein

---

[4] Exemplarisch listet die Plattform „online.casinocity.com" 93 französischsprachige, 152 deutschsprachige, 307 englischsprachige und 97 Webseiten in portugiesischer Sprache auf, die Sportwetten von Luxemburg aus in der Euro-Währung erlauben. Unter Berück-sichtigung anderer Glücksspielformen und Währungen kann aus Luxemburg auf 2273 von insgesamt 4147 gelisteten Webseiten online gespielt werden (Abruf 13.01.2021).

Umsatz von 1,8 Mrd. US$ vorhergesagt[5]. In der Adoleszenz spielen zudem informelle, privat organisierte Sportwetten in der Peer-Gruppe eine bedeutsame Rolle (Fiedler und Hayer 2016).

Ein Erstkontakt findet häufig zunehmend über *simulierte Glücksspiele* statt, die zwar keinen direkten Einsatz von echtem Geld erfordern, ansonsten aber aufgrund des Einsatzes virtueller Währung und eines als zufallsbedingt wahrgenommenen Spielausgangs strukturell identisch mit klassischen Glücksspielformaten sind. Durch gezielte Werbung verstärkt erhöhen sie die Wahrscheinlichkeit für einen späteren Umstieg zu klassischem Glücksspiel und fördern, durch spielimmanente Faktoren wie gesteuerte Spielausgänge, Spiellust und kognitive Verzerrungsmuster (Meyer et al. 2015; Fiedler und Hayer 2016; Hayer und Brosowski 2016).

Die Einführung *glücksspielartiger Elemente in Computerspielen* stellt eine neue Dimension in der aktuellen Entwicklung dar, der Einzug von In-Game-Kaufsystemen (z. B. Mikrotransaktionen, „Lootboxes") hat diese bedeutsam verändert.

Eine *Lootbox* enthält eine zufällige Auswahl virtueller Items und kann wiederholt unter Einsatz echten Geldes gekauft werden. Die geringe Wahrscheinlichkeit, das gewünschte Item (z. B. eine bestimmte Waffe, die einem im Spiel weiterbringt) zu erhalten bedeutet, dass der Spieler eine unbestimmte Anzahl von Lootboxes erwerben muss, um das Item zu erhalten. Der von implementierten Mechanismen her klare Glücksspielcharakter ist strukturell z. B. mit Slotmachines oder Rubbellosen identisch, jedoch wird in vielen Ländern kontrovers diskutiert, inwieweit es sich juristisch um finanzielle „Verluste" und „geldwerte Vorteile" handelt (King und Delfabbro 2018). So scheitert in Luxemburg die Subsumtion unter den Glücksspielbegriff an dessen juristischer Definition (Reding 2019).

In den vergangenen Jahren hat sich vor allem im Mobilmarktsegment *Free-to-Play* – eine von der Spieleindustrie selbst gewählte, Kostenlosigkeit suggerierende Bezeichnung – als dominierendes Geschäftsmodell entwickelt (Schaack et al. 2017). Da Gewinne nur über die Animation zum regelmäßigen Bezahlen erwirtschaftet werden können, werden Spielende in einer langfristig angelegten Strategie per Design über einen längeren Zeitraum ins Spiel eingeführt. Ihnen wird der Freiraum gelassen, das Spiel zu explorieren und sich „ein-

---

zuleben". Gerade dann, wenn es besonders spannend wird, werden sie z. B. über Limitierung der täglichen Spieldauer oder der Menge verfügbarer Inhalte durch eine Paywall[6] ausgebremst, die jederzeit durch Bezahlen einer Ingamewährung umgangen werden kann, die durch echtes Geld erworben werden kann. Zudem lassen sich im Ingame-Shop oft kostenpflichtige Extras erwerben. Das Verrechnen von realem Geld und virtueller Währung erfolgt allerdings in einer fragwürdigen Mechanik nach „krummen" Faktoren, welche den tatsächlichen Wert verschleiern und suggerierte „Schnäppchen" durch Einkauf gleich größerer Mengen der virtuellen Währung schwerer beurteilen lassen. In Deutschland müssen mittlerweile an Kinder gerichtete Aufforderungen von Spieleanbietern, besonders schnell oder günstig kostenpflichtige Angebote zu erwerben oder Dienstleistungen in Anspruch zu nehmen, nach einem Urteil des BGH vom 18.09.2014 (AZ.: I ZR 34/12) unterbleiben.

Nach Dreier et al. (2017) haben 37 % aller Jugendlichen im Alter zwischen 12 und 18 Jahren bereits Erfahrungen mit Free-to-Play-Spielen, wobei die rasante Verbreitung des Geschäftsmodells einen mittlerweile höheren Anteil nahelegt. In Supermärkten, Tankstellen und Postfilialen zu erwerbende Prepaidkarten erlauben jungen Menschen nahezu barrierefrei echtes Geld in eine virtuelle Geldbörse laden und damit innerhalb von Gaming-Apps kaufen zu können. Sowohl süchtig, als auch riskant spielende Gamer weisen ein erhöhtes Risiko auf, in Spielen mit Monetarisierungsstrategien mehr Zeit und reales Geld zu verlieren als nichtproblematische Nutzer. In Fachstellen hilfesuchende junge Gamer gaben 2016 hierfür durchschnittlich 2.601,02 € aus (Schaack et al. 2017). Nicht von ungefähr bezeichnet die Gamingbranche in Analogie zu Begriffen im Poker Gamer solche Gamer, die über längere Zeitbeträge mit hohen Geldbeträgen spielen, als „Whales" (dt. Wale).

King et al. (2019) charakterisieren in ihrer Analyse verschiedener Patente für In-Game-Kaufsysteme einige aufgrund der implementierten Taktiken als unfair oder ausbeuterisch. In-Game-Kaufsysteme implementieren nach King et al. (2019) mitunter unfaire oder ausbeuterische Taktiken, indem sie gezielt Informationsvorteile durch Verfolgen von Nutzeraktivitäten am PC und Möglichkeiten der Datenmanipulation ausnutzen, indem z. B. zur Maximierung der Wahrscheinlichkeit kontinuierlicher In-Game-Käufe damit ein individuell zugeschnittener Kaufpreis „optimiert" wird (Preis, Kontext, Timing). Auf der

---

[6] Eine Paywall (Bezahlschranke) blockiert, ähnlich wie beim kostenpflichtigen Zugang bestimmter Inhalte einer Online-Zeitung, dauerhaft oder temporär das Weiterspielen insgesamt oder den Zugang zu bestimmten Spielbereichen oder Inhalten.

anderen Seite werden nur eingeschränkte oder keine Garantien oder Schutzmechanismen (z. B. Anrecht auf Erstattung) implementiert. Aufgrund der Gefahr
für vulnerable Spieler empfehlen die Autoren, Richtlinien eines ethisches Game-
Designs und weitere Verbraucherschutzmaßnahmen entgegenzusetzen. Kriterien
zur Alterseinstufung und eine klare und unmissverständliche Kennzeichnung
digitaler Spiele mit Glücksspielelementen könnten Erziehungsberechtigte über
eine dadurch nahegelegte achtsame Begleitung ihrer Kinder in ihrer suchtpräventiven Kompetenz stärken (Schaack et al. 2017). Insgesamt stellt die Einführung von Monetarisierungsstrategien in Computerspielen in der aktuellen
Entwicklung aus suchtpräventiver Perspektive eine kritische neue Dimension dar.

10   Fazit und praktische Implikation für die Prävention

Häufiges bis tägliches Computerspielen ist in den meisten Fällen unbedenk-
lich und Teil der Alltagsgestaltung besonders männlicher Jugendlicher. Mit dem
hohen Anteil Computerspielender an der jugendlichen Gesamtpopulation geht
allerdings einher, dass eine substanzielle Minderheit problematisch und süchtig
spielt, mit entsprechenden leistungsmäßigen, psychosozialen und gesundheitlichen Folgen auf individueller, sowie sozialen und wirtschaftlichen Kosten auf
gesellschaftlicher Ebene. Die aktuelle Literatur betont daher die höchste klinische
und gesundheitspolitische Relevanz der Verhinderung oder Verzögerung des Aus-
bruchs internetbezogener und komorbider Störungen durch Prävention, sowie
die Verkürzung der Krankheitsdauer durch Frühintervention (Szász-Janocha
et al. 2019). Welche längerfristigen Auswirkungen der deutliche Anstieg der
durchschnittlichen täglichen Spielzeiten während der aktuell noch andauernden
Corona-Pandemie diesbezüglich mit sich bringt, beginnt sich gerade abzu-
zeichnen (DAK 2020).

Im Gegensatz zum Konsum legaler oder illegaler Drogen stellt Computerspielen allerdings an sich keinen Problemcharakter dar, sondern kann bei
moderater Nutzung zur Steigerung des Wohlbefindens beitragen und je nach
Spielcharakter potenziell selektive kognitive Fähigkeiten fördern. Daher ist ein
Gleichsetzen mit Drogenkonsum weder zielführend, noch praktikabel. Im Alltag der Erziehung und der Jugendarbeit kann eine konsequente Unterscheidung
zwischen temporär exzessivem, problematischem und süchtigem Spielen
(Gaming Disorder) einer inflationären Verwendung des Suchtbegriffs entgegenwirken, die Gefahr birgt, dass Hinweise auf „Suchtgefahren" von Jugendlichen
letztlich weniger ernst genommen werden oder verstärkt Reaktanz auslösen,

sowie die Kluft zwischen Panikmache und Herunterspielen zu vergrößern. Bei Eltern und professionell mit Jugendlichen Arbeitenden kann ferner eine Sensibilisierung und gesteigerte Achtsamkeit für den dimensionalen Charakter und die gesamte Bandbreite möglicher Symptome problematischen Spielens einer kategorialen oder in der Praxis oft vorgefundenen Fixierung auf das problematische Kriterium der mit Spielen verbrachten Zeit entgegenwirken und eine differenziertere Wahrnehmung von Unterschieden fördern. Dies unterstützt sowohl das frühere Erkennen problematischer Entwicklungen, als auch die feinstufigere Wahrnehmung und Rückmeldung positiver Veränderungen. Auf dieser Basis wiederum können Nutzungszeiten durchaus hilfreich zur Verlaufskontrolle und Anzeige der vom Betroffenen ausgeübten Selbstkontrolle über das gestörte Spielverhalten sein (Stavrou 2018).

Bereits Betroffene bzw. für diese Verantwortliche suchen meistens spät, oft erst nach Einbruch schulischer Leistungen, professionelle Hilfe auf. Neben Sensibilisierung und Information über möglichst niederschwellige Hilfsangebote könnte daher ein regelmäßiges Screening nach auffälligem Nutzungsverhalten, sowie bei dessen Vorliegen nach psychopathologischer Symptomatik auch außerhalb klinischer Settings sinnvoll und nützlich sein, um betroffenen Jugendlichen und deren Bezugspersonen möglichst zeitnah passende Angebote anbieten bzw. kooperativ gemeinsam mit diesen gegenregulierenden Maßnahmen ergreifen zu können. Jugendliche zeigen ein deutlich höheres Bewusstsein für Auswirkungen, die das Spielen auf sie selbst hat, als für solche auf ihre Beziehungen zur Umwelt, insbesondere auf Schule und Familie (Bonnaire und Phan 2017). Wer Nebeneffekte weniger ernst nimmt, spielt zudem exzessiver (Allahverdipour et al. 2010). Dies betont die Bedeutung des sozialen Umfelds als Frühwarnsystem. Dieses steht oft vor der Herausforderung, die Problematik auf eine Reaktanz minimierende Weise anzusprechen, die vorbestehende Konflikte nicht weiter verschärft. Dabei ist in der Regel hilfreich, dass statt einer sorgengetriebenen Verteufelung das Gaming zunächst als grundsätzlich legitime Freizeitbeschäftigung mit für die Entwicklung einiger kognitiver Fähigkeiten sogar potenziell förderlichem Charakter anerkannt wird. Bei der erneuten Etablierung einer „Game-Life-Balance" bzw. in klinischen Fällen einer möglichen Spieleabstinenz ist ferner die Unterstützung beim Verständnis der individuell zugrunde liegenden Nutzungsmotive bedeutsam, für die auch offline hinreichend Möglichkeiten der Befriedigung zur Verfügung stehen sollten (Scerri et al. 2019), sowie klar zwischen kurz- und langfristigen Konsequenzen des Spielens zu unterscheiden und diese für sich selbst identifizieren zu können (Von der Heiden et al. 2019).

Suchtentwicklung beginnt auch bei Computerspielabhängigen meist bereits im Jugendalter, wobei Minderjährige aufgrund der altersbedingten Unterentwicklung kognitiver Kontrolle besonders anfällig sind (Sugaja et al. 2019). Ihnen gegenüber steht eine Gaming-Industrie, welche im Rahmen aktuellen Monetarisierungsstrategien anhand permanent gesammelter Daten zum Online-verhalten die Nutzungszeiten in aller Regel zu verlängern sucht. Primärpräventiv können Maßnahmen der lebensweltorientierten und kompetenzfördernden Sucht-prävention Spielende und Betreuende bei der Entwicklung eines bewussten und kompetenten Umgangs mit Computerspielen, dem Aufbau psychosozialer Ressourcen, sozialer Kompetenzen und solcher zur Stressbewältigung, sowie dem Angebot alternativer Freizeitaktivitäten unterstützen. Vor dem Hintergrund der Zusammenhänge zwischen mit Gaming verbrachter Zeit und verringerter körperlicher Aktivität und sedentärem Lebensstil, kommt dabei insbesondere Interventionsprogrammen zur Förderung körperlicher und sportlicher Aktivität während des Teenageralters eine hohe Bedeutung zu. Vor dem Hintergrund einer breiten Erreichbarkeit und der dort verbrachten Lebenszeit bietet sich vor allem die Schule dafür als ideales Setting an.

Ein verbreiteter Mangel an zeitlichen Vorgaben und elterlicher Kontrolle der Mediennutzung (König und Steffgen 2015; DAK 2020) fördert eine ungünstige Mediensozialisation und legt auch Eltern als Zielgruppe primärpräventiver Bemühungen nahe, um diese bei der Entwicklung und Etablierung von Nutzungs-regeln in der Familie zu unterstützen. Um der während der Pubertät bestehenden generellen Rhythmusverschiebung (Exelmans und Van den Bulck 2017) und mangelndem Schlaf nicht weiter Vorschub zu leisten, sollte wegen des erhöhten psychophysiologischem Erregungsniveaus beim Spielen und der bildschirm-induzierten Melatoninsuppression vor allem die abendliche Nutzung adressiert werden. Das oft höhere Kompetenzniveau im Vergleich zur Erwachsenenwelt erlaubt Kindern und Jugendlichen das schnelle Umgehen von Maßnahmen, die für sie verantwortliche Erwachsenen zur Regulation des Mediennutzungsver-haltens ergriffen haben, ohne dass diese davon Kenntnis nehmen (Evers-Wölk und Opielka 2016). Insofern bietet sich auch eine Stärkung deren technischer Kompetenz an. Regulierung und verbesserte Kontrollmöglichkeiten sind allerdings kein Ersatz dafür, stets mit Kindern und Jugendlichen in Beziehung zu bleiben und ein authentische Interesse für ihre Onlineaktivitäten zu zeigen, um sie angemessen beim Aufbau eines gesunden Nutzungsverhaltens begleiten und bei Auffälligkeiten ein Gespräch über etwaige psychische und soziale Probleme aktiv aufzusuchen zu können, sowie diese bei Bedarf zu ermutigen, professionelle Hilfsangebote in Anspruch zu nehmen – oder dies mit gutem Beispiel voraus-gehend selbst zu tun.

Literatur

Allahverdipour, H., Bazargan, M., Farhadinasab, A. & Moeini, B. (2010). Correlates of video games playing among adolescents in an Islamic country. *BMC Public Health, 10 (286)*, 2–7.

Allison, S. E., von Wahlde, L., Shockley, T. & Gabbard, G. O. (2006). The development of the self in the era of the Internet and role-playing fantasy games. *The American Journal of Psychiatry, 163(3)*, 381–385.

Anderson, E.L., Steen, E. & Stavropoulos, V. (2016). Internet use and Problematic Internet Use: A systematic review of longitudinal research trends in adolescence and emergent adulthood. *International Journal of Adolescence and Youth, 22(4)*, 430-454.

Altenburg, T.M., Singh, A.S., van Mechelen, W., Brug, J. & Chinapaw, M.J.M. (2012). Direction of the association between body fatness and self-reported screen time in Dutch adolescents. *International Journal of Behavioral Nutrition and Physical Activity* 9, 4. https://doi.org/10.1186/1479-5868-9-4

Batthyány, D., Müller, K.W., Benker, F. & Wölfling, K. (2009). Computerspielverhalten: Klinische Merkmale von Abhängigkeit und Missbrauch bei Jugendlichen. *Wiener Klinische Wochenschrift, 121*, 502–509.

Bell, V., Bishop, D.V & Przybylski, A.K. (2015). The debate over digital technology and young people. *BMJ 2015; 351*. https://doi.org/10.1136/bmj.h3064

Bonnaire, C. & Phan, O. (2017). Negative Perceptions of the Risks Associated With Gaming in Young Adolescents: An Exploratory Study to Help Thinking About a Prevention Program. *Archives de Pédiatrie, 24(7): 607–617.*

Brand, M., Rumpf, H.-J., King, D.L., Potenza, M.N. & Wegmann, E. (2020). Clarifying terminologies in research on gaming disorder and other addictive behaviors: distinctions between core symptoms and underlying psychological processes. *Current Opinion in Psychology. 36*, 49–54.

Brand, M., Wegmann, E., Stark, R., Müller, A., Wölfling, K., Robbins, T. W., & Potenza, M.N. (2019). The Interaction of Person-Affect-Cognition-Execution (I-PACE) model for addictive behaviors: Update, generalization to addictive behaviors beyond internet-use disorders, and specification of the process character of addictive behaviors. *Neuroscience and Biobehavioral Reviews, 104, 1–10.*

Brand, M., Young, K. S., Laier, C., Wölfling, K., & Potenza, M. N. (2016). Integrating psychological and neurobiological considerations regarding the development and maintenance of specific Internet-use disorders: An Interaction of Person-Affect-Cognition-Execution (I-PACE) model. *Neuroscience and Biobehavioral Reviews, 71,* 252–266.

Burleigh, T.L., Griffiths, M.D., Sumich, A. et al. (2019). A systematic review of the co-occurrence of gaming disorder and other potentially addictive behaviors. Current Addiction Reports. *Current Addiction Reports, 6,* 383–401.

Calado, F., Alexandre J., & Griffiths, M.D. (2016). Prevalence of Adolescent Problem Gambling: A Systematic Review of Recent Research. *Journal of Gambling Studies, 33,* 397–424.

Cappuccio, F. P., Taggart, F. M., Kandala, N. B., Currie, A., Peile, E., Stranges, S., & Miller, M. A. (2008). Meta-analysis of short sleep duration and obesity in children and adults. *Sleep, 31(5).* 619–626. https://doi.org/10.1093/sleep/31 5.619

Carli, V., Durkee, T., Wasserman, D., Hadlaczky, G., Despalins, R., Kramarz E., et al. (2013). The association between pathological internet use and comorbid psychopathology: a systematic review. *Psychopathology. 46(1)*, 1–13. doi:https://doi. org/10.1159/000337971.

Coyne, S. M., Stockdale, L. A., Warburton, W., Gentile, D. A., Yang, C., & Merrill, B. M. (2020). Pathological video game symptoms from adolescence to emerging adulthood: A 6-year longitudinal study of trajectories, predictors, and outcomes. *Developmental Psychology, 56(7)*, 1385–1396.

Chang, F., Chiu, C.H., Lee, C., Chen, P., & Miao, N. (2014). Predictors of the initiation and persistence of internet addiction among adolescents in Taiwan. *Addictive behaviors, 39 (10)*, 1434–1440.

Chen, M. Y., Wang, E. K., & Jeng, Y. J., (2006). Adequate sleep among adolescents is positively associated with health status and health-related behaviors: BMC. Public Health, v. 6, p. 59.

Cho, S., Sung, M., Shin, K.M., Lim, K.Y., & Shin, Y.M. (2013). Does Psychopathology in Childhood Predict Internet Addiction in Male Adolescents? *Child Psychiatry & Human Development, 44*, 549–555.

DAK (2020). *Gaming und Social Media in Zeiten von Corona. DAK-Längsschnittstudie: Befragung von Kindern, Jugendlichen (12 – 17 Jahre) und deren Eltern.* https://www. dak.de/dak/download/internetsucht-studie-pdf-2106324.pdf (Abruf 30.12.2020)

Davis, R. A. (2001). A cognitive–behavioral model of pathological internet use. *Computers in Human Behavior, 17*, 187–195.

Dahl, R. E. (2006). Sleeplessness and aggression in youth [Editorial]. Journal of Adolescent Health, 38(6), 641–642. https://doi.org/10.1016/j.jadohealth.2006.03.013

Deci, E.L. & Ryan, R.M. (2000). The „What" and „Why" of Goal Pursuits: Human Needs and the Self-Determination of Behavior, *Psychological Inquiry 11(4)*, 227–268.

Delfabbro, P., King, D.L. & Derevensky, J.L. (2016). Adolescent gambling and problem gambling: Prevalence, current issues, and concerns. Current Addiction Reports, 3 (2), 268-274.

Demetrovics, Z., Urbán, R., Nagygyörgy, K., Farkas, J., Zilahy, D., Mervó, B., Reindl, A., Ágoston, C., Kertész, A. & Harmath, E. (2011). Why do you play? The development of the motives for online gaming questionnaire (MOGQ). *Behavior Research Methods, 43*, 814–825.

Deutsche Hauptstelle für Suchtfragen (2020). *Ergebnisse der gemeinsamen Arbeitsgruppe „Problematisches Computerspielen und Computerspielstörung (Gaming Disorder)" der Deutschen Hauptstelle für Suchtfragen e.V. und des Fachverbands Medienabhängigkeit e.V.. Bestandsaufnahme und Positionierung in den Bereichen Prävention und Frühinter- vention, Beratung, Behandlung und Rehabilitation sowie Forschung.* https://www.dhs. de/fileadmin/user_upload/pdf/news/Ergebnispapier_AG_Problematisches_Computer- spielen_und_Gaming_Disorder.pdf (Abruf: 15. September 2020).

Drachen, A., Nacke, L. E., Yannakakis, G., & Pedersen, A. L. (2010). Correlation between heart rate, electrodermal activity and player experience in first-person shooter games. 5th ACM SIGGRAPH Symposium on Video Games, Los Angeles. 49–54.

Dreier, M., Wölfling, K., Duven, E., Giralt, S., Beutel, M. E., & Müller, K. W. (2017). Free-to-play: About addicted Whales, at risk Dolphins and healthy Minnows. Monetarization design and Internet Gaming Disorder. *Addictive behaviors, 64*, 328-333.

Drummond, A. & Sauer, J.D. (2014). Video-Games Do Not Negatively Impact Adolescent Academic Performance in Science, Mathematics or Reading. *PLoS ONE 9(4): e87943.* https://doi.org/10.1371/journal.pone.0087943

Eichenberg, C. (2014). Internetsucht geht mit unsicherer Bindung einher. *Deutsches Ärzteblatt, 6,* 269–271.

Evers-Wölk, M. & Opielka, M. (2016). *Neue elektronische Medien und Suchtverhalten.* Berlin: Büro für Technikfolgen-Abschätzung beim Deutschen Bundestag.

Exelmans, L., & Van den Bulck, J. (2017). Bedtime, shuteye time and electronic media: Sleep displacement is a two-step process. *Journal of Sleep Research, 26,* 363–370.

Feierabend, S., Rathgeb, T. & Reutter, T. (2020). *JIM-Studie 2019. Jugend, Information, Medien: Basisuntersuchung zum Medienumgang 12- bis 19-Jähriger.* Stuttgart: Medienpädagogischer Forschungsverbund Südwest. https://www.mpfs.de/fileadmin/ files/Studien/JIM/2019/JIM_2019.pdf

Fam, J.Y. (2018). Prevalence of internet gaming disorder in adolescents: A meta-analysis across three decades. *Scandinavian Journal of Psychology, 59(5),* 524–531. doi:https:// doi.org/10.1111/s op.12459.

Feng, W., Ramo, D. E., Chan, S. R., & Bourgeois, J. A. (2017). Internet Gaming Disorder: Trends in Prevalence 1998-2016. *Addictive Behaviors 75,* 17–24. https://doi. org/10.1016/j.addbeh.2017.06.010

Fiedler, I. & Hayer, T. (2016). Sportwetten und Jugendliche: Spielangebote und Suchtgefahren. *Pro Jugend: Fachzeitschrift der Aktion Jugenaschutz Landesarbeitsstelle Bayern e.V..* 4–9.

Figueiro, M.G., Wood, B., Plitnick, B., & Rea, M.S. (2011). The impact of light from computer monitors on melatonin levels in college students. *Neuroendocrinology Letters* 32(2): 158-163.

Fotheringham, M.J., Wonnacott, R.L. & Owen, N. (2000). Computer use and physical inactivity in young adults: Public health perils and potentials of new information technologies. *Annals of Behavioral Medicine, 22 (4),* 269–275.

Fountas, E.,Stratinaki, M., Kyrzopoulos, S., Tsiapras, D., Iakovou, I., Athanasopoulos, G. & Voudris, V. (2018). Relationship between sleep duration and cardiovascular disease: a meta-analysis, *European Heart Journal,* 39 (1), P2540, doi:https://doi.org/10.1093/ eurheartj/ehy565.P2540

Fredriksen, K., Rhodes, J., Reddy, R., & Way, N. (2004). Sleepless in Chicago: tracking the effects of adolescent sleep loss during the middle school years. Child Development, 75(1), 84 – 95.

Fritz, J., Lampert, C., Schmidt J.H. & Witting, T. (2011). *Kompetenzen und exzessive Nutzung bei Computerspielern – gefordert, gefördert, gefährdet.* Berlin: Vistas,

Gervasi, A.M., La Marca, L., Costanzo, A., Pace, U., Guglielmucci, F., & Schimmenti, A. (2017). Personality and Internet Gaming Disorder: a Systematic Review of Recent Literature. *Current Addiction Reports, 4,* 293–307.

Gentile, D.A., Choo, H., Liau, A., Sim, T., Li, D., Fung, D. & Khoo, A. (2011). Pathological video game use among youths: a two-year longitudinal study. *Pediatrics, 127,* 318–330.

Gnambs, T., Stasielowicz, L., Wolter, I., & Appel, M. (2020). Do computer games jeopardize educational outcomes? A prospective study on gaming times and academic achievement. *Psychology of Popular Media, 9, 69–82.* doi:https://doi.org/10.1037/ppm0000204

Granic, I., Lobel, A., & Engels, R. (2014). The benefits of playing video games. *American Psychologist, 69,* 66–78.

Grescher M., Lindenberg K., Reck C., et al. (2013). Bindungsstile bei Probanden mit und ohne pathologischen Internetgebrauch. Poster auf dem DGPPN Kongress, 28.11.2013, Berlin.

Griffiths, M. D., van Rooij, A. J., Kardefelt-Winther, D., Starcevic, V., Király, O., Pallesen, S., Müller, K., Dreier, M., Carras, M., Prause, N., King, D. L., Aboujaoude, E., Kuss, D. J., Pontes, H. M., Lopez Fernandez, O., Nagygyorgy, K., Achab, S., Billieux, J., Quandt, T., Carbonell, X., … Demetrovics, Z. (2016). Working towards an international consensus on criteria for assessing internet gaming disorder: a critical commentary on Petry et al. (2014). *Addiction (Abingdon, England), 111(1), 167–175.*

Hale, L., & Guan, S. (2015). Screen time and sleep among school-aged children and adolescents: a systematic literature review. *Sleep medicine reviews, 21,* 50-58.

Hartmann, T., & Klimmt, C. (2006). Gender and Computer Games: Exploring Females' Dislikes. *Journal of Computer-Mediated Communication, 11,* 910–931.

Hayer, T. (2012). Jugendliche und glücksspielbezogene Probleme: Risikobedingungen, Entwicklungsmodelle und Implikationen für präventive Handlungsstrategien. Frankfurt/M.: Peter Lang.

Hayer, T. & Brosowski, T. (2016). Simuliertes Glücksspiel im Internet: Anmerkungen zu möglichen (Sucht-) Gefahren aus psychologischer Sicht. *Praxis Klinische Verhaltensmedizin und Rehabilitation, 97,* 4–12.

Ho, R.C., Zhang, M.W.B., Tsang, T.Y., Toh, A.H., Pan, F., Lu, Y. et al. (2014). The association between internet addiction and psychiatric co-morbidity: A meta-analysis. *BMC Psychiatry, 14, 183.* doi:https://doi.org/10.1186/1471-244X-14-183.

Hu, J., Zhen, S., Yu, C., Zhang, Q., & Zhang, W. (2017). Sensation Seeking and Online Gaming Addiction in Adolescents: A Moderated Mediation Model of Positive Affective Associations and Impulsivity. *Frontiers in psychology, 8,* 699. https://doi.org/10.3389/fpsyg.2017.00699

Huang, C. (2010). Internet use and psychological well-being: A meta-analysis. *Cyberpsychology, Behavior and Social Networking, 13(3),* 241–249.

Hysing, M., Pallesen, S., Stormark, K. M., Jakobsen, R., Lundervold, A. J., & Sivertsen, B. (2015). Sleep and use of electronic devices in adolescence: results from a large population-based study. *BMJ open, 5(1),* e006748. https://doi.org/10.1136/bmjopen-2014-006748

Jeong, J. E., Rhee, J. K., Kim, T. M., Kwak, S. M., Bang, S. H., Cho, H., Cheon, Y. H., Min, J. A., Yoo, G. S., Kim, K., Choi, J. S., Choi, S. W., & Kim, D. J. (2017). The association between the nicotinic acetylcholine receptor α4 subunit gene (CHRNA4) rs1044396 and Internet gaming disorder in Korean male adults. *PloS one, 12(12),* e0188358. https://doi.org/10.1371/journal.pone.0188358

King, D. & Delfabbro, P. (2018). Video Game Monetization (e.g., 'Loot Boxes'): a Blueprint for Practical Social Responsibility Measures. *International Journal of Mental Health and Addiction, 10,* doi:1007/s11469–018–0009–3.

King, D. L., Delfabbro, P. H., Gainsbury, S. M., Dreier, M., Greer, N., & Billieux, J. (2019). Unfair play? Video games as exploitative monetized services: An examination of game patents from a consumer protection perspective. *Computers in Human Behavior, 101,* 131–143. https://doi.org/10.1016/j.chb.2019.07.017

König, A. & Steffgen, G. (2015). Mediennutzung Jugendlicher in Luxemburg. Aktueller Überblick zur Nutzung von Internet und Computerspielen und erste Prävalenzdaten zur dysfunktionalen Nutzung. Luxembourg: University of Luxembourg.

Ko, C.H., Yen, J.Y., Yen, C.F., Chen, C.S. & Chen, C.C. (2012). The association between Internet addiction and psychiatric disorder: a review of the literature. *European Psychiatry, 27(1),* 1–8.

Ko, C.H., Yen, J.Y., Chen, C.S., Yeh, Y.C. & Yen, C.F. (2009). Predictive values of psychiatric symptoms for internet addiction in adolescents: a 2-year prospective study. *Archives of pediatrics & adolescent medicine, 163*(10): 937–943.

Koepp, M. J., Gunn, R. N., Lawrence, A. D., Cunningham, V. J., Dagher, A., Jones, T., Brooks, D. J., Bench, C. J., & Grasby, P. M. (1998). Evidence for striatal dopamine release during a video game. *Nature, 393*(6682), 266–268. https://doi.org/10.1038/30498

Kuss, D.J. & Griffiths, M.D. (2012). Online gaming addiction in adolescence: A literature review of empirical research. *Journal of Behavioural Addiction, 1,* 3–22.

Kuss, D.J., Griffiths, M.D., Karila, L., & Billieux, J. (2014). Internet addiction: a systematic review of epidemiological research for the last decade. *Current pharmaceutical design, 20* (25), 4026–4052.

Lampen-Imkamp, S., te Wildt, B. (2009). Phänomenologie, Diagnostik und Therapie der Internet- und Computerspielabhängigkeit. In: Hardt J, Cramer-Düncher U, Ochs, M (Hrsg.): *Verloren in virtuellen Welten. Computerspielsucht im Spannungsfeld von Psychotherapie und Pädagogik,* 120–131. Göttingen: Vandenhoeck & Ruprecht.

Latham, A. J., Patston, L. L., & Tippett, L. J. (2013). The virtual brain: 30 years of video-game play and cognitive abilities. *Frontiers in Psychology, 4* (629), 1–10.

Lei, L., & Wu, Y. (2007). Adolescents' paternal attachment and Internet use. *Cyberpsychology & behavior: the impact of the Internet, multimedia and virtual reality on behavior and society, 10*(5), 633–639. https://doi.org/10.1089/cpb.2007.9976

Lemmens, J. S., Valkenburg, P. M., & Peter, J. (2011). Psychosocial causes and consequences of pathological gaming. *Computers in Human Behavior, 27,* 144–152.

Lindenberg, K., Halasy, K., Szász-Janocha, C., & Wartberg, L. (2018). A Phenotype Classification of Internet Use Disorder in a Large-Scale High-School Study. *International Journal of Environmental Research and Public Health, 15(4).* doi:https://doi.org/10.3390/ijerph15040733

Lindenberg, K., Szász-Janocha, C., Schoenmaekers, S., Wehrmann, U., & Vonderlin, E. (2017). An analysis of integrated health care for Internet Use Disorders in adolescents and adults. *Journal of Behavioral Addictions, 6(4),* 579–592.

Mehroof, M., & Griffiths, M. D. (2010). Online gaming addiction: The role of sensation seeking, self-control, neuroticism, aggression, state anxiety, and trait anxiety. *Cyberpsychology, Behavior, and Social Networking, 13(3),* 313–316.

Mérelle, S. Y. M., Kleiboer, A. M., Schotanus, M., Cluitmans, T. L. M., Waardenburg, C. M., Kramer, J., van de Mheen, D., & van Rooij, A. J. (2017). Which Health-Related Problems Are Associated with Problematic video-gaming or social media use in adolescents? A large cross-sectional study. *Clinical Neuropsychiatry: Journal of Treatment Evaluation, 14(1),* 11–19.

Meyer, G., Brosowski, T. von Meduna, M. & Hayer, T. (2015). Simuliertes Glücksspiel. Analyse und Synthese empirischer Literaturbefunde zu Spielen in internetbasierten sozialen Netzwerken, in Form von Demoversionen sowie Computer- und Videospielen. *Zeitschrift für Gesundheitspsychologie, 23 (4),* 153–168.

Monacis, L., De Palo, V., Griffiths, M.D. & Sinatra, M. (2017). Exploring Individual Differences in Online Addictions: the Role of Identity and Attachment. *International journal of mental health and addiction 15 (4),* 853–868.

Montag, C., Schivinski, B., Sariyska, R., Kannen, C., Demetrovics, Z. & Pontes, H.M. (2019). Psychopathological symptoms and gaming motives in disordered gaming – a psychometric comparison between the WHO and APA diagnostic frameworks. *Journal of Clinical Medicine, 8,* 1–18.

Müller, K.W., Beutel, M.E., Dreier, M., & Wölfling, K. (2019). A clinical evaluation of the DSM-5 criteria for Internet Gaming Disorder and a pilot study on their applicability to further internet-relateddisorders. *Journal of Behavioral Addictions, 8(3),* 1–9.

Müller, K. W., Janikian, M., Dreier, M., Wölfling, K., Beutel, M. E., Tzavara, C., Richardson, C., & Tsitsika, A. (2015). Regular gaming behavior and internet gaming disorder in European adolescents: results from a cross-national representative survey of prevalence, predictors, and psychopathological correlates. *European child & adolescent psychiatry,* 24(5), 565–574. https://doi.org/10.1007/s00787-014-0611-2

Müller, K.W. & Wölfling, K. (2017a). Both sides of the story: addiction is not a pastime activity: commentary on: scholars' open debate paper on the World Health Organization ICD-11 Gaming Disorder proposal (Aarseth et al.). *Journal of Behavioral Addictions, 6,* 118–120. doi: https://doi.org/10.1556/2006.6.2017.038

Müller, K.W. & Wölfling, K. (2017b). *Pathologischer Mediengebrauch und Internetsucht.* Stuttgart: Kohlhammer.

Nightingale, C.M., Rudnicka, A.R., Donin, A.S., Sattar, N., Cook, D.G., Whincup, P.H. & Owen, C.G. (2017). Screen-time is associated with adiposity and insulin resistance in children. *Archives of Disease in Childhood, 102 (7),* 612–616.

Park, J., Sung, J.Y., Kim, D.K., Kong, I.D., Hughes, T.L. & Kim, N. (2018). Genetic Association of Human Corticotropin-Releasing Hormone Receptor 1 (CRHR1) With Internet Gaming Addiction in Korean Male Adolescents. *BMC Psychiatry, 18(1):*396. doi: https://doi.org/10.1186/s12888-018-1974-6.

Paulus, F. W., Ohmann, S., von Gontard, A., & Popow, C. (2018). Internet gaming disorder in children and adolescents: a systematic review. *Developmental medicine and child neurology, 60(7),* 645–659. https://doi.org/10.1111/dmcn.13754

Porter G., Starcevic V., Berle D. &, Fenech P. (2010). Recognizing problem video game use. *Australian and New Zealand Journal of Psychiatry, 44(2),* 120–128.

Reding, L. (2019). *Der gesetzliche Rahmen des Glücksspiels in Luxemburg.* Spills De? 15 ans de l'asbl «Anonym Gléckspiller» 25. September 2019, Hesperange, Luxemburg.

Rehbein, F. & Baier, D. (2013). Family-, Media-, and School-Related Risk Factors of Video Game Addiction. *Journal of Media Psychology,25(3),*118–128.

Rehbein, F., Hayer, T., Baier, D. & Mößle, T. (2015). Psychosoziale Risikoindikatoren regelmäßiger und riskanter Glücksspielnutzung im Jugendalter: Ergebnisse einer bundesland-repräsentativen Schülerbefragung. *Kindheit und Entwicklung, 24,* 171 – 180.

Ra, C.K., Cho, J., Stone, M.D., De La Cerda, J. Goldenson, N.I., Moroney, E., Tung, I., Lee, S.S. & Leventhal, A.M. (2018). Association of digital media use with subsequent symptoms of attention-deficit/hyperactivity disorder among adolescents. *Journal of the American Medical Association, 320(3)*, 255–263.

Rho, M.J., Jeong, J.E., Chun, J.W., Cho, H., Jung,D.J., Choi, I. Y., & Kim, D.-J. (2016). Predictors and patterns of problematic Internet game use using a decision-tree model. *Journal of Behavioral Addictions 5 (3)*, 500–509.

Rothmund, T., Klimmt, C. & Gollwitzer, M. (2018). Low Temporal Stability of Excessive Video Game Use in German Adolescents. *Journal of Media Psychology, 30*, 53–65.

Russoniello, C., O'Brien, K. & Parks, J.M. (2009). The effectiveness of casual video games in improving mood and decreasing stress. *Journal of Cyber Therapy and Rehabilitation 2(1)*, 53–66.

Ryan, R.M. & Dec, E.L. (2000). Self-Determination Theory and the Facilitation of Intrinsic Motivation, Social Development, and Well-Being, *American Psychologist 55*, 68–78.

Sarchiapone, M., Mandelli, L., Carli, V., Iosue, M., Wasserman, C., Hadlaczky, G., Hoven, C.W., Apter, A., Balazs, J., Bobes, J., Brunner, R., Corcoran, P., Cosman, D., Haring, C., Kaess, M., Keeley, H., Keresztény, A., Kahn, J.P., Postuvan, V., Mars, U., Saiz, P.A., Varnik, P., Sisask, M. & Wasserman, D. (2014). Hours of sleep in adolescents and its association with anxiety, emotional concerns, and suicidal ideation. *Sleep Medicine, 15(2):* 248–54.

Schaack, C., Dreier, M. & Wölfling, K. (2017). *Glücksspielelemente in Computerspielen. Wie ein Trend aus Japan bedenkliche Standards setzt.* Landeszentrale für Gesundheitsförderung Rheinland-Pfalz e.V.

Schneider, L. A., King, D. L., & Delfabbro, P. H. (2017). Family factors in adolescent problematic Internet gaming: A systematic review. *Journal of Behavioral Addictions, 6(3)*, 321–333.

Schulte-Markwort, M., Plaß, A., & Barkmann, C. (2002) *Internet und familiäre Beziehungen.* In W. Hantel-Quitmann & P. Kastner (Eds.), Die Globalisierung der Intimität. Gießen, Germany: Psychosozial-Verlag.

Scerri, M., Anderson, A., Stavropoulos, V. & Hu, E. (2019). Need fulfilment and internet gaming disorder: A preliminary integrative model. *Addictive Behaviors Reports, 9*, 100158. https://doi.org/10.1016/j.abrep.2018.100158

Shi, L., Wang, Y., Yu, H.,Wilson, A., Cook, S., Duan, Z., Peng, K., Hu., Z., Ou, J., D, S., Yang, Y., Ge, J., Wang, H., Chen, L., Zhao, K. & Chen, R (2020). The relationship between childhood trauma and Internet gaming disorder among college students: A structural equation model. *Journal of Behavioral Addiction, 9(1)*, 175–180.

Starcevic, V. & Billieux, J. (2017). Does the construct of internet addiction reflect a single entity or a spectrum of disorders? *Clinical Neuropsychiatry, 14(1)*, 5–10.

Stavrou, P.D. (2018). Addiction to video games: A case study on the effectiveness of psychodynamic psychotherapy on a teenager addict struggling with low self-esteem and aggression issues. *Psychology, 9*, 2436–2456. doi https://doi.org/10.4236/psych.2018.91014C.

Sugaya, N., Shirasaka. T., Takahashi, K., & Kanda, H. (2019). Bio-psychosocial factors of children and adolescents with Internet gaming disorder: A systematic review. *BioPsychoSocial Medicine, 13(1).* doi: https://doi.org/10.1186/s13030-019-0144-5

Sweetser, P. & Wyeth, P. (2005). GameFlow: A Model for Evaluating Player Enjoyment in Games. *Computers in Entertainment, 3. (3)*, 1–24.

Szász-Janocha, C., Halasy, K., Kindt, S. & Lindenberg, K. (2019). Prävention und Frühintervention bei Internetbezogenen Störungen - (inter-)nationaler Stand der Forschung, *Suchtmedizin, 21 (4)*, 259–271.

Thomasius, R. (2018). Nachrichten aus der DG-Sucht. *Sucht 64 (4)*, 225–227. doi: https://doi.org/10.1024/0939-5911/a000554

Tsitsika, A., Critselis, E., Louizou, A., Janikian, M., Freskou, A., Marangou, E., Kormas, G., & Kafetzis, D. (2011). Determinants of Internet addiction among adolescents: a case-control study. *The Scientific World Journal, 11*, 866–874. https://doi.org/10.1100/tsw.2011.85

Valkenburg, P.M. & Peter, J. (2009). Social Consequences of the Internet for Adolescents: A Decade of Research. Current Directions in Psychological Science, 18 (1), 1–5.

Van Rooij, A.J., Kuss, D.J., Griffiths, M.D., Shorter, G.W., Schoenmakers, T.M. & Van de Mheen, D. (2014). The (Co-)Occurrence of Problematic Video Gaming, Substance Use, and Psychosocial Problems in Adolescents. *Journal of Behavioral Addictions, 3(3)*, 157–165

Van Rooij, A. J., Schoenmakers, T. M., Vermulst, A. A., Van den Eijnden, R. J., & Van de Mheen, D. (2011). Online video game addiction: identification of addicted adolescent gamers. *Addiction (Abingdon, England), 106*(1), 205–212. https://doi.org/10.1111/j.1360-0443.2010.03104.x

von der Heiden, J. M., Braun, B., Müller, K. W., & Egloff, B. (2019). The association between video gaming and psychological functioning. Frontiers in Psychology, 10, 1721: https://doi.org/10.3389/fpsyg.2019.01731

Wartberg, L., Kriston, L., Kammerl, R., Petersen, K. U., & Thomasius, R. (2015). Prevalence of pathological internet use in a representative German sample of adolescents: results of a latent profile analysis. *Psychopathology, 48*(1), 25–30. https://doi.org/10.1159/000365095

Wartberg, L., Kriston, L., & Thomasius, R. (2017). The Prevalence and Psychosocial Correlates of Internet Gaming Disorder. *Deutsches Arzteblatt International, 114(25)*, 419–424. https://doi.org/10.3238/arztebl.2017.0419

Wang, J.-L., Jackson, L. A., & Zhang, D.-J. (2011). The mediator role of self-disclosure and moderator roles of gender and social anxiety in the relationship between Chinese adolescents' online communication and their real-world social relationships. *Computers in Human Behavior, 27(6)*, 2161–2168. https://doi.org/10.1016/j.chb.2011.06.010

Wang, J.L., Jackson, L.A., Gaskin, J. & Wang, H.Z. (2014). The effects of Social Networking Site (SNS) use on college students'friendship and well-being. *Computers in Human Behavior, 37*, 229–236.

Wright, J. (2011). The effects of video game play on academic performance. *Modern Psychological Studies, 17(1)*, 37–44.

Yen, J.Y., Yen, C.F., Chen, C.C., Chen, S.H. & Ko, C.H. (2007). Family factors of internet addiction and substance use experience in Taiwanese adolescents. *Cyberpsychology, Behavior and Social Networking, 10(3)*, 323–329. doi: https://doi.org/10.1089/cpb.2006.9948.

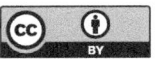

Geschlechterbezogene Rollen und Stereotype und ihre Auswirkungen auf das Leben Jugendlicher und junger Erwachsener

Miriam-Linnea Hale, Elisabeth Holl und André Melzer

1   Wohlbefinden und Soziale Medien

Wohlbefinden stellt ein komplexes und multidimensionales Konzept dar, das unterschiedlich definiert werden kann. Allgemein wird Wohlbefinden als Balance zwischen den Ressourcen einer Person und den sich ihr stellenden Herausforderungen verstanden. Bestehen in einer gegebenen Situation, die psychisch, sozial und/oder körperlich herausfordernd ist, jedoch keine entsprechend ausreichenden Ressourcen, ist das Wohlbefinden einer Person bedroht (Dodge et al. 2012). Keyes et al. (2002) unterscheiden zwei Betrachtungsweisen von Wohlbefinden. Hedonistisch subjektiv ist Wohlbefinden durch Lebenszufriedenheit, positive Affekte und weitgehende Abwesenheit negativer Emotionen definiert. Demgegenüber berücksichtigt die eudaimonische Sicht das psychologische Wohlbefinden, und damit nicht nur um das Erleben von Glück, sondern zudem um die Verwirklichung von Potenzialen, die als grundlegende psychologische Bedürfnisse Kompetenz, Autonomie und soziale Eingebundenheit umfassen (Deci und Ryan 2000). Die hedonistischen und eudaimonischen Aspekte von Wohlbefinden

M.-L. Hale (✉) · E. Holl · A. Melzer
Department of Behavioural and Cognitive Sciences, University of Luxembourg,
Esch-sur-Alzette, Luxembourg
E-Mail: miriam-linnea.hale@uni.lu

E. Holl
E-Mail: elisabeth.holl@uni.lu

A. Melzer
E-Mail: andre.melzer@uni.lu

© Der/die Autor(en) 2022
A. Heinen et al. (Hrsg.), *Wohlbefinden und Gesundheit im Jugendalter*,
https://doi.org/10.1007/978-3-658-35744-3_19

425

werden nach Su et al. (2014) unter dem Begriff des *Thriving* zusammengefasst, der als Zustand positiven Funktionierens mentale, psychische und soziale Elemente einschließt. *Thriving* beinhaltet nach Su et al. (2014) mit Beziehung, Engagement, Können, Autonomie, Sinn, Optimismus und subjektivem Wohlbefinden insgesamt sieben Komponenten.

Vor dem Hintergrund der ständig steigenden Popularität sozialer Medien wird in der Forschung seit einiger Zeit die Frage nach dem Zusammenhang zwischen der zunehmend intensiveren Nutzung dieser Medien und dem Wohlbefinden der Nutzerinnen und Nutzer gestellt. Allerdings sind die derzeit vorliegenden Ergebnisse uneinheitlich. So werden etwa Studien berichtet, in denen insbesondere die nächtliche Nutzung sozialer Medien sowie ein hohes Maß an emotionaler Involviertheit in diese Medienangebote zu schlechterem Schlafverhalten, geringerem Selbstwertgefühl sowie größerer Ängstlichkeit und Depression führte (Woods und Scott 2016). Andere Studien sehen speziell die Nutzungshäufigkeit von Instagram negativ an depressive Symptome, Selbstwert, das generelle und körperliche Erscheinungsbild sowie Körperzufriedenheit gekoppelt, wobei insbesondere einer starken sozialen Vergleichsorientierung eine vermittelnde Funktion zukommen soll (Sherlock und Wagstaff 2019). Durchaus beeindruckend sind die Befunde zweier repräsentativer Studien mit insgesamt über 500.000 Adoleszenten in den Vereinigten Staaten, die starke Zusammenhänge zwischen der Nutzung neuer Medien und psychischen Gesundheitsproblemen nahelegen (Twenge et al. 2018). Demgegenüber liegt jedoch auch eine Reihe an Befunden vor, die eine solche negative Korrelation nicht nachweisen konnten. So erwies sich die generelle Nutzung sozialer Medien nicht als signifikanter Prädiktor für psychische Gesundheit (Berryman et al. 2018). Zudem wiesen Orben und Przybylski (2019) mithilfe eines statistischen Verfahrens (Specification Curve Analysis) nach, dass der korrelative Nachweis aus den vorstehenden Befunden einer genaueren Analyse nicht standhält. Die Autoren gehen daher davon aus, dass der negative Zusammenhang zwischen der Nutzung digitaler Technologien und dem Wohlbefinden von Jugendlichen tatsächlich zu klein ausfällt, um entsprechende Warnungen bezüglich der Nutzung auszusprechen.

Allen genannten Studien gemein ist jedoch ihre querschnittliche, wenn auch z. T. repräsentative Natur, die zudem keine kausalen Inferenzen erlaubt. Demgegenüber bietet die Studie von Heffer et al. (2019) eine längsschnittliche Betrachtung. Anhand zweier Stichproben, in denen Jugendliche bzw. junge Bachelorstudierende über zwei bzw. sechs Jahre beobachtet wurden, konnte keinerlei Zusammenhang zwischen der Nutzung sozialer Medien und depressiver Symptomatik nachgewiesen werden. Dieser Befund zeigte sich unabhängig vom Geschlecht der Teilnehmer*innen. Im Unterschied zudem ausgebliebenen

Sozialisationseffekt konnten die Autor*innen jedoch einen Selektionseffekt nachweisen, nach dem das Vorliegen einer depressiven Symptomatik mit einer stärkeren sozialen Mediennutzung bei adoleszenten Mädchen einherging.

2 Videospiele und Wohlbefinden

Neben der Nutzung sozialer Medien steigt seit mehreren Jahren weltweit auch die Zahl an (insbesondere jungen) Menschen, die sich in ihrer Freizeit mit Videospielen beschäftigen (Entertainment Software Association 2018). Im Jahr 2018 spielten in Deutschland 58 % der 12- bis 19-Jährigen mindestens mehrmals pro Woche, und zwar durchschnittlich 103 min pro Wochentag (Medienpädagogischer Forschungsverbund Südwest 2018). Die steigende Nutzung von Videospielen veranlasste auch die psychologische Forschung sich hauptsächlich mit den negativen, aber auch den positiven Aspekten von Gaming im Zusammenhang mit jugendlichem Wohlbefinden zu beschäftigen. Insbesondere Kinder und Jugendliche wurden hinsichtlich ihrer Videospielgewohnheiten befragt, da sie als Hochrisikogruppe für dysfunktionale psychosoziale Entwicklungen gesehen werden.

Am bekanntesten ist diesbezüglich sicher die fortgesetzte Debatte um Transfereffekte gewalthaltiger Videospiele auf Aggression und Sozialverhalten (Anderson et al. 2010; Ferguson 2015; Prescott et al. 2018), die aufgrund widersprüchlicher Befunde weiterhin ungeklärt ist. So konnte eine längsschnittliche Studie zwar zeigen, dass eine längere Spielzeit mit erhöhten emotionalen Problemen bei Kindern zusammenhängt, aber keine Beziehung zwischen gewalthaltigen Videospielen und psychosozialen Veränderungen bei Kindern nachweisbar ist (Lobel et al. 2017). Andere Studien belegen zwar den Zusammenhang zwischen Bildschirmzeiten und Verhaltensproblemen bei Kindern, allerdings nur für längeren Fernsehkonsum, nicht aber für Videospiele (Parkes et al. 2013).

Eine Vielzahl von Studien beschäftigt sich außerdem mit dem Suchtpotential von Videospielen (z. B. Gentile et al. 2017), welches schließlich 2019 zu einer eigenständigen Klassifizierung als Abhängigkeitserkrankung unter dem Namen „Gaming disorder" im ICD-11 führte (World Health Organization 2019). Dabei schwankt die Prävalenz von Computerspielabhängigkeit je nach untersuchter Population (Allgemeinbevölkerung vs. Gamern) zwischen 0.7 % bis 27.5 % (Feng et al. 2017; Mihara und Higuchi 2017). Insgesamt scheinen Männer, junge Menschen und asiatische Populationen stärker betroffen zu sein (Sussman et al. 2018). Am Beispiel des beliebten Online-Multiplayer-Spiel *World of Warcraft* (Blizzard Entertainment 2004) ließ sich zeigen, das

Spieler*innen dieses bevorzugt bei geringerem Wohlbefinden (d. h. hoher Stress und ein niedriges Selbstwertgefühl) nutzen, um vor Problemen im Alltag in die virtuelle Welt zu entfliehen (Kardefelt-Winther 2014). Dass diese eskapistische Motivation wiederum einen direkten Einfluss auf das Wohlbefinden der Spieler hat, konnte ebenfalls für Online-Multiplayer gezeigt werden (Kaczmarek und Drazkowski 2014). Zusammen mit fehlender Selbstregulation könnte diese ungünstige Form des Coping durch Eskapismus als Negativspirale wiederum zu exzessiver Nutzung und sogar Abhängigkeitssymptomatik führen (Kardefelt-Winther 2014; LaRose et al. 2003).Demgegenüber belegen empirische Studien aber auch einen positiven Effekt der Videospielnutzung auf die Entwicklung von Jugendlichen. Bei einer Befragung von Highschool-Schüler*innen schnitten regelmäßige Spieler*innen besser bei Variablen wie schulischem Engagement, psychischer Gesundheit, Selbstkonzept, familiärer Nähe, Freundschaften und Freizeitaktivitäten ab als Nicht-Spieler*innen (Durkin und Barber 2002). Weiterhin fanden Studien mit Stichproben aus dem asiatischen Raum Indizien für eine Aufwärtsspirale von prosozialen und kooperativen Videospielen und realem prosozialem Verhalten bei Jugendlichen (Gentile et al. 2009). Andere Untersuchungen belegen Zusammenhänge zwischen verschiedenen Videospielgenres und erhöhter Kreativität, Problemlösefähigkeit, räumlicher Wahrnehmung und Aufmerksamkeitsleistungen, positiven Emotionen und Entspannung sowie sozialen Kompetenzen und Prosozialität (Granic et al. 2014). Weiterhin konnte durch die motivierende und ablenkende Wirkung von lernorientierten Spielen, den sogenannten Serious Games[1], im Medizinsektor eine Verbesserung für Krebs, Schmerz- und Angstpatient*innen erreicht werden (Kato 2010). Schließlich bestätigte Jugendforschung zu Exergames[2] den positiven Effekt der Nutzung solcher aktivierender Spiele auf die Gesundheit sowie die sozialen und schulischen Fähigkeiten (Staiano und Calvert 2011).

Diese gemischte Studienlage verdeutlicht, dass generelle Aussagen zum Zusammenhang von Videospielen und jugendlichem Wohlbefinden derzeit nicht möglich sind. Vielmehr müssen unterschiedliche Variablen genauer betrachtet werden: Aus welcher Motivation heraus spielen Kinder und Jugendliche? Welches Spiel wird wie gespielt (online vs. offline, kooperativ vs. kompetitiv,

---

[1] dt. ernsthafte Spiele, d. h. Videospiele, die nicht allein der Unterhaltung, sondern auch der Vermittlung von Lerninhalten dienen.

[2] dt. Fitnessspiele, d. h. Videospiele, die körperliche Bewegungen und Reaktionen als hauptsächliche Spielmechanik nutzen.

gewalthaltig vs. prosozial, etc.)? Welche Charakteristiken und Persönlichkeit bringen Spieler*innen mit?

Trotz der relativ umfangreichen Studienlage zu positiven und negativen Einflüssen von Videospielen sind Untersuchungen, die konkret das Wohlbefinden der Spieler*innen erfassen, bemerkenswert unterrepräsentiert. Nur eine der hier aufgeführten Studien erhebt subjektives Wohlbefinden durch ein direktes Maß (Steen Happiness Index; Kaczmarek und Drazkowski 2014). Häufig wird stattdessen indirekt von Drittvariablen (z. B., Aggression und prosoziales Verhalten: Anderson et al. 2010; Impulsivität: Gentile et al. 2012) auf das vermeintliche Wohlbefinden geschlossen. Daher empfiehlt es sich, diese Erkenntnislücke durch künftige Studien unter Einbeziehung des Wohlbefindens von Kindern und Jugendlichen als direkte Variable zu schließen.

3 Die Rolle von Geschlechterstereotypen

Nicht nur soziale Medien oder interaktive Medienangebote und deren Nutzung können eine Herausforderung für die individuelle Lebenszufriedenheit und das psychologische Wohlbefinden einer Person darstellen, sondern auch verallgemeinernde und stereotypisierende Zuschreibungen. Insbesondere Geschlechterstereotype sind in der Gesellschaft heutzutage weit verbreitet. Im Folgenden werden die Begriffe *Genderstereotype* oder *Geschlechterstereotype* sowie deren Auswirkungen auf die Lebensrealität und das Wohlbefinden junger Menschen beschrieben.

Genderstereotype werden in der Psychologie als kognitive Strukturen definiert, die sozial geteiltes Wissen über die charakteristischen Merkmale von Frauen und Männern beinhalten (Eckes 2004). Vermittelt werden diese Schemata durch Eltern, Schule, Freunde, Medien, politische Vorgaben und gesellschaftliche Haltungen. Eingesetzt werden sie, um Personen in unserer Wahrnehmung als Teil einer sozialen Gruppe zu kategorisieren. Eigenschaften werden dabei einer ganzen Gruppe („die Frauen"), sowie einzelnen Individuen innerhalb der Gruppe („typisch Mann") zugeschrieben, während zugunsten der Gruppenzugehörigkeit individuelle Eigenschaften ignoriert werden (Jussim et al. 1995).

Schon von Kindheit an wird unsere Wahrnehmung von gesellschaftlich-normativen Konzepten der Maskulinität und Femininität beeinflusst (Zosuls et al. 2011). Strampelanzüge sind entweder blau, oder rosa, der Ritter rettet die Prinzessin und „Jungs weinen nicht!". Im Rahmen der Sozialisierung werden geschlechterspezifische Normen und Werte von der Familie, den Medien und weiteren Bezugspersonen gelernt. Die Entwicklung von genderstereotypen

Überzeugungen von Hilflosigkeit und Macht bzw. Dominanz wird durch solche Sozialisierungsprozesse unterstützt (Martin et al. 2002).

Im Rahmen individueller Entwicklungsprozesse werden soziale Stereotype aufgenommen und über die Zeit als kulturelle Normen, Überzeugungen und Erwartungen internalisiert und zum Bestandteil der Identität. Die Aktivierung von Geschlechterrollen und Gendersstereotype erfolgt in der Regel unbewusst (z. B. was als „typisches" Verhalten von Männern und Frauen bezüglich ihrer Rolle in Beruf und Familie oder ihrer äußeren Erscheinung gilt, Gill und Gill 2007). Menschen sehen sowohl sich selbst wie auch andere durch diesen Filter der aktivierten Stereotype, so dass sowohl Fremd-, als auch Selbstwahrnehmung beeinträchtigt werden. In den Sozialwissenschaften werden solche Prozesse oft auch als *unconscious bias* (unbewusste Verzerrung; z. B. Easterly und Ricard 2011) bezeichnet. Nachweise für die Auswirkungen von Stereotypen finden sich beispielsweise in den Bereichen Wahrnehmung und Bewertung anderer (z. B. Heilman 2012), Selbstwert und Körperbild (z. B. Pennell und Behm-Morawitz 2015), Stigmatisierung und Prävalenz von sexuellen Übergriffen (z. B. Hill und Marshall 2018), Verhalten gegenüber anderen sowie Entscheidungen bezüglich der eigenen Studien- und Berufswahl (z. B. Cheryan et al. 2013).

Als eine Form geteilten sozialen Wissens sind Stereotype nicht statisch und unveränderbar, zudem sind solche Vorstellungen nicht überall dieselben. Vorherrschende Stereotype und ihre Repräsentation in den Medien verändern sich über die Zeit und Kulturen hinweg (Valentova 2013). Zusammenfassend entstehen geschlechterbezogene Stereotype im frühen Entwicklungsalter, können von etlichen Einflussfaktoren geprägt werden und sich über die Jahre entfalten und verfestigen. Die spezifischen Inhalte von solchen Stereotypen mögen sich verändern, die negativen Konsequenzen persistieren jedoch (z. B. Hill und Marshall 2018).

Aus diesem Grund wurde im Jahr 2018 in Luxemburg eine psychologische Studie durchgeführt, mit dem Ziel spezifische Ansatzpunkt für präventive Maßnahmen insbesondere für die jüngere Generation zu ermitteln. Aufgrund der jungen Zielgruppe lag der Schwerpunkt dieser Studie zusätzlich auf dem medialen Konsum und den Neuen und Soziale Medien. Der jährlichen Studie des Medienpädagogischen Forschungsverbundes Südwest (2018) zufolge, haben so gut wie alle Menschen im jugendlichen und jungen Erwachsenenalter täglich Umgang mit diesen Medien. 97 % der Jugendlichen besitzen ein Smartphone, während 66 % eine Spielkonsole benutzen. Durchschnittlich sind Jugendliche unter der Woche 214 min online. Mädchen verbringen diese Zeit statistisch gesehen vorwiegend mit Kommunikation und sozialen Medien, während Jungs eher Interesse an Spielen und Unterhaltung zeigen. Sieht man die heutige

Omnipräsenz und nahezu grenzenlose Verfügbarkeit neuer Medien im Alltag junger Menschen, ist es kaum überraschend, dass ein Fokus der Grundlagen- und Anwendungsforschung auf der Rolle von digitalen und sozialen Medien liegt, wenn es um den Kontext von Lernen und entwicklungsbezogenen Fragestellungen geht.

Die Forschung identifizierte Medien als einer der wichtigsten Faktoren für das soziale Lernen von Stereotypen (Scharrer 2013; Signorielli 2001). Dies geschieht über mediale Unterrepräsentation von Frauen (z. B. Greenberg und Worrell 2007; Signorielli 2001), sowie unrealistische Darstellungen der Geschlechter, was nachweislich zu negativen Konsequenzen für sowohl Männer und Frauen in den verschiedensten Bereichen führen kann, wie etwa Selbstbild und Körperwahrnehmung (Barlett et al. 2008; Groesz et al. 2002), sowie Beruf und Karrierechancen (World Bank 2011). Entsprechende Befunde liegen für verschiedene Medienformen von Fernsehen und Musikvideos (Turner 2011), bis hin zu Videospielen (Beasley und Collins Standley 2002; Melzer 2019) vor. In Anbetracht der stark zunehmenden Bedeutung sozialer Medien gerade für die jüngere Generation überrascht die für diese Medien eher geringe Menge an Forschung in diesem Bereich.

4   #Lëtzstereotype18 Studie[3]

Für die Untersuchung der Entstehung geschlechterbezogener Stereotype bietet sich der luxemburgische Kulturraum, geprägt von unterschiedlichen kulturellen Hintergründen, ganz besonders an. Deswegen wurde hierzu im Jahre 2018 im Auftrage des luxemburgischen Ministeriums für die Gleichstellung von Frauen und Männern (Ministère de l'Égalité des Chances) eine Studie zur Beurteilung der aktuellen Sachlage in Luxemburg durchgeführt. Nicht nur eine Erfassung des aktuellen Standes der vorherrschenden Rollenbilder und Stereotype in Bezug auf Geschlecht bei Jugendlichen und jungen Erwachsenen war das Ziel

---

[3] Im Rahmen der Beschreibung dieser Studie wird durchgängig von Teilnehmer*innen, Jungen/Mädchen oder Frauen/Männern berichtet. Die Studie beinhaltete selbstverständlich auch Teilnehmende, die sich nicht mit dem Genderbinär männlich-weiblich identifizierten. Jedoch war die Anzahl dieser Personen zu gering (Anzahl = 6) um im Rahmen einer Studie mit quantitativen Methoden statistisch aussagekräftige Ergebnisse zu ermöglichen. Eine genauere Beschreibung der Ergebnisse dieser Gruppe kann dem Bericht der Studie (Melzer et al. 2019) entnommen werden.

der Studie #Lëtzstereotype18 (Melzer et al. 2019), sondern auch eine Analyse der Einflussfaktoren, wie z. B. Eltern, Peers, Medienkonsum, oder sozioökonomischer Hintergrund. Des Weiteren wurde geprüft, welche Alltagsbereiche die jungen Teilnehmer*innen am stärksten von diesen Stereotypen und Rollenbildern betroffen sehen.

Somit ergaben sich folgende Hauptfragen für die #Lëtzstereotype18 Studie:[4]

1. *Wie ist das Geschlechterbild junger Luxemburgerinnen und Luxemburger? Welche Einstellungen und Erwartungen haben sie in Bezug auf die unterschiedlichen Geschlechter?*
2. *Welche Konsequenzen ergeben sich aus Sicht der befragten Jugendlichen und jungen Erwachsenen aus den wahrgenommenen geschlechtsbezogenen stereotypen Geschlechterüberzeugungen?*
3. *Was sind die von den Jugendlichen und jungen Erwachsenen wahrgenommenen Haupteinflussfaktoren dieser Genderstereotype und Geschlechterrollen, und welches Gewicht ordnen ihnen die Teilnehmerinnen und Teilnehmer zu?*

Vom 8. November bis zum 31. Dezember 2018 wurden im Rahmen der Studie unter dem Titel *#Lëtzstereotype18* Daten von insgesamt 396 Versuchspersonen erhoben, die online sowie auf Papierfragebögen in vier verschiedenen Sprachversionen (luxemburgisch, deutsch, französisch, portugiesisch) erfasst wurden. Tab. 1 zeigt die Alters- und Geschlechtsverteilung.

Zusätzlicher Bestandteil der Studie war es, dass Versuchsteilnehmer*innen einen vermeintlich echten Post auf dem sozialen Netzwerk *Instagram* sahen. So sah die eine Hälfte der Teilnehmer*innen zufallszugewiesen ein Foto mit zwei Personen in „traditioneller" stereotyper Verteilung der Rollen im Haushalt (d. h. der Mann trinkt Bier, während die Frau bügelt), wohingegen die andere Hälfte dieselbe Situation sah, in diesem Fall jedoch mit „vertauschter", also nicht-stereotyper Verteilung der Rollen (d. h. die Frau trinkt Bier, während der Mann bügelt, vgl. Abb. 1). Beide Bilder waren als typische Social Media-Beiträge mit Hashtags versehen. Bei der Betrachtung des jeweiligen Bildes wurden individuelle emotionale Reaktionen (positiv und negativ) der Teilnehmer*innen auf das Foto erfasst. Hierzu wurden in einer Pilotstudie ausgewählte Items des *Positive and Negative Affect Schedule* (PANAS) (Watson et al. 1988) verwendet. Ziel dieser

---

[4] Melzer et al. (2019, S. 7).

Tab. 1 Alters- und Geschlechtsverteilung der #Lëtzstereotype18 Studie. (Eigene Darstellung)

		Häufigkeit	%
Alter	14 bis 17 Jahre	40	11.1
	18 bis 23 Jahre	253	70.1
	24 bis 30 Jahre	68	18.8
Geschlecht	Weiblich	272	75.3
	Männlich	89	24.7

experimentellen Manipulation war es, Stereotype und Soziale Medien in einem typischen Kontext miteinander zu verbinden, indem stereotype beziehungsweise nicht-stereotype Rollenverteilungen in einem Bild dargestellt wurden, auf die spontan reagiert werden sollte, ohne dass explizit auf Stereotype verwiesen wurde. Dieses explorative Vorgehen diente der Erweiterung der im Folgenden beschriebenen expliziten Messung stereotyper Einstellungen: Inwieweit rufen Stereotype auch in einem solchen Kontext unterschiedliche Reaktionen hervor?

Während die emotionale Reaktion auf verschiedene Bilder von Geschlechterrollen ein eher implizites Maß darstellt, wurden die expliziten Geschlechterrollenbilder und Geschlechterstereotype in dieser Studie unter anderem mithilfe des Social Role Questionnaire (SRQ; Baber und Tucker 2006) erhoben, der Einstellungen zu sozialer Rollenverteilung in Bezug auf das Geschlecht misst (z. B. Verteilung der Tätigkeiten im Haushalt).

Es wurde außerdem erfragt, welche Lebensbereiche Jugendliche und junge Erwachsene in welchem Ausmaß durch geschlechterbezogene Stereotype beeinflusst sehen. Hierbei wurde unterschieden zwischen den *eigenen* Stereotypen und den Stereotypen *anderer Menschen*. Nicht nur die betroffenen Lebensbereiche waren von Interesse, sondern auch, welchen Ursprung junge Menschen ihren Stereotypen zuschreiben. Sie wurden gefragt, welchen subjektiv empfundenen

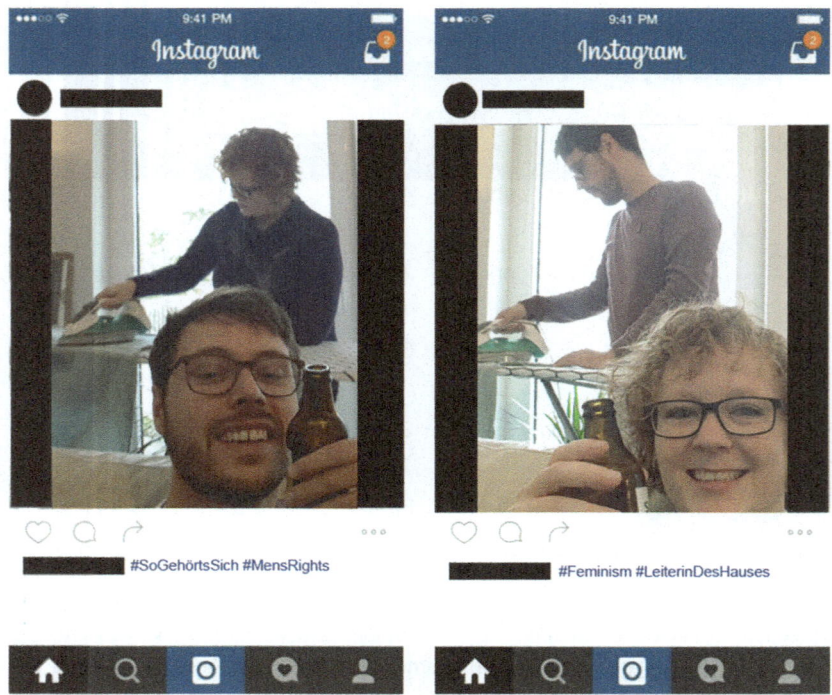

Abb. 1 Instagram Post der #Lëtzstereotype18 Studie Version 1 mit stereotyper Rollenverteilung und Version 2 mit „vertauschter" Rollenverteilung. (Eigene Abbildung)

Einfluss Faktoren wie etwa Eltern, Kultur, Religion oder soziale Medien auf ihre persönlichen Einstellungen in diesem Bereich haben.

Schließlich wurden Teilnehmer*innen nach ihrem Mediennutzungsverhalten gefragt. Neben der Häufigkeit der Nutzung diverser Medien, von Büchern bis Video-Streaming, wurden sie insbesondere nach Ihrer Nutzung bestimmter Social Media Plattformen sowie der Häufigkeit und dem Lieblingsgenre von Video-spielen gefragt.

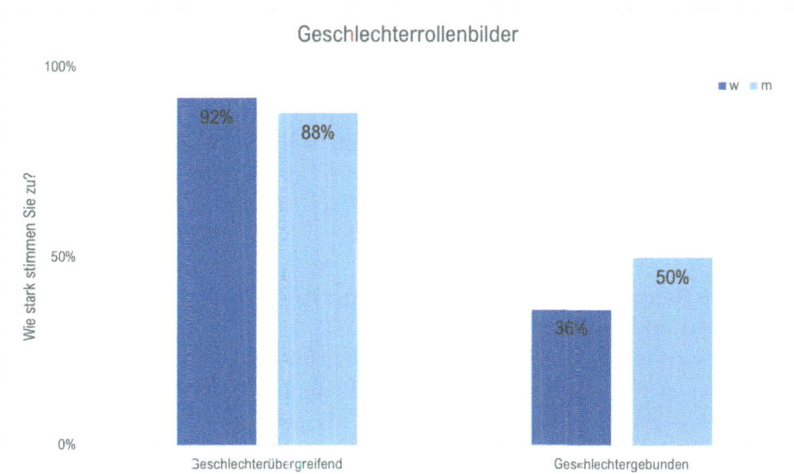

Abb. 2 Stärke der mittleren Zustimmung in % (0 = Lehne voll und ganz ab; 100 = Stimme voll und ganz zu) von weiblichen (w) und männlichen (m) Teilnehmer*innen zu geschlechterübergreifenden (z. B., „Aufgaben am Haushalt sollen net nom Geschlecht verdeelt ginn") und geschlechtergebundenen (z. B., „Männer sin méi sexuell wie Fraen") Aussagen. (Eigene Abbildung)

4.1 Ergebnisse[5]

4.1.1 Wahrgenommenes Geschlechterbild, Einstellungen und Erwartungen in Bezug auf die unterschiedlichen Geschlechter

Die Ergebnisse des SRQ zeigen, dass im Mittel geschlechterübergreifende Aussagen ($M = 5.55$, $SD = .50$) signifikant größere Zustimmung fanden als geschlechtergebundene ($M = 2.24$, $SD = .90$). Allerdings unterschieden sich die Geschlechter deutlich (vgl. Abb. 2), da weibliche Versuchspersonen geschlechterübergreifenden Aussagen stärker zustimmten als männliche. Bei geschlechtergebundenen Aussagen lag ein umgekehrtes Meinungsbild vor, da männliche Teilnehmer hier signifikant höhere Zustimmung zeigten als weibliche.

---

[5]Folgende Ergebnisse sind Auszüge des Abschlussberichts der #Lëtzstereotype18 Studie (Melzer et al. 2019).

Bei der Betrachtung der einzelnen Aussagen zeigten sich interessanterweise vor allem bei den geschlechtergebundenen Items der Erfassung des Grades der Zustimmung zu geschlechterstereotypen Aussagen signifikante Unterschiede zwischen männlichen und weiblichen Befragten. So stimmten männliche Teilnehmer der Aussage „*Manche Arten von Arbeit sind für Frauen einfach nicht angemessen*" am stärksten zu ($M = 3.30$, $SD = 1.71$), während dies bei den Teilnehmerinnen für die Aussage „*Männer sind sexorientierter als Frauen*" galt ($M = 3.22$, $SD = 1.63$).

Emotionale Reaktionen auf Darstellung von stereotypen Rollenbildern in Sozialen Medien

Bei der Auswertung der Reaktionen auf den angeblichen Instagram Post zeigten Personen bei stereotyper Genderrollendarstellung im Durchschnitt eine deutlich größere negative ($M = 2.50$, $SD = 1.14$) als positive ($M = 1.26$, $SD = .46$) emotionale Reaktion. Im umgekehrten Fall zeigten Personen, die das Bild mit den "umgekehrten", d. h. nicht-stereotypen Geschlechterrollen sahen, im Durchschnitt eine stärkere positive ($M = 2.07$, $SD = 1.05$) als negative emotionale Reaktion ($M = 1.55$, $SD = .81$; vgl. Abb. 3). Obwohl der Durchschnitt der Antworten etwa bei den negativen Emotionen zu dem Bild der stereotypen

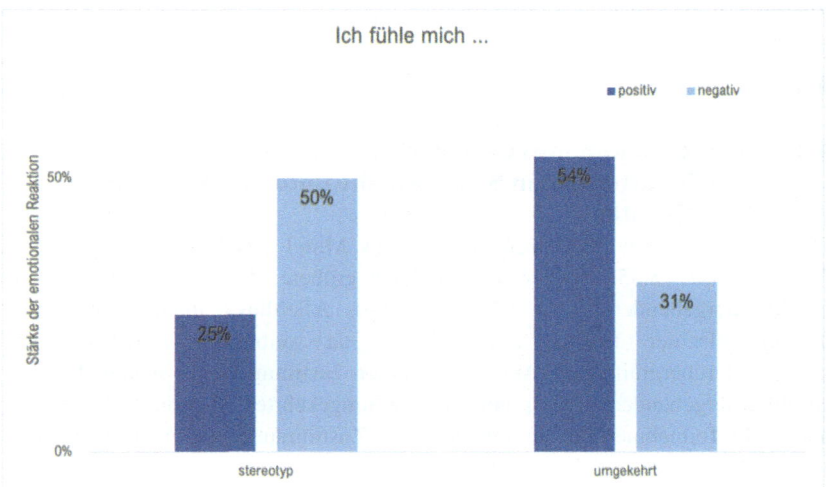

Abb. 3 Stärke der mittleren positiven (z. B., interessiert, stolz, stark) und negativen (z. B., feindselig, bekümmert, beschämt) emotionalen Reaktion in % (0 = Gar nicht; 100 = Äußerst) auf stereotype und umgekehrte Geschlechterrollen. (Eigene Abbildung)

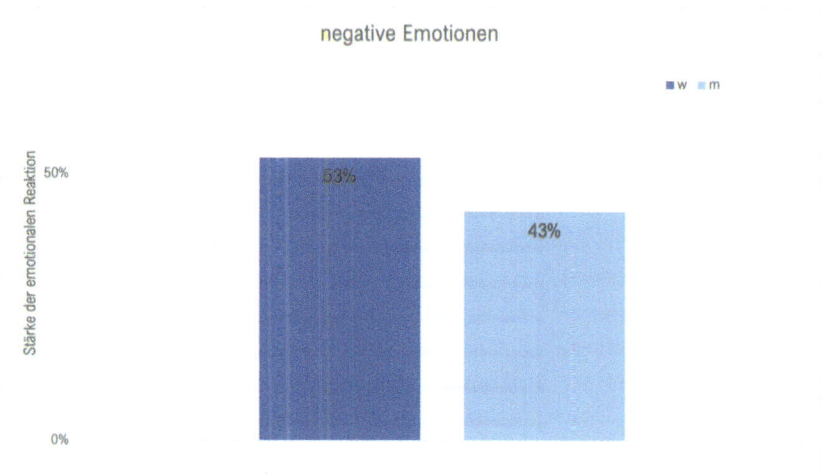

Abb. 4 Stärke der mittleren negativen (z. B., feindselig, bekümmert, beschämt) emotionalen Reaktion von weiblichen (w) und männlichen (m) Teilnehmer*innen in % (0 = Gar nicht; 100 = Äußerst) auf stereotype Geschlechterrollen. (Eigene Abbildung)

Geschlechterrollen zwischen „ein bisschen" und „einigermaßen" lag, variierten die Antworten trotzdem, da einige Personen eher in Richtung „erheblich" antworteten.

Für die genauere Betrachtung dieser Ergebnisse wurden beide Versuchsbedingungen (stereotypes vs. „umgekehrtes" Bild) bezüglich möglicher Geschlechterunterschiede untersucht. Beim Betrachten des Bildes nicht-stereotyper Geschlechterrollen fiel die emotionale Reaktion der Frauen im Durchschnitt sowohl bei positiven als auch negativen Emotionen numerisch stärker aus als bei männlichen Teilnehmern.

Wurde der Instagram Post mit der stereotypen Geschlechterrollenverteilung gesehen, gaben Frauen im Durchschnitt deutlich stärkere negative Emotionen an ($M = 2.63$, $SD = 1.14$) als Männer ($M = 2.15$, $SD = 1.11$; vgl. Abb. 4).

4.1.2 Einschätzung der Konsequenzen wahrgenommener, geschlechtsbezogen stereotyper Geschlechterüberzeugungen

Hinsichtlich der wahrgenommenen Folgen „typischer" Geschlechterüberzeugungen wurden die Antworten für die verschiedenen Lebensbereiche in Bezug

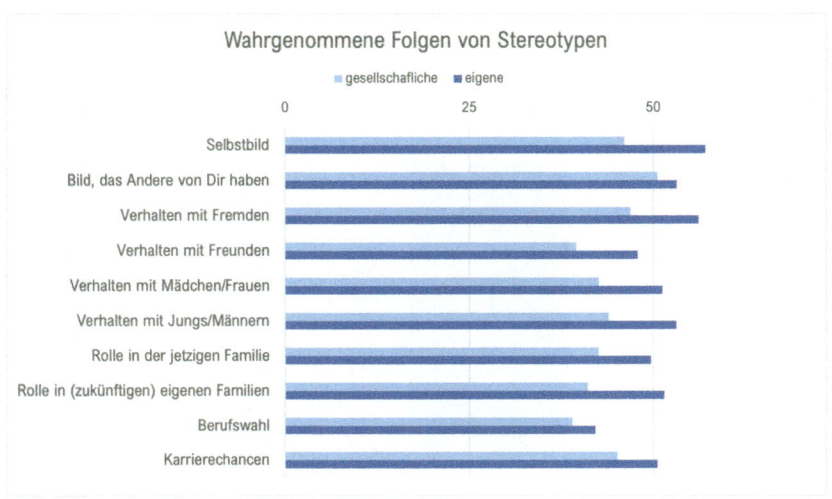

Abb. 5 Mittlere wahrgenommene Folgen von gesellschaftlichen und eigenen Stereotypen für verschiedene Bereiche in % (0 = hat keinen Einfluss; 100 = hat einen sehr starken Einfluss). (Eigene Abbildung)

auf die eigenen Stereotype denen auf den in der Gesellschaft vorherrschenden entgegengestellt (vgl. Abb. 5). Hierbei zeigte sich, dass die Befragten den Einfluss ihrer eigenen geschlechterbezogenen Stereotype auf sämtliche Lebensbereiche signifikant höher einschätzten als denen, die sie der Gesellschaft zuschrieben.

Während die Teilnehmerinnen ihr Selbstbild durch ihre *eigenen* Stereotypen am stärksten betroffen sahen ($M = 3.47$, $SD = 1.71$), galt dies für die männlichen Befragten in ihrem *Verhalten gegenüber Fremden* ($M = 3.49$, $SD = 1.49$; vgl. Abb. 10). Beide Geschlechter waren sich hingegen einig, dass gesellschaftliche Stereotype am stärksten das Bild beeinflussen, das andere von ihnen haben ($M_{m=w} = 3.07$, $SD_m = 1.57$ und $SD_w = 1.63$).

Bei der geschlechtergetrennten Betrachtung der Alltagsfolgen eigener Stereotype gab es lediglich einen signifikanten Geschlechterunterschied. Frauen sahen ihre Karrierechancen deutlich stärker durch ihre eigenen Stereotype beeinflusst ($M = 3.19$, $SD = 1.58$) als Männer ($M = 2.67$, $SD = 1.60$; vgl. Abb. 6). Interessanterweise war der Geschlechterunterschied in Bezug auf die Wahl des Berufs statistisch nicht signifikant. Während sich Frauen durch Stereotype nicht stärker als Männer bei der Berufswahl behindert sehen, sehen sie ihre Aufstiegs-

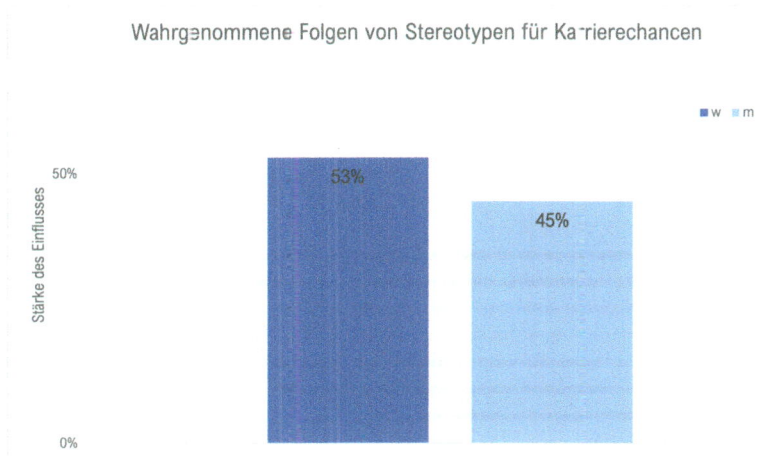

Abb. 6 Mittlere wahrgenommene Folgen von eigenen Stereotypen für Karrierechancen in % (0 = hat keinen Einfluss; 100 = hat einen sehr starken Einfluss) aufgeschlüsselt für weiblichen (w) und männliche (m) Teilnehmer*innen. (Eigene Abbildung)

chancen durch geschlechtsbezogene Vorurteile deutlich gefährdeter als Männer dies tun.

Einen solchen signifikanten Geschlechterunterschied gab es nur in Bezug auf die Alltagsfolgen der *eigenen* Stereotype, bei den Folgen der Stereotype *anderer* antworteten Frauen und Männer im Durchschnitt recht ähnlich.

Wie Abb. 5 zeigt, wurden *sämtliche* Lebensbereiche, die im Fragebogen als möglicherweise von Stereotypen betroffen vorgeschlagen wurden, auch von den Teilnehmerinnen und Teilnehmern als durch Stereotype beeinflusst wahrgenommen.

4.1.3 Die Entstehung von Gendersstereotypen und Geschlechterrollen: Wahrgenommene Haupteinflussfaktoren und deren Gewichtung

Die Befragten schrieben hier ihren *Eltern* den stärksten Einfluss auf die eigenen geschlechterbezogenen Stereotype zu ($M = 4.13$, $SD = 1.58$), während sie *Religion* ($M = 1.91$, $SD = 1.48$) und *Videospielen* ($M = 1.91$, $SD = 1.44$) den geringsten Einfluss unterstellten (vgl. Abb. 7). Bemerkenswert ist erneut, dass alle

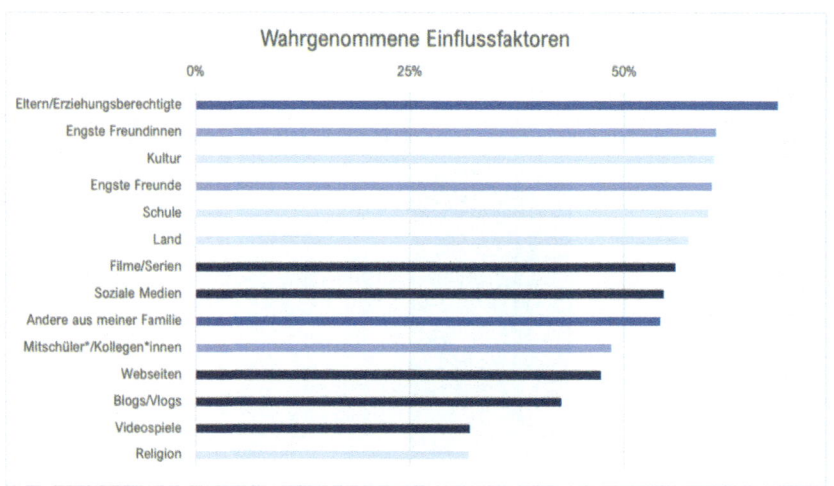

Abb. 7 Mittlerer wahrgenommener Einfluss verschiedenen Kategorien auf Stereotype in % (0 = hat keinen Einfluss; 100 = hat einen sehr starken Einfluss). (Eigene Abbildung)

Mittelwerte deutlich über dem Minimalwert 1 lagen, sodass alle zu beurteilenden Größen als prinzipiell relevante Einflussfaktoren wahrgenommen wurden.

Bei der getrennten Betrachtung der Geschlechter zeichneten sich einige signifikante Unterschiede ab (vgl. Abb. 8). Männer schrieben ihren Mitschülern*innen und Kollegen*innen einen größeren Einfluss zu ($M = 3.33$, $SD = 1.47$) als es Frauen taten ($M = 2.82$, $SD = 1.41$). Darüber hinaus fühlten sich Männer ($M = 2.20$, $SD = 1.55$) auch deutlich stärker durch Videospiele in ihren Stereotypen beeinflusst als Frauen ($M = 1.81$, $SD = 1.40$).

Der größte Geschlechterunterschied bei der Bewertung der Einflussfaktoren lag für den Faktor *Soziale Medien* vor, dem Teilnehmerinnen signifikant größeren Einfluss in Bezug auf ihre Geschlechterstereotypen zuweisen ($M = 3.46$, $SD = 1.67$) als männliche Teilnehmer ($M = 2.79$, $SD = 1.60$).

Obwohl die befragten Teilnehmer*innen Videospielen und Sozialen Medien subjektiv einen Einfluss auf ihre Stereotype zuschrieben, gab es keine signifikante Korrelation zwischen der Nutzungshäufigkeit von Sozialen Medien oder Videospielen und den stereotypen und egalitären Einstellungen (gender-linked und gender-transcendent Subskalen des SRQ). Dies galt sowohl für weibliche, als auch für männliche Teilnehmende.

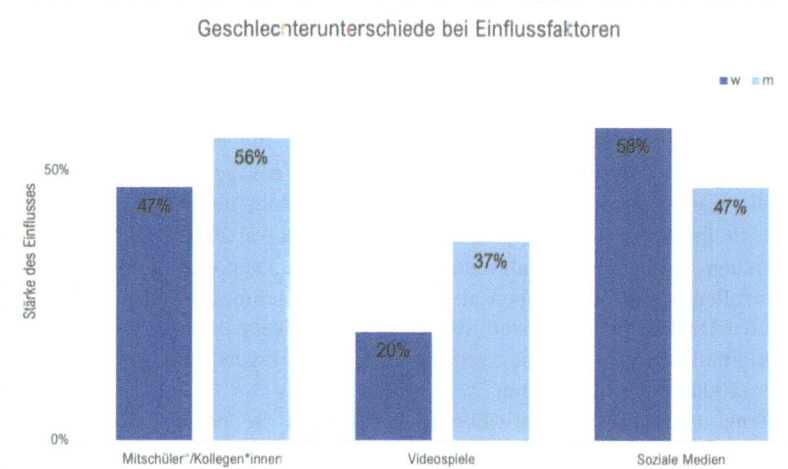

Abb. 8 Mittlerer wahrgenommener Einfluss von Mitschüler*innen und Kollegen*innen auf Stereotpye in % (0 = hat keinen Einfluss; 100 = hat einen sehr starken Einfluss) aufgeschlüsselt für weibichen (w) und männliche (m) Teilnehmer*innen. (Eigene Abbildung)

Mediennutzung

Angesichts der Befunde zu Medien als Einflussfaktor überraschte es nicht, dass die Teilnehmerinnen angaben, soziale Medien generell signifikant häufiger zu nutzen als männliche. Einer im Durchschnitt *„sehr häufigen"* Nutzung sozialer Medien durch die Teilnehmerinnen steht eine im Durchschnitt nur *„häufige"* Nutzung der männlichen Befragten gegenüber. Zudem sahen Jungen/Männer Videospiele nicht nur als stärkeren Einflussfaktor auf Stereotype, sondern nutzen diese signifikant häufiger ($M = 3.85$, $SD = 1.82$) als Frauen ($M = 2.13$, $SD = 1.52$).

Auch bei den Fragen zur Nutzung spezifischer Sozialer Medien gab es klare Geschlechterunterschiede. So wird die Videostreaming-Plattform *YouTube* beispielsweise im Durchschnitt bedeutend häufiger von Männern ($M = 5.32$, $SD = .82$) genutzt als von Frauen ($M = 4.90$, $SD = 1.18$). Dasselbe gilt für die Streaming-Plattform *Twitch*, (Männer: $M = 1.82$, $SD = 1.36$; Frauen: $M = 1.24$, $SD = .84$). Dies ist jedoch aufgrund der verschiedenen Nutzungshäufigkeiten von Videospielen wenig überraschend, da es sich hierbei um eine Social Media Plattform für das Streaming von Videospielen handelt. Frauen wiederum berichteten im Durchschnitt deutlich häufiger, das speziell auf das Teilen von Bildmaterial spezialisierte *Instagram* zu benutzen ($M = 4.92$, $SD = 1.61$) als Männer ($M = 3.50$,

SD = 2.06). Auch die Online-Pinnwand *Pinterest* für Grafiken und Fotos nutzen Frauen signifikant häufiger (*M* = 2.61, *SD* = 1.55) als Männer (*M* = 1.57, *SD* = 1.11).

Die Ergebnisse der *#Lëtzstereotype18*-Studie zeigen, dass ein eher egalitäres und weniger stereotypes Geschlechterrollenbild Jugendlicher und junger Erwachsener in Luxemburg vorherrscht. Aufgrund des gesellschaftspolitischen Wandels sind ähnliche Ergebnisse in anderen Ländern des westlichen Kulturraums zu finden (Sani und Quaranta 2017; Valentova 2013). Dass Mädchen und Frauen dazu neigen, traditionellere, stereotype Denkweisen in Bezug auf Genderrollen stärker abzulehnen als männliche Teilnehmer und diesen auch im egalitären Denken in voraus sind, ist nicht neu und spiegelt auch die Ergebnisse der Originalstichprobe des hier verwendeten SRQ Fragebogens von Baber und Tucker (2006) vor fast 16 Jahren.

Offenkundig geht die Entwicklung generell in die positive Richtung hin zu mehr egalitärem Denken und weg vom Denken in veralteten traditionellen Rollenbildern, die gerade für junge Menschen schwerwiegende Folgen für ihr körperliches und geistiges Wohlbefinden sowie ihre Lebenslaufbahn haben kann. Jedoch zeigen die Ergebnisse auch, dass sich einige Stereotype noch beharrlich in den Köpfen auch der jüngeren Generation halten. So halten selbst im Jahre 2018 viele männliche Teilnehmer der Studie nicht *alle Arten von Arbeit für Frauen angemessen.*[6]

Solche moralisch-normative Konnotationen, dass sich manche Dinge oder Verhaltensweisen für das ein oder andere Geschlecht „nicht gehören", bringen geschlechterbezogene Stereotype grundsätzlich mit sich, da die Gesellschaft dem jeweiligen Geschlecht entsprechende typische soziale Normen und Rollen zuweist (Gill und Gill 2007). Die Befunde zeigen auch, dass trotz positiver Veränderungen insbesondere bei männlichen Personen noch Entwicklungspotential vorhanden ist, was eine wichtige Information und einen Ansatzpunkt für Arbeit im Bereich der Prävention und Intervention liefert – gerade auch vor dem Hintergrund ihrer Bedeutung für Lebenszufriedenheit und psychologische Wohlbefinden. Um solche Informationen und Ansatzpunkte auch für eine spezifisch jüngere Zielgruppe zu haben, wurden in der #Lëtzstereotype18 Studie auch Daten zur Mediennutzung erhoben. Die diesbezüglichen Befunde stehen im Einklang mit Ergebnisse der JIM Studie (Medienpädagogischer Forschungsverbund

---

[6]Männliche Teilnehmer stimmten dieser Aussage im Durchschnitt stärker zu als Teilnehmerinnen.

Südwest 2018), einer der bekanntesten jährlichen Studien zur Mediennutzung Jugendlicher im Nachbarland Deutschland. Darüber hinaus zeigt sich in der luxemburgischen Studie, dass Teilnehmer*innen interessanterweise auch selbst einen Bezug zwischen ihrer Mediennutzung und der Entwicklung ihrer eigenen Stereotype herstellen. So nutzen Jungs nicht nur Videospiele und soziale Medien mit Videospielbezug (z. B. Twitch) häufiger als Mädchen, sondern bewerten diese auch als größere Einflussfaktoren, wenn es um die Entstehung eigener Stereotype geht. Diese Einsicht ist insofern bedeutsam, da besonders in Videospielen die Darstellung von weiblichen Charakteren oft sehr problematisch ist. Vor allem in den Spielen, die am häufigsten genutzt werden (wie Action- und Adventure Spiele, die auch in dieser Studie zu den beliebtesten gehörten), sind weibliche Charaktere stark unterrepräsentiert und werden meist in übersexualisierter Darstellung gezeigt (z. B. Glaubke et al. 2001; Jansz und Martis 2007). Solche stereotypen Darstellungen finden sich auch in der Wahrnehmung junger Menschen; sie tragen überdies wesentlich zur Sozialisierung der Geschlechterbilder bei (z. B. Dill und Thi.l 2007).

Die Teilnehmerinnen der Studie hingegen nutzen stärker soziale Medien als männliche Teilnehmer und schreiben diesen auch einen stärkeren Einfluss zu, wenn es um ihre Geschlechterstereotype geht. Jedoch werden Frauen und Mädchen in diesem Kontext oft als nach männlicher Aufmerksamkeit strebende, sexualisierte Objekte präsentiert (Bailey et al. 2013). Das ist insofern problematisch, als dass stereotype Selbstdarstellungen im sozialen Medien Kontext von Frauen oder Mädchen selbst als vielversprechend für sozialen Erfolg und Popularität gesehen werden (Bailey et al. 2013). Leider befinden sich Frauen und Mädchen in der Onlinewelt in einer Zwickmühle, ca sie häufig mit Kritik konfrontiert werden, nämlich dann, wenn sie den stereotypen Erwartungen nicht gerecht werden, aber auch, wenn sie online in ihrer Selbstdarstellung zu offen sind (z. B. öffentliches Profil, Preisgabe von persönlichen Informationen,...; Bailey et al. 2013). Dies hat auch eine negative Auswirkung auf ihr Wohlbefinden, da gerade bei weiblichen Jugendlichen der Selbstwert oft stark mit der sozialen Akzeptanz einhergeht (Hagborg 1993).

Dass sich der Einfluss von Videospielen und Sozialen Medien zwar in der Selbsteinschätzung, jedoch nicht im Zusammenhang mit der angegebenen Nutzungshäufigkeit zeigt, muss nicht bedeuten, dass keine Korrelation zwischen der Nutzung moderner Medien und der Entwicklung von Stereotypen besteht. Wie oben erläutert, gibt es sowohl theoretische Überlegungen wie auch empirische Belege, die einen Zusammenhang nahelegen. Die Messung in der vorliegenden Studie beschränkte sich jedoch auf die reine Nutzungshäufigkeit. Neuere Studien in der Medienpsychologie deuten darauf hin, dass gerade in Bezug auf Soziale Medien die Qualität und Motivation der Nutzung in vielen Bereichen viel entscheidender sind als die reine Quantität der Nutzung (z. B. Stein et al. 2019). Daher ist für die Stereotypentwicklung zu vermuten, dass das *Wie* und das *Wieso* der Mediennutzung einen sehr viel bedeutenderen Einfluss auf die Entwicklung von Stereotypen hat als das *Wieviel*.

Ein weiterer wichtiger Bereich, in dem sich die jungen Teilnehmerinnen selbst stark negativ durch ihre eigenen Stereotype beeinträchtigt sehen, ist der Beruf. Hier sehen sie jedoch weniger ihre Berufswahl, sondern vielmehr ihre späteren Chancen für einen Karriereaufstieg eingeschränkt. Dies könnte mitunter daran liegen, dass junge Frauen durchschnittlich ein geringeres Selbstwertgefühl besitzen als junge Männer, etwa in Bezug auf ihre eigenen Leistungen (Hackett et al. 1989; Maiano et al. 2004).

Die Tatsache, dass Frauen und Mädchen den sozialen Medien eine solch große Bedeutung und starken Einfluss beimessen, stellt aufgrund der dort präsentierten Stereotype eine Herausforderung mit möglichen negativen Folgen in Bezug auf ihr allgemeines Wohlbefinden dar. So ist nicht nur eine negative Beeinträchtigung des Selbst- und Körperbilds durch Stereotype denkbar, sondern auch ihrer beruflichen Bestrebungen sowie ihrer Überzeugungen hinsichtlich tatsächlich erbrachter Leistungen. Ein Teufelskreis selbsterfüllender Prophezeiungen kann wiederum dazu führen, dass sich die negativen Einstellungen in Bezug auf ihre Karrierechancen tatsächlich bestätigen. Vor diesem Hintergrund ist Grundlagenforschung vor allem im Bereich der neuen Medien überaus wichtig, speziell im Hinblick auf effektive Präventions- und Interventionsmaßnahmen.

Doch soziale Medien sind nicht per se *schlecht, böse,* oder *gefährlich* für junge Menschen, im Gegenteil. Beispiele wie die *Fridays-for-Future-* oder die *#MeToo*[7] Bewegung zeigen deutlich, wie gut junge Menschen heutzutage in großer Zahl und flächen-, sowie plattformübergreifend durch Online-Bewegungen und -Kampagnen erreicht werden können. Vor diesem Hintergrund ist es auch nicht verwunderlich, dass eine stereotype „Sexorientiertheit" der Männer bei weiblichen Teilnehmerinnen der *#Lëtzstereotype18*-Studie auf die größte Zustimmung traf. Sowohl soziale Medien als Werkzeug und Kontext, als auch spezifische Stereotype, wie die in der vorliegenden Studie untersuchten, sollten in Hinblick auf Aufklärungskampagnen oder Interventionsmaßnamen unbedingt weiter erforscht und in Betracht gezogen werden. Auch die starken

---

[7] Eine Online Bewegung gegen sexuelle Übergriffe von Männern gegen Frauen, gestartet im Jahr 2017, vor allem geprägt und bekannt geworden durch Aktivistin Tarana Burke und Schauspielerin Alyssa Milano.

emotionalen Reaktionen auf die in der Studie verwendeten stereotypen (vermeintlichen) Instagram-Posts sprechen als Indikator hierfür. Besonders Frauen reagierten stark verärgert auf diese stereotypen sozialen Medieninhalte, während sie mit Interesse und teilweise sogar Begeisterung auf die Version mit *vertauschten* Rollen reagierten.

Nicht zuletzt, da diese Studie auch deutlich gezeigt hat, wie viele Lebensbereiche junger Menschen von Stereotypen beeinträchtigt sind, sollte der Forschungsfokus darauf liegen, wie moderne Medien genutzt werden können, um Stereotype erfolgreich aufzubrechen und ein egalitäreres Geschlechterrollenbild junger Menschen zu fördern und dessen Bedeutung für das Wohlbefinden zu erfassen.

Besonders interessant und relativ unerwartet war das Ergebnis, dass es vor allem die *eigenen* Stereotype der Teilnehmer*innen sind, denen der größte Einfluss auf die verschiedenen Lebensbereiche zugesprochen wurde. Dass alle vorgeschlagenen Lebensbereiche als sowohl von eigenen, als auch von gesellschaftlichen Stereotypen beeinträchtigt gesehen werden zeigt, wie bewusst es den jungen Menschen ist, welche große Bedeutung Stereotype für ihr Leben und Wohlbefinden haben. Der Fakt, dass sie zudem den eigenen Stereotypen eine größere Bedeutung beimaßen, belegt ein hohes Maß an Selbstbestimmtheit und Selbstwirksamkeit. Dieser Befund stellt einen vielversprechenden Ansatzpunkt für mögliche Präventions- und Interventionskampagnen dar.

Auch wenn das Denken im westlichen Kulturraum immer egalitärer wird, sind Stereotype offensichtlich immer noch präsent im Alltag und spielen eine wichtige Rolle im Leben von jungen Menschen. Somit beeinträchtigen sie auch weiterhin ihr Wohlbefinden. Für die zukünftige Forschung wäre es im nächsten Schritt zielführend, weitere Methoden zu implementieren, um Stereotype und die zugrunde liegenden Prozesse genauer ergründen und besser verstehen zu können. Über die kognitive und emotionale Ebene hinaus, ist das Erfassen weiterer Daten auf der physiologischen sowie der Verhaltensebene sinnvoll. Auch experimentelle Variationen verschiedener Bedingungen, ähnlich wie die in der vorliegenden Studie vorgenommene Variation der Instagram-Posts, könnten an dieser Stelle einen signifikanten Mehrwert an Informationen bringen. Ein tieferes Verständnis dieser Prozesse ist vor allem wichtig, da sie stark abhängig von rapiden und dynamischen Verläufen, wie medien- und gesellschaftspolitischen Entwicklungen sind. Nur wenn junge Menschen auf der aktuellen Ebene in ihrer Entwicklung und zielgerecht im relevanten Kontext erreicht werden können, sind Interventionsmaßnahmen und präventive Arbeit wirklich erfolgreich. Die hier besprochene Datengrundlage zeigt, dass neben dem Elternhaus, der Schule und

Peers, insbesondere auch Soziale Medien als Zielfaktor vielversprechend sein können. Dieses Potenzial sollte unbedingt genutzt werden.

Wie zu Beginn bereits erläutert, ist Wohlbefinden ein Zustand, in dem es eine Balance gibt, zwischen den Ressourcen einer Person und den sich ihr stellenden Herausforderungen. Moderne Medien sind Teil der Lebensrealität der jungen Generationen und werden in Zukunft eher an Bedeutung und Einfluss gewinnen, als verlieren. Um im Zeitalter der neuen Medien also nach Wohlbefinden zu streben, sollten wir diese Medien nicht nur unter dem Aspekt der Herausforderungen sehen, die sie in vielen Bereichen mit sich bringen, sondern auch als mögliche Ressourcen, zum Beispiel im Kampf gegen Stereotype und ihre Auswirkungen.

Literatur

Anderson, C. A., Shibuya, A., Ihori, N., Swing, E. L., Bushman, B. J., Sakamoto, A., Rothstein, H. R., & Saleem, M. (2010). Violent video game effects on aggression, empathy, and prosocial behavior in Eastern and Western countries: A meta-analytic review. *Psychological Bulletin, 136*(2), 151–173. https://doi.org/10.1037/a0018251

Baber, K. M., & Tucker, C. J. (2006). The social roles questionnaire: A new approach to measuring attitudes toward gender. *Sex Roles, 54*(7–8), 459–467. https://doi.org/10.1007/s11199-006-9018-y

Bailey, J., Steeves, V., Burkell, J., & Regan, P. (2013). Negotiating with gender stereotypes on social networking sites: From "bicycle face" to Facebook. *Journal of Communication Inquiry, 37*(2), 91–112. https://doi.org/10.1177/0196859912473777

Barlett, C. P., Vowels, C. L., & Saucier, D. A. (2008). Meta-analyses of the effects of media images on men's body-image concerns. *Journal of Social and Clinical Psychology, 27*(3), 279–310. https://doi.org/10.1521/jscp.2008.27.3.279

Beasley, B., & Collins Standley, T. (2002). Shirts vs. skins: Clothing as an indicator of gender role stereotyping in video games. *Mass Communication & Society, 5*(3), 279–293. https://doi.org/10.1207/S15327825MCS0503_3

Berryman, C., Ferguson, C. J., & Negy, C. (2018). Social media use and mental health among young adults. *Psychiatric Quarterly, 89*(2), 307–314. https://doi.org/10.1007/s11126-017-9535-6

Blizzard Entertainment. (2004). *World of Warcraft.*

Cheryan, S., Drury, B. J., & Vichayapai, M. (2013). Enduring influence of stereotypical computer science role models on women's academic aspirations. *Psychology of Women Quarterly, 37*(1), 72–79. https://doi.org/10.1177/0361684312459328

Deci, E. L., & Ryan, R. M. (2000). The "What" and "Why" of Goal Pursuits: Human Needs and the Self-Determination of Behavior. *Psychological Inquiry, 11*(4), 227–268. https://doi.org/10.1207/S15327965PLI1104_01

Dill, K. E., & Thill, K. P. (2007). Video game characters and the socialization of gender roles: Young people's perceptions mirror sexist media depictions. *Sex Roles, 57*(11–12), 851–864. https://doi.org/10.1007/s11199-007-9278-1

Dodge, R., Daly, A., Huyton, J., & Sanders, L. (2012). The challenge of defining wellbeing. *International Journal of Wellbeing, 2*(3), 222–235. https://doi.org/10.5502/ijw.v2i3.4

Durkin, K., & Barber, B. (2002). Not so doomed: Computer game play and positive adolescent development. *Journal of Applied Developmental Psychology, 23*(4), 373–392. https://doi.org/10.1016/S0193-3973(02)00124-7

Easterly, D. M., & Ricard, C. S. (2011). Conscious efforts to end unconscious bias: Why women leave academic research. *Journal of Research Administration, 42*(1), 61–73. https://eric.ed.gov/?id=EJ955003

Eckes, T. (2004). Geschlechterstereotype: Von Rollen, Identitäten und Vorurteilen. In *Handbuch Frauen -und Geschlechterforschung* (pp. 165–176). Springer.

Entertainment Software Association. (2018). *Essential facts about the computer and video game industry.* http://www.theesa.com/wp-content/uploads/2018/05/EF2018_FINAL.pdf

Feng, W., Ramo, D. E., Chan, S. R., & Bourgeois, J. A. (2017). Internet gaming disorder: Trends in prevalence 1993–2016. *Addictive Behaviors 75*, 17–24. https://doi.org/10.1016/j.addbeh.2017.06.010

Ferguson, C. J. (2015). Do angry birds make for angry children? A meta-analysis of video game influences on children's and adolescents' aggression, mental health, prosocial behavior, and academic performance. *Perspectives on Psychological Science, 10*(5), 646–666. https://doi.org/10.177/1745691615592234

Gentile, D. A., Anderson, C. A., Yukawa, S., Ihori, N., Saleem, M., Lim Kam Ming, Shibuya, A., Liau, A. K., Khoo, A., Bushman, B. J., Rowell Huesmann, L., & Sakamoto, A. (2009). The Effects of Prosocial Video Games on Prosocial Behaviors: International Evidence From Correlational, Longitudinal, and Experimental Studies. *Personality and Social Psychology Bulletin, 35*(6), 752–763. https://doi.org/10.1177/0146167209333245

Gentile, D. A., Bailey, K., Bavelier, D., Brockmyer, J. F., Cash, H., Coyne, S. M., Doan, A., Grant, D. S., Green, C. S., Griffiths, M., Markle, T., Petry, N. M., Prot, S., Rae, C. D., Rehbein, F., Rich, M., Sullivan, D., Woolley, E., & Young, K. (2017). Internet Gaming Disorder in Children and Adolescents. *Pediatrics, 140*(Supplement 2), S81–S85. https://doi.org/10.1542/peds.2016-1758H

Gentile, D. A., Swing, E. L., Lim, C. G., & Khoo, A. (2012). Video game playing, attention problems, and impulsiveness: Evidence of bidirectional causality. *Psychology of Popular Media Culture, 1*(1), 62–70. https://doi.org/10.1037/a0026969

Gill, R., & Gill, R. M. (2007). *Gender and the Media.* Polity.

Glaubke, C. R., Miller, P., Parker, M. A., & Espejo, E. (2001). *Fair play? Violence, gender and race in video games.* https://eric.ed.gov/?id=ED463092

Granic, I., Lobel, A., & Engels, R. C. M. E. (2014). The benefits of playing video games. *American Psychologist, 69*(1), 66–78. https://doi.org/10.1037/a0034857

Greenberg, B. S., & Worrell, T. R. (2007). New faces on television: A 12-season replication. *The Howard Journal of Communications, 18*(4), 277–290. https://doi.org/10.1080/10646170701653651

Groesz, L. M., Levine, M. P., & Murnen, S. K. (2002). The effect of experimental presentation of thin media images on body satisfaction: A meta-analytic review. *International Journal of Eating Disorders, 31*(1), 1–16. https://doi.org/10.1002/eat.10005

Hackett, G., Esposito, D., & O'Halloran, M. S. (1989). The relationship of role model influences to the career salience and educational and career plans of college women. *Journal of Vocational Behavior, 35*(2), 164–180. https://doi.org/10.1016/0001-8791(89)90038-9

Hagborg, W. J. (1993). Gender differences on Harter's self-perception profile for adolescents. *Journal of Social Behavior and Personality, 8*(1), 141.

Heffer, T., Good, M., Daly, O., MacDonell, E., & Willoughby, T. (2019). The longitudinal association between social-media use and depressive symptoms among adolescents and young adults: An empirical reply to twenge et al. (2018). *Clinical Psychological Science, 7*(3), 462–470. https://doi.org/10.1177/2167702618812727

Heilman, M. E. (2012). Gender stereotypes and workplace bias. *Research in Organizational Behavior, 32*, 113–135. https://doi.org/10.1016/j.riob.2012.11.003

Hill, S., & Marshall, T. C. (2018). Beliefs about sexual assault in India and Britain are explained by attitudes toward women and hostile sexism. *Sex Roles, 79*(7–8), 421–430. https://doi.org/10.1007/s11199-017-0880-6

Jansz, J., & Martis, R. G. (2007). The Lara phenomenon: Powerful female characters in video games. *Sex Roles, 56*(3–4), 141–148. https://doi.org/10.1007/s11199-006-9158-0

Jussim, L., Nelson, T. E., Manis, M., & Soffin, S. (1995). Prejudice, stereotypes, and labeling effects: Sources of bias in person perception. *Journal of Personality and Social Psychology, 68*(2), 228–246. https://doi.org/10.1037/0022-3514.68.2.228

Kaczmarek, L. D., & Drazkowski, D. (2014). MMORPG Escapism Predicts Decreased Well-Being: Examination of Gaming Time, Game Realism Beliefs, and Online Social Support for Offline Problems. *Cyberpsychology, Behavior, and Social Networking, 17*(5), 298–302. https://doi.org/10.1089/cyber.2013.0595

Kardefelt-Winther, D. (2014). The moderating role of psychosocial well-being on the relationship between escapism and excessive online gaming. *Computers in Human Behavior, 38*, 68–74. https://doi.org/10.1016/j.chb.2014.05.020

Kato, P. M. (2010). Video games in health care: Closing the gap. *Review of General Psychology, 14*(2), 113–121. https://doi.org/10.1037/a0019441

Keyes, C. L. M., Shmotkin, D., & Ryff, C. D. (2002). Optimizing well-being: The empirical encounter of two traditions. *Journal of Personality and Social Psychology, 82*(6), 1007–1022. https://doi.org/10.1037/0022-3514.82.6.1007

LaRose, R., Lin, C. A., & Eastin, M. S. (2003). Unregulated Internet Usage: Addiction, Habit, or Deficient Self-Regulation? *Media Psychology, 5*(3), 225–253. https://doi.org/10.1207/S1532785XMEP0503_01

Lobel, A., Engels, R. C. M. E., Stone, L. L., Burk, W. J., & Granic, I. (2017). Video Gaming and Children's Psychosocial Wellbeing: A Longitudinal Study. *Journal of Youth and Adolescence, 46*(4), 884–897. https://doi.org/10.1007/s10964-017-0646-z

Maiano, C., Ninot, G., & Bilard, J. (2004). Age and gender effects on global self-esteem and physical self-perception in adolescents. *European Physical Education Review, 10*(1), 53–69. https://doi.org/10.1177/1356336X04040621

Martin, C. L., Ruble, D. N., & Szkrybalo, J. (2002). Cognitive theories of early gender development. *Psychological Bulletin, 128*(6), 903. https://doi.org/10.1037//0033-2909.128.6.903

Medienpädagogischer Forschungsverbund Südwest. (2018). JIM-Studie 2018: Jugend, Information, Medien. Basisstudie zum Medienumgang 12-bis 19-Jähriger in Deutschland. *Stuttgart, 13*(6). https://www.mpfs.de/fileadmin/files/Studien/JIM/2018/Studie/JIM_2018_Gesamt.pdf

Melzer, A. (2019). Cf princesses, paladins, and player motivations: Gender stereotypes and gendered perceptions in video games. In J. Breuer, D. Pietschmann, B. Liebold, & B. P. Lange (Eds.), *Evolutionary psychology and digital games. Digital hunter-gatherers.* Routledge.

Melzer, A., Hale, M.-L., & Hall, M. (2019). *Abschlussbericht des Projekts #LËTZSTEREOTYPE18—Geschlechterbezogene Rollen und Geschlechterstereotype bei Jugendlichen und jungen Erwachsenen in Luxemburg.* University of Luxembourg, Ministry for Equality Between Women and Men.

Mihara, S., & Higuchi, S. (2017). Cross-sectional and longitudinal epidemiological studies of Internet gaming disorder: A systematic review of the literature: Review of epidemiological studies of IGD. *Psychiatry and Clinical Neurosciences, 71*(7), 425–444. https://doi.org/10.1111/pcn.12532

Orben, A., & Przybylski, A. K. (2019). The association between adolescent well-being and digital technology use. *Nature Human Behaviour, 3*(2), 173–182. https://doi.org/10.1038/s41552-018-0506-1

Parkes, A., Sweeting, H., Wight, D., & Henderson, M. (2013). Do television and electronic games predict children's psychosocial adjustment? Longitudinal research using the UK Millennium Cohort Study. *Archives of Disease in Childhood, 98*(5), 341–348. https://doi.org/10.1136/archdischild-2011-301508

Pennell, H., & Behm-Morawitz, E. (2015). The empowering (super) heroine? The effects of sexualized female characters in superhero films on women. *Sex Roles, 72*(5–6), 211–220. https://doi.org/10.1007/s11199-015-0455-3

Prescott, A. T., Sargent, J. D., & Hull, J. G. (2018). Metaanalysis of the relationship between violent video game play and physical aggression over time. *Proceedings of the National Academy of Sciences, 115*(40), 9882–9888. https://doi.org/10.1073/pnas.1611617114

Sani, G. M. D., & Quaranta, M. (2017). The best is yet to come? Attitudes toward gender roles among adolescents in 36 countries. *Sex Roles, 77*(1–2), 30–45. https://doi.org/10.1007/s11199-016-0698-7

Scharrer, E. L. (2013). Representations of gender in the media. In *The Oxford handbook of media psychology* (pp. 267–284). Oxford University Press.

Sherlock, M., & Wagstaff, D. L. (2019). Exploring the relationship between frequency of Instagram use exposure to idealized images, and psychological well-being in women. *Psychology of Popular Media Culture, 8*(4), 482–490. https://doi.org/10.1037/ppm0000182

Signorielli, N. (2001). Television's gender role images and contribution to stereotyping: Past, present, future. In D. G. Singer & J. L. Singer (Eds.), *Handbook of children and the media* (pp. 341–358). Thousand Oaks.

Staiano, A. E., & Calvert, S. L. (2011). Exergames for Physical Education Courses: Physical, Social, and Cognitive Benefits: Exergames for Physical Education Courses. *Child Development Perspectives*, *5*(2), 93–98. https://doi.org/10.1111/j.1750-8606.2011.00162.x

Stein, J.-P., Krause, E., & Ohler, P. (2019). Every (Insta)Gram counts? Applying cultivation theory to explore the effects of Instagram on young users' body image. *Psychology of Popular Media Culture*. https://doi.org/10.1037/ppm0000268

Su, R., Tay, L., & Diener, E. (2014). The Development and Validation of the Comprehensive Inventory of Thriving (CIT) and the Brief Inventory of Thriving (BIT): Comprehensive and Brief Inventory of Thriving. *Applied Psychology: Health and Well-Being*, *6*(3), 251–279. https://doi.org/10.1111/aphw.12027

Sussman, C. J., Harper, J. M., Stahl, J. L., & Weigle, P. (2018). Internet and Video Game Addictions. *Child and Adolescent Psychiatric Clinics of North America*, *27*(2), 307–326. https://doi.org/10.1016/j.chc.2017.11.015

Turner, J. S. (2011). Sex and the spectacle of music videos: An examination of the portrayal of race and sexuality in music videos. *Sex Roles*, *64*(3–4), 173–191.

Twenge, J. M., Joiner, T. E., Rogers, M. L., & Martin, G. N. (2018). Increases in Depressive Symptoms, Suicide-Related Outcomes, and Suicide Rates Among U.S. Adolescents After 2010 and Links to Increased New Media Screen Time. *Clinical Psychological Science*, *6*(1), 3–17. https://doi.org/10.1177/2167702617723376

Valentova, M. (2013). Age and sex differences in gender role attitudes in Luxembourg between 1999 and 2008. *Work, Employment and Society*, *27*(4), 639–657.

Watson, D., Clark, L. A., & Tellegen, A. (1988). Development and validation of brief measures of positive and negative affect: The PANAS scales. *Journal of Personality and Social Psychology, 54*(6), 1063–1070.

Woods, H. C., & Scott, H. (2016). #Sleepyteens: Social media use in adolescence is associated with poor sleep quality, anxiety, depression and low self-esteem. *Journal of Adolescence, 51*, 41–49. https://doi.org/10.1016/j.adolescence.2016.05.008

World Bank. (2011). Gender differences in employment and why they matter. In *World Development Report 2012: Gender Equality and Development*. World Bank. http://siteresources.worldbank.org/INTWDR2012/Resources/7778105-1299699968583/7786210-1315936222006/chapter-5.pdf

World Health Organization. (2019). *International classification of diseases for mortality and morbidity statistics* (11th Revision). https://icd.who.int/browse11/l-m/en

Zosuls, K. M., Miller, C. F., Ruble, D. N., Martin, C. L., & Fabes, R. A. (2011). Gender development research in sex roles: Historical trends and future directions. *Sex Roles, 64*(11–12), 826–842. https://doi.org/10.1007/s11199-010-9902-3

Cybermobbing und die gesundheitlichen Folgen für Kinder und Jugendliche

Georges Steffgen und Matthias Böhmer

1   Einleitung

Die Nutzung der neuen elektronischen Medien findet derzeit einen rasanten Anstieg insbesondere bei Jugendlichen. Die virtuelle Welt des World Wide Web ist für viele zu einer zweiten Heimat geworden (KIM-Studie 2009; Smith und Steffgen 2013; Steffgen et al. 2010). Diese verstärkte Mediennutzung mit deren inhärenten Gefahren und Risiken beschäftigt nicht nur Eltern, Pädagogen und Politiker, sondern auch die breite Öffentlichkeit. Insbesondere die Gesundheitsgefahren und -risiken des Mobbings mittels moderner Kommunikationstechnologien, das Cybermobbing, erlangen hierbei in jüngster Vergangenheit von wissenschaftlicher Seite verstärkte Aufmerksamkeit (Davidson und Martellozzo 2008; Steffgen 2014; Vaillancourt et al. 2017).

Im folgenden Beitrag werden, aufbauend auf einer Begriffsklärung von Cybermobbing unter Berücksichtigung der relevanten Prävalenzraten, die potenziellen gesundheitlichen Folgen analysiert und diskutiert. Hierzu wird vorab traditionelles Mobbing von Cybermobbing abgegrenzt sowie eine Phänomenologie des Cybermobbings vorgestellt, zudem sowohl das „Happy Slapping" als auch das „Online Grooming" gehört. Neben Angaben zur Prävalenz insbesondere in Luxemburg werden die wesentlichen gesundheitlichen Auswirkungen von

G. Steffgen (✉) · M Böhmer
Department of Behavioural and Cognitive Sciences, University of Luxembourg,
Esch-sur-Alzette, Luxembourg
E-Mail: georges.steffgen@uni.lu

M. Böhmer
E-Mail: matthias.boehmer@uni.lu

Cybermobbing herausgearbeitet. Abschließend werden unterschiedliche Möglichkeiten der Prävention des individuell schädigenden Einflusses von Cybermobbing
aufgezeigt.

2 Cybermobbing – eine definitorische Eingrenzung

2.1 Abgrenzung zwischen Mobbing und Cybermobbing

Das klassische Mobbing unter Kindern und Jugendlichen ist mittlerweile ein
vielfältig untersuchtes und fest etabliertes Forschungsfeld in der Aggressions-
forschung, dessen Gefährdungspotenzial weitgehend belegt ist (Böhmer und
Steffgen 2020; Huberty und Steffgen 2008; Scheithauer et al. 2003). Mobbing
wird nach Olweus als Spezialfall aggressiven Verhaltens definiert: „Ein Schüler
oder eine Schülerin wird gemobbt, wenn er oder sie wiederholt und im Laufe
der Zeit negativen Handlungen seitens eines oder mehrerer anderer Schüler oder
Schülerinnen ausgesetzt ist" (1996, S. 266). Folgende Merkmale sind dabei
zentral (Huberty und Steffgen 2008):

1. Bei Mobbing handelt es sich um negative Handlungen – aggressive Verhaltensweisen, Gewalt –, die eine Person oder Personengruppe (Täter) gegenüber einer anderen Person (Opfer) ausübt. Hierbei ist die Intentionalität von
   großer Bedeutung, d. h., dass eine Handlung *zielgerichtet* ausgeführt wird, um
   einen anderen zu schädigen. Dies impliziert, dass das aggressive Verhalten
   auch vom Opfer als verletzend empfunden wird.
2. In der Beziehung zwischen Täter und Opfer besteht ein ungleiches, asym-
   metrisches Kräfte- bzw. Machtverhältnis, wobei der Täter dem Opfer über-
   legen ist. Das Machtungleichgewicht kann sowohl auf physischen (z. B.
   Größe), kognitiven (z. B. Intelligenz) als auch sozialen Faktoren (z. B. sozialer
   Status) beruhen. Das Opfer, das den negativen Handlungen ausgesetzt ist, hat
   Mühe sich zu verteidigen und ist somit dem Täter eher hilflos ausgeliefert.
3. Mobbing wiederholt sich (z. B. einmal pro Woche oder mehrmals am Tag),
   über einen längeren Zeitraum (z. B. über mehrere Wochen oder über mehrere
   Jahre) und erfolgt systematisch. Opfer werden ausgesucht, um regelmäßig
   schikaniert zu werden. Daher werden einzelne „Ausraster" und negative Handlungen, die einmal gegen eine Person und ein anderes Mal gegen eine andere
   Person gerichtet sind, nicht als Mobbing verstanden.

4. Das vierte Merkmal bezieht sich auf die Erscheinungsformen des Mobbings. Die Begrenzung von Mobbing auf direkte körperliche Angriffe werden dem Phänomen nicht gerecht. Olweus (2002) unterscheidet stattdessen mittelbare Gewalt von unmittelbarer Gewalt. Unter unmittelbarer Gewalt versteht er direkte, offene Angriffe (physisches oder verbales Mobbing), unter mittelbarer Gewalt jeden Versuch, eine Person sozial auszugrenzen (relationales Mobbing).

Bei diesen vier Mobbing-Kriterien handelt es sich um die geläufigsten Aspekte, die sich in jeweils leicht veränderter Form in der Literatur wiederfinden (vgl. Kulis 2005; Olweus 2002; Scheithauer et al. 2003; Wolke und Stanford 1999). Als darüberhinausgehendes Definitionsmerkmal erweist sich nach Schäfer und Korn (2001) sowie Smith und Morita (1999):

5. dass Mobbing meist in sozialen Kontexten auftritt, denen man sich nicht ohne weiteres entziehen kann und die durch eine starre Gruppenstruktur geprägt sind. Schule repräsentiert hierbei solch ein soziales Umfeld. Da Schülerinnen und Schüler schulpflichtig sind und täglich zur Schule gehen müssen, sind die Fluchtmöglichkeiten von (potenziellen) Opfern stark begrenzt. Zusätzlich bewegen sich Schulpflichtige über Jahre hinweg in gleichen sozialen Umwelten, was dazu führt, dass über die Zeit hinweg veränderungsresistente Gruppengefüge entstehen. Einmal angenommene soziale Rollen (z. B. die des Opfers) sind dann nur noch schwer abzulegen. Daher kann aus Opfersicht von einem Zustand des „Ausgeliefertseins" gesprochen werden, bei dem eigene Handlungsmöglichkeiten stark eingeschränkt sind. Auch die virtuelle Welt des Internets, insbesondere die sogenannten Sozialen Netzwerke, erfüllt diese Kriterien.

Cybermobbing, das Mobbing via moderner Kommunikationstechnologien, steht in engem Zusammenhang mit dem traditionellen Begriff des Mobbings. Es ist insbesondere das Nutzen von elektronischen Kommunikationsmitteln zum Zwecke des Mobbings, welches die beiden Verhaltensweisen voneinander abgrenzt. Neben diesem Aspekt können jedoch weitere Unterschiede benannt werden, die es erschweren, Cybermobbing als verdecktes psychologisches Mobbing zu betrachten (Hinduja und Patchin 2009). Da der Täter meist anonym bleibt, liegt die Kontrolle über die Situation verstärkt in seinen Händen. Er fühlt sich vor Sanktionen geschützt und die aggressiven Handlungen durchdringen noch stärker die Privatsphäre des Opfers. An jedem Ort, zu jeder Zeit können Mobbinghandlungen durchgeführt werden (Smith et al. 2008). Daneben wird bei Cybermobbing auch betont, dass a) neben der Intention des Täters zu schädigen, insbesondere der negative Effekt auf das Opfer auschlaggebend ist, b) der Aspekt der Wiederholung der Tat nicht immer gegeben ist, c) eine potenziell sehr große Reichweite der Handlungen erkennbar ist, d) die Angriffe allgegenwärtig sein können und e) die Verstärkung des Täters häufig verzögert erfolgt, da beispielsweise das Opfer eine negative Handlung nicht unmittelbar, sondern erst mit Zeitverzögerung wahrnimmt (Schenk 2020).

Insgesamt weist eine Vielzahl von Befunden darauf hin, dass Opfer von traditionellem Mobbing häufig auch Opfer von Cybermobbing sind (Hinduja und Patchin 2009; Smith und Steffgen 2013; Steffgen und König 2009). Zudem erweisen sich Mobbing-Opfer zum Teil auch als potenzielle Cybermobbing-Täter (König et al. 2010). Neben Opfer und Täter besitzen darüber hinaus auch Außenstehende, sogenannte Bystander, beim Cybermobbing eine bedeutsame Rolle (Salmivalli 2010; Machackova et al. 2018). Die Außenstehenden nehmen insofern am Mobbinggeschehen teil, als sie a) problematische Inhalte, d. h. die negativen Handlungen des Täters, betrachten, weiterleiten und/oder liken oder b) den Täter oder das Opfer beispielsweise mit Nachrichten direkt unterstützen.

2.2 Unterschiedliche Formen von Cybermobbing

Es lassen sich viele unterschiedliche Formen von Cybermobbing differenzieren. Die von Smith et al. (2006) aufgestellte Typologie basiert auf dem jeweils verwendeten elektronischen Kommunikationsmittel mithilfe dessen Cybermobbing durchgeführt wird:

- Cybermobbing durch Textnachrichten: zum Beispiel das Versenden von beleidigenden SMS
- Cybermobbing durch Fotos oder Videos: normalerweise werden diese mit den Kameras der Mobiltelefone gemacht und anschließend auf Fotoseiten im Internet verteilt
- Cybermobbing durch Telefonanrufe, besonders mithilfe von Mobiltelefonen
- Cybermobbing durch E-Mails
- Cybermobbing in Chatrooms
- Cybermobbing durch Instant Messenger
- Cybermobbing auf Webseiten

Dementsprechend finden sich in der Literatur mittlerweile eine Vielzahl von Begrifflichkeiten, die dieser Differenzierung Rechnung tragen (electronic mobbing, e-mobbing, sms mobbing, mobile mobbing, online mobbing, digital mobbing und Internetmobbing).

Andere Autoren wiederum differenzieren Cybermobbing anhand der Ausrichtung der durchgeführten Handlungen (vgl. zusammenfassend Hinduja und Patchin 2009). So unterscheidet Willard (2006) zwischen:

- Flaming: Streitigkeiten, hitzige Online-Diskussionen mit Hilfe von elektronischen Nachrichten, bei denen vulgäre und beleidigende Worte verwendet werden. An diesen meist kurzlebigen Streitigkeiten sind zwei oder mehr Personen beteiligt sowie manchmal auch Bystander, die Einfluss auf den Verlauf der Diskussion nehmen. Wesentlich ist außerdem, dass Flaming Gewaltdrohungen enthalten kann (aber nicht muss), welche auch zu physischer Gewalt führen können. Bei Flaming befinden sich die beteiligten Personen auf der gleicher Machtebene, weshalb es teilweise nicht als Cybermobbing im engeren Sinne angesehen wird.
- Belästigung: Wiederholtes Senden von beleidigenden und/oder bedrohlichen Nachrichten. Hierbei ist vor allem das Andauern über die Zeit hervorzuheben; im Gegensatz zu Flaming handelt es sich bei Belästigung um das wiederholte Senden von negativen Nachrichten/Informationen über einen längeren Zeitraum. Beim Opfer kann, sobald es online ist, eine ständige Angst vor Belästigung bestehen. Die Belästigung ist meist einseitig; antwortet das Opfer seinerseits mit beschimpfenden Nachrichten, dann nur in der Absicht, das Verhalten des Täters zu beenden.
- Verunglimpfung: Jemanden durch die Verbreitung von Gerüchten oder Lügen im Internet beleidigen oder diffamieren. Das Opfer ist dabei nur indirekt beteiligt, da die Empfänger der Nachrichten andere Personen sind, wobei es sich entweder um dem Opfer bekannte Personen oder aber um sämtliche Nutzer des Kommunikationsmittels handeln kann (z. B. beim Veröffentlichen von Gerüchten in sozialen Netzwerken). Verunglimpfung im Internet kann Sprache beinhalten, die als Beleidigung oder Verleumdung strafbar ist.
- Personifikation: Durch Auftreten als eine andere Person im Internet (Rollenübernahme mit Hilfe von Benutzernamen, Passwörtern etc.) wird versucht, diese andere Person durch unangemessenes Verhalten schlecht aussehen zu lassen und sie vorzuführen. Das Ziel besteht darin, dem Ansehen dieser anderen Person zu schaden.
- Outing und Verrat: Geheimnisse, intime oder peinliche Informationen oder Bilder einer Person online verbreiten (outing). Dabei ist meist eine Gruppe von Personen beteiligt. Um Verrat handelt es sich z. B., wenn ein Täter ihm anvertraute private Informationen beispielsweise per E-Mail an andere weiterleitet oder andere Personen seine Onlineunterhaltung mit dem Opfer mitlesen lässt.

- Ausschluss: Jemanden bewusst aus einer Online-Gruppe ausschließen (Chats, Freundeslisten, thematische Foren etc.). Dies geschieht besonders häufig unter Jugendlichen, die eine sogenannte In-Group und deren Außenseiter definieren. Gerade im Schulsetting führt der Ausschluss von Online-Aktivitäten meist auch zu einem Ausschluss aus dieser Gruppe im täglichen Leben, was bedeutende emotionale Konsequenzen für das Opfer haben kann.
- Cyberstalking: Wiederholtes Senden von Nachrichten, die Bedrohungen und eventuell auch Erpressungen enthalten oder verstörend wirken. Dabei soll das Opfer eingeschüchtert und/oder ihr Ruf oder ihre Freundschaften zerstört werden. Der Unterschied zwischen Belästigung und direktem Cyberstalking ist zum Teil schwierig festzulegen, jedoch ist insbesondere die Furcht des Opfers um die eigene Sicherheit ein deutlicher Indikator dafür, dass es sich um Cyberstalking handelt. Indirektes Cyberstalking nimmt meist die Form von Verunglimpfung oder Personifikation an (siehe oben). Wesentlich ist, dass Opfer von Cyberstalking aus Angst vor den Konsequenzen oftmals zögern dieses zu berichten, vor allem, wenn sie selbst dem Täter das Material (z. B. Fotos aus einer vorherigen intimen Beziehung) geliefert haben.

Eine weitere spezifische Form von Cybermobbing stellt das „Happy Slapping" dar. Darunter wird eine meist unerwartete Attacke auf ein Opfer verstanden, wobei Unterstützer des Täters das Vorgehen filmen, oftmals mit der Kamera eines Mobiltelefons, um es danach im Internet zu verbreiten. Dier Täter und seine Unterstützer versuchen die gewalthaltige Tat meist wie ein Spiel erscheinen zu lassen. Bei Happy Slapping werden mindestens zwei Täter benötigt: der eigentliche Täter, der die Attacke vornimmt sowie eine Person, die die Tat filmt. Der meist stattfindende körperliche Missbrauch wird hier einer breiten Öffentlichkeit gezeigt und zur Verfügung gestellt.

Auch „Online Grooming", die systematische, gezielte Anbahnung von Kontakten von Erwachsenen mit dem Ziel der sexuellen Ausbeutung von Minderjährigen, kann als eine spezifische Form des Cybermobbings angesehen werden. Diese Form des Cybermobbings geht über Belästigung hinaus, Kinder und Jugendliche erhalten hier z. B. unaufgefordert pornographisches Bildmaterial zugesandt, werden zu Treffen animiert und für Fotoshootings angeworben (Derr 2009; Katzer 2008). Dabei bauen Täter über das Internet (z. B. im Chat) über einen längeren Zeitraum Vertrauen zu ihrem minderjährigen Opfer auf, oftmals indem sie sich ebenfalls als Teenager ausgeben und sich als verständnisvoller Zuhörer darstellen. Durch Geschenke und Aufmerksamkeit wird diese Beziehung gestärkt. Die Anonymität im Internet, die geringere Hemmschwelle und die relativ hohe Verfügbarkeit von Opfern erleichtern es den Tätern, das aufgebaute Vertrauen auszunutzen und sexuelle Gewalt auszuüben (Katzer 2008). Im Weiteren kann es dann zu sexuellen Übergriffen im Chat, bis hin zu Treffen und Übergriffen im realen Leben kommen. Der Zugang der Täter zu ihren Opfern erweist sich in der virtuellen Welt als insgesamt leichter und unauffälliger umsetzbar (Derr 2009).

Zusammenfassend lassen sich nach Weitzmann (2017) Online-Verhaltensweisen als Cybermobbing kennzeichnen, wenn sie als massive Belästigung, Bloßstellung, Diffamierung, Demütigung und/oder Bedrohung wahrgenommen werden.

3   Ausmaß des Problems Cybermobbing

Aufgrund starker methodischer (z. B. Stichprobenwahl, Messmethode) und definitorischer Differenzen in den derzeit vorliegender Studien zur Prävalenz des Cybermobbings erweist es sich als äußerst schwierig, das Ausmaß der Problematik zu quantifizieren (Schenk 2020; Smith und Steffgen 2013).

Thorp (2004) berichtet in einer der ersten Studien zur Erforschung des Auftretens von Cybermobbing in den USA, dass während des Jahres 2000 6 % der befragten Jugendlichen Opfer von Cybermobbing wurden. Auch Oliver und Candappa (2003) belegen, dass 4 % der Schüler zwischen 12 und 13 Jahren mit aggressiven Textnachrichter auf ihren Mobiltelefonen konfrontiert wurden. In einer von Burgess-Proctor (vgl. Patchin und Hinduja 2006) durchgeführten Studie in den USA gaben 38,3 % der Jugendlichen an, schon einmal Opfer von Cybermobbing gewesen zu sein. 16 % der Stichprobe führen an, schon einmal andere Online angegriffen zu haben. Eine telefonische Befragung, die von Ybarra und Mitchell (2004) mit Jugendlichen zwischen 10 und 17 Jahren durchgeführt wurde, ergab, dass 19 % bei einem Cybermobbingvorfall entweder als Opfer oder als Täter beteiligt waren.

In Kanada erreichte der Anteil der Internetnutzer, die bereits über Internet schikaniert und bedroht wurden 25 % (MNet 2001). 69 % geben an jemanden zu kennen, der bereits Opfer von Cybermobbing wurde (Beran und Li 2005). In einer weiteren Studie belegt Li (2006), dass fast 25 % Opfer von Online-aggressionen wurden, während 17 % angaben, schon einmal jemanden auf diese Art und Weise angegriffen zu haben (Vaillancourt et al. 2017).

Auch für Europa liegen vergleichbare Daten vor. In einer repräsentativen Untersuchung des National Children's Home, einer britischen Wohltätigkeitsorganisation für Kinder, von 2005 geben 20 % der Befragten an, Opfer von Cybermobbing gewesen zu sein, wobei 14 % durch Textnachrichten, 5 % in

Chatrooms und 4 % durch E-Mails bedroht wurden. Smith et al. (2006) belegen einen noch höheren Anteil an Schülern, die bereits Erlebnisse mit Cybermobbing hatten (22 %), wobei 6,6 % der Schüler angaben, in den letzten zwei Monaten längere Zeit unter Angriffen gelitten zu haben.

Für Deutschland berichten Katzer und Fetchenhauer (2007), dass über 40 % aller befragten Chatter von anderen Chatteilnehmern bereits beleidigt, gehänselt, geärgert oder beschimpft, 14 % von anderen erpresst, unter Druck gesetzt oder bedroht und fast ein Viertel aller Chatter von anderen in Gesprächen ausgegrenzt, nicht beachtet oder isoliert wurden. Weiterhin zeigen sie, dass 38 % der befragten Chatter schon gegen ihren Willen nach sexuellen Dingen gefragt wurden oder ihnen über sexuelle Erfahrungen anderer berichtet wurde. 11 % der chattenden Jugendlichen erhielten unaufgefordert Nacktfotos und 5 % Pornofilme, zudem wurden 8 % zu sexuellen Handlungen vor der Webcam aufgefordert. Weiterhin zeigt Oppenheim (2008) auf, dass 15 % der 10- bis 15-Jährigen bereits sexuell im Netz bedrängt wurden, indem sie beispielsweise aufgefordert wurden, sexuelle Handlungen vorzunehmen, über Sex zu reden, oder sexuelle Erfahrungen im Chat zu teilen.

In Luxemburg geben 3,8 bis 4,4 % der Schüler an, regelmäßig Opfer von Cybermobbing und 3,9 bis 5 % andere regelmäßig online zu mobben (Steffgen et al. 2010).

Fasst man die derzeit vorliegenden Studien aus unterschiedlichen Europäischen Ländern, den USA, Kanada und Australien zusammen, so sind Prävalenzraten der Cyberviktimisierung von 3 % bis 26 %, und des Cybermobbings von 6 % bis 17 % anzunehmen (Li et al. 2012; Smith und Steffgen 2013). Insgesamt unterstreichen die Prävalenzraten, dass es sich bei Cybermobbing um ein relevantes und ernstzunehmendes Problem handelt.

4   Gesundheitliche Folgen von Cybermobbing

Werden in der Forschung insbesondere die Folgen des Cybermobbings für Opfer thematisiert, so lassen sich auch negative gesundheitliche Folgen für Täter von Cybermobbing belegen (Campbell et al. 2013). Die gesundheitlichen Konsequenzen für Bystander wurden bisher kaum untersucht (Steffgen et al. 2018).

So weisen Täter erhöhte Depressionswerte (Selki et al. 2015) sowie höhere Ängstlichkeit (Lam et al. 2013) bei geringerem Selbstwertgefühl (Patchin und Hinduja 2010) auf. Dies verdeutlicht, dass auch das Handeln der Täter einen direkten Bezug zu ihrer Gesundheit hat.

Insbesondere jedoch weisen Opfer kurz- und langfristige physische und psychische Gesundheitsprobleme aufgrund des erfahrenen Cybermobbings auf (Vaillancourt et al. 2017). Dabei treten als Folge des Cybermobbings sowohl akute, direkte Belastungen (sich verletzt fühlen, verängstigt sein) als auch dauerhafte Belastungen (psychische und gesundheitliche Probleme) auf (Gradinger et al. 2012). Vielfältige negative Auswirkungen sind belegt, wie z. B. psychosomatische Beschwerden (Schlafstörungen, Kopf- und Bauchschmerzen, Bettnässen oder gestörtes Essverhalten), Gefühle der Hilflosigkeit, Traurigkeit, persönliche Abwertungen, negative Selbstwertgefühle, Selbstmitleid, Selbstbeschuldigungen, sozialer Rückzug, Isolation, Beziehungsprobleme, Leistungsabfall in der Schule bis hin zum Meiden der Schule (Smith und Steffgen 2013; Sourander et al. 2010; Steffgen und König 2009; Willard 2006). Insbesondere die sexuelle Viktimisierung im Chat stellt für die Opfer eine starke emotionale Belastung dar, die mit zum Teil dauerhaften negativen psychischen Folgen einhergeht (Katzer und Fetchenhauer 2007). Neben einem erhöhten Depressionsrisiko (Machmutow et al. 2012), einem verstärktem Angsterleben (soziale Angst und Schulangst, Juvonen und Cross 2008) sind selbstverletzendes (Lam et al. 2013) bis hin zu suizidalem Verhalten (Weitzel et al. 2020) Folgen von Cybermobbing (Schenk 2020).

Auch Ybarra und Mitchell (2004) legen dar, dass Jugendliche, die Cybermobbing erlebt haben, mit höherer Wahrscheinlichkeit depressive Verstimmungen und andere Verhaltensprobleme zeigen, und auch häufiger Opfer von Mobbing außerhalb des Internets werden, was wiederum die Gesundheitsproblematik weiter verstärkt (Li et al. 2012). Im Vergleich zwischen klassischem Mobbing und Cybermobbing belegen Smith et al. (2006), dass:

- Cybermobbinghandlungen wie ungewollt verbreitete Fotos, Filme ebenso wie Telefonanrufe von Opfern als belastender wahrgenommen werden als klassische Mobbinghandlungen,
- die Verbreitung von Aggressionen über Webseiten und durch Textnachrichten von Opfern als genauso belastend empfunden werden wie klassische Mobbinghandlungen.

Die Studie von msn.uk (2006) zeigt zudem auf, dass 11 % der Befragten angaben, dass die Auswirkungen des Cybermobbings ernster sind als erlebte körperliche Angriffe.

Anzunehmen ist, dass, vergleichbar mit klassischem Mobbing, die in der Kindheit und Jugend erlebten Cybermobbingerfahrungen, sich auch noch im späteren Erwachsenenalter negativ auswirken werden (Takizawa et al. 2014).

5   Präventions- und Interventionsansätze

Die psychologisch-pädagogische Fachliteratur hat mittlerweile eine Vielzahl anwendbarer Interventionskonzepte zu klassischem Mobbing dokumentiert (Smith et al. 1999). Diese werden von einer Vielzahl von Schulen angewendet und für deren spezifische Bedürfnisse adaptiert. Insgesamt gewinnen in Bezug auf Mobbing-Interventionen schulweite Mehr-Ebenen-Konzepte zunehmend an Bedeutung (Scheithauer et al. 2003). Ttofi und Farrington (2011) konnten anhand einer Meta-Analyse belegen, dass derartige Konzepte bis zu 23 % an Mobbing-verhalten und bis zu 20 % an Viktimisierung reduzieren können.

Diese Konzepte sind auch als Ansatzpunkte für Interventionen gegen-über Cybermobbing zu nutzen. Jedoch ist davon auszugehen, dass gegenüber den Mobbingansätzen zusätzliche Aspekte zu berücksichtigen sind, z. B. hin-sichtlich der Kenntnisse über die Funktionsmöglichkeiten von technischen Kommunikationsmitteln. So verfügen Lehrer und Eltern zum Teil über geringere Kenntnisse über die Nutzung neuer Kommunikationstechnologien als Kinder und Jugendliche.

Erste empirische Befunde in diesem Bereich belegen, dass es Schülern ins-gesamt an angemessenen Strategien und Verhaltensweisen fehlt, um mit erlebtem Cybermobbing umzugehen (Li 2005). Daher zielen unterschiedliche Ansätze darauf, den Mangel an Problembewusstsein bei Eltern und Schulpersonal zu minimieren. Erste Richtlinien für Eltern, Erzieher und Lehrer wurden vorgelegt, die Schüler dazu auffordern über ihre Erfahrungen zu berichten. Zudem wird gefordert (Hinduja und Patchin 2009), dass:

- Schulen Einfluss auf die Eltern nehmen sollen,
- vertrauensvolle Beziehungen zwischen Schülern und Lehrern aufgebaut werden,
- angemessene soziale Normen sowie sozial-emotive Kompetenzen (z. B. Empathie, siehe Steffgen et al. 2011) entwickelt und
- Medienkompetenz vermittelt werden.

Cross et al. (2012) benennen darüber hinaus fünf Strategien, welche sich als effektiv zur Reduzierung von Cybermobbing erweisen sollen. Es gilt:

1. Problemverständnis/Bewusstsein sowie Handlungskompetenzen über (Cyber-)Mobbing bei Lehrern, Schülern und Eltern zu entwickeln,
2. proaktive Schulpolitik, Handlungspläne und Praktiken zu entwickeln, um auf den unterschiedlichen Ebenen angemessen zu reagieren,

3. ein unterstützendes soziales Umfeld herzustellen,
4. eine schützende physikalische bzw. technische Umwelt zu gestalten,
5. eine Vernetzung zwischen Schule, Familie und Gemeinschaft/Gemeinde zu etablieren.

Insgesamt ist festzustellen, dass bisher kaum wissenschaftlich evaluierte Interventionsprogramme zu Cybermobbing vorliegen. Das Programm „Medienhelden" stellt hier ein erster theoriebasierter präventiver Ansatz zur Reduktion von Cybermobbing und zur Förderung der Medienkompetenz von Schülern dar (Schultze-Krumbholtz et al. 2012). Ziele des Programms sind es, Problembewusstsein zu erarbeiten, Informationen/Wissen zu vermitteln sowie angemessene soziale Normen zu etablieren. Neben dem Erlernen von Perspektivenübernahme und Empathie sollen ebenso Einstellungen angepasst werden. Zudem sollen die Schüler lernen, ihre Mediennutzung bzw. ihr Medienverhalten kritisch zu hinterfragen, angemessene Handlungskompetenzen herauszubilden, sowie das Klassenklima zu verbessern und zufriedenstellende Peerbeziehungen zu entwickeln. Erste Befunde der Wirksamkeitsevaluation des Programms weisen darauf hin, dass die einzelnen Programmelemente sehr positiv von Lehrern und Schülern aufgenommen und beurteilt werden (Jäkel et al. 2012).

Als wesentlich erweist es sich, dass neben Maßnahmen auf pädagogischer Ebene (Schule, Lehrer, Eltern) sowie individueller Ebene (Opfer, Täter, Bystander; vgl. Pfetsch et al. 2011), auch Maßnahmen auf technischer (Provider) sowie juristischer und polizeilicher Ebene erforderlich sind. Insbesondere das Happy Slapping sowie das Online-Grooming erfordern es, dass weitere Schritte im Jugendmedienschutz vorzunehmen sind. Insgesamt sollte bei Cybermobbing-Interventionen sowohl auf der individuellen (z. B. psychosoziale Charakteristiken berücksichtigend), der familiären (z. B. die durch die Familie vermittelten Werte), der schulischen (z. B. dem Schulklima und den Schüler-Lehrer-Beziehungen), der öffentlichen (z. B. der gesellschaftlichen Kommunikation von Cybermobbing) als auch der technischen (z. B. der Umgang mit Online-Medien) Ebene angesetzt werden (Papatraiancu et al. 2014).

6   Fazit

Cybermobbing in seinen unterschiedlichen Formen, dessen relevante Prävalenz und weitreichenden gesundheitlichen Folgen (bis hin zu suizidalem Verhalten der Opfer) verweisen deutlich auf einen konkreten Handlungsbedarf in diesem Bereich.

Neben Interventionen auf pädagogischer sowie individueller Ebene sind auch Maßnahmen auf technischer (Provider) sowie juristischer und polizeilicher Ebene erforderlich. Erste spezifische Präventionsprogramme für Cybermobbing wurden vorgelegt, eine nötige Wirksamkeitsevaluation steht jedoch noch weitgehend aus.

Literatur

Beran, T., & Li, Q. (2005). Cyber-harassment: A study of a new method for an old behavior. *Journal of Educational Computing Research, 32(3)*, 265–277.

Böhmer, M., & Steffgen, G. (Eds.). (2020). *Mobbing an Schulen. Maßnahmen zur Prävention, Intervention und Nachsorge.* Berlin: Springer.

Campbell, M.A., Slee, P.T., Spears, B., Butle, S., & Kift, S. (2013). Do cyberbullies suffer too? Cyberbullies' perceptions of the harm they cause to others and their own mental health. *School Psychology International, 34*, 613-629.

Cross, D., Li, Q., Smith, P.K., & Monks, H. (2012). Understanding and preventing cyberbullying: Where have we been and where should we be going? In Q. Li, D. Cross, & P.K. Smith (Eds.), *Cyberbullying in the global playground* (pp. 287–305). Malden, MA: Wiley-Blackwell.

Davidson, J., & Martellozzo, E. (2008). Protecting vulnerable young people in cyberspace from sexual abuse: raising awareness and responding globally. *Police Practice and Research, 9(4)*, 277–289.

Derr, R. (2009). Sexuelle Gewalt in den neuen Medien. Herausforderungen für den Kinder- und Jugendschutz. *Monatsschrift Kinderheilkunde, 5*, 449–455.

Ttofi, M.M., & Farrington, D.P (2011). Effectiveness of school-based programs to reduce bullying: a systematic and meta-analytic review. *Journal of Experimental Criminology, 7*, 27–56.

Gradinger, P., Strohmeier, D., & Spiel, C. (2012). Motives for bullying others in cyberspace: A study on Bullies and Bully-Victims in Austria. In Q. Li, D. Cross, & P.K. Smith (Eds.), *Cyberbullying in the global playground* (pp. 263–284). Malden, MA: Wiley-Blackwell.

Hinduja, S., & Patchin, J.W. (2009). *Bullying. Beyond the schoolyard.* Thousand Oaks, CA: Corwin Press.

Huberty, Y. & Steffgen, G. (2008). *Bullying in Schulen. Prädiktoren zivilcouragierten Verhaltens.* Saarbrücken: VDM.

Jäkel, A., Schultze-Krumbholtz, A., Zagorscak, P., & Scheithauer, H. (2012). Das Medienhelden-Programm. *Forum Kriminalprävention, 12(1)*, 16-20.

Juvonen, J., & Gross, E.F. (2008). Extending the school grounds? Bullying experiences in cyberspace. *Journal of School Health, 78(9)*, 496–505.

Katzer, C. (2008). Tatort Internet: Cyberbullying und sexuelle Viktimisierung von Kindern und Jugendlichen in Chatrooms. *Forum Kriminalprävention, 8(3)*, 26–33.

Katzer, K., & Fetchenhauer, D. (2007). Cyberbullying: Aggression und Viktimisierung in Chatrooms. In M. Gollwitzer, J. Pfetsch, V. Schneider, A. Schulz, T. Steffke & C. Ulrich (Hrsg.), *Gewaltprävention bei Kindern und Jugendlichen* (pp. 104–122). Göttingen: Hogrefe.

KIM-Studie. (2009). *Kim-Studie 2008: Kinder und Medien, Computer und Internet*. Stuttgart: Medienpädagogischer Forschungsverbund Südwest.

König, A., Gollwitzer, M., & Steffgen, G. (2010). Cyberbullying as an act of revenge? *Australian Journal of Guidance and Counselling, 20*, 210–224.

Kulis, M. (2005). *Bullying als Gruppenphänomen: der Beitrag der Mitschüler für die Stabilisierung von Bullying*. München: Dr. Hut.

Lam, L.T., Cheng, Z., & Liu, X. (2013). Violent online games exposure and cyberbullying/ victimization among adolescents. *Cyberpsychology, Behavior, and Social Networking, 16*, 159–164.

Li, Q. (2005). *Cyberbullying in schools: Nature and extent of adolescents' experience*. Paper presented at the Annual American Educational Research Association Conference, Montreal.

Li, Q. (2006). Cyberbullying in schools: A research of gender differences. *School Psychology International, 27*, 157–170.

Li, Q., Cross, D., & Smith, P.K. (Eds.). (2012). *Cyberbullying in the global playground*. Malden, MA: Wiley-Blackwell.

Machmutow, K., Perren, S., Sticca, F., & Alsaker, F.D. (2012). Peer victimization and depressive symptoms: Can specific coping strategies buffer the negative impact of cybervictimization? *Emotional and Behavioral Difficulties, 17*(3-4), 403–420.

Machackova, H., Pfetsch, J. & Steffgen, G. (2018). Editorial: Special issue on bystanders of online aggression. *Cyberpsychology: Journal of Psychosocial Research on Cyberspace, 12*(4), 1–7

MNet. (2001). *Young canadians in a wired world-Mnet Survey*. Available from http://www. media-awareness.ca/English/special_initiatives/surveys/index.cfm

NCH. (2005). *Putting U in the picture – Mobile phone bullying survey 2005*. Available from http://www.nch.org.uk/uploads/documents/Mobile_bul ying_%20report.pdf/.

Oliver, C., & Candappa, M. (2003). *Tackling bullying: Listening to the views of Children and Young People* Department for Education and Skills, Nottingham.

Olweus, D. (1996). Bullying at school. Knowledge base and an effective intervention program. In C.G. Ferris & T. Grisso (Eds.), *Understanding aggressive behaviour in children. Annals of the New York Academy of Sciences, Vol. 794* (pp. 265–276). New York: The New York Academy of Sciences.

Olweus, D. (2002). Gewalt in der Schule. *Was Lehrer wissen sollten – und tun können* (3. korr. Aufl.). Bern: Huber.

Oppenheim, K. (2008). Social Networking Sites: Growing Use Among Tweens and Teens, but a Growing Threat As Well? *Trends & Tudes, 7*(3), 1–4.

Papatraianou, L.H., Levine, D., & West, D. (2014). Resilience in the face of cyberbullying: an ecological perspective on young people's experiences of online adversity. *Pastoral Care in Education, 32*(4), 264–283.

Patchin, J.W., & Hinduja, S. (2006). Bullies move beyond the schoolyard: A preliminary look at cyberbullying. *Youth Violence and Juvenile Justice, 4*, 148–169.

Patchin, J.W., & Hinduja, S. (2010). Cyberbullying and self-esteem. *Journal of School Health, 80*, 614–621.

Pfetsch, J., Steffgen, G., Gollwitzer, M., & Ittel, A. (2011). Prevention of aggression in schools through a bystander intervention training. *International Journal of Developmental Science, 5*, 139–149.

Salmivalli, C. (2010). Bullying and the peer group: A review. *Journal of Aggression and Violent Behavior, 115,* 112–120.

Schäfer, M. & Korn, S. (2001). Bullying – eine Definition. *Psychologie in Erziehung und Unterricht, 51,* 236–237.

Scheithauer, H., Hayer, T. & Petermann, F. (2003). *Bullying unter Schülern. Erscheinungsformen, Risikobedingungen und Interventionskonzepte.* Göttingen: Hogrefe.

Schenk, L. (2020). Was ist Cybermobbing? In M. Böhmer, & G. Steffgen (Hrsg.), *Mobbing an Schulen. Maßnahmen zur Prävention, Intervention und Nachsorge* (pp. 273–301). Berlin: Springer.

Schultze-Krumbholtz, A., Zagorscak, P., Siebenbrock, A., & Scheithauer, H. (2012). *Medienhelden: Unterrichtsmaterial zur Förderung von Medienkompetenz und Prävention von Cybermobbing.* München: Reinhardt Verlag

Selkie, E.M., Kota, R., Chan, Y.F., & Moreno, M. (2015). Cyberbullying, depression, and problem alcohol use in female college students. A multisite study. *Cyberpsychology, Behavior, & Social Networking, 18,* 79-86.

Smith, P.K. & Morita, Y. (1999). Introduction. In P.K. Smith, Y. Morita, J. Junger-Tas, D. Olweus, R. Catalano & P. Slee (Eds.), *The nature of school bullying. A cross-national perspective* (S. 1–4). London: Routledge.

Smith, P.K., Pepler, D., & Rigby, K. (1999). *Bullying in schools. How succesful can interventions be?* Cambridge: Cambridge University Press

Smith, P.K., Mahdavi, J., Carvalho, M., & Tippett, N. (2006). *An investigation into cyberbullying, its forms, awareness and impact, and the relationship between age and gender in cyberbullying.* Unit for school and family studies, Goldsmiths College, University of London.

Smith, P.K., Mahdavi, J., Carvalho, M., Fisher, S., Russell, S., & Tippett, N. (2008). Cyberbullying: Its nature and impact in secondary school pupils. *Journal of Child Psychology and Psychiatry, 49(4),* 376–385.

Smith, P.K., & Steffgen, G. (Hrsg.). (2013). Cyberbullying through the new media: findings from an international network. Hove: Psychology Press.

Sourander, A., Klomek, A.B., Ikonen, M., Lindroos, J., Luntamo, T., Koskelainen, M., Ristkari, T., & Helenius, H. (2010). Psychological risk factors associated with cyberbullying among adolescents: a population-based study. *Archives of General Psychiatry, 67(7),* 720–728.

Steffgen, G. (2014). Cyberbullying. Missbrauch mittels neuer elektronischer Mittel. In H. Willems & D. Ferring (Hrsg.), Macht und Missbrauch in Institutionen (pp. 133–148). Wiesbaden: Springer VS.

Steffgen, G. Costa, A.P., & Slee, P. (2018). The coping of bystanders with cyberbullying in an adolescent population. In P. Slee, G. Skrzypiec & C. Cefai (Eds.), *Child and adolescent wellbeing and violence prevention in schools* (pp. 129–137). London: Routledge.

Steffgen, G., & König, A. (2009). Cyber bullying: The role of traditional bullying and empathy. B. Sapeo, L. Haddon, E. Mante-Meijer, L. Fortunati, T. Turk & E. Loos (Eds.), *The good, the bad and the challenging. Conference Proceedings* (Vol. II; pp. 1041–1047). Brussels: Cost office.

Steffgen, G., Pfetsch, J., König, A. & Melzer, A. (2011). Are cyber bullies less empathic? Adolescents' cyber bullying behavior and empathic responsiveness. *Cyberpsychology, Behavior, and Social Networking, 14,* 643–648.

Steffgen, G., Vandebosch, H., Völlink, T., Deboutte, G., & Dehue, F. (2010). Cyberbullying in the Benelux-Countries: First findings and ways to address the problem. In J. Mora-Merchan & T. Jäger (Eds.), *Cyberbullying: a cross-national comparison* (pp. 35–54). Landau: Verlag Empirische Pädagogik.

Takizawa, R., Maughan, B., & Arseneault, L. (2014). Adult health outcomes of childhood bullying victimization: Evidence from a five-decade longitudinal British birth cohort. *American Journal of Psychiatry, 171*(7), 777–784.

Thorp, D. (2004). *Cyberbullies on the prowl in schoolyard.* The Australian, 15 July. Available from http://www.australianit.news.com.au/.

Vaillancourt, T., Faris, R., & Mishna, F. (2017). Cyberbullying in children and youth: Implications for health and clinical practice. *The Canadian Journal of Psychiatry, 62*(6), 368–373.

Weitzel, L., Albert, L., & Steffgen, G. (2020). The paradoxical effect of social support on suicidal ideation in bullying involvement in different cultural contexts. *Journal of Child and Adolescent Behavior, 8*(2), 1–11.

Weitzmann, J.H. (2017). Cyber-Mobbing und was man dagegen tun kann (I): Erscheinungsformen, Gründe und Auslöser. https://irights.info/artikel/cyber-mobbing-cyberbullying-und-was-man-dagegen-tun-kann-2/6919. Zugegriffen: 31.01.2020

Willard, N. (2006). *Cyberbullying and cyberthreats: responding to the challenge of online social cruelty, threats, and distress.* Eugene, Oregon: Center for safe and Responsible Internet Use.

Wolke, D., & Stanford, K. (1999). *Bullying in schoolchildren.* London: Arnold.

Ybarra, M., & Mitchell, K. (2004). Online aggressor/targets, aggressors, and targets: A comparison of associated youth characteristics. *Journal of Child Psychology and Psychiatry and Allied Disciplines, 45*(7), 1308–1316.

Praxisansätze zur Förderung von Wohlbefinden und Gesundheit in Luxemburg

Die Förderung von Gesundheit und Wohlbefinden in der Offenen Jugendarbeit – aus der Sicht der Träger der Luxemburger Jugendstrukturen

Caroll Kremer, Jérôme Mailliet und Simone Grün

1 Einleitung

Die Weltgesundheitsorganisation sieht Gesundheitsförderung im Sinne der Ottawa-Charta[1] als einen Prozess, der Menschen dazu in die Lage versetzen soll, mehr Einfluss auf ihren Gesundheitszustand zu entwickeln und ihre Gesundheit aktiv zu verbessern. Ziel ist die Erreichung eines Zustandes vollständigen körperlichen, geistigen und sozialen Wohlbefindens, der dadurch erreicht werden soll, dass Individuen und Gruppen unterstützt werden, eigene Wünsche wahrzunehmen und zu realisieren, Bedürfnisse zu befriedigen sowie die Umgebung zu verändern oder sich an diese anzupassen. Gesundheit ist demnach ein positives Konzept, das sowohl soziale und individuelle Ressourcen als auch körperliche Fähigkeiten betont. Aus diesem Grund ist Gesundheitsförderung nicht nur im Kompetenzbereich des Gesundheitssektors anzusiedeln, sondern Gesundheitsförderung geht weiter als ein gesunder Lebensstil zum Wohlbefinden.

---

[1] https://www.who.int/teams/health-promotion/enhanced-wellbeing/first-global-conference.

C. Kremer (✉) · J. Mailliet
Daachverband vun de Lëtzebuerger Jugendstrukturen, Luxembourg, Luxembourg
E-Mail: caroll.kremer@dlj.lu

J. Mailliet
E-Mail: jerome.mailliet@dlj.lu

S. Grün
Centre Biergop, Betzdorf, Luxembourg
E-Mail: simone.gruen@biergop.lu

© Der/die Autor(en) 2022
A. Heinen et al. (Hrsg.), *Wohlbefinden und Gesundheit im Jugendalter*,
https://doi.org/10.1007/978-3-658-35744-3_21

Insofern werden unter Gesundheitsförderung die Förderung von Verhaltens- und Handlungsweisen verstanden, welche einen positiven Einfluss auf die Gesundheit des Menschen haben, und die Unterbindung jener Verhaltensweisen, welche negative Auswirkungen auf die Gesundheit haben. Die Gesundheitsförderung zielt auf Ansätze zur Verbesserung und Stärkung des Gesundheitspotenzials des Menschen ab. Dabei geht es zum einen um die Stärkung von Wissen und Kenntnissen jedes Einzelnen, seine Gesundheit zu verbessern, aber auch um die Bearbeitung von Umweltfaktoren, Gesellschaft und Politik. Die Ottawa-Charta umfasst Prinzipien, die auch in der Jugendarbeit vorkommen. Jugendarbeit bietet sich daher als Ansatzpunkt für Förderung von Gesundheit und Wohlbefinden an und zielt dabei auf eine Verbindung von Wissen, Handeln und Erleben ab. Mit diesem Ansatz lässt sich Gesundheitsförderung und insbesondere Gesundheitsbildung prozesshaft und langfristig in die Jugendarbeit integrieren (Landesjugendring Baden-Württemberg 2007).

Zahlreiche theoretische Modelle legen dar, auf welchen Ebenen eine Maßnahme ansetzen muss, um eine Veränderung der Verhaltensweisen zu bewirken, damit eine optimale Gesundheitsförderung erreicht werden kann (CePT 2020).

Im Nachfolgenden wird die Förderung von Gesundheit und Wohlbefinden in der Offenen Jugendarbeit aus der Sicht der Träger der Luxemburger Jugendstrukturen näher beleuchtet.

Im Rahmen einer seiner Haupt-Missionen ist der „Daachverband vun de Lëtzebuerger Jugendstrukturen" (DLJ) als der Verband der Träger der Jugendstrukturen unter anderem zuständig für die Sensibilisierung zu den meisten Inhalten der Jugendarbeit. Schon seit einigen Jahren finden daher seitens der Träger von Jugendstrukturen zusammen mit dem Jugenddienst des luxemburgischen Bildungsministeriums wie auch dem Nationalen Jugenddienst (Service National de la Jeunesse) Fortbildungen, Seminare und (inter-)nationale Konferenzen zu unterschiedlichen Themen und somit auch zur Gesundheit statt.

2 Gesundheitsförderung und Wohlbefinden junger Menschen als anerkanntes Ziel der Jugendarbeit in Luxemburg

In den vergangenen Jahren wurden in der Jugendarbeit in Luxemburg der Aufgabenbereich der Einrichtungen stark erweitert und vermehrt auch Maßnahmen der Qualitätssicherung eingeführt. Diese Entwicklung hält bis dato an und

kulminiert in der Einführung des neuen Jugendgesetzes[2] und der damit verbundenen Verpflichtung zur systematischen Qualitätssicherung der pädagogischen
Prozesse in Kinder- und Jugendstrukturen sowie der Orientierung am nationalen
Bildungsrahmenplan für die non-formale Bildung im Kindes- und Jugendalter. Der nationale Rahmenplan schreibt in erster Linie die grundlegenden
pädagogischen Ziele in den Jugendstrukturen vor, die vom Staat finanziell unterstützt werden.

Die Zielsetzungen des nationalen Rahmenplans sind in sieben Handlungs-
felder integriert und setzen einen Rahmen, welcher in der jeweiligen Einrichtung
sowohl als Richtlinie wie auch als Impulsgeber angesehen werden kann. Der
Rahmen lässt Jugendeinrichtungen viel Raum, ihre eigenen Konzepte und Leitlinien einzubeziehen (MENJE & SNJ 2018).

Im Hinblick auf die Gesundheitsentwicklung und -förderung sieht der
nationale Bildungsrahmenplan für die non-formale Bildung im Kinder- und
Jugendbereich vor, dass die Strukturen der Offenen Jugendarbeit jungen
Menschen zeigen, wie sie auf ihren Körper, ihre Gesundheit und ihr allgemeines
Wohlbefinden achten sollen. Angebote, bei denen sich junge Menschen freiwillig
und abseits vom gesellschaftlichen Leistungsdruck ausprobieren können, sowie
die Vermittlung von Freude an Bewegung gehören ebenso zu den Bildungsauf-
gaben der Offenen Jugendarbeit wie das Informieren und Beraten über alle
gesundheitsrelevanten Themen junger Menschen.

Die Offene Jugendarbeit spricht auch gesundheitliche Themen rund um die
körperliche Entwicklung im Rahmen der sexuellen Bildung und der Prävention
an. Sie sensibilisiert Jugendliche dahin gehend, ein positives Körperbewusstsein
zu entwickeln und die motorischen und sensorischen Fähigkeiten ihres Körpers
wahrzunehmen. Ziel ist es, Jugendliche in ihren zentralen Entwicklungsaufgaben,
wie sexuelle Selbstbestimmung und geschlechtliche Identität, zu unterstützen und
zu begleiten.

Weiterhin strebt der nationale Rahmenplan eine ressourcenorientierte Prävention als Lernstrategie an Prävention im Rahmen Offener Jugendarbeit wird
in diesem Zusammenhang als ganzheitliche und subjektorientierte Form der
Bildung von jungen Menschen verstanden, um eine offene und positive Auseinandersetzung mit sozialen und gesellschaftlichen Werten, Normen und
Handlungsweisen zu ermöglichen. Offene Jugendarbeit begegnet den Krisen und

---

[2] Vgl. Loi du 24 avril 2016 portant modification de la loi modifiée du 4 juillet 2008 sur la
jeunesse.

Konflikten in den Entwicklungsphasen junger Menschen und ihrem riskanten und abweichenden Handeln mit positiven, ressourcen- und kompetenzorientierten Präventionsansätzen, um so das Selbstwertgefühl und die Bewältigungsstrategien der Jugendlichen zu stärken (MENJE & SNJ 2018).

3 Zielbeschreibungen, in denen sich die Förderung von Gesundheit und Wohlbefinden in der Offenen Jugendarbeit niederschlägt

3.1 Zielsetzungen auf lokaler, regionaler und nationaler Ebene

Die gesundheitsbezogenen Zielsetzungen finden sich in den Handlungskonzepten CAG (Concept d'action général) der Jugendhäuser wieder. Ein Handlungskonzept beinhaltet zum einen ein pädagogisches Konzept der Praxis mit der Umsetzung der allgemeinen Zielsetzungen und grundlegenden pädagogischen Prinzipien auf lokaler oder regionaler Ebene. Darüber hinaus umfasst es die Maßnahmen der Selbstevaluation, die Festlegung derjenigen Bereiche, in denen Projekte zur pädagogischen Qualitätssicherung entwickelt werden, und den Weiterbildungsplan des Personals.

Das Jugendhaus ist ein Ort der Freizeitgestaltung, der pädagogischen Arbeit und der jugendlichen Entfaltung und dient als Anlaufstelle und zweites Zuhause. Die dort geleistete pädagogische Arbeit stellt sich den Herausforderungen, die sich aus den Lebenslagen und Erfahrungen junger Menschen ergeben. Die persönlichen und sozialen Gegebenheiten der Besucher:innen bestimmen die Inhalte, Methoden und Angebotsformen der pädagogischen Arbeit. Die pädagogische Arbeit im Jugendhaus orientiert sich an der Lebenswelt der Jugendlichen. Der Fokus liegt auf: Familie, Schule, Ausbildung und Beruf, konkreter Hilfe zur Lebensbewältigung, Engagement für benachteiligte junge Menschen, Mitbestimmung, Mitverantwortung und Partizipation sowie personalem Angebot. Das Jugendhaus ist nicht nur ein Bildungsort, sondern bietet auch Angebote im Bereich der Gesundheitsförderung sowie Entwicklung und Reflexion von Geschlechtsidentität und Geschlechterverhältnissen (DLJ asbl 2017a).

Alles in allem wird Jugendlichen im Rahmen der Gesundheitsförderung bewusstgemacht, dass Bewegung und gesunde Ernährung zu einer verantwortungsbewussten Lebensführung gehören. Auch Themen wie Sexualität gehören zu diesem Handlungsfeld. Einige Jugendhäuser verfügen darüber hinaus bereits über Handlungsstrategien zur Drogenprävention und Suchtprävention oder sind dabei, entsprechende Konzepte auszuarbeiten.

Auch im Rahmen von *Outreach Youth Work* wird die Förderung der Gesundheit und des Wohlbefindens junger Menschen in einer sogenannten NEET-Situation (Not in Education, Employment or Training) berücksichtigt. Die erwerbslosen Jugendlichen in NEET-Situationen, die von *Outreach Youth Work* angesprochen werden, befinden sich meist in prekären Situationen und sind nicht in der Lage, sich mit eigenen Mitteln zu reaktivieren. Damit stellt *Outreach Youth Work* ein in dieser Form neues Angebot der Offenen Jugendarbeit in Luxemburg dar, welches das bestehende non-formale Bildungsangebot ergänzt. *Outreach Youth Work* ermöglicht es, Jugendliche in schwierigen Lebenslagen aufzufangen und ihnen bei der Integration in die Gesellschaft zur Seite zu stehen. Die Jugendlichen sollen dabei unterstützt werden, auf ihre Gesundheit und ihr psychisches Wohlbefinden zu achten, z. B. durch Hygieneaufklärung, gesunde Ernährung und Bewegung.

Vor dem Hintergrund oftmals unsicherer Lebensbedingungen verfügen Jugendliche, die in mehreren Lebensbereichen gescheitert sind, nur über ein geringes Maß an Selbstvertrauen, Motivation und Selbstwirksamkeit. Hinzu kommen geringe Sozialkompetenzen sowie bei manchen auch gesundheitliche Probleme (z. B. Suchterkrankungen, Depressionen). Dies kann dazu führen, dass sie oftmals keinen Arbeits- oder Ausbildungsplatz finden bzw. diesen schnell wieder verlieren (DLJ asbl 2018).

Das Ziel von *Outreach Youth Work* ist es, als Instrument auf lokaler Ebene, diese Jugendlichen ausfindig zu machen, eine Beziehung zu ihnen aufzubauen und ihnen die individuelle Betreuung und Unterstützung zu bieten, die sie dringend benötigen. Durch Empowerment in Form von Gesprächen sowie Einzel- und Gruppenaktivitäten sollen die Jugendlichen so gestärkt werden, dass sie wieder Motivation, Selbstvertrauen und Handlungsfähigkeit erlangen und Mut finden, ihr Leben selbst aktiv zu gestalten. *Outreach Youth Work* steht für aufsuchende Jugendarbeit. Im Konkreten bedeutet dies, dass sich die Jugendarbeiter:innen in den jeweiligen Gemeinden aktiv in den Sozialraum der Jugendlichen begeben und sich deren Lebenswelt annähern.

Das bedeutet aber nicht, dass sich *Outreach Youth Work* für alle Probleme zuständig sieht – im Gegenteil. *Outreach Youth Work* respektiert die Kompetenzen anderer Dienste und auch die eigenen Grenzen des pädagogischen Handlungsfelds. Bei schwerwiegenden gesundheitlichen und psychischen Problemen oder bei Suchtproblemen werden die Jugendlichen von Jugendarbeiter:innen an kompetente Stellen weitervermittelt.

3.2   Zielsetzungen auf europäischer Ebene

Auch auf europäischer Ebene sind Zielbeschreibungen verankert, in denen sich die Förderung von Gesundheit und Wohlbefinden in der Offenen Jugendarbeit niederschlägt. Luxemburg ist in den meisten Gremien der internationalen Jugendarbeit vertreten und involviert, damit Jugendarbeit auf lokaler Ebene den aktuellsten Trends und Entwicklungen folgen kann.

In den Jahren 2017 und 2018 wurden im Dialog mit jungen Menschen in ganz Europa 11 Europäische Jugendziele (Youth Goals) ausgearbeitet. Die Youth Goals fassen zusammen, welche Themen junge Menschen in Europa bewegen und welche politischen Schwerpunkte ihnen wichtig sind. Als Teil der EU-Jugendstrategie sollen die Jugendziele zur Verwirklichung der Vision dieser jungen Menschen beitragen. Die aktuelle EU-Jugendstrategie läuft noch bis 2027. Verantwortliche aus Politik und Gesellschaft können in dieser Zeit die Jugendziele als Anregung nutzen, um Politik im Sinne junger Menschen zu gestalten.

Die Nationalen Arbeitsgruppen (National Working Groups, NWG) leiten diesen partizipativen Prozess auf nationaler Ebene und setzen sich aus im Jugendbereich tätigen Organisationen, Jugendministerien, Jugendräten und anderen interessierten Parteien zusammen.

Die NWG Luxemburg setzt sich für einen regelmäßigen Dialog zwischen Jugendlichen und politischen Entscheidungsträgern in Luxemburg und in Europa ein und verpflichtet sich, die Jugend des Landes regelmäßig zu konsultieren, um ihre spezifischen Bedürfnisse, Ideen und Anforderungen zu identifizieren.

Des Weiteren verpflichtet sich die NWG, die Themen des Dialogs durch das breite Spektrum der Aktivitäten von ständigen Mitgliedern sowie Partnern aus dem Jugendsektor umzusetzen. Die NWG setzt sich für eine Sensibilisierungsarbeit und die Förderung von Youth Goals ein, um sie bei den verschiedenen Partnern und Interessengruppen hervorzuheben.

Darüber hinaus setzt sich die NWG dafür ein, die Ergebnisse und Empfehlungen junger Menschen im Umgang mit politischen Entscheidungsträgern zu vermitteln, und verpflichtet sich, die Ergebnisse des Dialogs und der vergangenen Zyklen zu bewerten und zu überwachen.

Im Hinblick auf die Youth Goals liegt für den luxemburgischen Kontext ein zentrales Ziel der NWG in der Sensibilisierung für die psychische Gesundheit und das Wohlbefinden junger Menschen. Dieses europäische Jugendziel wurde im Rahmen der Versammlungen der NWG priorisiert und diente als zentrales Thema des „Jugenddësch" am 20. Mai 2021 mit dem Ziel, Politik im Sinne junger Menschen zu gestalten.

Viele junge Menschen sind besorgt über die Zunahme von psychischen Gesundheitsproblemen wie extremem Stress, Angstzuständen, Depressionen und anderen psychischen Erkrankungen bei ihren Altersgenoss:innen, die teilweise unter sehr hohem sozialem Druck leiden.[3]

Die Umsetzung dieses Jugendziels soll dazu beitragen, die Verbesserung des psychischen Wohlbefindens zu erreichen, die Stigmatisierung psychischer Krankheiten zu beenden und damit die gesellschaftliche Inklusion aller jungen Menschen zu fördern.

Dabei soll Folgendes besonders berücksichtigt werden:

- „Die Entwicklung von Selbstbewusstsein und eines weniger konkurrenzorientierten Denkens zu unterstützen, indem die Wertschätzung für individuelle Fähigkeiten und Stärken gefördert wird.
- Das Recht auf Arbeit und Lernen für Menschen mit psychischen Krankheiten während und nach ihrer Erkrankung zu schützen, um sicherzustellen, dass sie weiterhin ihre Ziele verfolgen können.
- Einen inklusiven, sektorübergreifenden Ansatz im Umgang mit der Gesundheitsversorgung bei psychischen Erkrankungen zu entwickeln, insbesondere für gesellschaftlich benachteiligte Gruppen.
- Qualitativ hochwertiges „Erste-Hilfe-Training für psychische Erkrankungen" anzubieten für alle, die beruflich mit jungen Menschen zu tun haben, aber auch für Familien und Freund*innen.
- Inklusive, respektvolle und gut finanzierte Behandlungsmöglichkeiten durch eine integrierte, qualitativ hochwertige Gesundheitsversorgung für psychische Erkrankungen in allen medizinischen Einrichtungen bereitzustellen.
- Den Schwerpunkt auf vorbeugende Maßnahmen zu setzen, die sicherstellen, dass junge Menschen das Wissen und die Fähigkeiten erwerben, die sie für ein besseres psychisches Wohlbefinden brauchen.
- Programme zu entwickeln, die die Stigmatisierung von psychischen Erkrankungen bekämpfen und ein Bewusstsein dafür schaffen."[4]

---

[3] Vgl. https://jugenddialog.de/youth-goals/psychische-gesundheit-und-wohlbefinden/.
[4] https://jugenddialog.de/youth-goals/psychische-gesundheit-und-wohlbefinden/.

4 Zugrunde liegendes Verständnis von Gesundheit und Wohlbefinden

Die Offene Jugendarbeit in Luxemburg fördert Gesundheit, schafft gesundheitsförderliche Lebenswelten für junge Menschen und bietet unterschiedlichste Lern- und Erfahrungsmöglichkeiten zur Förderung und Stärkung der persönlichen Gesundheitskompetenz. Jugendarbeiter:innen nehmen dabei eine wichtige Vorbildfunktion ein.

Der DLJ engagiert sich dafür, jungen Menschen gesundheitsförderliche Lebens- und Lernbedingungen zu ermöglichen, indem er den Jugendstrukturen relevante Werkzeuge und Ressourcen zur Verfügung stellt. Die Mitglieder des DLJ orientieren ihre Arbeit an den Prinzipien der non-formalen Bildung, setzen an den Bedürfnissen der Jugendlichen unter Berücksichtigung ihrer jeweiligen Lern- und Entwicklungsmöglichkeiten an und leisten durch die Entwicklung und Förderung wichtiger Schlüsselkompetenzen einen wesentlichen Beitrag zu einer positiven Sozialisation von jungen Menschen.

Das Gesundheitsverständnis beruht im Kern auf einem Gesundheitsbegriff, dessen Bedeutung medizinische, soziale, biologische und psychische Sichtweisen gleichermaßen umfasst.

Der DLJ versteht unter Gesundheitsförderung nicht nur die Förderung von Gesundheit und Wohlbefinden junger Menschen, sondern sieht sie auch als wichtigen Bestandteil der Arbeit und Organisationskultur innerhalb der ehrenamtlich geführten Jugendstrukturen in Luxemburg. Das Personal zählt zu den wichtigsten Ressourcen, über die Organisationen und Einrichtungen in der Jugendarbeit verfügen. Die Mitarbeitenden prägen die Außendarstellung einer Jugendstruktur ganz wesentlich und bestimmen die Qualität der Jugendarbeit mit. Die Gesundheit und das Wohlbefinden der Mitarbeitenden sind wichtige Voraussetzungen dafür, dass die Jugendarbeit in den Jugendstrukturen gelingt und junge Menschen in ihrer Identitätsentwicklung und in ihren Bildungsprozessen Unterstützung finden (DLJ asbl 2017b).

Ein besonderes Augenmerk legt der DLJ dabei auf das Konzept der Salutogenese, das sich an den individuellen Ressourcen orientiert, die jedem persönlich zur Verfügung stehen. Sie soll das Kohärenzgefühl stärken und Strategien liefern, die letztlich der Gesamtgesundheit einer Person zuträglich sind (Fröhlich-Gildhoff et al. 2009).

5 Strategien im Hinblick auf die Gesundheitsförderung aus Sicht der Träger der Jugendstrukturen

Wohlbefinden und Gesundheit in der Einrichtung sind entscheidend für die Arbeitszufriedenheit des Personals und insbesondere für die Umsetzung einer guten und gelingenden Jugendarbeit.

Der Jugendsektor in Luxemburg zeichnet sich durch eine relativ hohe Fluktuation des Personals aus. Vor diesem Hintergrund hat der DLJ im Jahre 2019 einen Fragebogen entwickelt, der sich vor allem mit dem subjektiven Stresspotenzial des erzieherischen Personals in den Jugendhäusern in Luxemburg befasst und dessen Erkenntnisse darauf abzielen, die Gesundheit und das Wohlbefinden des Personals zu verbessern. Das subjektive Stresspotenzial aufseiten des Personals kann laut Auswertung der Umfrage als eher gering eingeschätzt werden.

Um in Einzelfällen unterstützend zur Seite zu stehen, hat der DLJ folgende Unterstützungsmaßnahmen vorgesehen: Die Zusammenarbeit und Vernetzung zwischen Arbeitgebern und Beratungsstellen soll ausgebaut werden. Beratungsstellen und andere psychosoziale Dienste sind in diesem Zusammenhang von großer Bedeutung und können betroffenen Personen Bewältigungsstrategien zur Überwindung von Belastungen liefern.

Der DLJ hat zum Ziel, das Bewusstsein der Mitgliedsstrukturen für gesamtgesundheitliche Themen zu schärfen und Informationen über Hilfs- und Unterstützungsangebote bereitzustellen. Im Sinne einer umfassenden Sensibilisierung sollen passende Schulungen und Mini-Seminare für Arbeitgeber und Personal angeboten werden, in denen die verschiedenen Fragestellungen behandelt und thematisiert werden (DLJ asbl 2019).

Eine weitere Strategie im Hinblick auf die gesundheitliche Förderung in der Jugendarbeit liegt insbesondere in der Organisation der Führungsarbeit und im zugrunde liegenden Führungsverständnis der Träger von Jugendstrukturen. Wie ehrenamtliche Träger in der Offenen Jugendarbeit ihre Leitungs- und Führungsaufgaben wahrnehmen, hängt stark von der Größe des Trägers ab und davon, in welcher Gemeinde sich eine Jugendstruktur befindet. Da sich die Risikolagen und individuellen Bewältigungsaufgaben junger Menschen von Gemeinde zu Gemeinde unterscheiden, stehen auch die einzelnen Jugendhäuser vor jeweils unterschiedlichen Herausforderungen.

Maßnahmen, Instrumente und Planungen bezüglich des eigenen Personals sind zentrale Schlüsselprozesse, die zum Erfolg einer Jugendstruktur beitragen.

Da die Wirkung in der Jugendarbeit in besonderer Weise von der Motivation, dem Engagement, der Qualifikation und der Gesundheit des Personals abhängt, wird die Relevanz einer ganzheitlichen Führungsarbeit in Organisationen und Einrichtungen der Jugendarbeit besonders deutlich.

Im Rahmen der Personalarbeit kann die Förderung der Gesundheit und des Wohlbefindens der Jugendarbeiter:innen als eine präventive und stärkende Maßnahme zum psychischen und physischen Gesundheitsschutz gesehen werden (Friedrich 2010).

Eine zentrale Aufgabe der ehrenamtlichen Träger ist, dafür zu sorgen, dass die strukturellen und personellen Rahmenbedingungen im Jugendhaus stimmen und das hauptamtliche Personal in der Lage ist, seine Alltagsarbeit zu bewältigen. Eine wesentliche Aufgabe liegt darin, das Personal zu motivieren und in seiner beruflichen Weiterentwicklung zu unterstützen.

Führungsarbeit ist also notwendig, damit die jugendpolitischen Zielsetzungen der Jugendarbeit erreicht werden und die Aufgaben und Zielsetzungen des Trägers ihre Wirkung im Hinblick auf die jugendliche Zielgruppe zeigen können.

Zahlreiche Studien zeigen, dass insbesondere Personen, die soziale und erzieherische Berufe ausüben, oftmals hohe Ansprüche an sich selbst stellen und eine erhöhte Verausgabungsbereitschaft aufweisen. Gehen erzieherische Fachkräfte anhaltend über ihre physischen und psychischen Grenzen hinaus, so können reduzierte Erholungszeiten zu psychischer und körperlicher Ermüdung führen, mit der Folge, dass die Leistungsfähigkeit rapide abnimmt (Friedrich 2010). Ein ganzheitliches und gesundheitsförderndes Denken und Handeln ist daher in den Führungsebenen der Jugendstrukturen unabdingbar. Im Rahmen der Führungsarbeit gilt es insbesondere das selbstwirksame Verhalten der Mitarbeitenden zu stärken. Hierfür regt der DLJ seine Mitglieder an, gesundheitsfördernde Rahmenbedingungen und Maßnahmen zu schaffen, die das Erlernen eines selbstreflektierenden und selbstsicheren Verhaltens ermöglichen, die Arbeitsmotivation stärken und bei drohender Berufsmüdigkeit im Sinne einer Work-Life-Balance vorbeugende Wirkungen haben (Friedrich 2010).

Hierfür bietet der DLJ seinen Mitgliedsstrukturen ein umfassendes und praxisnahes Beratungs- und Weiterbildungsangebot an, welches sich dadurch auszeichnet, dass es den Bedürfnissen der Träger entspricht und ihnen beim Ausführen ihrer alltäglichen Aufgaben hilft.

Diese Unterstützungsangebote erfolgen zum einen individuell und sind maßgeschneidert für die Bedürfnisse der Struktur, wie beispielsweise durch die Begleitung und Beratung im Hinblick auf die Integration der Gesundheitsförderung in das personalpolitische Konzept der Jugendstruktur.

Zum anderen bietet der DLJ zahlreiche gesundheitsbezogene Fort- und Weiterbildungen für seine Mitglieder an. Im Konkreten handelt es sich dabei unter anderem um:

* Mini-Seminare zu spezifischen Themen, die für die Jugendarbeit und die Führungsarbeit relevant sind. (Themen: Krebsvorsorge, Rauchen, Sex Education, Suchtprävention, Konsequenzen von Cannabis-Legalisierung usw.)
* Gesundheitsbezogene Schulungen, wie etwa der Erste-Hilfe-Kurs oder die Schulung zum Beauftragten für Sicherheit und Gesundheit am Arbeitsplatz, welche in Kooperation mit Partnerorganisationen angeboten werden.

Dieses breite Angebot an Unterstützungsmaßnahmen wird zudem durch das Bereitstellen von Materialien und das Ausarbeiten von geeigneten Instrumenten und Methoden zum Qualitäts- und Personalmanagement ergänzt. Das Handbuch „Vademecum" enthält alle für die Führung einer Jugendstruktur relevanten Informationen (EGMJ asbl 2017).

6 Aktivitäten und Programme, die in der Praxis der Jugendarbeit zum Einsatz kommen

Die Analyse der Handlungskonzepte der Jugendhäuser sowie eine kürzlich durchgeführte Erhebung seitens des DLJ zeigen auf, dass die Jugendstrukturen in Luxemburg zahlreiche Angebote bereitstellen, die in Form von Informations- und Sensibilisierungskampagnen, Workshops, Ausflügen oder Aktivitäten stattfinden. Allen gemein ist das übergeordnete Ziel, die Gesundheit im Rahmen einer ganzheitlichen Stärkung der psychischen, physischen und sozialen Kompetenzen junger Menschen durch Präventions- und Beratungsarbeit zu stärken und zu fördern.

Nachfolgend werden einige Angebote der Mitgliedsstrukturen des DLJ exemplarisch dargestellt:

Im Echternacher Jugendhaus fördern und stärken die erzieherischen Mitarbeiter:innen des Jugendhauses im Rahmen verschiedener Projekte und Aktivitäten das Körperbewusstsein, die Bewegung und die Gesundheit der Jugendlichen.

Regelmäßige Koch- und Sportaktivitäten tragen hierzu bei (Eechternoacher Jugendhaus asbl 2019).

Das Jugendhaus Wiltz bietet zur Förderung des öffentlichen Erscheinungsbildes des Hauses das Tanzprojekt Young DaWo an. Diese Tanzgruppe besteht aus über 40 Jugendlichen, die auf zahlreichen öffentlichen Veranstaltungen in der Region auftreten. Im Mittelpunkt stehen hier insbesondere Aspekte wie: Körperbewusstsein, Fitness, Bewegung und Gesundheit (Jugendhaus Wooltz asbl 2019). Die Nordstadjugend bietet über das ganze Jahr zahlreiche bewegungsfördernde Aktivitäten an, um unter anderem dem „Abhängen" entgegenzuwirken und junge Menschen für körperliche Aktivitäten zu motivieren. Zudem wird in den Jugendhäusern der Nordstadjugend regelmäßig gemeinsam gekocht und gebacken mit dem Ziel, Jugendlichen eine bewusste, gesunde und abwechslungsreiche Ernährung näherzubringen (Nordstadjugend asbl 2019).

Das Schifflinger Jugendhaus strebt insbesondere eine starke Vernetzung und eine enge Zusammenarbeit zwischen dem Jugendhaus und den in der Gemeinde ansässigen Sport- und Kulturvereinen an. Im Sinne eines komplementären Ansatzes soll jungen Menschen dadurch eine große Anzahl an gesundheits- und sportbezogenen Aktivitäten angeboten werden (Schëfflenger Jugendhaus asbl 2019).

Das Jugendhaus „Jugendwave Remich" bietet jede Woche sportliche Aktivitäten in der Einrichtung an. Gymnastikübungen, Yoga, Pilates oder Muskelaufbauübungen werden den Jugendlichen gezeigt und gemeinsam ausprobiert. Zusätzlich werden externe Experten eingeladen, um den Jugendlichen weitere Sportarten näherzubringen. Auf dem Multisport-Gelände vor dem Jugendhaus können zudem Parkour, Skateboarding und andere Outdoor-Sportarten angeboten werden. Die verfolgten Ziele sind dabei einerseits, dass die Jugendlichen ihr Körperbewusstsein weiterentwickeln, und andererseits, dass sie den Fair-Play-Gedanken beim Spiel respektieren (Jugendwave Remich 2019).

Auf nationaler Ebene verfolgt das CNAPA (Centre national de prévention des addictions) zahlreiche Ideen und Strategien, um einen gesunden und positiven Lebensstil zu fördern und zu verbreiten, insbesondere durch die Verhinderung von Verhaltensweisen, die zu den verschiedensten Formen von Sucht und anderen Abhängigkeiten führen können.

An dieser Stelle soll insbesondere kurz auf das Projekt „Localize It!" eingegangen werden, welches das CNAPA in Kooperation mit den Jugendhäusern in Mondorf-Les-Bains und Düdelingen von 2017 bis 2019 durchgeführt hat.

Bei dem Projekt geht es um die Entwicklung lokaler Strategien zur Prävention vor erhöhtem Alkoholkonsum. Im Mittelpunkt stehen verschiedene Settings der Alkoholprävention: Schulen, Kinder aus alkoholbelasteten Familien, Alkohol im öffentlichen Raum, Party-Szenen, Festivals, Handel und Gastronomie sowie Alkohol im Straßenverkehr. Hintergrund des „Localize It!"-Projektes ist die Annahme, dass Rauschtrinken und übermäßiger Alkoholkonsum von Jugendlichen zwischen 12 und 25 Jahren am besten durch Maßnahmen reduziert werden können, die dort ansetzen, wo der Konsum stattfindet: auf der lokalen Ebene. Deswegen sollten solche Vorhaben auch durch Behörden und Akteure durchgeführt werden, die vor Ort bekannt und vernetzt sind.

Teil von „Localize It!" ist auch die Ausarbeitung eines Handbuchs zur lokalen Alkoholprävention, das Instrumente und Tools zur Verfügung stellt sowie spezifische Handlungsorientierungen für die verschiedenen Settings liefern und diese durch Good-Practice-Beispiele verdeutlichen soll (CePT 2020).

7 Gesundheitsbezogene Probleme und Sorgen junger Menschen

Ein kurzer Blick auf die aktuelle Lage der Jugend in Europa macht deutlich, dass angesichts unsicherer ökonomischer und sozialer Verhältnisse die Lebenswirklichkeiten vieler Jugendlicher brüchig geworden sind und immer mehr jungen Menschen berufliche und persönliche Perspektiven fehlen. Der Übergang von der Schule in den Arbeitsmarkt ist heute differenzierter und auch mit größeren Ängsten und Unsicherheiten verbunden als früher. Gestiegene Anpassungs- und Flexibilisierungserfordernisse, die selbstständig gemeistert werden müssen, führen dazu, dass die eigene Biografie zunehmend zu einem gestaltbaren und gestaltungsbedürftigen Prozess wird (Sting und Sturzenhecker 2013). Jungen Menschen wird in zunehmendem Maße eigenverantwortliches Handeln und aktive Gestaltung ihres eigenen Werdegangs abverlangt. Die Lebensphase Jugend löst sich dadurch mehr und mehr auf und die Kluft zwischen den gesellschaftlichen Erwartungen und Anforderungen an junge Menschen einerseits und den Interessen und Bedürfnissen der Jugendlichen andererseits wird immer größer (Frosch 2010).

Diese gestiegenen gesellschaftlichen Leistungsanforderungen oder Sorgen um die eigene berufliche und persönliche Zukunft werden häufig in intensiven Konflikten mit sich selbst und anderen ausgetragen. Komplizierte Lebensumstände, wie fehlender Bildungsabschluss, Überschuldung oder Wohnungslosigkeit, gehen oft mit Beeinträchtigungen des gesundheitlichen Wohlbefindens, mit mangelnden sozialen Kompetenzen und Ressourcen sowie einem niedrigen sozialen Status einher. Ein geringes Einkommen erschwert zudem eine gesunde Lebensführung und Ernährung. Junge Menschen, die unter wenig gesundheitsförderlichen Bedingungen aufwachsen, müssen in ihrer Entwicklung einen deutlich größeren Kraftaufwand leisten und sowohl die Folgen ihrer prekären Lebenslage meistern als auch ihre altersrelevanten Entwicklungsanforderungen bewältigen (Ziethen et al. 2011).

Die Auswertung der Handlungskonzepte der Jugendhäuser, der sozio-demo-grafischen Merkmale junger Menschen in einer NEET-Situation sowie eine Befragung seitens des DLJ in Bezug auf die gesundheitliche Situation junger Menschen machen deutlich, dass insbesondere junge Menschen, die in prekären Lebenslagen aufwachsen, oftmals multiplen Problemlagen ausgesetzt sind und sich der Übergang in das Erwachsenenalter häufig risikoreicher und problem-behafteter gestaltet:

- Sie sind häufiger von Übergewicht, Adipositas oder Essstörungen betroffen.
- Sie haben häufiger emotionale und psychische Probleme, die sich u. a. in Störungen der Konzentration und Aufmerksamkeit oder in stressbedingten Erkrankungen wie Depressionen zeigen können.
- Sie leiden häufiger unter allgemeinen Erkrankungen (Erkältungen, Kopf-schmerzen, Rückenschmerzen usw.).
- Sie sind häufiger von Suchtproblematiken betroffen (Tabak-, Alkohol- und Drogenkonsum).
- Sie treiben oftmals weniger Sport und verbringen viel Zeit vor dem Smart-phone, Fernseher oder Computer (exzessiver Medienkonsum).

8   Herausforderungen und Perspektiven im Hinblick auf die Förderung von Gesundheit und Wohlbefinden in der Offenen Jugendarbeit

Die Jugendstrukturen in Luxemburg entwickeln ihre eigenen gesundheits-bezogenen Aktivitäten und Projekte, die an den nationalen Bildungsrahmen-plan für die non-formale Bildung im Kinder- und Jugendbereich angelehnt sind. Allerdings ist der gesetzliche Rahmenplan sehr weit gefasst und überlässt den einzelnen Strukturen einen großen Spielraum und viele Handlungsmöglichkeiten. Diese Wahrung der Autonomie der einzelnen Jugendstrukturen ist eine große Stärke der Offenen Jugendarbeit in Luxemburg, führt jedoch auch dazu, dass nicht in allen Jugendstrukturen ein klarer Bezug zur Gesundheitsförderung oder gesundheitsbezogenen Prävention erkennbar ist. Darüber hinaus fehlt es in vielen Fällen an einer Nachhaltigkeit der Angebote oder an einer effektiven und ganz-heitlichen Zusammenarbeit aller Akteure aus Sozialwesen, Gesundheit, Bildung und Politik.

Der DLJ regt daher die Entwicklung eines ganzheitlichen nationalen Hand-lungskonzeptes zur Gesundheitsförderung junger Menschen in der Offenen

Jugendarbeit an, welches darauf abzielt, das Gesundheitspotenzial junger Menschen zu verbessern und zu stärken (Lehmann et al. 2010):

- **Prävention und Gesundheitsförderung sind konzeptionell verankert**
  Gesundheitsförderung und -kompetenz werden als wichtiger Bestandteil der Arbeit und Organisationskultur verstanden und sind in den Leitbildern der Jugendstrukturen verankert.
- **Nachhaltige Vernetzung und Kooperationen**
  Die Jugendstrukturen beziehen alle relevanten Stakeholder und Zielgruppen in die Planung, Entwicklung, Umsetzung und Evaluierung von gesundheitsbezogenen Angeboten und Maßnahmen mit ein und setzen auf langfristige und nachhaltige Kooperationen.
- **Schulung der Jugendarbeiter:innen für gesundheitskompetente Kommunikation**
  Die Jugendarbeiter:innen sind über aktuelle gesundheitsrelevante Trends und Angebote im Hinblick auf die jugendliche Zielgruppe auf dem Laufenden und verfolgen in ihrer Arbeit hohe Qualitätsmaßstäbe in Bezug auf die gesundheitliche Förderung junger Menschen.
- **Niedrigschwellige Arbeitsweise**
  Offene Jugendarbeit ist niederschwellig und für alle jugendlichen Zielgruppen offen und arbeitet sowohl standortbezogen als auch mobil.
- **Gesundheit als Querschnittsthema und ganzheitlicher Gesundheitsbegriff**
  Gesundheitsthemen werden in den Praxisalltag der Offenen Jugendarbeit eingebaut und als Querschnittsthema verstanden. Die Jugendstrukturen stellen einen positiven Zugang zum Thema Gesundheit und vermitteln eine gesundheitsbewusste Haltung, die authentisch ist. Den Jugendarbeiter:innen kommt hier eine besondere Vorbildfunktion zu.
  Zudem folgen die Jugendstrukturen einem ganzheitlichen Gesundheitsbegriff, der an der Lebenswelt junger Menschen orientiert ist und sowohl physische als auch psychische und soziale Faktoren umfasst und sich auf Gesundheitsförderung, Prävention und Information bezieht.
- **Die Gesundheit der Mitarbeitenden als Voraussetzung gelingender Jugendarbeit**
  Die Jugendstrukturen bieten gesundheitsförderliche Rahmenbedingungen für ihre Beschäftigten und unterstützen sie bei der Bewältigung berufsbedingter Gesundheitsbelastungen. Der Ausgestaltung der Führungsarbeit und dem zugrunde liegenden Führungsverständnis der Träger von Jugendstrukturen kommt in diesem Zusammenhang eine hohe Relevanz zu.

- **Qualitätsmanagement**
  Qualitätsmanagement, Dokumentation und Evaluation tragen zu einem kontinuierlichen Anpassungs- und Verbesserungsprozess bei. Sie sind wesentliche Bestandteile eines ganzheitlichen Handlungskonzeptes zur Gesundheitsförderung junger Menschen in der Offenen Jugendarbeit und unterstützen darüber hinaus dessen Nachhaltigkeit.

9 Schlussfolgerungen und Ausblick

Dieser Beitrag hat gezeigt, dass die Strukturen der Offenen Jugendarbeit in Luxemburg verstärkt gesundheitsbezogene Aktivitäten und Projekte anbieten, die sich am nationalen Bildungsrahmenplan für die non-formale Bildung orientieren. Durch vielfältige Lern- und Erfahrungsmöglichkeiten fördern und stärken sie die persönliche Gesundheitskompetenz junger Menschen. Jugendarbeiter:innen nehmen dabei eine wichtige Vorbildfunktion ein.

Die Rolle der Jugendarbeit in Bezug auf gesundheitliche Themen wird besonders in Zeiten der COVID-19-Pandemie deutlich, deren Folgen sich auch auf die psychische Verfassung von jungen Menschen auswirken können. Jugendliche müssen daher in ihrer körperlichen, geistigen und seelischen Entwicklung unterstützt werden und dazu brauchen sie Räume und Möglichkeiten, in denen sie sich verwirklichen können.

Da der gesetzliche Rahmenplan den einzelnen Jugendstrukturen einen großen Spielraum und viele Handlungsmöglichkeiten überlässt, kann dies dazu führen, dass nicht in allen Einrichtungen ein konzeptioneller Bezug zu gesundheitsbezogenen Themen erkennbar ist.

Der DLJ hat sich als wichtiges Ziel den Austausch zwischen Akteuren aus Gesundheits- und Sozialwesen auf nationaler und europäischer Ebene gesetzt, um die Entwicklung eines ganzheitlichen Handlungskonzeptes sowie Strategien zur Gesundheitsförderung junger Menschen in der Offenen Jugendarbeit anzustoßen und weiterzuentwickeln.

Literatur

CePT (Centre de Prévention des Toxicomanies) (2020). Aktivitätenbericht. Luxembourg (unveröffentlichtes Dokument).
DLJ asbl (2017a). Ziele der offenen Jugendarbeit in den Jugendhäusern (unveröffentlichtes Dokument).

DLJ asbl (2017b). Studie zum Führungsverständnis sowie den Möglichkeiten und Grenzen ehrenamtlichen Engagements in luxemburgischen Jugendhäusern und Jugenddiensten (unveröffentlichtes Dokument).

DLJ asbl (2018). Soziodemografische Merkmale der Jugendlichen Teilnehmer und die pädagogische Intervention – Auswertung der Projektdatenbank „Profil des bénéficiaires" (unveröffentlichtes Dokument).

DLJ asbl (2019). «Avis Stress-Enquête» vom 8.November 2019 (unveröffentlichtes Dokument).

Eechternoacher Jugendhaus asbl (2019). CAG – Concept d'Action Générale CIRJE (unveröffentlichtes Dokument).

EGMJ asbl (2017). VADEMECUM. Sammlung vu wichtegen Texter a Recommendatioune vun der EGMJ fir hier Memberen (unveröffentlichtes Dokument).

Friedrich, Andrea (2010). Personalarbeit in Organisationen Sozialer Arbeit - Theorie und Praxis der Professionalisierung. Wiesbaden: VS Verlag für Sozialwissenschaften.

Fröhlich-Gildhoff, Klaus, Baier-Hartmann, Marianne, Geissler, Frank & Kraus, Björn (Hrsg.) (2009). Lebensphasen - Entwicklung aus interdisziplinärer Sicht. Band 3. Verlag FEL.

Frosch, Ulrike (2010). Bastelbiographie, Patchwork-Identität und Co. Atypische Erwerbsbiographien aus gegenwärtiger Forschungsperspektive. In Berufs- und Wirtschaftspädagogik, Ausgabe Nr. 18.

Jugendhaus Wooltz asbl (2019). CAG – Conceps d'Action Cénérale (unveröffentlichtes Dokument).

Jugendwave Remich (2019). CAG – Concept d'Action Générale (unveröffentlichtes Dokument).

Landesjugendring Baden-Württemberg e.V. (2007). Mehr als Dauerlauf und Salat –Arbeitshilfe zur Gesundheitsbildung in der Jugendarbeit. Stuttgart.

Lehmann, Frank et al. (2010). (Kriterien guter Praxis in der Gesundheitsförderung bei sozial Benachteiligten. Bundeszentrale für gesundheitliche Aufklärung (BZgA). Köln.

Ministère de l'Éducation nationale, de l'Enfance et de la Jeunesse (MENJE) & Service National de la Jeunesse (SNJ) (2018). Nationaler Rahmenplan zur non-formalen Bildung im Kindes- und Jugendalter. Luxembourg.

Nordstadjugend asbl (2019). CAG – Concept d'Action Générale (unveröffentlichtes Dokument).

Schëfflenger Jugendhaus asbl (2019). CAG – Concept d'Action Générale (unveröffentlichtes Dokument).

Sting, Stephan & Sturzenhecker, Benedikt (2013). Bildung und Offene Kinder- und Jugendarbeit. Wiesbaden: VS Verlag für Sozialwissenschaften.

Ziethen, Peggy et al. (2011). Gesundheit – (k)ein Thema für die Jugendsozialarbeit? Prävention und Gesundheitsförderung in der sozialen Arbeit mit benachteiligten Kindern und Jugendlichen. Berlin: Deutsches Rotes Kreuz e.V.

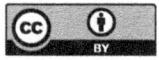

KJT ein „Seismograf" für das Wohlbefinden von Kindern und Jugendlichen in Luxemburg

Barbara Gorges-Wagner, Aline Hartz, Cathy Reuter und Sally Stephany

> *Safety and security don't just happen; they are the result of collective consensus and public investment. We owe our children, the most vulnerable citizens in our society, a life free of violence and fear.*
> Nelson Mandela

1 Einleitung

Dieser Artikel beschreibt die Aufgaben, Arbeitsweisen und Konzepte des Kanner-Jugendtelefon (KJT) und berichtet von den Erfahrungen aus der Beratungspraxis. Der Artikel beruht auf Daten von Kontakten mit Kindern und Jugendlichen an den unterschiedlichen Helplines im Jahr 2018. Die Daten geben Aufschluss über das Wohlbefinden der Kinder und Jugendlichen in Luxemburg und zeigen deren Sorgen und Probleme auf. In einem gesonderten Unterpunkt gehen wir auf die Zeitspanne während und kurz nach dem Lockdown in der Coronakrise 2020 ein. Hier fokussieren wir die Themen, welche Kinder und Jugendliche während dieser

B. Gorges-Wagner (✉) · A. Hartz · C. Reuter · S. Stephany
KJT, Hesperange, Luxembourg
E-Mail: bgorgeswagner@kjt.lu

A. Hartz
E-Mail: ahartz@kjt.lu

C. Reuter
E-Mail: creuter@kjt.lu

S. Stephany
E-Mail: sstephany@kjt.lu

© Der/die Autor(en) 2022
A. Heinen et al. (Hrsg.), *Wohlbefinden und Gesundheit im Jugendalter*,
https://doi.org/10.1007/978-3-658-35744-3_22

489

Phase beschäftigt haben. Diese Angaben interpretieren wir und ordnen sie anhand wissenschaftlicher Literatur ein. Des Weiteren skizzieren wir, mit dem Blick auf die Probleme und Belastungen der Kinder und Jugendlichen, die aktuellen und zukünftigen Herausforderungen aus Sicht des KJT.

2 Aufgaben, Arbeitsweisen und Konzepte des KJT zur Verbesserung der Gesundheit und des Wohlbefindens von Kindern und Jugendlichen

Das KJT ist ein nationales Beratungsangebot für Kinder, Jugendliche, Eltern wie auch Professionelle, die mit Kindern oder Jugendlichen zu tun haben. Getragen wird dieser Dienst von *Croix-Rouge luxembourgeoise, Ligue Médico Sociale* und der *Fondation Kannerschlass* und steht unter der Federführung von *Caritas Jeunes et Familles a.s.b.l.* Das Beratungsangebot ist 1992 im Kontext der Ratifizierung der UN-Kinderrechtskonvention von 1989 auf den Weg gebracht worden. Zentrale Aufgabe ist es, Wohlergehen und Gesundheit von Kindern und Jugendlichen zu schützen. Gesundheit „ist ein Zustand vollständigen körperlichen, seelischen und sozialen Wohlbefindens und nicht nur das Freisein von Krankheit und Gebrechen" (WHO 2012). In ihrem Faktenblatt zum neuen Rahmenkonzept „Gesundheit 2020" benennt die WHO das Wohlbefinden als „entscheidendes Element von Gesundheit". Wohlbefinden wird in diesem Kontext aus zwei Sichten betrachtet – aus der objektiven und aus der subjektiven. Maßgeblich für das objektive Wohlbefinden sind die Lebensbedingungen von Menschen und ihre Chancen auf Nutzung ihres Potenzials. Wesentliche Faktoren für objektives Wohlbefinden sind Gesundheit, Bildung, Arbeitsplatz, soziale Beziehungen, Umwelt, Sicherheit, Bürgerbeteiligung, Politikgestaltung, Wohnbedingungen und Freizeit. Subjektives Wohlbefinden hingegen steht in direktem Zusammenhang mit den Lebenserfahrungen von Menschen.

Objektive Maßstäbe für Wohlbefinden lassen sich aus psychologischer Perspektive mit grundlegenden Bedürfnissen von Kindern und Jugendlichen identifizieren, wie Maslow sie in seiner Bedürfnispyramide benennt: physiologische Bedürfnisse, Bedürfnis nach Sicherheit, soziale Bedürfnisse (Zugehörigkeit, Freundschaft etc.), Bedürfnis nach Anerkennung und Wertschätzung (Individualbedürfnisse) sowie das Bedürfnis nach Selbstverwirklichung (Maslow 1943).

Da, wo grundlegende Bedürfnisse von jungen Menschen in Familie, Schule und Umfeld eingeschränkt oder verletzt werden, gibt das KJT Kindern und

Jugendlichen eine Stimme. Es unterstützt Kinder und Jugendliche darin, sich zu entwickeln und ihre Chancen und Rechte wahrzunehmen.

Das KJT hat sich über die Jahre hinweg den gesellschaftlichen Anforderungen und den sich entsprechend verändernden Lebenslagen von Kindern und Jugendlichen gestellt und angepasst. Das hat zu einer Ausweitung und Differenzierung der Aufgaben geführt.

Das älteste Beratungsangebot ist das Kanner-Jugendtelefon 1 1 6 1 1 1, an das Kinder und Jugendliche sich seit 1992 gratis, anonym und vertraulich wenden können. Seit 2005 wird das Beratungsangebot durch die Online Help ergänzt. Kinder und Jugendliche können seitdem auch schriftlich – anonym und vertraulich – Kontakt aufnehmen. Seit 2015 ist das Angebot in englischer Sprache verfügbar, sodass auch englischsprachige Kinder, Jugendliche und Eltern die Möglichkeit haben, die Online Help zu nutzen.

Da immer mehr Eltern sich mit ihren Fragen an das 1 1 6 1 1 1 Kanner-Jugendtelefon gewandt haben, wurde das Beratungsangebot im Jahre 2007 durch das Elterentelefon 26 64 05 55 erweitert.

Im gleichen Jahr wurde auch die BEE SECURE Helpline 8002 1234 ins Leben gerufen, da die sichere Nutzung der digitalen Medien ein immer größeres Thema wurde. Seit 2007 können zudem illegale Inhalte, denen man im Internet begegnet, anonym über die BEE SECURE Stopline gemeldet werden.

In Situationen, die spezielle fachliche Hilfe erfordern, werden die Ratsuchenden gezielt weiterorientiert und ermutigt, die weiterführenden Angebote zu nutzen.

2.1   Konzepte und Strategien

Unser Beratungsverständnis basiert darauf, dass (junge) Menschen sich mit ihren Fragen, Sorgen und in akuten Krisen über die angebotenen Kommunikationskanäle an uns wenden. Folglich immer dann, wenn ihre Gesundheit und ihr Wohlbefinden beeinträchtigt und gefährdet sind. Telefon-, Online, und Chatberatung sind ein ergänzendes und alternatives Angebot zu anderen Beratungsformaten im Land. Insbesondere junge Menschen greifen auf digitale Kommunikationsformen zurück. Dabei kommen Kindern und Jugendlichen die besonderen Merkmale der Begleitung per Telefon und der webbasierten Onlineberatung entgegen. Die zeitliche Erreichbarkeit (eine Nachricht kann zu jeder Tages- und Nachtzeit geschrieben und gesendet werden) und die jederzeit direkte Zugänglichkeit machen das Beratungsformat Onlineberatung besonders bei unserer Zielgruppe beliebt. Herausforderungen der Beratungsformate liegen im Wegfall des visuellen

Zugangs und der nonverbalen Kommunikation, die im direkten Gespräch eine wichtige Funktion haben, abe auch in der Zeitversetzung der Onlineberatung (asynchron).

Die drei besonderen Merkmale der medienvermittelten Beratung und Begleitung, nämlich Anonymität, Nähe durch Distanz und Niederschwelligkeit, erleichtern Kindern und Jugendlichen den Zugang.

1. *Anonymität* meint, dass niemand, der sich an uns wendet, namentliche Angaben zu seiner Person zu machen braucht. Zudem sind auch die Mitarbeiterinnen und Mitarbeiter und der Ort der Beratung anonym. Alle Mitarbeiterinnen und Mitarbeiter unterliegen der Schweigepflicht. Es werden keinerlei Informationen weitergegeben. Die zugesicherte Anonymität ermöglicht es, Angst und Scham zu überwinden, Probleme zu benennen und Hilfe in Anspruch zu nehmen. Da weder Name noch andere Daten von Anrufern oder Usern erfasst werden, kann eine erste Klärung und Orientierung ohne die Angst vor direkter Intervention erfolgen. Im Schutz der Anonymität können junge Menschen ihre Autonomie und Entscheidungsfreiheit bewahren. So bietet die Anonymität die Chance, sich zu öffnen, und gleichzeitig einen Schutzraum vor (erneutem) Kontrollverlust. Das Gespräch und die Klärung stehen im Mittelpunkt. Die Entscheidung darüber, ob ein Kontakt konkrete Folgen hat und welcher Art diese sind, bestimmt ganz allein der Anrufer. Wir unterstützen ihn bei seiner Suche nach eigenen Lösungen und zeigen gegebenenfalls den Weg zu weiterführenden Beratungsstellen oder Hilfseinrichtungen auf.

2. *Nähe durch Distanz* beschreibt, dass die besonderen Beratungsformate Telefon- und Onlineberatung Kommunikationssituationen ermöglichen, in denen durch die garantierte Distanz Nähe entstehen und zugelassen werden kann. So gestalten sich Kontakte vor dem Hintergrund gerade dieses Spezifikums intensiv und emotional. Wird ein Gespräch oder ein Online-Kontakt zu nah oder unangenehm, kann er jederzeit ohne Begründung abgebrochen werden. Dieser Effekt ermöglicht Offenheit und den Mut, persönliche Probleme anzusprechen. Kinder und Jugendliche, deren Wohlbefinden aus welchem Grund auch immer aus der Balance ist, bestimmen selbst, wann, wie lange und worüber sie sprechen wollen. Das gilt für den Jungen, der einsam ist und niemanden hat, mit dem er sprechen kann, genauso wie für ein Mädchen, das sexuell vom Vater missbraucht wird. Es können tabuisierte Themen, wie Fragen zur Sexualität, Gewalterfahrungen, selbstverletzendem Verhalten oder der Wunsch zu sterben, ausgesprochen oder aufgeschrieben werden (Knatz &

Schumacher 2019, S. 5). Kinder und Jugendliche rufen gerade beim KJT an oder schreiben weil sie noch nicht bereit zu konkreten Handlungen sind und wissen, dass die Berater nicht direkt in ihre Situation eingreifen können. Auch verängstigte oder scheue Kinder und Jugendliche können sich so geschützt herantasten und ausprobieren. Da der Jugendphase Verunsicherungen immanent sind, sind die genannten Merkmale der medienvermittelten Kommunikation Türöffner, um Unangenehmes auszusprechen, auch wenn es schwerfällt.

3. *Niederschwelligkeit* meint, dass (fast) jeder junge Mensch die Möglichkeit hat, die Beratungsangebote zu nutzen. 100 % der Jugendlichen ab 16 Jahren haben heute Zugriff aufs Internet und 88 % davon verfügen über ein Smartphone (STATEC 2019). Damit haben sie extrem niederschwellige Möglichkeiten, den Kontakt zur Telefon-Helpline oder Onlineberatung vor Ort zu suchen. Die Anwendung ist einfach, der Aufwand gering, die Kontaktaufnahme kann von jedem Ort geschehen, wie z. B. vom Bus. Es gibt keine Wartelisten und das Angebot ist gratis.

Einhergehend mit den drei spezifischen Merkmalen der medialen Kommunikation verstehen wir Beratung als Prozess, der darauf angelegt ist, mit Jugendlichen und Kindern, deren Wohlbefinden oft erheblich gestört ist, eigene Lösungswege zu erarbeiten. Dabei respektieren wir die individuelle Situation jedes Anrufers mit dem Ziel, die je eigenen Ressourcen zu entdecken und zu entfalten. Der Anrufer/User steht mit seinen Fragen und Problemen im Mittelpunkt, auch wenn andere Personen wie Eltern, Lehrer oder Freunde beteiligt sind. Unser Beratungskonzept basiert auf den drei Basisvariablen Empathie (einfühlendes Verstehen), Wertschätzung (Akzeptanz und Anteilnahme) sowie Authentizität (Echtheit, Stimmigkeit). Wir implizieren damit die Variablen der klientenzentrierten Gesprächspsychotherapie nach Carl R. Rogers (Rogers 1951), die für den Beziehungsaufbau und die Entwicklung einer Beratungsbeziehung notwendig sind. Zuhören ermöglicht die Lebenswelt von Kindern und Jugendlichen wahrzunehmen und zu begreifen, was die Voraussetzung für Interaktion ist. Es geht also immer um die Frage: Wie kann ich junge Menschen so begleiten, dass sie die Erfahrung machen können, wirklich verstanden zu werden? Die sechs Eigenschaften des Beratungsgesprächs (Empathie, emotionale Stabilität, aktives Zuhören, Respekt, Gesprächsführung und Ressourcenaktivierung) sind essentielle Voraussetzungen für gutes Zuhören und aufmerksames Lesen, und orientieren sich am europäischen „EmPoWEring-Projekt" (Pädagogischer Weg für emotionales Wohlbefinden), (Knatz und Schumacher 2019, S. 11).

Eine weitere maßgebliche Ergänzung des Konzepts basiert auf dem Grund-lagenwissen des systemischen Denkens und Handelns, um im Beratungs- und Begleitungsprozess individuelle und interaktionelle Muster zu unterbrechen und Ressourcen hin zu einer Lösung zu aktivieren (von Schlippe und Schweitzer 2016).

Gleichzeitig komplementiert Grundlagenwissen zur Entwicklung im Kindes- und Jugendalter, wie auch zu spezifischen wiederkehrenden Themen, z. B. Dynamik in Trennungs- und Scheidungsfamilien, Sexualität, Gewalterfahrungen und sexueller Missbrauch, Cyberbullying, Umgang mit Krisen (Suizidalität), Gefahren im Internet, das Konzept.

2.2 Aktivitäten und Programme

Die Eine der Hauptaktivitäten von KJT im Kontext von Gesundheit und Wohl-befinden zielt darauf ab, die Dienste bei Kindern und Jugendlichen, in den Familien und bei Professionellen aus dem pädagogischen und psychologischen Raum bekannt zu machen. Nur dann, wenn die niederschwelligen Dienste 1 1 6 1 1 1 und Online Help www.kjt.lu elementar bekannt und vertraut sind, stehen sie Kindern und Jugendlichen als Ressource für den Ernstfall zur Verfügung. Um das zu gewährleisten, müssten Kinder und Jugendliche eine systematische Ein-führung und Information über das Hilfsangebot erhalten. KJT hat seine Präsenz vor Ort in den letzten Jahren in Form von Teilnahme an Jugendevents, Workshops an Schulen und der Teilnahme an Elternabenden erheblich ausgebaut. Dies wurde möglich durch den Aufbau eines Botschafterteams, das das professionelle Team unterstützt. Zudem erstellt KJT alljährlich einen Kommunikationsplan, um zu gewährleisten, dass die Angebote der Dienste im Bewusstsein der Bevölkerung ankommen. Über das Jahr verteilt finden analog zum Kommunikationsplan ver-schiedene Aktivitäten statt: Veröffentlichung des Jahresberichts, Veröffentlichung von Fachartikeln in der Presse, Interviews im Fernsehen und Radio, Präsenz auf verschiedenen sozialen Medien (Facebook, Twitter, Instagram, YouTube), Erstellung und Einsatz von Videos sowie Plakat- und Materialversand.

Mit unseren Aktivitäten im öffentlichen Bereich leisten wir einen Beitrag dazu, Themen wie Cyberbullying, Gewalt in Familien usw. zu enttabuisieren; diese entfalten ja in der Regel ihre Macht dadurch, dass in ihrem Wohlergehen geschädigte Kinder und Jugendliche (zu) lange schweigen. Gerade hier setzt das Angebot des KJT mit seinen beschriebenen spezifischen Merkmalen an.

Im November 2018 hat das KJT die BOD-Kampagne gestartet, um seine Angebote, besonders die 1 1 6 1 1 1 Kanner-Jugendtelefons, bekannter zu machen. Mit neuen Plakaten und der neuen Maskotte, genannt BOD, ist KJT deutlich erkennbar. Parallel zur BOD-Kampagne wurde auch die BOD-Fortbildung entwickelt. Ziel der Fortbildung ist es, Pädagogen und Psychologen Schlüsselkompetenzen für den Umgang mit Gefühlen zu vermitteln. Die Fortbildung greift die Frage vieler Pädagogen auf: Was passiert, wenn ich Gefühle anspreche? Kann ich da etwas falsch machen? In dieser Fortbildung bringt KJT sein Wissen über Gefühle ein. Wenn ich die Gefühle eines Menschen einordnen und verbalisieren kann, fühlt er sich verstanden und es entsteht ein guter Kontakt (Knatz und Schumacher 2019, S. 24). Zudem findet die Maskotte des KJT und damit die Nummer 1 1 6 1 1 1 über die validierte, praxisorientierte Fortbildung den Weg in die Maisons Relais. Auch bietet die Puppe BOD für alle, die pädagogisch arbeiten, eine Hilfe und Unterstützung, um Kontakt herzustellen.

3   Ein Blick auf die Sorgen und Probleme von Kindern und Jugendlichen an Hand von Daten und Erfahrungen des KJT

Im Jahr 2018 haben sich 767 Kinder und Jugendliche in Luxemburg an die 1 1 6 1 1 1 gewandt. 221 Erwachsene haben das Elterntelefon kontaktiert und 218 Kinder, Jugendliche und Eltern haben das Angebot der Online Help wahrgenommen. An die BEE SECURE Helpline haben sich 412 Personen jedes Alters gewandt, und bei der BEE SECURE Stopline sind insgesamt 2.180 Meldungen eingegangen. Das 1 1 6 1 1 1 Kanner-Jugendtelefon wird eher von den unter 15-Jährigen genutzt, gleichermaßen von Jungen und Mädchen. Die Online Help wird zunehmend von 13- bis 15-Jährigen genutzt, Hauptgruppe sind die 16- bis 25-Jährigen. Hier sind die Nutzer überwiegend Mädchen, beziehungsweise junge Frauen. Die Zahlen, die ja nur die Spitze des Eisbergs darstellen, verweisen darauf, dass man sich um das Wohlergehen und Wohlbefinden einer doch großen Gruppe junger Menschen sorgen muss.

Sie verdeutlichen eindringlich, wie wichtig es für Kinder und Jugendliche ist, jemanden zu haben, mit dem sie reden können, wenn es ihnen nicht so gut oder gar schlecht geht.

Psychosoziale und psychische Gesundheit (Einsamkeit, Ängste, Beziehungen zwischen Gleichaltrigen, Fragen zur Sexualität, Konflikte in familiären Beziehungen, Missbrauch und Gewalt) sowie Probleme in der Schule (Versagensängste, Leistungsdruck, Cyberbullying, Sexting, ...), Abhängigkeit und Sucht, Rechtsangelegenheiten, Diskriminierung, körperliche Gesundheit und Behinderung/Entwicklungsstörung sind Themen, mit denen sich Kinder und Jugendliche beim KJT melden.

Die Zahlen zeigen, dass sich Fragen und Sorgen, die im direkten oder indirekten Zusammenhang mit Gesundheit und Wohlbefinden der jüngsten Bewohner Luxemburgs stehen, häufen und im direkten Umfeld vorerst unbeantwortet und unbeachtet bleiben. Die Anonymität und die Vertraulichkeit – Prinzipien, nach denen die Dienste des KJT funktionieren – machen Mut und schaffen Raum zum Sprechen, oft zum ersten Mal. Dabei macht es keinen Unterschied, ob übers Telefon gesprochen oder online geschrieben wird.

Aufgefallen ist 2018, dass es eine Zunahme an konkreten Fragen in Bezug auf Rechtsangelegenheiten gab (z. B. hinsichtlich Trennungs- und Scheidungssituationen).

Die Themen am Elterntelefon decken sich mit denen der anderen Dienste, eben aus dem Blickpunkt des Vaters oder der Mutter. Hier ist 2018 besonders aufgefallen, dass Gespräche rund um das Thema Schule vom fünften auf den dritten Platz vorgerückt sind. Eltern fühlen sich hilflos, überfordert und alleingelassen.

Erfahrungen von Missbrauch und Gewalt, der Umgang mit suizidalen Gedanken und Absichten (latent oder akut) sowie Erfahrungen mit Trennung/Scheidung können für Kinder und Jugendliche, aber auch für Eltern, einen extrem hohen Stressfaktor darstellen, wie unsere Gespräche zeigen. Allgemein fühlen sich immer mehr junge Menschen unter Druck und gestresst. Sichtbar ist auch, dass die Gründe dafür vielfältig sind.

Unsere zentralen Themen, wegen denen Jugendliche uns kontaktieren, zeigen auf, in welchen konkreten Bereichen das Wohlbefinden von Kindern und Jugendlichen beeinträchtigt ist. Der Kontakt mit den Jugendlichen ermöglicht auch das Verstehen der direkten Konsequenzen für Kinder und Jugendliche in den genannten Bereichen.

3.1   Psychische Gesundheit

Die Gespräche zeigen die großen Herausforderungen, denen Kinder und Jugendliche ausgesetzt sind und ihre Auswirkungen auf das psychisches Wohlergehen. Dabei wird deutlich, dass Jugendliche objektive Faktoren als sehr wichtig für ihr Wohlergehen beschreiben, dazu gehören z. B. Sicherheit, Umwelt, Wohnbedingungen, soziale Beziehungen und Freizeit. Jugendliche äußern in den Gesprächen ihre Unsicherheit in Bezug etwa auf die Arbeitsplatzsuche, Wohnungssuche oder auch den Klimawandel. Im Zusammenhang mit den Schwierigkeiten bei der Wohnungssuche und dem späteren Auszug aus dem Elternhaus berichten Jugendliche von Konflikten in der Familie.

Die Unsicherheit bezüglich zentraler Lebensumstände, die für das objektive Wohlergehen von Bedeutung sind, hindert Jugendliche oft daran, selbstständig zu werden, eigene Lebensziele und Lebensperspektiven zu entwickeln. Häufig werden Versagensängste thematisiert.

Das Erleben der Unsicherheit hat einen Einfluss auf die Lebenserfahrungen der Jugendlichen und damit auf das subjektive Wohlbefinden. Jugendliche erleben einerseits eine größere Freiheit in Bezug auf ihre persönlichen Lebensentwürfe, andererseits aber auch mehr Unsicherheiten und Risiken (wie z. B. Schwierigkeiten bei der Arbeitssuche nach dem Studium). Das macht Entscheidungen schwierig und wird teilweise als Druck und Belastung erlebt (KJT, Atelier 2019).

Die Unsicherheit bezüglich der Zukunftsperspektive setzt Jugendliche unter hohen Leistungsdruck. Schule sowie Eltern fordern die Jugendlichen. Durchschnittliche Noten werden weniger akzeptiert. Prüfungsangst ist die Folge und wird durch Zukunftsängste verstärkt. Daraus ergibt sich nicht zuletzt ein selbstauferlegter Leistungsdruck. Dass dieser zum Alltag der Jugendlichen gehört, wurde schließlich auch beim Jugendkonvent 2019 deutlich. KJT war an diesem Event mit einem Atelier zur mentalen Gesundheit und Wohlbefinden aktiv beteiligt. Die Reduktion des Leistungsdrucks war eine der Hauptforderungen, die Jugendliche im Atelier „Mentale Gesundheit und Wohlbefinden" ausgewählt hatten und den Ministern im Parlament darlegten. Die Konsequenz sei mangelndes Selbstvertrauen und das Risiko der Suche nach einer Flucht aus dem Alltag (mit dem Risiko der Sucht, Isolation, Depression, …). Die Jugendlichen äußerten des Weiteren ihren Missmut darüber, wie mit psychischen Problemen umgegangen wird und wie Jugendliche mit psychischen Erkrankungen im schulischen Kontext in Luxemburg aufgefangen werden.

Ein weiterer oft genannter Stressfaktor am KJT ist die Veränderung von familiären Strukturen. Das Erleben von Trennungen, Scheidungen sowie Patchwork-Familien wird oftmals krisenhaft erlebt.

Jugendliche berichten regelmäßig von Konflikten mit den im Jugendalter so wichtigen „Peers". Soziale Beziehungen werden neu organisiert. Jugendliche lösen sich langsam von der Familie, den Eltern und orientieren sich stärker nach außen. Sie versuchen Anschluss zu finden, von ihren Freunden angenommen und akzeptiert zu werden. Diese Suche nach sozialer Anerkennung wurde als konstanter Druck beim Jugendkonvent formuliert.

Besonders über unsere Online Help erreichen uns Jugendliche, die von ihrem Unwohlsein und ihrer Unzufriedenheit mit ihrem Erscheinungsbild berichten. Sie fühlen sich nicht wohl in ihrem Körper. Die körperlichen Veränderungen müssen verarbeitet, integriert und letztendlich akzeptiert werden. Das eigene

Erscheinungsbild zu akzeptieren, ist nicht immer einfach. Der Vergleich mit den anderen liegt nahe. Durch die sozialen Netzwerke wird der Vergleich mit anderen quantifizierbar. Der Selbstwert wird gemessen durch „Likes" und Kommentare zu den „Posts". Die Selbstdarstellung online ist eine zusätzliche Herausforderung. Durch die Vergleiche mit den anderen wird hier eine weitere Druckquelle erzeugt, „gut aussehen zu müssen", „reinpassen zu müssen", „dabei sein zu müssen".

Dieses Unwohlsein im Körper kann manche Jugendliche dazu verleiten, ihr Körpergewicht und ihr Erscheinungsbild kontrollieren zu wollen. Dies kann zu Essstörungen führen wie Anorexie oder Bulimie. Oft berichten Jugendliche, dass sie unter Selbstwertproblemen leiden.

3.2 Suizidale Gedanken und selbstverletzendes Verhalten

Ein nicht unerheblicher Teil der Anfragen über Telefon oder auch über die Online Help betrifft suizidale Gedanken und selbstverletzendes Verhalten von Kindern und Jugendlichen.

Suizidale Gedanken sowie selbstverletzendes Verhalten sind besonders schwierig anzusprechen und sich einzugestehen. Durch die Anonymität und Vertraulichkeit bietet unsere Telefon- und Onlineberatung eine äußerst niederschwellige Möglichkeit der Kontaktaufnahme. Die Anonymität ermöglicht Angst, Schuld, Hilflosigkeit und Scham anzusprechen.

In den Gesprächen berichten Kinder und Jugendliche von Gefühlschaos, Druckgefühl, Stress und Leistungsdruck. Manche fühlen sich alleingelassen oder unverstanden. Auch berichten Kinder und Jugendliche regelmäßig davon, dass sie keine Vertrauensperson haben, mit der sie über Persönliches sprechen können. Sie berichten, dass ihre Eltern selbst gestresst sind, keine Zeit haben, nicht zugänglich oder überfordert sind. Manche Kinder und Jugendliche erleben Eltern, die sie ständig kritisieren, bemängeln oder „nicht da sind". Die Besprechung schulischer Themen in der Familie ist konfliktbesetzt.

Latente oder akute suizidale Gedanken tauchen oft auch in Verbindung mit Cyber-Mobbing auf. Mobbingopfer berichten davon, dass sie von anderen ausgeschlossen und öffentlich (online und offline) bloßgestellt werden. Sie fühlen sich wertlos, nicht akzeptiert und allein. Die Opfer schämen sich und trauen sich oft nicht mit Außenstehenden zu reden. Sie fühlen sich hilflos und sind von der Angst getrieben, dass sich ihre Situation verschlimmern könnte. In vielen Fällen führt dies zu Schuldgefühlen, da sie das Gefühl haben, dieMobbingsituationen selbst herbeizuführen oder sogar zu provozieren. Oft wissen sie keinen Ausweg mehr. Suizidale Gedanken koppeln sich bei manchen mit selbstverletzendem Verhalten; es löst dieses schwer zu fassende Druckgefühl und wandelt es in fühlbaren und fassbaren Schmerz.

Suizidale Gedanken werden auch thematisiert in Verbindung mit depressiven Verstimmungen. Kinder und Jugendliche empfinden sich als energielos, antriebslos und lustlos. So beschreiben einige, dass sie am liebsten einfach im Bett liegen bleiben würden. Sie geben ihre Hobbys auf, ziehen sich zurück und brechen ihre sozialen Kontakte ab, wodurch ihr Wohlbefinden und ihre Gesundheit beeinträchtigt werden.

Besonders bei der Online Help berichten suizidale Kinder und Jugendliche von hochkomplexen Situationen. Sie mussten verschiedenste und manchmal hochtraumatisierende Erfahrungen erleben: hoch strittige Trennungs-/Scheidungssituationen und eskalierte Familiensituationen; häufiger Wechsel der Partner der Eltern; sexueller Missbrauch; psychische Probleme eines Elternteils; Suchtproblematik eines Elternteils; Verlust eines Elternteiles oder einer anderen Bindungsperson; schwerwiegende Cyber-Mobbingsituationen; wirtschaftliche Not der Familie.

3.3   Mobbing und Cybermobbing

Mobbing geschieht heute sowohl online als auch offline. Waren früher Kinder und Jugendliche zu Hause vor Mobbing meist geschützt, ist dies heute nicht mehr so. Kinder und Jugendliche erleben wiederholte und regelmäßige Verletzungen durch andere in vielfältigen Formen: Beleidigungen, Erniedrigungen, Verletzungen, Schikanen, Belästigungen, Demütigungen, üble Nachrede, Verbreitung falscher Tatsachen, Zuweisung sinnloser Aufgaben, ständige und unangemessene Kritik, soziale Isolation, Gewaltandrohungen oder physische Gewalt. Nicht selten berichten Kinder von konkreten Situation, z. B. dass sie durch den Schlamm gezogen werden, ihnen Sand in den Schulranzen gesteckt wird, ihnen ihr Pausenbrot jeden Morgen weggenommen oder ihnen Gewalt angedroht wird. Jugendliche berichten von Drohungen, Beleidigungen und regelrechtem Psychoterror: „Alle lachen immer, wenn ich morgens in die Klasse komme, rempeln mich an, stoßen mich immer in der Kantine, wenn ich mein Essen hole". Oder: „ich bekomme regelmäßig Nachrichten wie ‚Keiner braucht dich, du wärst am besten tot‘".

Besonders nach Schulschluss und bei außerschulischen Aktivitäten nehmen digitale Medien überhand und verstärken die psychische Belastung des Opfers. Kinder und Jugendliche berichten von beleidigenden Nachrichten, die sie persönlich oder öffentlich in den sozialen Netzwerken erhalten, von beleidigenden und bloßstellenden Fake-Accounts, gestohlenen und/oder veränderten Fotos mit verletzenden Kommentaren, Kritiken oder der Verbreitung falscher Tatsachen. Dies erleben die betroffenen Kinder und Jugendlichen als sehr belastend, weil sie sich ausgeliefert und hilflos fühlen. Sie finden keine Ruhe, keinen sicheren Ort. Pausenlos werden sie von eingehenden Nachrichten überschwemmt. Opfer leiden oft unter mangelndem Selbstwertgefühl, empfinden sich als Versager, als dumm und wenig anziehend. Oft sind sie einsam, haben keine Freundin oder keinen Freund, die oder der für sie da ist. Sie reagieren immer sensibler auf ihr Umfeld, werden unsicher und wissen nicht, wie sie reagieren sollen, um nicht noch mehr in den Fokus des oder der Bullys zu geraten. Kinder und Jugendliche, die unter Cyber-Mobbing leiden, berichten von Schuld und Schamgefühlen.

Oft haben sie die Erfahrung gemacht, dass sie von ihrem Umfeld nicht unterstützt werden: Keiner hört richtig hin, keiner hat Zeit, das Geschehen wird bagatellisiert. Ratschläge wie „Hör doch nicht hin", „Geh denen doch aus dem Weg", „Du bist doch stärker/größer/älter als die" sind häufig. So manche Lehrer oder Erzieher gehen dem Opfer aus dem Weg oder sagen, sie hätten nichts mitbekommen. Diese Art von Reaktionen macht es dem Opfer besonders schwer, sich Hilfe zu holen.

Die Opfer werden durch den Bully in eine untergeordnete Position gedrängt, dadurch demonstriert der Bully ein Machtgefälle. Es sind genau diese Gefühle von Hilflosigkeit, Angst, Scham und Schuld, die das Opfer lähmen und es ihm so schwerer machen, sich helfen zu lassen, um aus diesem Teufelskreis auszubrechen. Aus Angst, selbst in den Fokus des oder der Bullys zu geraten, trauen sich die Unbeteiligten (passive Supporter) oft nicht, das Opfer offen zu unterstützen. Dies benötigt Zivilcourage. Je länger Mobbing andauert, desto festgefahrener wird die Situation. Kinder und Jugendliche sowie deren Eltern berichten oft von auftretenden psychosomatischen Symptomen, wie etwa Kopf- oder Bauchschmerzen oder Übelkeit am Morgen vor der Schule. Des Weiteren berichten sie von Schlaflosigkeit, Appetitlosigkeit, Gereiztheit oder depressiven Verstimmungen.

Durch Cybermobbing ziehen falsche Behauptungen oder öffentliche Beleidigungen (Veröffentlichung von geklauten, nicht einvernehmlich geschossenen oder veränderten Fotos, Fotos besetzt mit Stink-Emojis, Erstellen von falschen Accounts „Wer hasst …") immer größere Kreise. Kinder und Jugendliche außerhalb der Klasse, der Schule oder der Gemeinde sehen die Veröffentlichungen. Dies führt zu einer noch größeren und verstärkten Demütigung und Bloßstellung des Opfers.

3.4   Emotionen und Gefühle

Gefühle und Emotionen aller Art haben beim KJT einen Platz und finden Gehör.
Sie dürfen sein. Über Sorgen, Fragen und Gefühle zu sprechen hilft. Egal, ob ein
Kind gerade nicht einschlafen kann, weil es Angst vor dem Dunkeln hat, oder ob
ein Kind zum ersten Mal erzählt, dass es geschlagen oder sexuell missbraucht
wird: Gefühle wie Scham, Hilflosigkeit, Schuld, Angst können ausgesprochen
werden. Dies ist sehr wichtig und hilfreich, sowohl für Kinder als auch für
Jugendliche.

3.5   Belastungen und Beratungsbedarf während der Coronazeit

Während des Lockdowns (16.03.–31.03.2020) haben sich 179 Kinder und
Jugendliche an das KJT gewandt (158 telefonische Kontakte und 21 über die
Online Help). In der Zeit danach (01.04.–19.05.) nahmen im April 78 Kinder
und Jugendliche (43 über Telefon sowie 35 über die Online Help) Kontakt auf.
Anfang Mai waren es 55 Kinder und Jugendliche (42 über Telefon sowie 13 über
die Online Help).

   In einigen Gesprächen wurde die Angst thematisiert sich selbst mit Corona
anzustecken. Manche Kinder entwickelten psychosomatische Symptome wie
Bauchschmerzen, Panikattacken, hatten das Gefühl, keine Luft zu bekommen,
obwohl sie negativ getestet worden waren. Öfter wurde die Angst thematisiert,
andere anstecken zu können, wie z. B. die Großeltern.

   Andere Themen waren Konflikte und Stress zu Hause. Kinder und Jugendliche waren gereizt und genervt von den anderen Familienmitgliedern wie Eltern,
aber auch Geschwistern und beschwerten sich z. T. über mangelnde Privatsphäre. Manche waren genervt, dass die anderen keine Lust auf gemeinsame
Unternehmungen hatten. Konflikte mit Freunden war auch Thema: Es gab
Kommunikationsprobleme, Missverständnisse und Streit und es fehlten
Erfahrungen, diese über soziale Netzwerke zu klären.

   Kinder und Jugendliche haben eskalierte Konflikte zu Hause in der Familie
thematisiert. In manchen Fällen kam es zu Gewalt in der Familie:

- sexuelle Gewalt
- psychische Gewalt (Eltern, die dauernd kritisieren, dauernd kontrollieren,
  beschimpfen, einen runtermachen, ...)

- physische Gewalt (eskalierte Konflikte, bei denen Eltern handgreiflich geworden sind, das Kind die Treppe runterstoßen, umherschubsen, schlagen, …)
- Vernachlässigung (keine gemeinsamen Aktivitäten, sich selbst um alles kümmern müssen)

Manche Jugendliche äußerten den Wunsch, von zu Hause auszuziehen. In vielen Gesprächen am KJT und an der Online Help wurde die psychische Gesundheit thematisiert. Manche, die schon vorher unter psychischen Problemen gelitten hatten, berichteten von Verschlimmerungen der Symptome. Sie erlebten diese Zeit als sehr belastend. Einsamkeit und sich im eigenen Körper nicht wohlfühlen waren weitere Themen. Wir führten Gespräche mit Jugendlichen, die unter depressiven Verstimmungen litten, die von Panikattacken und/oder großen Ängsten berichteten. Viele hatten suizidale Gedanken. Manche hatten sich schon vorher geritzt und taten dies nun verstärkt wieder.

Andere Anrufer berichteten, dass sie vor kurzem stationär behandelt wurden, dann kurzfristig entlassen worden waren und keinen Kontakt mehr zu ihrem Therapeuten hatten. Manche wollten einen neuen Kontakt herstellen und sich Hilfe holen, sie wollten wissen, wohin sie sich wenden könnten (manche waren verwirrt aufgrund der vielen unterschiedlichen Helplines, die während des Lockdowns ins Leben gerufen wurden), andere wollten keinen weiteren Kontakt mehr aufsuchen. Auf dem Hintergund des Beschriebenen ergibt sich die Notwendigkeit ein Konzept zu erstellen, in dem festgelegt ist, wie psychiatrische Kliniken Klienten in „solchen spezifischen" Krisenzeiten ambulant oder stationär begleiten können.

In der Phase 2 (Zeitnach dem Lockdown) haben Beratungen zu Themen wie Mobbing und Cybermobbing wieder an Bedeutung gewonnen. Schüler berichteten davon, dass sie Angst hatten, wieder zurück in die Schule zu gehen. Grundschulkinder waren traurig, dass sie ihre beste Freundin bzw. ihren besten Freund nicht mehr wiedersehen konnten, weil diese nicht in ihrer Halbgruppe waren. Jugendliche wurden in Gruppen aufgeteilt, in denen manchmal nur Mitschüler waren, mit denen sie nicht so gut klar kamen; mitunter war ihr Bully dabei.

Einige Grundbedürfnisse, wie das Bedürfnis nach Sicherheit, Kontrolle, Privatsphäre, Ruhe, gut schlafen zu können, sozial anerkannt und eingebettet zu sein, wurden gar nicht oder nur teilweise befriedigt. Deshalb ist es nicht verwunderlich, dass sich bereits existierende psychische Probleme in Krisenzeiten wie dieser intensivierten.

Menschen brauchen Halt. Die fehlende Zukunftsperspektive, wann ein Ende der Pandemie in Sicht ist, bringt Unsicherheit und fällt insbesondere Jugendlichen zur Last. Die entwicklungsspezifischen Aufgaben der Jugendlichen, wie u. a. die Abgrenzung von den Eltern, der Kontakt mit der Peergruppe, die Suche nach Autonomie und Freiheit, waren in dieser Zeit gehemmt. Die Pandemie hat bestehende Probleme verstärkt.

## 4	Interpretationen und Einordnung der Daten des KJT anhand der wissenschaftlichen Literatur

Die Jugendlichen sind in der Schule und in der Freizeit gefordert. Die Ausbildung dauert länger, die Berufsanfänge sind prekärer und hemmen die Entfaltung der Autonomie der Jugendlichen. Hurrelmann bestätigt diesen verlängerten Prozess: „Jugendzeit dauert immer länger." (Hurrelmann und Quenzel 2016, S. 17).

Die Gespräche am KJT zeigen, dass die Unsicherheit bezüglich der Zukunftsperspektiven und die gleichzeitig große Auswahl an Möglichkeiten die Jugendlichen mit zunehmendem Alter stärker unter Druck setzt. Die Freiheit, zu wählen, ist gleichzeitig auch ein Zwang, zu wählen (Gahleitner et al. 2013, S. 113–120). Diese Ungewissheit und geforderte Flexibilität haben einen wesentlichen Einfluss auf die Entfaltung und Entwicklung der Jugendlichen. Im schlimmsten Fall kann diese Unsicherheit zu einer psychischen Instabilität sowie Entwicklungshemmung der Jugendlichen führen.

Adoleszenz umfasst wichtige Entwicklungsaufgaben wie die psychische Entwicklung zur Selbstständigkeit und des Verantwortungsbewusstseins, die Aufnahme und den Aufbau intimer Beziehungen, die Entwicklung von Identität, Zukunftsperspektiven, Selbstsicherheit, Selbstkontrolle und von sozialen Kompetenzen.

Dies stellt die Jugendlichen vor große Herausforderungen, und dies ganz besonders in der bewegten Zeit der Adoleszenz, wo es gleichzeitig zu einer grundlegenden Reorganisation des Gehirns kommt. Laut Konrad et al. (2013) besteht ein Ungleichgewicht zwischen dem früher reifenden limbischen System und dem Belohnungssystem und einem noch nicht voll ausgereiften präfrontalen Kontrollsystem. Dieses Ungleichgewicht könnte den für die Adoleszenz typischen emotionalen Reaktionsstil und die risikoreichen Verhaltensweisen der Jugendlichen begünstigen. Dies bedeutet, dass „in emotionalen Situationen die Wahrscheinlichkeit zunimmt, dass Belohnung und Emotionen stärker die Handlung beeinflussen als rationale Entscheidungsprozesse" (Konrad et al. 2013, S. 428). Gleichzeitig ist „Adoleszenz- typisches Verhalten die Basis der Autonomieentwicklung Jugendlicher und fördert die Emanzipation von ihrer Primär-familie" (Konrad et al. 2013, S. 429). „Diese Reorganisation eröffnet Chancen für Bildung und Erziehung. Jugendliche können insbesondere von Lernerfahrungen profitieren, die in einem positiven emotionalen Kontext stattfinden und die gezielt eine Emotionsregulation trainieren." Jedoch ergibt sich auch eine „erhöhte Vulnerabilität". Manche Jugendliche geraten in eine große Instabilität. In den Gesprächen am KJT zeigt sich dies in Themen wie geschilderten Panikattacken, Prüfungsängsten, Zukunftsängsten, depressiven Verstimmungen, aber auch in suizidalen Gedanken oder selbstverletzendem Verhalten.

Suizidgedanken sind „Ausdruck einer großen Not, einer Ambivalenz zwischen Leben und Tod" (Knatz und Schumacher 2019, S. 71). Rein statistisch ist Suizid in Deutschland, nach Unfällen, die zweithäufigste Todesursache in der Alters-gruppe der 15- bis unter 30-Jährigen. Suizide bei Jugendlichen sind oft Kurz-schlussreaktionen. Knatz und Schumacher führen dies auf die mangelnde Krisenkompetenz zurück (Knatz und Schumacher 2019, S. 70). Jugendliche berichten von Überforderung, die sie stoppen wollen, aber nicht wissen, wie. Sie sind hilflos und ihre Situation erscheint ihnen in dem Moment als aussichts-los. Hier kann ein Gespräch oder das Schreiben mit einer Beraterin oder einem Berater des KJT sehr hilfreich sein. „Anonymität hat einen enthemmenden Effekt und bietet gleichzeitig einen Schutzraum." Knatz und Schumacher (2019, S. 4) sprechen von „Nähe durch Distanz". Anonymität verhindert eine direkte mögliche Intervention und wahrt die Autonomie und Entscheidungsfrei-heit des Anrufers (Schaeffer und Schmidt-Kaehler 2011 zitiert von Knatz und Schumacher 2019, S. 4).

Des Weiteren erleben Kinder und Jugendliche einen „Verlust struktureller Geborgenheit" (Gahleitner et al. 2013). Familiäre Strukturen verändern sich. „Es entstehen Wahlgemeinschaften und neue Formen des Zusammenlebens. Statt ein-gespielter Regeln sind kommunikative Kompetenzen gefordert, um unterschied-liche Bedürfnislagen auszuhandeln. Kinder und Jugendliche haben es heute vermehrt mit wechselnden Bezugspersonen, einem erweiterten Verwandtschafts-system sowie biologischen und sozialen Eltern zu tun. Gleichzeitig bleibt jedoch ein inneres Bild von Familie erhalten, das durchaus einer konservativen Aus-richtung folgt, wobei sich eine Umsetzung dieser Sehnsüchte immer schwieriger gestaltet." (Gahleitner et al. 2013).

Der Jugendforscher Philipp Ikrath (Ikrath, 2012) formulierte in einem Inter-view diese gelebten Ambivalenzen in der Jugendzeit so: „Man könnte sie als eine Generation verhinderter Spießer bezeichnen. Sie sehnen sich nach einem Leben mit heiler Familie, Haus im Grünen und Golden-Retriever-Welpen. In der Reali-tät sind sie aber mit überzogenen Mobilitätsanforderungen, ständigem Leistungsdruck und beinhartem Konkurrenzkampf konfrontiert, was ein unauffälliges, dafür aber zufriedenes Leben für sie zunehmend utopisch erscheinen lässt."

Kinder und Jugendliche erleben sich unter Stress und Druck. „Stress entsteht, wenn ein Mensch vor Aufgaben steht und nicht mehr glaubt, dass er sie bewältigen kann. Kurze Phasen von Stress sind normal, können sogar antreiben. Wenn ein Mensch aber dauerhaft unter Stress steht, kann das zu psychischen Erkrankungen führen. Chronischer Stress wird als Risikofaktor für psychische Erkrankungen angesehen." (KJT, Jahresbericht 2018, S. 46).

Allgemein ist bekannt, dass die Hälfte aller psychiatrischen Erkrankungen im Alter von 14 Jahren beginnen, zwei Drittel spätestens mit 24 Jahren (Hintenberger 2018). Dies bestätigt die Dringlichkeit einer guten Präventionsarbeit und von Unterstützungsangeboten in dieser Alterskategorie.

Die Benennung von starken und blockierenden Gefühlen wie Scham, Hilflosigkeit, Schuld und Angst ist sehr wichtig für die Entwicklung eines ausgewogenen Stresssystems. Wir wissen, dass durch Zuwendung, Trost und Besänftigung sowie die Gewissheit des Schutzes durch ihre Eltern und Fürsorger Kinder lernen, Gefahren besser einzuschätzen und gemäßigter darauf zu reagieren. Sie werden resistenter gegenüber Stress. Das körperliche Stresssystem und die beteiligten Hirnstrukturen lernen einen „Zustand körperlicher Grundgelassenheit (Vagatonie) herzustellen" und sich „schnell und adäquat nach einer Stresssituation wieder zu normalisieren" (Hoffmann und Michaux 2018). Hoffmann und Michaux (2018) sprechen von einem „emotionalen Pflaster", durch das „das vagale System lernt, wie es die überschießenden Emotionen wieder eindämmen kann". Falls Kinder hingegen die Erfahrung machen, dass ihre Eltern sie nicht schützen, sondern sie im Gegenteil anschreien, vor anderen blamieren oder ihnen in den Rücken fallen, so kann es zu einer Art gelernter Schutzlosigkeit kommen. Fehlen Trost und Besänftigung „sind emotionale Überdrehungen und sprunghafte Impulsivität mehr oder weniger vorprogrammiert" (Hoffmann & Michaux, 2018, S. 62). Hier kann auch das KJT junge Menschen entlasten.

Auf jeden Fall ist es hilfreich sowohl für Kinder als auch für Jugendliche, über ihre Gefühle zu sprechen und sich so weiter zu entwickeln. Besonders in Situationen, in denen Schuld, Scham oder Angst im Vordergrund stehen, ermöglicht ein Gespräch Kindern und Jugendlichen, die Situation besser zu verstehen und zu verarbeiten. Manchmal können Ambivalenzen bearbeitet werden.

Durch aktives Zuhören und die Annahme, dass der Anrufer selbst Experte seiner eigenen Situation ist, stärken wir die Selbstwirksamkeit des Anrufers oder Users. Wir machen uns mit dem Anrufer zusammen auf den Weg und suchen gemeinsam nach Ideen. Der Anrufer entscheidet, was und wann für ihn das

Richtige ist. Dies stärkt Selbstwirksamkeit und Autonomie. Mit jemandem über etwas zu reden hilft. Keiner muss allein bleiben.

5 Aktuelle und zukünftige Herausforderungen mit Blick auf die Probleme und Belastungen von Kindern und Jugendlichen

Digitale Kommunikationsmöglichkeiten verändern und erweitern die Kommunikationswege, über die sich Kinder und Jugendliche mitteilen. So ist „Chatten" ein zunehmend beliebtes Kommunikationsformat bei den Jugendlichen. Vor diesem Hintergrund befindet sich das KJT in der Vorbereitung eines chatbasierten Beratungsangebots, das das telefonische und Online- Angebot ergänzen soll. In vielen europäischen Ländern können sich Jugendliche bereits auch per Chat an ein ausgebildetes Beraterteam wenden. Mit Blick auf die Erfahrungen im Jahr 2020 plant das KJT das Hilfs- und Kommunikationsangebot zu erweitern. Die Beratung im Chatformat wird zunächst in einer Pilotphase erprobt. In diesem Kontext ist es auch eine vorrangige Aufgabe, die Website, Eingangstür des KJT, der Zeit anzupassen und zu aktualisieren.

Die BEE SECURE Stopline und BEE SECURE Helpline, die beide im Kontext eines EU-Projekts gemanagt und operiert werden, haben sich etabliert, was steigende Zahlen signalisieren. Hier ist das KJT gefordert, mit ständig neuen Herausforderungen umzugehen, wie z. B. Hypersexualisierung von Jugendlichen und der sich immens schnell weiterentwickelnden Digitalisierung.

Die Schulung und Stärkung von Professionellen im Umgang mit Gefühlen von Kindern und Jugendlichen sowie die systematische Information über das Angebot des KJT bleiben auch zukünftig absolut notwendig.

Literatur

Gahleitner, S., Hintenberger, G. & Leitner, A. (2013). Biopsychosoziale Versorgung von Kindern und Jugendlichen heute – eine zunehmende Herausforderung. Resonanzen. *E-Journal für biopsychosoziale Dialoge in Psychotherapie, Supervision und Beratung*, S. 113–120.
Hintenberger, G. (2018). Interne Weiterbildung. Luxemburg. (unveröffentlichtes Manuskript)
Hoffmann, M. & Michaux, G. (2018). *Grenzenlos emotional. Von impulsiv bis Borderline. Balance Ratgeber.* Medienverlag.

Ikrath, P. (29. August 2012). *Eine Generation verhinderter Spießer*. (N. Lisa, Interviewer). Von https://www.derstandard.at/story/1345165571598/eine-generation-verhinderter-spiesser, abgerufen 27. November 2020.

Kanner-Jugendtelefon. (2018). *Jahresbericht*. Kanner-Jugendtelefon.

Kanner-Jugendtelefon. (15. November 2019). Atelier *Mentale Gesundheit und Wohlbefinden*. Jugendkonvent, Luxemburg.

Knatz, B. & Schumacher, S. (2019). *Mediale Dialogkompetenz.Umgang mit schwierigen Gesprächssituationen am Telefon und im Chat*. Berlin: Springer.

Konrad, K., Firk, C. & Uhlhaas, P. (2013). Brain development during adolescence: neuroscientific insights into this developmental period. *Deutsches Arzteblatt international*. 110(25): 425-431.

Maslow, A. H. (1943). A Theory of Human Motivation. *Psychological Review 50(4)*, S. 370–396.

Hurrelmann, K. & Quenzel, H. (2016). *Lebensphase Jugend*. Eine Einführung in die sozialwissenschaftliche Jugendforschung. Weinheim Basel: Beltz Verlag.

Rogers, C. (1951). Client-centered therapy: its current practice, implications, and theory. London: Constable & Robinson.

STATEC (2019). *Regards. Au Luxembourg, 100% des jeunes et 82% des 65 à 74 ans ont un accès internet*. Von https://statistiques.public.lu/catalogue-publications/regards/2019/PDF-12-2019.pdf, abgerufen 26. September 2019.

von Schlippe, A. & Schweitzer, J. (2016). *Lehrbuch der systemischen Therapie und Beratung I: Das Grundlagenwissen*. Göttingen: Vandenhoeck & Ruprecht.

World Health Organisation (WHO) (2012). *Gesundheit 2020 und die Bedeutung der Messung von Wohlbefinden. Faktenblatt*. Von https://www.euro.who.int/__data/assets/pdf_file/0018/185310/Health-2020-and-the-case-Fact-Sheet-Ger-final.pdf, abgerufen 26. September 2019.

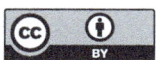

Gesundheitsförderung und Wohlbefinden in der Fremdunterbringung: eine Herausforderung auf allen Ebenen für das „Institut étatique d'aide à l'enfance et à la jeunesse" (AITIA)

René Schmit

1 Einleitung

In einer im Jahr 2005 veröffentlichten Studie zum Wohlbefinden der Jugendlichen in Luxemburg (Wagener et al. 2005, S. 26) haben 11- bis 12-jährige Jugendliche positive Aspekte des Wohlbefindens folgendermaßen ausgedrückt: „ein Zuhause haben, eine Familie haben, sich geborgen fühlen", „zuhause in meinem Zimmer fühle ich mich sehr wohl"; negative Aspekte hingegen sind: „allein sein, traurig sein, sich schämen"; „in einem anderen Haus, in der Gesellschaft bei anderen Menschen, die mich nicht mögen, fühle ich mich schlecht".

Zum Wohlbefinden in der Familie gehören vor allem mit den Eltern scherzen, diskutieren, sich an familiären Aufgaben und Entscheidungen beteiligen (ebd., S. 50). Im Kommentar betont die Studie die Wichtigkeit der Gewohnheiten und Verhaltensweisen Lebensarten, Lebensgewohnheiten innerhalb der Familie, die die Kinder prägen. Das „Vertrauen, die Kommunikation, die Beziehungen" innerhalb der Familie „beeinflussen maßgeblich das psychosoziale Gleichgewicht und die Beziehungsfähigkeit" der Jugendlichen. „Die Familie spielt eine wesentliche Rolle in der Persönlichkeitsentfaltung jedes Jugendlichen. Defizite an dieser Stelle gehören oft zu den Hauptursachen für Beeinträchtigungen des Wohlbefindens zu einem späteren Zeitpunkt." (ebd., S. 75).

R. Schmit (✉)
Luxemburg, Luxemburg
E-Mail: rene.schmit@education.lu

© Der/die Autor(en) 2022
A. Heinen et al. (Hrsg.), *Wohlbefinden und Gesundheit im Jugendalter*,
https://doi.org/10.1007/978-3-658-35744-3_23

509

Die gleiche Studie beschreibt Gesundheit als „wichtigen Faktor für die individuelle, soziale und wirtschaftliche Entwicklung eines Menschen. (…) Anerkennung, Ablehnung, Selbstwertgefühl, Stress, Einsamkeit, Ausgrenzung, Gewalt, Solidarität, Armut, Lebensperspektive (…) bestimmen das Wohlbefinden oder das Missempfinden eines Menschen" (ebd., S. 15).

Ein 2010 veröffentlichter Bericht über die seelische Gesundheit der Jugendlichen in Luxemburg (Louazel et al. 2010) definiert im Einklang mit der Weltgesundheitsorganisation (WHO) die seelische Gesundheit als eine individuelle und eine kollektive Ressource, sie entspricht einem Zustand von Wohlbefinden, in dem die Person sich verwirklichen, normale Spannungen des Lebens überwinden, eine produktive und erfolgreiche Arbeit bewältigen und zum Leben in Gemeinschaft beitragen kann. Seelische Gesundheit ist viel mehr als das Fehlen von psychischer Krankheit (Zermatten 2005).

Der Beitrag zeigt auf, wie Kinder und Jugendliche mit belastenden Erfahrungen und Erlebnissen umgehen und inwiefern ein Leben im Kinderheim für diese Kinder und Jugendlichen eine Chance auf eine bessere Zukunft sein kann. Dabei richtet der Beitrag auch den Blick auf die professionelle Praxis in Heimstrukturen und diskutiert die zentralen Konzepte und Methoden, mit denen die Einrichtungen ihren gesetzlichen Auftrag umsetzen. Die Grundlage der Darstellungen, Analysen und Interpretationen in diesem Beitrag bilden die Praxiserfahrungen im Institut AITIA.

Im ersten Kapitel geht es um die geschichtliche Entwicklung der Einrichtung, von den Anfängen bis hin zu den Konzepten der Traumapädagogik und deren Implementierung in einer partizipativen Vorgehensweise. Das zweite Kapitel erläutert die Neuerungen des Gesetzes vom 01.08.2019 und deren Folgen für die Einrichtung. Im dritten Kapitel stehen die Menschen, Arbeitsprozesse und Strukturen im Dienst des Wohlbefindens von Kindern und Jugendlichen im Mittelpunkt. Das vierte Kapitel zeigt die Arbeitsprozesse im Institut AITIA anhand einiger konkreter Beispiele. Abschließend skizziert das fünfte Kapitel die möglichen Folgen einer zunehmenden Ökonomisierung auf die Soziale Arbeit.

2 Historischer Rückblick

Fremdunterbringung beruhte im 19. und weit bis ins 20. Jahrhundert hinein auf einem bestimmten gesellschaftlichen Problemverständnis, wonach dem Kindeswohl am besten begegnet werden konnte durch Herausnahme des Kindes aus einem schlechten Milieu und seine Verpflanzung in ein gesundes Milieu. Das Kind wird nicht gefragt, es hat keine Meinung (zu haben), es hat sich anzupassen und dankbar zu sein. Fragen nach Sicherheit, Geborgenheit und Wohlbefinden waren kein Thema.

Erst die große Reformbewegung der 1970er Jahre ermöglichte die Entwicklung anderer Vorstellungen des Umgangs mit verwahrlosten und gefährdeten Kindern. Sie entsprachen eher dem „Staffellaufmodells". wonach die Einrichtung die gefährdeten Kinder zu einem bestimmten Moment von der Familie übernimmt, zeitlich begrenzt und mit dem Ziel, es wieder zurück in die Obhut der Familie geben zu können. Die Aufnahme eines Kindes schreibt sich hier ein in die Lebens- und Familiengeschichte des Kindes, die Aufnahme ist nicht zeitlos. Das Kind ist nicht genötigt, sich anzupassen, es geht darum, dass es sich entfalten kann. Die Beziehungen des Kindes rücken in den Mittelpunkt und damit auch das subjektive Erleben des Kindes und sein Wohlbefinden (Schmit 2010).

Das „Institut étatique d'aide à l'enfance et à la jeunesse – AITIA" hat diese Entwicklung seit der Gründung der Einrichtung im Jahre 1884 selbst durchlaufen (Staatlech Kannerheemer 1994; Schmit 2009). Vor diesem Hintergrund soll hier nur ein kurzer Blick auf die Entwicklung der letzten 10 Jahre geworfen werden, als versucht wurde, ein Leitbild und handlungsfähige Konzepte der „Staatlichen Kinderheime" zu erstellen.

Dies erwies sich als schwieriges Unterfangen, da das damalige Rahmengesetz von 2004 keine klaren Rahmenbedingungen vorgab und das ASFT-Gesetz von 1998 eigentlich nur rein formale Kriterien zum Erlangen eines *Agréments* enthielt[1].

Ebenso schwierig gestaltete sich eine Bestandsaufnahme der Stärken und Schwächen der Einrichtung in den Jahren 2002 bis 2005. Der Versuch der Formalisierung eines Institutionskonzeptes fand seine Grenzen in der Tatsache, dass Erzieher, Sozialpädagogen und Sozialarbeiter ihren Beruf als einen Beruf der Aktion, des Handelns mit den Kindern verstanden und keine eigene Sprache zum Reflektieren ihrer Arbeit hatten. Jede Art der Formalisierung hatte demnach den Charakter des Fremden.

Gleichzeitig und vielleicht genau aus diesem Grund zeigte sich jedoch, dass die Arbeitsbedingungen in der Einrichtung sich veränderten und dass die Problematik der Kinder und Jugendlichen die Professionellen vor immer größere Herausforderungen stellten.

Die Betreuung dieser Kinder und Jugendlichen verlangt eine Unterstützung der interdisziplinären Teams, institutionelle Rahmenbedingungen

---

[1] Vgl. Projet de loi portant création d'un Institut public d'aide à l'enfance et à la jeunesse, doc. parl. n° 7189/00 du 16.10.2017, S. 3.

und Ermutigungen, um berufliche Spannungen und Segmentierungen zu überwinden. Es braucht interaktive Zusammenarbeit zwischen den erzieherischen,
therapeutischen und schulischen Bereichen, dies in einer Perspektive von Pflege.

In Anlehnung an diese Stellungnahme und in Anbetracht eines generell entstandenen Gefühls der Überforderung, der steigenden Ohnmacht und Müdigkeit
der Mitarbeiter hat das Institut AITIA im Jahr 2012 ein „Atelier de réflexion"
ins Leben gerufen, mit dem Ziel, alle Karten auf den Tisch zu legen. In einem
Prozess des permanenten Dialoges der Leitung und der (gewählten) Vertreter
des „Atelier de réflexion" mit den Mitarbeitern des „Département Hébergement"
konnen auf diese Art und Weise alle Fragen, Sorgen, Ängste, Herausforderungen,
Hoffnungen und Zukunftsperspektiven offen und gemeinsam besprochen und
nach Lösungen gesucht werden.

Aus dieser gemeinsamen Arbeit ergab sich die Notwendigkeit der Suche nach
einem gemeinsamen Referenzmodell und einer gemeinsamen Sprache für die
institutionelle Arbeit mit den Kindern und Jugendlichen sowie die Notwendigkeit
einer Überarbeitung des bestehenden Gesetzes, das die Existenz und den Auftrag/das
Mandat der staatlichen Einrichtung regelt. Gemeinsam wurde sich auf die Traumapädagogik als Referenzmodell für das „Département Hébergement" verständigt.

Konkrete Schritte waren zunächst eine systematische Fortbildung vor Ort für
alle betroffenen Mitarbeiter über 3–4 Jahre, eine Implementierung der traumapädagogischen Konzepte als permanenten Prozess, garantiert durch die Schaffung
eines Fachdienstes, das Ausarbeiten eines spezifischen Rahmenkonzeptes
durch die Leitung und zunehmende Partizipation der Kinder und Jugendlichen.
Die traumapädagogische Arbeitsweise wird u. a. daran zu messen sein, wie sie
ermöglicht, dass der „Fremdzwang" zurückgenommen wird und das Kind „Mit-
gestalter" des erzieherischen Alltags wird (Wolf 2008, S. 102).

3   Das Gesetz vom 01.08.2019

Am ersten August 2019 ist das neue Rahmengesetz „concernant l'institut étatique
d'aide à l'enfance et à la jeunesse"[2] in Kraft getreten. Es stellt einen Meilenstein
in der Geschichte dieser staatlichen Einrichtung dar, deren Gründung in die Mitte
des 19. Jahrhunderts zurückführt.[3]

---

[2]Vgl. Mémorial A-N°541 du12 août 2019: Loi du 1er août 2019 concernant l'Institut
étatique d'aide à l'enfance et à la jeunesse. Dieses Gesetz ersetzt das Gesetz „Loi modifiée
du 18 avril 2004 portant organisation des Maisons d'Enfants de l'Etat".

[3]Vgl. Doc. Parl. 7189–7 du 09.07.2019, Rapport de la commission parlementaire.

Das neue Gesetz wurde notwendig, um die Struktur und die Organisation der Einrichtung „Staatliche Kinderheime" an die neuen Gegebenheiten anzupassen. Es ging darum, eine transversale Politik zu fördern und Konzepte zu entwickeln, welche die erzieherischen, sozialen, schulischen, psychologischen, therapeutischen, und medizinischen Dimensionen miteinander verbinden und eine ganzheitliche und personenzentrierte Betreuung der Jugendlichen ermöglichen können. Desweiteren wird hier ein Schritt in Richtung Entgrenzung („décloisonnement") gegangen, welche im Bericht „Pour une stratégie nationale en faveur de la santé mentale des enfants et des jeunes au Luxembourg" (Louazel et al. 2010) als ein wichtiger Schritt auf dem Weg zu einer globalen, holistischen Betreuung dargestellt wird.

Ein wesentlicher Aspekt dieser Vorgehensweise besteht darin, dem Staat als Träger und Initiator der sozialen Arbeit die Möglichkeit zu geben, eigene Strukturen zu schaffen, neue Vorgehensweisen zu initiieren respektive modellhaft neue, innovative Wege zu gehen. Der Staat gibt sich so die Möglichkeit, aktiv in der Rolle eines Regulierers zu bleiben.

Im Gesetz ist die Umsetzung dieser Missionen (Aufträge, Mandate) durch die Aufteilung des Instituts in verschiedene „Départements"[4] vorgeschrieben. Es definiert klare Vorgaben im Sinn einer „Assurance-Qualité" sowie durch das Verständnis des Mandates als eines dreifachen Mandates.

Assurance-qualité: Zurzeit gibt es (noch) keinen rationalen Referenzkader für den Bereich der „Aide à l'enfance". Das Gesetz vom 1. August 2019 gibt Vorgaben für das staatliche Institut AITIA: So wird ein Rahmenkonzept („Projet institutionnel") für die gesamte Einrichtung gefordert, eine Beschreibung der Zielsetzung und der Orientierung der Arbeit in den verschiedenen Bereichen, sowie Transversalität und Öffnung zum Arbeitsfeld der Santé mentale, Interdisziplinarität sowie eine Arbeitsweise, welche differenzierte, modulierbare und an die Betroffenen angepasste Strukturen und Prozesse vorsieht. Ein „Projet d'accompagnement personnalisé" für alle betreuten Menschen garantiert und verlangt eine partizipative Arbeitsweise, die den Kindern und Jugendlichen sowie ihren Familien einen wesentlichen Platz in der Ausarbeitung und der Umsetzung aller Hilfemaßnahmen einräumt.

Das dreifache Mandat: Das im Gesetz eingeschriebene Mandat (mission) wird, in Anlehnung an Staub-Bernasconi (2007), als ein dreifaches Mandat verstanden. Die Einrichtung erhält ein erstes Mandat von den Kindern und Jugend-

---

[4] Doc. Parl. 7189–7 du 09.07.2019, Rapport de la commission parlementaire, S. 3.

lichen und ihren Familien, die eine Hilfe erbitten. Die Einrichtung bemüht sich, ihnen als einzigartigen Menschen zu begegnen und sie nicht als „Objekte" der Pflege und Fürsorge zu sehen. Die Einrichtung kann dieses Mandat auch von den Justizbehörden erhalten, welche die institutionelle Betreuung eines Kindes anhand eines gerichtlichen Beschlusses entscheiden. Die Institution erhält ein zweites Mandat von der Gesellschaft. Der Staat hat die Pflicht, eine Sozialpolitik umzusetzen, die allen Bürgern, und insbesondere den Kindern, die in der staatlichen Einrichtung betreut werden, zugutekommt. Es ist Aufgabe des Staates, die nötigen Voraussetzungen und Rahmenbedingungen zu schaffen, damit diese Institution ihren verschiedenen Aufträgen gerecht werden kann. Dies geschieht u. a. durch das oben genannte Gesetz. Ein drittes Mandat ergibt sich auf der Ebene der Fachleute selbst, aus deren fachlicher Verantwortlichkeit und deren Berufsethos. Dies bedeutet für die Mitarbeiter, die Arbeit auf der Grundlage ihrer beruflichen und deontologischen Regeln zu begreifen und die Arbeit nach institutionellen Richtlinien zu organisieren. Wichtig ist, die Arbeit nach Maßstäben sozialer Einbeziehung (inclusion sociale) zu verstehen und nicht so sehr nach Maßstäben sozialer Integration oder Anpassung (intégration ou adaptation sociale). Dies kann durch eine Vorgehensweise der Interdisziplinarität, des Zusammentragens von Sichtweisen und Praktiken, und nicht durch das Aufzwingen eines Wissens um das Beste für den Anderen, erreicht werden.

So gilt es auch, aufmerksam zu bleiben, damit nicht eine Fachrichtung zu dominant wird und den anderen Fachrichtungen keinen Platz mehr lässt. Echte Interdisziplinarität verlangt interaktive Zusammenarbeit sowie die Bereitschaft, die anderen Fachkräfte in das eigene Berufsfeld einzuladen.

4 Konzepte und Methoden des staatlichen Instituts AITIA zur Förderung des Wohlbefindens von Kindern und Jugendlichen: das Kind im Mittelpunkt, Interdisziplinarität und Traumpädagogik

Die pädagogische Arbeit des staatlichen Instituts AITIA gründet auf verschiedenen Konzepten und Methoden. Sie zielen auf eine Förderung des Wohlbefindens der in den Einrichtungen untergebrachten Kindern und Jugendlichen.

4.1 Das Kind im Mittelpunkt

Ein zentrales Prinzip der Arbeit ist die Orientierung an den Bedürfnissen des Kindes, das in eine Einrichtung aufgenommen wird. Das Kind braucht einen Platz zur Begleitung und Pflege durch Erwachsene, die ihm Kontinuität, Verlässlichkeit und Betreuung und Pflege „maßgeschneidert" zusichern, wobei auch den Eltern und den Betreuern Rechnung zu tragen ist. Es braucht keinen Ort, an dem es „aufbewahrt" wird, in Erwartung einer Lösung. Der psychischen Realität soll Rechnung getragen werden, das heißt die Mitarbeiterinnen und Mitarbeiter müssen über Fakten und objektive Tatsachen hinaus aufmerksam sein für die Art und Weise, wie die betroffene Person, ob Junge oder Mädchen, Mann oder Frau, ein Geschehen erlebt hat. Es gilt, anzuerkennen, dass ein Mensch nicht reduzierbar ist auf ein Objekt des Bemühens anderer, der Erzieher zum Beispiel, sondern vielmehr Subjekt seines eigenen Wortes und Handelns ist. Es gilt, die Einzigartigkeit jedes Kindes und jedes Jugendlichen zu erkennen und anzuerkennen.

Ein Heim kann für Kinder und Jugendliche ein förderlicher oder ein verhindernder Ort des Aufwachsens sein, so wie es auch für die Fachkräfte gesundheitsfördernde oder krankmachende Arbeitsplätze bieten und für die Eltern eine bedeutsame Unterstützungseinrichtung oder eine „Einrichtung der Missachtung" sein kann.

4.2 Interdisziplinarität

Interdisziplinarität impliziert das Zusammentragen von verschiedenen Sichtweisen, Aufgaben und Interventionen auf Basis gemeinsamer Reflexion und Erarbeitung, mit dem Ziel, eine einheitliche konzeptionelle Rahmenstruktur aufzubauen und gemeinsame Lösungsstrategien zu erarbeiten. Interdisziplinarität verlangt von allen Mitarbeitern, die eigene Arbeit mit den Sichtweisen und Praktiken der anderen Disziplinen zu einem gemeinsamen Arbeitsprozess zu verknüpfen und auf dieser Basis ein Arbeitsbündnis mit den Kindern und Familien auszuarbeiten. Das verlangt u. a., dass alle Mitarbeiter ihre eigene Praxis in eine Teamarbeit einschreiben und die Sichtweisen und die Arbeit aller Teammitglieder wertschätzen und unterstützen. Eine solche Herangehensweise ermöglicht es allen Beteiligten, sich der emotionalen Erfahrungen der Kinder und Jugendlichen bewusst zu werden und somit deren symptomatische Äußerungen und die daraus entstehenden Widerstände zu erkennen, auszuhalten und adäquat darauf zu reagieren. Diese gemeinsame Haltung ermöglicht den Kindern und Jugendlichen, aus den ihnen bekannten, sich wiederholenden Verhaltensmustern auszusteigen und andere Seiten an sich zu entdecken.

Diese Art der institutionellen Arbeit erweist sich als ein komplexer Prozess, dessen Umsetzung im Alltag für alle Beteiligten anspruchsvoll ist und die Bereitschaft zu konflikthaften Auseinandersetzung voraussetzt. Die Mitarbeiter sind dafür verantwortlich, sich der Anforderung von Selbstreflexion zu stellen, der eigenen Person als Werkzeug gewahr zu werden, mit Widersprüchen und Ambivalenzen leben zu können und sich der Prinzipien der Übertragung und Gegenübertragung bewusst zu werden.

In der interdisziplinären institutionellen Arbeit ist es von großer Bedeutung, einen Raum der Vertraulichkeit zu schaffen, der es ermöglicht, dass ein Kind, ein Jugendlicher sich einer Vertrauensperson öffnen kann, mit der Gewissheit, dass nicht alle Teammitglieder über alles genauestens informiert sind.

4.3   Traumapädagogik

Im Jahr 2012 wurde beschlossen, das Rahmenkonzept des „Département Hébergement" nach den traumapädagogischen Standards der BAG Traumapädagogik auszurichten (BAG Traumapädagogik 2011; Lang et al. 2013). Traumapädagogik bildet damit ein wichtiges Konzept der pädagogischen Arbeit in den Einrichtungen. Sie ist heute eine eigenständige Fachdisziplin geworden, die Kindern hilft, gemeinsam mit Betreuern Antworten zu suchen auf die Frage, wie sie zu welcher Zeit selbstbemächtigt ihren eigenen Lebensweg finden können. Des Weiteren hilft Traumapädagogik der Institution, Konzepte zu entwickeln, welche in Haltungen, Arbeitsprozesse und institutionelle Strukturen implementiert werden, so dass sie eine reale Hilfe sowohl zum Verstehen von Kindern und Jugendlichen mit lebensgeschichtlich belasteten Erfahrungen als auch zum pädagogischen Handeln bieten. Traumapädagogische Konzepte beziehen sich also auf alle Ebenen einer Institution.

Eine solche Vorgehensweise ist kohärent mit dem oben angeführten Modell des Staffellaufes. Sie beruht nicht auf einem vermeintlichen Wissen über andere Menschen, sondern geschieht in und durch ein wohlwollendes Zusammenfügen des Wissens von mehreren Professionalitäten, also auch dem eigenen Wissen der Kinder und Jugendlichen.

Eine traumapädagogische Vorgehensweise begnügt sich in keiner Hinsicht damit, „Rezepte" zu liefern. Sie soll vielmehr zu einem gemeinsamen, interdisziplinären Denken und Handeln anregen. Einige Hauptbegriffe der Traumapädagogik seien hier kurz erläutert (Maisons d'Enfants de l'État 2015).

Der Lebensort „Heim" als sicherer Ort
Die Kinder und Jugendlichen benötigen einen Ort, einen Lebensraum, der ihnen Sicherheit und Geborgenheit gibt, damit sie lernen, ihren alten, schmerzvollen Erfahrungen neue, korrigierende Beziehungserfahrungen entgegenzusetzen und so neue Beziehungsmuster zu entwickeln. Ein sicherer Ort zeichnet sich aus durch innere Sicherheit, ermöglicht und gerahmt durch äußere Sicherheit. Dazu braucht es eine adäquate räumliche Gestaltung, aber auch Fachkräfte, die sich den Kindern und Jugendlichen stellen, die zuverlässig da sind für die Kinder und Jugendlichen. Dann braucht es die Unterstützung durch haltgebende und sichernde Strukturen sowie die Unterstützung durch klare Arbeitsprozesse und fachliche Begleitung. Es gilt, den Kindern und Jugendlichen die Möglichkeit zu geben, bei sich selbst Sicherheit zu finden, sich selbst einen sicheren inneren Ort zu schaffen. Die Kinder und Jugendlichen lernen, wieder an sich selbst zu glauben und sich selbst zu vertrauen, sich selbst zur Ruhe zu bringen und ihre eigenen Emotionen zu regulieren.

Der sichere Ort ist ein Ort der Berechenbarkeit, der Transparenz, der Vorhersehbarkeit und der Selbstbemächtigung. Er ist eine Voraussetzung dafür, dass die betroffenen Kinder und Jugendlichen ihre Schutzmechanismen und Symptome aufgeben und sich neuen Beziehungserfahrungen öffnen können.

Die Grundhaltung
Die Traumapädagogik gründet auf einer wertschätzenden und verstehenden Grundhaltung. Dies gilt für die Arbeit aller Fachkräfte mit den Kindern und Jugendlichen sowie deren Familien und auch unter Professionellen auf allen Ebenen der Einrichtung. Ein fundiertes Wissen über Traumafolgestörungen ermöglicht ein (neues) Verständnis für das Verhalten der Kinder und Jugendlichen im Alltag, wie zum Beispiel die verminderte Belastbarkeit als Auswirkung von traumatischen Erlebnissen.

Eine solche Grundhaltung aller Teammitglieder ist auf Dauer nur möglich durch einen permanenten Prozess der Pflege und Unterstützung der Beteiligten.

Die Annahme des guten Grundes. „Alles, was ein Mensch zeigt, ergibt einen Sinn in seiner Geschichte!"
Viele der Verhaltensweisen, mit denen Jungen und Mädchen auf Traumatisierungen reagieren, sind für die Erzieher und die anderen Kinder und Jugendlichen der Gruppe belastend. Dabei geht die notwendige Wertschätzung und Würdigung der Verhaltensweisen der Kinder und Jugendlichen als Überlebensstrategien häufig verloren. Würdigung und Wertschätzung dieser notwendig gewordenen Verhaltensweisen sind aber ein entscheidender erster Schritt,

den Kindern und Jugendlichen zu ermöglichen, ihr belastendes Verhalten im Kontext seiner Notwendigkeit zu reflektieren und möglicherweise alternative Verhaltensweisen zu entwickeln. Ihr Verhalten als eine normale Reaktion auf eine außergewöhnliche Situation zu verstehen, entlastet die Kinder und Jugendlichen von Scham und Schuld. Wenn die Betreuer den eigenen „guten Grund" und den Sinn des eigenen Handelns kennen, so steigert dies ihre innere Sicherheit in ihren pädagogischen Handlungen. Und wenn die Kinder und Jugendlichen um die „guten Gründe" ihrer Erzieher wissen, steigert das ihr Vertrauen in diese Menschen und somit das Vertrauen in den „sicheren Ort" (Maisons d'Enfants de l'Etat 2016, S. 18–38).

Wertschätzung. „Es ist gut so, wie du bist!"
Das intensive und wiederholte Erleben von Hilflosigkeit, Ohnmacht und Willkür kann bei Kindern und Jugendliche dazu führen, dass sie kaum noch Sinn und Wert in sich und ihrem Handeln sehen. Sie übertragen Gefühle, Gedanken und Beziehungsinhalte der traumatisierenden Situationen immer wieder auf aktuelle. Sie müssen die Möglichkeit haben, sich und das, was sie tun, mehr und mehr wieder als wertvoll zu erleben. Dort anzusetzen, wo Stärken vorhanden sind, was gerne gemacht wird, ermöglicht es, sich selbst mit seinen Fähigkeiten zu erleben und sich selbst schätzen zu lernen. Die Traumapädagogik gestaltet einen sicheren Rahmen, in dem den Kindern und Jugendlichen der Aufbau eines positiven Selbstbildes ermöglicht wird, um ihr Selbstwertgefühl und ihr Selbstbewusstsein wachsen zu lassen. Neben dieser erforderlichen Korrektur nicht funktionaler Einstellungen und Überzeugungen besteht die Notwendigkeit, das Geschehen in die eigene Lebensgeschichte einzuordnen und traumatische Erinnerungsebenen selbst zu regulieren.

Partizipation. „Ich trau dir was zu und überfordere dich nicht."
Die Teilhabe an der Gestaltung der eigenen Lebensbedingungen zählt zu den wichtigen Einflussfaktoren, die zu seelischer Gesundheit führen. Kinder und Jugendliche bilden eine positive Motivation vor allem dann aus, wenn sie Erfahrungen auf folgenden drei Ebenen machen: 1) Erleben von Autonomie – ich kann etwas entscheiden, 2) Erleben von Kompetenz – ich kann etwas bewirken und 3) Erleben von Zugehörigkeit – ich gehöre dazu und werde wertgeschätzt.

In ihrem alten Lebensumfeld von Gewalt, Vernachlässigung und/oder Missbrauch haben traumatisierte Kinder und Jugendliche eine extreme, existentielle Form des Kontrollverlustes erfahren. Sie leben in der Erwartung, keinen Einfluss auf sich oder ihr Umfeld zu haben. Ihre Selbstwirksamkeitserwartung ist stark herabgesetzt, teilweise kaum vorhanden. Gerade für diese Mädchen und Jungen ist es unerlässlich. Strukturen und Ansätze zu schaffen, die, dem jeweiligen Entwicklungsstand entsprechend, die höchstmögliche Teilhabe gewährleisten.

Transparenz. „Jeder hat jederzeit ein Recht auf Klarheit."
Kinder und Jugendliche mit belastenden biographischen Erfahrungen haben in der Regel Macht und Hierarchie als etwas Missbräuchliches erlebt. Sie haben einen willkürlichen Umgang mit sichernden Strukturen erfahren. Es ist daher von großer Bedeutung, dass diese Kinder und Jugendlichen einen transparenten, verantwortungsvollen Umgang mit Hierarchien, Strukturen und Machtverhältnissen erleben. Der sichere Ort muss ein Ort der Berechenbarkeit sein und setzt somit ein Gegengewicht zur bisherigen Unberechenbarkeit des Lebensumfeldes. Kinder benötigen Erklärungsansätze, die ihr Verhalten positiv und begründend deuten. Kinder können hierdurch eine verstehende Haltung für die vielfach auch von ihnen selbst als negativ empfundene Verhaltensweise entwickeln.

Spaß und Freude. „Viel Freude trägt viel Belastung!"
Psychische Traumata gehen mit extremen Gefühlen der Angst, Ohnmacht, Scham, Trauer, Wut und Ekel einher. Die Belastungswaage der Emotionen zeigt ein erhebliches Ungleichgewicht. Es gilt daher, die Freudenseite zu beleben und ihr einen besonderen Schwerpunkt zu geben, um die Belastung und Widerstandsfähigkeit (Resilienz) ins Gleichgewicht zu bringen. Dieser die Gesundheit als Prozess verstehende Ansatz bringt Kopf und Körper in positives Erleben, das Konstruktivität, Lernen und Entwicklung nachhaltig unterstützt. Weiter unterstützen Spaß und Lachen die Serotoninausschüttung und setzen so ein Gegengewicht zur erhöhten Adrenalinausschüttung durch ein erhöhtes Stresslevel, das traumatisierte Kinder und Jugendliche erfahren. Kinder, die aus traumatisierenden familiären Bezügen kommen, sind in der Regel „Überlebenskünstler". Sie haben es geschafft, unter massiv vernachlässigenden Bedingungen eine oft beeindruckende Entwicklungsleistung zu vollbringen. Vor diesem Hintergrund erscheint es sinnvoll, die vorhandenen Ressourcen zu stärken und neue Ressourcen zu entdecken.

5   Konkrete Gestaltung auf den Weg gebracht

Im folgenden sollen einige zentrale Aktivitäten und Schritte des AITIA vorgestellt werden, mit denen die Einrichtung eine konzeptionelle und zielorientierte Neuausrichtung zum Wohle der Kinder umgesetzt hat.

5.1   Der Kinder- und Jugendrat als Instrument der Partizipation

Der Kinder- und Jugendrat (KJR) ist im Jahr 2015 aus dem Prozess der Implementierung der Traumapädagogik entstanden. Seit Jahren hat sich die Institution darum bemüht, die Partizipation der Kinder und Jugendlichen an den sie direkt betreffenden Entscheidungen, an der Gestaltung des Alltagslebens im Heim sowie an der Erarbeitung ihrer Hilfepläne zu beteiligen (Autorenband 2000; ADCA 2007). Verschiedene Initiativen, wie Kinderversammlungen in den Lebensgruppen, die Herausgabe eines Kinder-Info-Blattes sowie das Einbinden der Kinder und Jugendlichen in das Erarbeiten ihrer Hilfepläne, ermöglichten eine begrenzte Partizipation. Es gab jedoch keine allgemein anerkannte Kultur der Partizipation.

Nach einer Vorbereitungszeit wurde der KJR eingesetzt. Er wird von einem kleinen Team von Professionellen begleitet, welche nicht direkt im Alltag mit den Kindern und Jugendlichen in den Gruppen arbeiten. Ihre (neutrale) Aufgabe besteht darin, einen geregelten Ablauf der Sitzungen und eine respektvolle Kommunikation zu ermöglichen, Hilfe zu leisten bei der Vorbereitung der Sitzungen, bei der Aufstellung der Tagesordnung sowie bei der Berichterstattung. Diese Aufgabe war besonders in den ersten Jahren von großer Bedeutung.

Die Mitglieder des KJR vertreten die verschiedenen Wohngruppen und werden jeweils von diesen gewählt. Präsident und Sekretär werden im KJR in einer geheimen Wahl bestimmt. Die Vertreter der Heimgruppen vermitteln und garantieren den Dialog mit den Kindern und Jugendlichen in den Gruppen. Die Mitglieder des KJR werden für ihre Arbeit entlohnt.

Die Schaffung des KJR hat sich über ein gutes Jahr hingezogen. Es galt, Befürchtungen, Ängste, Zweifel (vor allem bei den Mitarbeiterinnen und Mitarbeitern) zu verstehen, eine eigene Arbeitsweise zu (er)finden und durch eine regelmäßige Evaluation die Arbeitsweise anzupassen. Heute hat sich der KJR einen festen Platz in der Institution erarbeitet.

Die Sitzungen werden mit großer Ernsthaftigkeit vorbereitet und durchgeführt. Das Arbeitsklima ist sehr positiv und respektvoll. Die Kinderversammlungen in den Wohngruppen sind auf Anfrage der Mitglieder des KJR neu geplant und strukturiert worden. Es gibt regelmäßig Treffen mit der Einrichtungsleitung. Mehrere Belange der Kinder und Jugendlichen sind von der Leitung angenommen und umgesetzt worden. So zum Beispiel der Zugang zu Internet über WiFi in allen Wohngruppen oder Zimmerschlüssel gratis für alle Kinder und Jugendlichen, was zu einer Besserung des Wohlfühlklimas der Kinder und Jugendlichen beigetragen hat. Andere Anfragen sind noch in Bearbeitung (was für die Kinder und Jugendlichen nicht immer nachvollziehbar ist), wie zum Beispiel eine größere Mitverantwortung und erweiterte Möglichkeiten beim Kleiderkauf. Es wurden viele Themen behandelt, wie u. a. das Thema der Traumapädagogik (was bedeutet Traumapädagogik für die Kinder und Jugendlichen, was bringt sie ihnen, wie können sie damit umgehen) oder die Beteiligung an der Planung und Gestaltung einer neuen Wohngruppe. Es wurden Umfragen in den Wohngruppen unternommen, um die Meinung der Kinder und Jugendlichen zu erfragen zu Themen wie der „sichere Ort", Umgarg mit Handy, Feste und Rituale, Begrüßungsmappe für neu ankommende Kinder und Jugendliche.

Die Schaffung des KJR hat in der Institution eine Dynamik ausgelöst und neue Akzente gesetzt, die heute zu festen Bestandteilen der Institution geworden sind.

So ist aus den Erfahrungen des KJR die Notwendigkeit erkannt worden, ein „Beschwerdemanagement"[5] zu schaffen, das heißt eine Anlaufstelle für Beschwerden und Anregungen sowie transparente Beschwerdebearbeitungswege, und das sowohl für die Kinder und Jugendlichen als auch für die Mitarbeiter. Es gilt, diesen Umgang mit Beschwerden in Einklang mit den Standards der Traumapädagogik zu bringen und die nötigen Voraussetzungen zu schaffen: wertschätzende und verstehende Haltung, positive Beschwerdekultur, Erlernen, dass Kinder, Jugendliche und Mitarbeiter sich beschweren dürfen, und dass dies ernstgenommen wird. Diese Vorgehensweise kann Erfahrungen von Selbstwirksamkeit herbeiführen.

Auf der Ebene der Mitarbeiter wurde eine Personalvertretung geschaffen, die als Hauptaufgaben hat: Beratung über Veränderungen, Vorschriften, Maßnahmen im Betrieb (Dienstzeiten, Arbeitsaufteilungen, Beförderungen, Arbeitsbedingungen), Förderung der Fortbildung der Mitarbeiter, Erarbeiten von Vorschlägen zur Verbesserung der Organisation und Unterstützung von Opfern jeglicher Diskriminetion am Arbeitsplatz. Die Personalvertretung wird eingebunden, wenn im Fall interpersoneller Probleme oder auch struktureller Probleme keine Lösung, über Dialog auf den verschiedensten Ebenen, möglich ist sowie im Fall von arbeitsrechtlichen Fragen.

Für die Kinder und Jugendlichen galt es, einen konkreten Beschwerdeweg mit der nötigen Dokumentation auszuarbeiten. Kinder und Jugendliche erhalten die Möglichkeit, über Brief, E-Mail, Beschwerdekasten, Telefon oder persönliche Gespräche Beschwerden einzureichen. Jede Beschwerde wird dokumentiert und

---

[5] Eigentlich sollte es hier „Umgang mit Beschwerden" heißen. um der sprachlichen Verschiebung durch die Ökonomisierung entgegenzutreten.

muss innerhalb einer Woche eine Antwort erhalten. Erster Ansprechpartner ist ein Erzieher, zweiter Ansprechpartner der Gruppensprecher im KJR usw. Es gibt zwei Vertrauenserzieher, die von den Kindern und Jugendlichen in diese Funktion gewählt werden. Eine Beschwerde kann innerhalb der Institution behandelt werden oder aber nach außen zum ORK (Ombuds-Komitee für die Rechte des Kindes) oder zum „Kanner- a Jugendtelefon" weitergereicht werden.

Eine große Herausforderung ist die Veränderung der Beschwerdekultur in der Institution (weg von Klagen hinter vorgehaltener Hand hin zu einer offenen Beschwerdekultur im Sinn einer Verbesserung der Lebens- und Arbeitsbedingungen). Es geht um Prävention gegen Missbrauch der Autorität in der Institution, also auch um Selbstschutz und Selbstfürsorge.

5.2 Traumafachberatung

Die Traumafachberatung ist in die institutionelle Struktur der AITIA fest eingeschrieben worden mit der Aufgabe, Fortbildung, evaluative Gespräche in den Gruppen, traumasensible Fallberatungen, Netzwerkarbeit, usw. zu garantieren.

Institutionelle Arbeit im Sinn der Traumapädagogik verlangt, dass alle Fachkräfte eine entsprechende Ausbildung erhalten und die Bereitschaft mitbringen zu einer wertschätzenden und verstehenden Haltung als Fundament ihrer Arbeit sowie zu einer interdisziplinären Zusammenarbeit und zur regelmäßigen Reflexion und Evaluierung. Des Weiteren ist eine strukturierte Implementierung der Traumapädagogik in die Arbeitsprozesse und in die institutionellen Strukturen sowie eine Anpassung der Rahmenbedingungen als permanenter Prozess notwendig.

Da Veränderungsprozesse in einer Institution viel Zeit brauchen, ist ein „Comité de pilotage" mit einem externen Fachberater geschaffen worden, das die Aufgabe erhalten hat, die Arbeit fachlich zu begleiten und zu beraten und damit die Implementierung auf eine breitere Basis zu stellen.

5.3 Geschwistergruppen

Das staatliche Institut AITIA bietet seit 2015 die Möglichkeit, Geschwister gemeinsam unterzubringen. Geschwisterbeziehungen sind von großer Bedeutung im Erleben, im Fühlen, in der Darstellung nach außen, und vor allem für das emotionale Gleichgewicht und die Identitätsentwicklung. Geschwisterbeziehungen stehen in der Regel für Kontinuität und Vertrautheit, sie bieten einander eine wichtige „Wir-Ebene", dies unabhängig von der Qualität der Beziehung.

„Zusammen sind wir stark", das gilt besonders, wenn die Elternfunktionen ausfallen, wenn Kinder von ihren Eltern getrennt leben müssen. Die Trennung von Geschwistern im Fall einer Fremdunterbringung bedeutet in den meisten Fällen einen zusätzlichen Schmerz durch das Entziehen der letzten noch Kontinuität sichernden Beziehung. Natürlich gilt es, im Vorfeld einer Platzierungsentscheidung von Geschwistern ein genaues Abwägen der Vor- und Nachteile einer gemeinsamen oder getrennten Einweisung in ein Kinderheim vorzunehmen. Auf keinen Fall aber sollten Geschwister aus rein administrativen oder finanziellen Gründen getrennt werden.

Grundsätzlich ist es wünschenswert, Geschwister gemeinsam unterzubringen. Stellt sich mit der Zeit heraus, dass das gemeinsame Leben in einer Heimgruppe erhebliche Nachteile mit sich bringt, kann es sinnvoll sein, an eine Trennung zu denken, wobei die Nachteile einer Trennung so weit wie möglich zu mildern sind. Es stellt sich manchmal mit der Zeit heraus, dass Geschwister, wenn sie älter werden, das Bedürfnis ausdrücken, mehr Distanz zueinander zu haben. Dann ergeben sich neue Formen von Geschwisterpädagogik, auf Basis eines gesamten Konzeptes und im Einklang mit den traumapädagogischen Standards.

Die Arbeit in Geschwistergruppen stellt eine besondere Herausforderung für die Fachkräfte dar, erweist sich aber für die betroffenen Kinder und Jugendlichen als besonders förderlich für die Identitätsfindung und das seelische Gleichgewicht.

5.4   Integration geflüchteter minderjähriger Jugendliche

Geflüchtete minderjährige Jugendliche werden in begrenzter Zahl in multikulturelle Gruppen des Instituts AITIA integriert. Alle geflüchteten Kinder und Jugendlichen haben in ihrer Heimat, auf der Flucht, im Exil traumatische Ereignisse erlebt und erfahren auch in Luxemburg angstbesetzte Situationen und Bedrohungen, etwa durch eine mögliche erzwungene Rückkehr.

Diese jungen Menschen brauchen dringend und zuallererst Sicherheit im Alltag (einen „sicheren Ort"), Sicherheit, was einen befristeten oder unbefristeten Aufenthalt anbelangt, Gewissheit, was ihre Familienangehörigen anbelangt. Sie brauchen Klarheit und Begleitung im Hinblick auf schulische und soziale Inklusion. Traumapädagogisch ausgerichtete Arbeit mit diesen Jugendlichen, wie sie im Institut AITIA angeboten wird, basiert auf einer Grundhaltung, die erkennt und zulässt, dass die Verhaltensweisen dieser Jugendlichen normale Reaktionen auf extreme Stressbelastungen sind, dass sie für ihre Reaktionen und Verhaltensweisen „einen guten Grund" haben, dass sie in ihrem Leben sehr viel überstanden und geleistet haben. Sie brauchen Unterstützung bei der Akzeptanz ihrer Verletzungen und Schwierigkeiten, sie brauchen Unterstützung und Hilfe, aber sie sind als Experten für ihr Bestehen in schwierigen Lebenslagen ernstzunehmen. Sie benötigen vonseiten der Fachkräfte Geduld, Gelassenheit, die Sicherheit von Zugehörigkeit, Rückzugsmöglichkeiten, möglichst stabile und verlässliche Beziehungen.

Die anderen Kinder und Jugendlichen benötigen im gleichen Maße Unterstützung der Fachkräfte, damit ein Zusammenleben mit geflüchteten Jugendlichen für alle lebenswert bleibt. Und die Fachkräfte sind hier in besonderem Maße auf Unterstützung der Traumafachberatung angewiesen.

5.5   Jugendliche, die großjährig werden

Das Institut AITIA hat Wohnstrukturen geschaffen, in denen junge Menschen auch über ihr 18. Lebensjahr hinaus bleiben können und Zeit zum Experimentieren haben. Dieses Angebot geht auf einen steigenden Bedarf an Begleitung und Unterstützung für Jugendliche im Übergang von der Heimversorgung zur Eigenverantwortung zurück, da diese Übergänge oft mit besonderen Unsicherheiten und Belastungen verbunden sind. Messmer (2013) hat in einer Studie die Vermutung formuliert, „dass in den Beziehungsstrukturen die Grundlagen für Selbstachtung und Selbstwirksamkeit angelegt sind, ohne die der Übergang in ein zufriedenstellendes und eigenständiges Erwachsenenleben kaum vorstellbar ist" (Messmer 2013, S. 437). „Bei den Faktoren, die Selbstachtung fördern, handelt es sich im Kern um die Aneignung derjenigen Kompetenzen, die notwendig sind, um authentisch mit sozial relevanten Umwelten in Beziehung zu treten und daraus Nutzen für sich selbst und seine Entwicklung zu ziehen" (Messmer 2013, S. 437). Kerviel (2015) bestätigt eine alltägliche Feststellung in der Praxis, dass junge Menschen, die ein Heim mit Erreichen des 18. Lebensjahres verlassen, sei es aus eigener Entscheidung oder gezwungenerweise, in der Regel nicht vorbereitet sind auf ein Leben in Eigenverantwortung. Sie benötigen Übergänge, Zeiten zum Experimentieren, zum Neubeginn im Fall eines Scheiterns, sie benötigen aber auch Unterstützung, materielle Ressourcen und Sozialkapital (Peters & Jaeger 2016). Nach Kerviel (2015) bedeutet Sozialkapital alle aktuellen und möglichen Ressourcen einer Person in Zusammenhang mit einem dauerhaften Netz von mehr oder weniger stabilen und wechselseitigen

Beziehungen und der Zugehörigkeit zu einer Gruppe von Menschen, die nicht nur gemeinsame Eigenschaften haben, sondern auch beständige und nützliche Bindungen untereinander leben.

Das Institut AITIA stellt zum Beispiel jungen Menschen, die im Ausland studieren möchten und keinen Rückhalt in ihrer Familie haben, ein Zimmer zur Verfügung, wo sie in den Ferienzeiten bleiben können. Der Erfolg des Experimentierens hängt einerseits von den Rahmenbedingungen ab, die das Institut den Jugendlichen anbietet, und andererseits von den pädagogischen Konzepten und den Haltungen, die die Institution vertritt und die die Mitarbeiter im Alltag vertreten. Die Rahmenbedingungen sind abhängig von den politischen Entscheidungen und dem Stellenwert, den die politisch Verantwortlichen diesen pädagogischen Konzepten zugestehen.

6   Ausblick: Rahmenbedingungen Sozialer Arbeit jenseits ökonomischer Effizienz

Das Institut AITIA hat sich die Möglichkeit gegeben, über das Département „Centre de Ressources" die Umsetzung der im Beitrag beschriebenen Handlungsweisen und Arbeitsprozesse zu begleiten, zu evaluieren und strukturell zu verankern. Dazu gehören gruppenübergreifende, spezifische Angebote an die Adresse der Kinder und Jugendlichen, aber auch Angebote an die Mitarbeiter (v. a. Fachberatung, pädagogische Begleitung, Fortbildung).

Die Institution stellt sich in den Dienst des Lebens der ihr anvertrauten Kinder und Jugendlichen. Dabei geht es notwendigerweise auch um die Gesundheit aller Mitarbeiter. Eine Institution ist nie gegen Auswüchse oder Missstände gewappnet, sie ist und bleibt in einem gewissen Sinn verwundbar. Das ist zugleich eine Chance: Eine Institution, die sich der eigenen Verwundbarkeit verschließt, entwickelt sich zu einem starren Gebilde, aus dem alles Leben entweicht, wo Kinder und Jugendliche nicht als Subjekte ihres eigenen Lebens gelten, sondern einzig und allein als Objekte der institutionellen Maßnahmen zählen, und das keine Öffnung nach außen zulässt. Nach Renders (2011, S. 67–68) ist eine Institution, die „gut funktioniert", eine Institution, in der gesprochen wird, in der entschieden wird und in der die Krankheiten ihrer Funktionsweise erkannt werden. In einer Institution arbeiten bedeutet mit Gegensätzlichkeiten und Widerspruch zu leben.

Dies zu ermöglichen, damit eine Institution ihrem Auftrag gerecht werden kann, liegt in der Verantwortung der Politik. Wenn man Institutionen als menschliche Gebilde/Strukturen definiert, erkennt man an, dass sie verschieden sein müssen. Die Verschiedenheit muss möglich sein, im Rahmen eines gemeinsam getragenen Referenzkaders, sie muss sich ausdrücken in verschiedenen Modellen, Konzepten und Finanzierungsmodellen.

Anders als im Fall der staatlichen Strukturen hat das durch das Gesetz vom 16. Dezember 2008[6] neu geschaffene Finanzierungsmodell für die privaten Träger zu einer Konzentration von Strukturen geführt, wobei die Lebendigkeit der Verschiedenheiten zu verschwinden droht. Die neuen großen Träger laufen viel eher die Gefahr, mit diesem Finanzierungsmodus einer marktwirtschaftlichen Logik zu verfallen, die im Sozialen eigentlich fehl am Platz ist, aber dem neoliberalen Zeitgeist entspricht. Darüber hinaus wirkt diese Entwicklung sich schleichend auf den gesamten sozialen Sektor aus.

Da, wo „die Übertragung von Marktprinzipien auf das Soziale (…) nach Ansicht der Marktgläubigen für noch mehr Effizienz bei gleichzeitig noch besserer Qualität sorgen" sollte, ist feststellbar geworden, dass der Charakter der „sozialen Dienstleistungen" sich verändert hat (Schneider 2014, S. 106). Wenn alles „in Geldwert umgerechnet" wird, wird letztendlich auch unsere Wertschätzung und werden unsere Bedürfnisse „nach Geldwert gefiltert und gelenkt" (ebd., S. 108). „Die Quantifizierung von Qualität ist Voraussetzung und Konsequenz der Ökonomisierung der sozialen Arbeit zugleich" (ebd., S. 110). Das wiederum führt dazu, dass „Leistungen völlig unabhängig von spezifischen Kontexten beschrieben werden", wobei das Spezifische, das Einzigartige, das Besondere, das Lebendige einer institutionellen Arbeit verlorengeht. Gesundheit und Wohlbefinden sind komplexe Realitäten, die nicht auf „quasi-objektive Messergebnisse und Kennzahlen" reduziert werden können (vgl. ebd., S. 114).

Soziale Arbeit ist und bleibt Beziehungsarbeit und folglich einzigartig, wobei die Fachlichkeit der Professionellen im Dienst der Menschen steht und nicht im Dienst von Effizienz oder Mehrwert.

Im Sozialsektor geht es um Humanisierung, um Menschlichkeit, wobei alle Mitarbeiter sich in ihrer Subjektivität den Herausforderungen stellen müssen und interdisziplinär zu arbeiten bereit sind.

Die Rahmenbedingungen müssen umfassende und gute Soziale Arbeit im oben beschriebenen Sinn ermöglichen, „die den Menschen als Ganzes in den Blick nimmt und eine vertrauensvolle Beziehung zu ihm aufbaut. Dazu brauchen die Fachkräfte Zeit, fachliche Freiräume und Vertrauen" (Schneider 2014, S. 134–135).

---

[6]Vgl. Memorial A-N°192 du 22 décembre 2008: Loi du 16 décembre 2008 relative à l'aide à l'enfance et à la famille.

Die heute schon weit verbreiteten sprachlichen Verschiebungen (der Mensch wird zum Klienten, die Soziale Arbeit zur Dienstleistung, die Institution zum Dienstleistungsanbieter und der Leiter zum Verwalter oder Manager) sind nicht so unbedeutend, wie sie oft dargestellt werden, sie zeigen den Einfluss der Ökonomisierung, sie haben die Ökonomisierung salonfähig gemacht. Gesundheit und Wohlbefinden sind mehr wert als Quantifizierung. Sie sind Herausforderung zu mehr Menschlichkeit.

Literatur

ADCA Luxembourg (2007). Vorstellung des ADCA-Dokumentes „Richtlinien zur Entwicklung von Qualitätsstandards in der Aufnahme und Betreuung von Kindern und Jugendlichen".

Autorenband (2000). Heimerziehung aus Kindersicht, Sozialpädagogisches Institut im SOD-Kinderdorf e.V., München.

BAG Traumapädagogik (2011). Standards für traumapädagogische Konzepte in der stationären Kinder- und Jugendhilfe: Ein Positionspapier der BAG Traumapädagogik. www.bag-traumapaedagogik.de//info@bag-traumapädagogik.de

Kerviel, A. (2015). Être adulte en sortant de structures d'Aide sociale à l'enfance, le capital social au cœur de la définition de l'autonomie. In. Vie sociale 2015 (12) 4. p. 107–127.

Lang, B., Schirmer, C., Lqang, T., Andrea de Hair, I., Wahlet, T., Bausum, J., Weiss, W. & Schmid, M. (Hrsg). (2013). Traumapädagogische Standards in der stationären Kinder- und Jugendhilfe. Eine Praxis- und Orientierungshilfe der BAG Traumapädagogik. Weinheim und Basel: Beltz Juventa.

Louazel, V., Wagener, Y. & Lair, M-L. (2010). Rapport de recommandations «Pour une stratégie nationale en faveur de la santé mentale des enfants et des jeunes au Luxembourg», Centre d'Etudes en Santé, CRP-Santé et Ministère de la Santé, Luxembourg.

Maisons d'Enfants de l'Etat (2016). Rahmenkonzept des « Département Hébergement ».

Messmer, H. (2013). Before Leaving Care. Eine Fallstudie zum fachlichen Handeln beim Übertritt aus der Heimerziehung in die selbstständige Lebensführung. Neue Praxis, 5/2013, S. 423–438.

Peters, U. & Jaeger, J. (2016). Beziehungen – Liens relationnels. Realitäten, Pertspektiven, Grenzen – réalités, perpectives et limites. Bericht zu einer Befragung von MitarbeiterInnen und Jugendlichen der Solidarité Jeunes asbl. Universität Luxemburg. Luxemburg.

Renders, X. (2011). Des fonctions et des rôles. In. Meynckens-Fourez M., Vander Borght, C. & Knoo, P. (Ed.): Eduquer et soigner en équipe. Manuel de pratiques institutionnelles. Bruxelles: De Boeck.

Schmit, R. (2010). La vie leur appartient, In. ARC N°118, Archiv fir sozial arbecht, bildung an erzéiung, ANCE, Luxembourg. S. 6–12.

Schmit, R. (2009): Quelles indications pour l'accueil en institution ? In. Willems. H. et al. (Hrsg.). Handbuch der sozialen und erzieherischen Arbeit in Luxemburg. Band 2., Luxembourg: éditions saint-paul. S.771–783.

Staatlech Kannerheemer (1994). 1884–1994 : 110 Joer Kanner op der Rhum. Luxembourg.

Staub-Bernasconi, S. (2007). Vom beruflichen Doppel- zum professionellen Tripelmandat. Wissenschaft und Menschenrechte als Begründungsbasis der Profession Soziale Arbeit. In. Zeitschrift für Sozialarbeit in Österreich, Wien. S. 8–17.

Schneider, U. (2014). Mehr Mensch! Gegen die Ökonomisierung des Sozialen. Frankfurt: Westend Verlag.

Wagener, Y., Henschen, M. & Petry, P. (2005). Das Wohlbefinden der Jugendlichen in Luxemburg. Ministère de la Santé & Ministère de l'Éducation nationale et de la Formation professionnelle. Luxembourg.

Wolf, K. (2008). Erziehung und Zwang. In. Widersprüche, Zeitschrift für sozialistische Politikk im Bildungs-, Gesundheits- und Sozialbereich, Heft 107. S. 93-108.

Zermatten, J. (2005). L'intérêt supérieur de l'enfant. Sion: IDE.

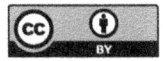

Konzepte, Strategien und Angebote des luxemburgischen Roten Kreuzes zur Förderung der Gesundheit und des Wohlbefindens von Jugendlichen

Marco Deepen

1 Einleitung

Im folgenden Artikel sollen unterschiedliche Angebote des luxemburgischen Roten Kreuzes dargestellt werden, die sich die Förderung von Gesundheit und Wohlbefinden von Jugendlichen als wesentliches Ziel setzen. Die Förderung von Gesundheit und Wohlbefinden spielt in der Sozialen Arbeit und Bildungsarbeit meist eine bedeutende Rolle. Mal stehen sie als direktes Ziel im Vordergrund, zum Beispiel in der Notfallhilfe. Mal sind Wohlbefinden und Gesundheit indirekte Ergebnisse mittel- oder langfristiger Projekte oder von präventiven Aktivitäten.

Vielen Jugendlichen in Luxemburg geht es gut. Sie profitieren von einem breiten sozio-kulturellen Angebot in einem der reichsten Länder der Erde. An diesem Angebot können sie erfolgreich teilhaben, weil sie auf etablierte personale, soziale und sozio-ökonomische Ressourcen zurückgreifen können. Sie durchlaufen die herausfordernde Jugendphase meist ohne intensive professionelle Unterstützung. Peers und Familie bieten ihnen ausreichend Orientierung und Hilfestellung.

Es gibt aber auch Jugendliche in Luxemburg, die nicht aus eigener Kraft die typischen Herausforderungen der Jugendphase bewältigen. Diese jugendtypischen Herausforderungen, Entwicklungsaufgaben und Transitionen sind zum

M. Deepen (✉)
Rotes Kreuz Luxemburg, Luxemburg, Luxemburg
E-Mail: marco.deepen@croix-rouge.lu

© Der/die Autor(en) 2022   529
A. Heinen et al. (Hrsg.), *Wohlbefinden und Gesundheit im Jugendalter,*
https://doi.org/10.1007/978-3-658-35744-3_24

Beispiel die Abnabelung von den Eltern, Selbstständigkeit beim Wohnen, eigenständige Sicherung des Lebensunterhalts, Aufbau von Partnerschaften sowie die schulische sowie berufliche Ausbildung und die gesellschaftliche Teilhabe. Je nach individueller Situation und Ressourcenausstattung gelingen diese typischen Entwicklungsaufgaben besser oder schlechter und einige Jugendliche benötigen dabei Unterstützung. In diesem Fall können spezifische professionalisierte Angebote greifen, die unterschiedliche Strategien und Intensitäten verfolgen.

Bei der Organisation seiner Angebote für Jugendliche verfolgt das Rote Kreuz im Wesentlichen vier Strategien: die Soziale Arbeit, die non-formale Bildung, die Jugend- und Familienhilfe sowie medizinische Beratung und Unterstützung. Diese vier Strategien münden jeweils in spezifische Aktivitätskonzepte. Das Rote Kreuz begleitet bedürftige Jugendliche ein Stück auf ihrem Weg zur Selbstständigkeit und trägt durch seine Aktivitäten zu deren Wohlbefinden und Gesundheit bei (CRL 2021a). Das bedeutet in diesem Zusammenhang, dass Jugendliche sich stark und gesund genug spüren, um ihr Leben selbstbestimmt, selbstverantwortlich, an der Gesellschaft teilhabend sowie ohne gesundheitliche, soziale und materielle Not gestalten zu können. Das Rote Kreuz geht davon aus, dass Jugendliche, die eine Ausbildung oder Arbeit beginnen können, erschwinglichen Wohnraum finden, eine gute Partnerschaft erleben, sozial integriert sind und an der Gesellschaft teilhaben, sich in der Regel besser und zufriedener fühlen.

2   Gesundheit und Wohlbefinden von Jugendlichen als Ziel der Arbeit des luxemburgischen Roten Kreuzes

Menschen helfen, auf Luxemburgisch: *Mënschen hëllefen,* das ist auf den Punkt gebracht die Mission des luxemburgischen Roten Kreuzes. Präziser: Der Auftrag des Roten Kreuzes ist es, bedürftigen Menschen in Notlagen zu helfen und Situationen materieller, gesundheitlicher und sozialer Not vorzubeugen. Um diesem Auftrag gerecht zu werden, existieren für vielfältige Problemlagen Konzepte, Programme und Aktivitäten für Menschen aller Alterskategorien, unabhängig von Herkunft, Geschlecht, sexueller Orientierung und Religion (CRL 2021b).

In Luxemburg befinden sich auch Jugendliche in materieller, gesundheitlicher oder sozialer Not. Ihre Notlagen können unterschiedlichste Ursachen und Ausprägungen haben, zum Beispiel ein zu geringes Einkommen, Obdachlosigkeit, Drogen- oder Alkoholsucht, keine oder nicht abgeschlossene Ausbildung, abgebrochene Schulbildung, alleinerziehende junge Mutter, fehlende

Sprachkenntnisse, schwieriger familiärer Hintergrund und traumatische Belastungen unterschiedlichsten Ursprungs.

Vor allem junge Menschen sind in Luxemburg auch einem Armutsrisiko ausgesetzt. Das Armutsrisiko (Definition: das Einkommen beträgt weniger als 60 % des Medianeinkommens) liegt bei der Gruppe der 18- bis 24-Jährigen in Luxemburg im Jahr 2019 bei 26,3 %. Das durchschnittliche Armutsrisiko in der Gesamtbevölkerung liegt dagegen bei 17,5 % (Statec 2020). Auch die Jugendarbeitslosigkeitsquote (Alter geringer als 25 Jahre) liegt in Luxemburg mit 16,6 % (im Dezember 2019) deutlich über der gesamten Arbeitslosenquote von 5,6 % (Eurostat 2020). Ein durch Spekulation getriebener Wohnungsmarkt macht es vielen Jugendlichen und jungen Erwachsenen zudem nahezu unmöglich, erschwinglichen Wohnraum zu finden.

Es ist die Mission des Roten Kreuzes, diejenigen Kinder und Jugendlichen auf ihrem Weg zu Selbstständigkeit und Teilhabe zu unterstützen, die die wesentlichen Transitionen und Entwicklungsaufgaben der Jugendphase nicht aus eigener Kraft bewältigen können. Dafür werden angepasste Aktivitäten für vielfältige Herausforderungen angeboten. Sei es im Kontext der non-formalen Bildung, der Kinder- und Familienhilfe, der Sozialen Arbeit oder im medizinischen Bereich. In der non-formalen Bildung begleiten die erzieherischen Fachkräfte die Kinder und Jugendlichen auf ihrem Weg zur Selbstständigkeit, in der Kinder- und Familienhilfe erhalten die Jugendlichen Beratung, Therapie oder Coaching, in der Sozialen Arbeit findet sozialpädagogische praktische Notfallhilfe statt, im medizinischen Bereich werden praktische medizinische Information, Beratung und Hilfe angeboten. Die Ansätze reichen von wenig intensiv bis sehr intensiv, von Bildungsarbeit über psychosoziale Beratung und Therapie, Betreutem Wohnen bis hin zu Notfallhilfe. Allen Ansätzen gemein ist die Notwendigkeit einer Beziehung, die die Fachkraft zum Jugendlichen aufbaut: Eine vertrauensvolle Beziehung zwischen Fachkraft und Klient ist ein wesentlicher Gelingensfaktor einer erfolgreichen Zusammenarbeit.

Als lernende Organisation entwickelt das Rote Kreuz seine Angebote permanent weiter und passt diese an aktuelle Entwicklungen der Gesellschaft an. Die Erfahrungen aus der internationalen Zusammenarbeit, kreative und angepasste Unterstützungsmaßnahmen in einem herausfordernden Umfeld zu entwickeln und zu implementieren, wirken sich positiv auf die Haltung und die Entwicklung von Maßnahmen in Luxemburg aus. Beispielhaft sei hier der Umgang mit der Flüchtlingskrise seit Ende 2015 genannt, in deren Kontext verschiedene Angebote bedarfsorientiert entwickelt und umgesetzt wurden.

Zunächst soll nun das Aktionsfeld Jugend kurz theoretisch beleuchtet werden: Wie verläuft die Jugendphase, was sind ihre wesentlichen Herausforderungen und wo setzt Unterstützung an?

Das Rote Kreuz betrachtet die Jugendphase einerseits als Wegstück hin zum Erwachsenensein (Jugend als Transition). Auf ihrem Weg bearbeiten die Jugendlichen Entwicklungsaufgaben (im Wesentlichen Qualifizierung, Bindung und Partizipation), um die Übergänge (Transitionen) in Arbeit, Partnerschaft, eigenständiges Wohnen und bürgerschaftliches Engagement zu bewältigen. Die Bewältigung der Entwicklungsaufgaben trägt dazu bei, Selbstständigkeit, Autonomie und Handlungsfähigkeit zu entwickeln. Je nach personaler, sozio-ökonomischer und sozialer Ausstattung gelingt die Jugendphase besser oder schlechter.

Nicht alle Transitionen sind gradlinig, einige dauern etwas länger, andere benötigen Unterstützung. Und da die Problemlagen der Jugendlichen vielfältig und unterschiedlich sind, hat das Rote Kreuz spezialisierte Dienste aufgebaut, die je nach Art und Intensität der Bewältigungslage eigene Zielsetzungen, Methoden und Programme verfolgen. Diese Dienste operieren im Kontext der non-formalen Bildung (zum Beispiel: *Maisons Relais,* Jugendhäuser, Jugendrotkreuz und andere), in der Kinder- und Familienhilfe (Kinder- und Jugendheime, Betreutes Wohnen, psychotherapeutische Beratung und Therapie und andere), im Bereich der Sozialen Arbeit (Streetwork, Nightshelter, Wanteraktioun, Migranten- und Flüchtlingsdienst und andere) und im medizinischen Bereich (HIV-Beratung).

Allerdings stellt die Jugend auch eine Lebensphase dar, in der eigen-ständige kulturelle und soziale Lebensformen existieren. Jugend ist nicht nur eine Durchgangszeit, in der Institutionen auf standardisierten Wegen auf den Beruf vorbereiten und angepasste Dienste Jugendliche mit Unterstützungsbedarf auffangen. Die Jugend braucht auch Freiraum, um in dieser Lebensphase zu experimentieren, zu testen und sich auszudrücken. In der Offenen Jugendarbeit wird Jugendlichen dieser Freiraum zur Verfügung gestellt und zugestanden.

Beide Perspektiven zusammen, a) Jugend als Phase der Bewältigung not-wendiger Entwicklungsaufgaben und Transitionen und b) Jugend als eigen-ständige Lebenskultur mit Freiraum für Experimente, ergeben die Sichtweise des Roten Kreuzes auf Jugend.

Ausgehend von den Entwicklungsaufgaben und den zu bewältigenden Transitionen der Jugendphase wird im Artikel der Frage nachgegangen, wie Gesundheit und Wohlbefinden die Bewältigung von Entwicklungsaufgaben, Transitionen und Hindernissen beeinflussen? Bremsen sie Entwicklungen aus oder beschleunigen und befähigen sie diese? In der Kindheit und Jugend werden nicht nur die Weichen zu Eigenständigkeit und zum Beruf gestellt, sondern auch zu Wohlbefinden und Gesundheit im ganzen Leben. Kindheit und Jugend prägen für das ganze Leben.

Die internationale HBSC-Studie, an der auch Luxemburg teilnimmt, erfasst seit mehr als 20 Jahren im 4-Jahres-Rhythmus gesundheitsrelevante Aspekte von Jugendlichen. Die aktuelle HBSC-Studie für Luxemburg (Heinz et al. 2018) zeigt einige interessante Ergebnisse auf:

- Die höchsten Werte für Gesundheit und Wohlbefinden weisen demnach Kinder zwischen 11 und 12 Jahren auf; in der folgenden Lebensphase (ab 13 Jahre) sind die Werte niedriger. Die Autoren folgern, dass diese Lebensphase besonders kritisch und prägend sei. Daraus lässt sich ableiten, dass gerade in diesem Altersabschnitt präventive und erzieherische Maßnahmen in Bezug auf Gesundheit sinnvoll sind, sicherlich auch bereits davor. Die Weichen scheinen sich in diesem Alter zu stellen.
- Die soziale Herkunft ist relevant: Je höher der Wohlstand, desto höher die Ergebnisse für Gesundheit und Wohlbefinden.
- Besonders hervorgehoben wird Mobbing in der Schule, das einen Risikofaktor für Schulleistungen darstellt sowie auch für Angststörungen im Erwachsenenalter.

Wohlbefinden und Gesundheit sind direkte Einflussfaktoren, die eine gelungene oder unterstützungsbedürftige Transitionen bedingen. Sie beeinflussen die Bewältigung von Entwicklungsaufgaben.

Sie sind aber auch als Ergebnis einer gelungenen Jugendphase zu betrachten, in der externe Einflüsse und Herkunftsindikatoren sich auf die Einstellung zu Gesundheit und Wohlbefinden im Erwachsenenleben auswirken. Verlaufen Kindheit und Jugend positiv, so werden Jugendliche wahrscheinlich auch gesunde und zufriedene Erwachsene. Sie können mit großer Wahrscheinlichkeit davon ausgehen, dass dieses Wohlbefinden und ihre gute Gesundheit sich positiv auf ihr weiteres Leben auswirken.

In Abb. 1 wird der Zusammenhang zwischen Transitionen, Entwicklungsaufgaben sowie Wohlbefinden und Gesundheit dargestellt und das Handlungsfeld des Roten Kreuzes in Bezug auf Unterstützungsmaßnahmen abgesteckt. Je nach Ausstattung mit personalen, sozialen und sozioökonomischen Ressourcen (siehe auch Schaubild 2) gelingt ihnen die Bewältigung von Entwicklungsaufgaben und den Herausforderungen im Zusammenhang mit der Transition besser oder schlechter.

Einige Indikatoren einer guten Bewältigung der Jugendphase sind (MENJE & UL 2015):

- Schulbildung abgeschlossen
- Ausbildung begonnen oder abgeschlossen
- Studium begonnen oder abgeschlossen
- eigene Wohnung oder ein Zimmer in einer Wohngemeinschaft
- Partnerschaft
- auskömmliches Einkommen und bewusster Umgang mit Geld
- bürgerschaftliches Engagement (Politik, Sport, Kultur, Soziales, Ehrenamt usw.)

Das Rote Kreuz geht davon aus, dass Jugendliche, die

- eine Ausbildung oder Arbeit beginnen können,
- erschwinglichen Wohnraum finden,
- eine gute Partnerschaft erleben,
- sozial integriert sind und
- an der Gesellschaft teilhaben,

sich in der Regel wohler und zufriedener fühlen.

Deutlich wird in Abb. 1, dass Wohlbefinden und Gesundheit einerseits Gelingensfaktoren für erfolgreiche Transitionen und erfolgreich bewältigte

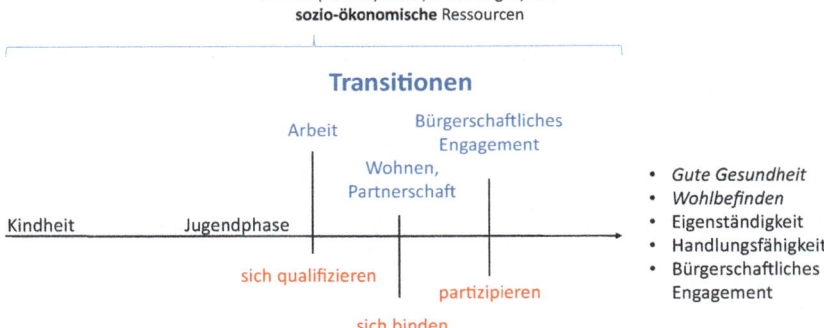

Abb. 1 Aktionsfeld Jugend. (Eigene Abbildung)

Entwicklungsaufgaben darstellen. Gleichzeitig sind sie auch Resultat einer erfolgreich bewältigten Jugendphase. Daraus folgt, dass die Herstellung von Wohlbefinden und Gesundheit im Rahmen sozio-pädagogischer Maßnahmen eine notwenige gesellschaftliche Aufgabe und ein sinnvolles Ziel ist.

3 Strategien, Konzepte und Aktivitäten des Roten Kreuzes

Im Folgenden sollen die vier Strategien des luxemburgischen Roten Kreuzes, die untergeordneten Konzepte der einzelnen Dienste sowie deren Angebote dargestellt werden. Dabei werden diejenigen Dienste aus den Bereichen der nonformalen Bildung, der Kinder- und Familienhilfe, der Sozialen Arbeit und der medizinischen Unterstützung dargestellt, die besonders die Förderung der Gesundheit und des Wohlbefindens von Jugendlichen fokussieren (siehe Abb. 2: Strategien des Roten Kreuzes).

Einige der dargestellten Dienste nehmen direkt Einfluss auf Gesundheit und Wohlbefinden, beispielsweise durch Erziehung zu gesunder Ernährung, Hygieneerziehung (Händewaschen, Zähneputzen), Workshops zu Verhaltensrisiken (Tabak, Alkohol, Drogen, Sexualität und Mobbing) oder die HIV-Beratung. Andere Dienste erreichen durch ihre Arbeit indirekte Resultate, indem sie bei akuten Unterstützungsbedürfnissen entsprechende Hilfeangebote sowie präventive Maßnahmen anbieten. Dadurch verbessern sich das Wohlbefinden und der Gesundheitszustand der Jugendlichen auch mittel- bis langfristig.

Abb. 2 zeigt die vier Strategien des Roten Kreuzes, die Einfluss auf die Gesundheit und das Wohlbefinden von Jugendlichen haben.

Für diejenigen Jugendlichen, die Unterstützung benötigen, bietet das luxemburgische Rote Kreuz vielfältige Dienste mit unterschiedlichen Strategien an: die non-formale Bildung, die Kinder- und Familienhilfe, die Soziale Arbeit und die medizinische Beratung und Unterstützung. Je nach Intensität und Ursprung der Situation wird ein spezifischer Dienst tätig Ansatzpunkte konkreter Unterstützung sind die jeweiligen Transitionen, Entwicklungsaufgaben und Gelingensfaktoren.

Die vier Strategien und die ihnen zugeordneten Rotkreuz-Dienste werden in Abb. 3 mit ihrem Rotkreuz-Namen dargestellt, eine exakte Beschreibung des Konzeptes und der Aktivität folgt dann weiter hinten in diesem Kapitel. Die ausgewählten Dienste, sortiert nach den vier Strategien, sind:

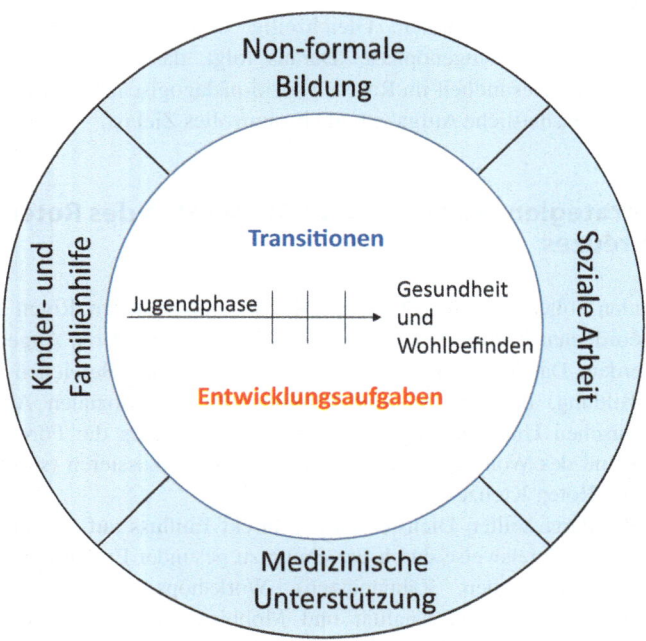

Abb. 2 Strategien des Roten Kreuzes in Bezug auf Gesundheit und Wohlbefinden von Jugendlichen. (Eigene Abbildung)

a) Non-formale Bildung	b) Kinder- und Familienhilfe	c) Soziale Arbeit	d) Medizinische Unterstützung
Maisons Relais	Perspectives	Migrants et Réfugiés	HIV Berodung
Jugendhäuser	Psy-Jeunes	LISKO	
Hariko	Centre d'accueil Norbert Ensch	DropIn	
Jugendwohnen		Abricoeur	
Jugendrotkreuz			

Abb. 3 Vier Strategien der Jugendarbeit mit einigen ausgewählten Diensten. (Eigene Abbildung)

Im Folgenden werden die vier Strategien mit den jeweiligen Diensten dargestellt. Pro Dienst werden Konzept, Zielgruppe und Aktivität beschrieben.

3.1   Non-formale Bildung

Die non-formale Bildung bietet Kindern und Jugendlichen auf freiwilliger Basis geplante pädagogische Programme an, die außerhalb des schulischen Kontextes stattfinden. Das Ziel der non-formalen Bildung ist die persönliche Entfaltung der Kinder und Jugendlichen, ihre soziale Bildung und Integration und ihre aktive Teilhabe an der Gesellschaft. Non-formale Bildung ergänzt sich mit der formalen Bildung (Schule) und der informellen Bildung. Der Staat legt per Rahmenplan für die non-formale Bildung die Aspekte Gesundheit und Wohlbefinden programmatisch fest (MENJE & SNJ 2018).

Seit einigen Jahren sammeln sich in Luxemburg Angebote zur außerschulischen Kinderbetreuung und Jugendarbeit unter dem Begriff der non-formalen Bildung. Lernorte sind: Kinderkrippen, *Maisons Relais,* Tageseltern, Jugendhäuser und andere Jugendaktivitäten. Vor allem die 2005 geschaffenen *Maisons Relais* verhalfen der non-formalen Bildung zunächst in quantitativer, später auch in qualitativer Hinsicht zum Erfolg: Heute verfügt jede Gemeinde in Luxemburg über eine *Maison Relais,* die von den meisten Grundschulkindern auch mehr oder weniger intensiv frequentiert wird. Betreuungsstrukturen haben sich heute in Bildungsstrukturen gewandelt. Im Gegensatz zur formalen Bildung (Schule) sind die Angebote der non-formalen Bildung jedoch nicht obligatorisch. Sie sind offen für alle Kinder und Jugendlichen und zielen nicht auf die Bearbeitung bestimmter Problemlagen ab. Dennoch profitieren von Ausgrenzung bedrohte Kinder und Jugendliche in besonderem Maß von diesen Angeboten. Inklusion, Mehrsprachigkeit, Partizipation und Freiwilligkeit sind einige Merkmale der non-formalen Bildung. Die höchst heterogene luxemburgische Gesellschaft verfügt dadurch über einen breiten Ansatz, zentralen Herausforderungen bereits ab dem Kleinkindalter zu begegnen. Allen Kindern soll die Chance auf Teilhabe an der Gesellschaft ermöglicht werden.

Die Qualität dieser Angebote wird staatlich kontrolliert. Das sogenannte ASFT-Gesetz (Chambre des Députés 1998) regelt Strukturbedingungen und das Jugendgesetz (Chambre des Députés 2016) regelt Elemente der Prozessqualität. Der Rahmenplan zur non-formalen Bildung beschreibt die grundsätzlichen pädagogischen Zielsetzungen. Regionale Agenten begehen die Einrichtungen und prüfen, ob staatliche Vorgaben (Fortbildung, Dokumentation, Konzept) umgesetzt werden. Gegebenenfalls finden Anpassungen statt.

Akteure im Kontext der non-formalen Bildung sind freie Wohlfahrtsträger wie das Rote Kreuz, aber auch Gemeinden und kommerzielle Anbieter, letztere eher im Kleinkindbereich. Das Rote Kreuz betreibt im Kontext der non-formalen Bildung 17 *Maisons Relais,* 6 Kinderkrippen, eine integrierte Ganztags-Maison-Relais für AsylbewerberInnen, 11 Jugendhäuser und zwei Hariko-Struktur. Das Jugendrotkreuz begleitet mehr als 250 ehrenamtlich tätige Jugendliche bei der Umsetzung sozialer Projekte und der Organisation von Ferienfreizeiten und bildet diese aus (Animateur-Ausbildung, Niveau b–f).

Die folgenden Dienste des Roten Kreuzes aus dem Bereich der non-formalen Bildung nehmen Einfluss auf Gesundheit und Wohlbefinden von Jugendlichen:

In den *Maisons Relais* des luxemburgischen Roten Kreuzes werden 2020 rund 3.800 Kinder betreut, davon viele 11- und 12-jährige, die sich im Übergang zum Jugendalter befinden. Eine *Maison Relais* ist ein Bildungsort für Kinder, der es den Eltern ermöglicht, Beruf und Familie zu vereinbaren. Ziel ist es, alle Kinder in ihrer Vielfalt und Einzigartigkeit zu begleiten, zu unterstützen und zu stärken, sodass diese nach ihren Bedürfnissen und Interessen in vielfältigen, altersangepassten und arrangierten Lernsituationen bestmöglich ihr Entwicklungspotenzial entfalten können. Pädagogische Ziele sind Eigenständigkeit, Autonomie, soziale Kompetenz und Partizipation. Es geht darum, die Kinder für die Bewältigung der Jugendphase und das Erwachsenenleben zu stärken. Die Kinder werden vom Team der *Maison Relais* auf ihrem Weg zu selbstverantwortlichen, selbstbestimmten und eigenständigen Menschen begleitet. Themen wie gesunde Ernährung, Gesundheit und Bewegung, die zum Wohlbefinden der Kinder und Jugendlichen beitragen, sind per Gesetz über die Qualitätssicherung verankert. Einige direkte Gesundheitsaktivitäten der *Maison Relais:*

- In allen *Maisons Relais* findet Erziehung zur gesunden Ernährung statt. Das tägliche Mittagessen entspricht den Kriterien einer gesunden Ernährung für Schulkinder des Gesundheitsministeriums, ErnährungsberaterInnen erarbeiten die Menüs. Die im Kinderrestaurant anwesenden ErzieherInnen begleiten die Kinder. Sie essen zusammen mit den Kindern und sorgen dabei für eine angenehme und ruhige Esssituation, in der Tischgespräche stattfinden können.
- Alle *Maisons Relais* des Roten Kreuzes verfügen über Bewegungsräume. Bewegung ist drinnen wie draußen jederzeit möglich.
- Bei Bedarf – wenn das Thema aufkommt – wird über Alkohol-, Tabak- und Cannabiskonsum gesprochen.
- In einigen *Maisons Relais* werden Kindermediatoren ausgebildet, um Konflikte zu bearbeiten und Mobbing vorzubeugen.
- In den Kinderkrippen werden die Zähne nach dem Essen geputzt.

In den *Jugendhäusern* des Roten Kreuzes wird Jugendlichen zwischen 12 und 26 Jahren ein geschützter Raum (Offener Treff) zur sinnvollen Freizeitgestaltung geboten. Es gibt regelmäßige Öffnungszeiten von 14 bis 19 Uhr, freitags und samstags auch länger. Ziel der Offenen Jugendarbeit ist die Unterstützung und Begleitung der Jugendlichen auf ihrem Weg zu verantwortungsbewussten, selbstständigen und aktiv mitwirkenden und teilhabenden Bürgern der Gesellschaft. Basis und Gelingensfaktor dieser Arbeit ist ein Vertrauensverhältnis zwischen JugendarbeiterInnen und Jugendlichen, welches sich durch eine stabile und kontinuierliche Interaktion auf Augenhöhe auszeichnet. Es gibt klare Regeln für ein Jugendhaus: Respekt, Toleranz und Gewaltfreiheit sind wesentliche Werte. Alkohol und Drogen werden nicht akzeptiert. Es findet keine Trennung nach Kriterien wie Geschlecht, Herkunft, Religion, sozialer Stellung, politischer Überzeugung, schulische oder sportliche Leistungen statt. Der Offene Treff ist die Basis eines freiwilligen und ungezwungenen Angebotes und die alltägliche Grundlage der Interaktion unter den Besuchern selbst sowie zwischen den Besuchern und dem pädagogischen Personal. Unterstützung findet in Form von Information, Beratung und Orientierung statt, vor allem in Hinsicht auf die wesentlichen Transitionen hin zu Arbeit, Wohnen, Partnerschaft und bürgerschaftlicher Teilhabe. Gegenseitiges Verständnis und Respekt im Umgang miteinander werden gefördert. Den Besuchern wird die Möglichkeit geboten, sich als individuelle Wesen oder als Teil einer sozialen Gemeinschaft zu erkennen und zu entwickeln. Jugendhäuser bieten eine niederschwellige Anlaufstelle für Hilfe und Beratung innerhalb der Gemeinde.

Einige direkte Gesundheitsaktivitäten der Jugendhäuser:
Jedes Jugendhaus des Roten Kreuzes verfügt über eine voll ausgestattete Küche und einen sehr großen Esstisch. Gemeinsames gesundes Kochen und gemeinsames Essen stellen wesentliche Aktivitäten dar. Die Jugendlichen genießen soziales Zusammensein. Die Fachkräfte beteiligen sich und greifen ein, wenn die Grundregeln des Jugendhauses verletzt werden.

In der Corona-Krise und vor allem während der Zeit der zweieinhalbmonatigen Schließung (Lockdown) von Mai bis Juli 2020 zeigte sich die enge Beziehung einiger Jugendlicher zu den MitarbeiterInnen der Jugendhäuser. Diese forderten die Weiterführung sozialer Kontakte untereinander und zu den Angestellten über digitale Angebote. Die Weiterführung der Jugendhausaktivitäten über digitale Angebote konnte die persönlichen Kontakte nicht ersetzen.

Eine Sonderform der Jugendhäuser des Roten Kreuzes stellt der Dienst *Hariko* dar. Von 2016 bis 2018 in Luxemburg-Stadt, dann seit 2018 in Esch/Alzette und ab Frühjahr 2021 in Ettelbrück, agiert Hariko ebenfalls im Kontext der Offenen Jugendarbeit, jedoch ausschließlich mit dem Medium Kunst als zentralem

Ausdrucksmittel der Jugendlichen. Kunst und Musik werden als mögliche Aus-
drucksformen jugendlicher Gefühle genutzt. Gesang und Musikinstrumente,
Graffiti, Schmuckherstellung sowie klassisches Malen und Zeichnen stehen hier
im Mittelpunkt. Künstlern wird in der Einrichtung ein Atelier zur Verfügung
gestellt, dafür engagieren diese sich, einmal pro Woche über einen längeren Zeitraum einen Workshop für die Jugendlichen anzubieten. Im Offenen Treff können
die Jugendlichen auch außerhalb der Workshops künstlerisch tätig sein, die
Öffnungszeiten ähneln denen der Jugendhäuser. Hariko ist bei den Jugendlichen
sehr beliebt, sie fühlen sich wohl und frei, ihren künstlerischen und musischen
Interessen und Bedürfnissen nachzugehen. Auch hier ist der Aufbau einer
Beziehung zwischen Besucher und pädagogischem Personal Grundlage einer
gelingenden Unterstützung.

Jugendwunnen Arboria bietet Jugendlichen, die bereits weitgehend autonom
ihr Leben bewältigen, erschwinglichen Wohnraum. Von allen Faktoren, die die
Transition Jugendlicher zum Erwachsenen erschweren, ist die Wohnungssuche
sicherlich der herausforderndste. Die Preise für Wohnraum steigen seit Jahren
kontinuierlich. Erschwinglicher Wohnraum wird in Luxemburg rarer und rarer.
Ob junge alleinstehende Mütter, Studenten, Arbeitslose, nicht in Ausbildung
befindliche junge Erwachsene oder Obdachlose – der Zugang zu angepasstem
und erschwinglichem Wohnraum ist heute eine schwierige Herausforderung in
Luxemburg. Junge Erwachsene mit niedrigem Einkommen und ohne Zugang zu
einem garantierten Mindesteinkommen (Revis) befinden sich oft in einer prekären
Situation, obwohl sie in der Schule, in einer Lehre oder in einem Arbeitsvertrag
sind. Diese Beobachtung, die seit mehreren Jahren zu verzeichnen ist, hat das
Luxemburger Rote Kreuz dazu veranlasst, eine koordinierte Wohnungsstrategie
zu entwickeln. So erweitert der Dienst *Perspectives,* seit mehreren Jahren
Hauptakteur im Bereich des Betreuten Wohnens für Jugendliche innerhalb des
Roten Kreuzes, das Spektrum seiner Zielgruppe, indem er sich an alle jungen
Menschen wendet, die nach erschwinglichem Wohnraum suchen: Das Konzept
Jugendwunnen ergänzt das Betreute Wohnen.

Im Gegensatz zum Ansatz der Jugendhilfe sind die BewohnerInnen hier ausreichend autonom, um ihre Transitionsaufgaben („Lebensprojekt") eigenständig
und ohne sozialpädagogische Unterstützung zu bewältigen. Daher ist der Ansatz
des Jugendwohnens auch näher an der Strategie der non-formalen Bildung als an
der Kinder- und Familienhilfe.

Jugendwunnen Arboria bietet in Differdange für bis zu 46 junge Erwachsene
zwischen 18 und 27 Jahren erschwinglichen Wohnraum. Das Gebäude ist ähnlich aufgebaut wie ein Studentenwohnheim mit kleinen Apartments. Einige davon
sind für Personen mit eingeschränkter Mobilität vorgesehen, andere für junge

Familien. Gemeinschaftsräume sollen sozialen Austausch fördern. Den Jugendlichen soll so die Teilnahme an schulischer Bildung, beruflicher Ausbildung, Eingliederung in die Arbeitswelt und soziale Integration erleichtert werden. Um die Unabhängigkeit und Selbstbestimmtheit der Jugendlichen zu fördern, findet mit den sozialen Akteuren vor Ort – vor allem mit den Jugenddiensten der Gemeinde – eine enge Zusammenarbeit statt. Eine intensivere Betreuung mittels ambulanter Jugendhilfemaßnahmen (Betreutes Wohnen) kann bei Bedarf gewährleistet werden.

Unter geschützten Rahmenbedingungen bietet das *Jugendrotkreuz* jedem Jugendlichen bzw. jungen Erwachsenen die Möglichkeit, seine Idee des sozialen Engagements zu realisieren und von dem bestehenden Angebot an Möglichkeiten des ehrenamtlichen Aktivwerdens zu profitieren. Der Dienst unterstützt Jugendliche, ihre eigene Identität zu entwickeln, indem sie Menschen in sozialer, materieller und gesundheitlicher Bedürftigkeit helfen. Die Aktionen, die von den Jugendlichen umgesetzt werden, richten sich an unterschiedliche Zielgruppen benachteiligter Personen. Im Rahmen der non-formalen Bildung und partizipativen Jugendarbeit wird den Jugendlichen ein Freiraum geboten. Hier können sie sich durch Übernahme von Verantwortung, Transparenz der Entscheidungen, regelmäßigen Austausch, eine intensive Form der Beteiligung und durch die Umsetzung ihrer eigenen Initiativen zu verantwortungsvollen Mitbürgern der Gesellschaft und zu aktiven Mitwirkenden des Jugendrotkreuzes entwickeln. Das Engagement ermöglicht dem Jugendlichen eine aktive Auseinandersetzung mit sich selbst und mit seinen Interessen. Das Zusammenbringen von Personen aus unterschiedlichen Verhältnissen, Empathie, Teilen und das Zusammenlernen steht für die Jugendlichen wie für die Teilnehmer im Mittelpunkt der Motivationen. Die Jugendlichen entwickeln ihr eigenes Normen- und Wertesystem.

Angebote des Jugendrotkreuzes:

- Ferienfreizeiten: Die Jugendlichen können als Begleiter oder als Hauptverantwortliche in den Ferienkolonien tätig sein.
- Fortbildung zum Animateur: Die Jugendlichen haben die Möglichkeit, eine Animateur- Fortbildung abzuschließen (Aide-Animateur, Animateur, Responsable, Formateur oder Animateur spécialisé).
- Projekte: Die Jugendlichen können Projekte selbst initiieren oder sich in die bestehenden Projekte des Jugendrotkreuzes einbringen.
- Aktionen: Die Jugendlichen können an jährlichen Aktionen für einen guten Zweck teilnehmen.

Es wird stets auf ein diversifiziertes Angebot geachtet, das den Interessen der Jugendlichen und den Bedürfnissen der Gesellschaft gerecht wird. Alle Jugendlichen können an den Aktivitäten des Jugendrotkreuzes teilnehmen. Grundeinstellung des Jugendrotkreuzes ist, jeden Jugendlichen, unabhängig von seinem Umfeld oder seiner derzeitigen sozialen, gesundheitlichen oder finanziellen Situation, als Ehrenamtlichen oder als Teilnehmer der Aktionen willkommen zu heißen. Es findet keine Trennung nach Kriterien wie schulische oder sportliche Leistungen, Herkunft, Sprache oder Religion statt. Die Jugendlichen können sich jede vertretbare Möglichkeit offenhalten, sich dort einzubringen, wo sie ihre Interessen hinführen. Auch neue Ideen für Projekte und Aktionen sind willkommen und werden gefördert.

Das Jugendrotkreuz fokussiert klar auf die Entwicklung bürgerschaftlicher Teilhabe. Die Jugendlichen engagieren sich aus freiem Willen für soziale oder ökologische Aktivitäten. In der Gruppe erfahren sie Anerkennung und entwickeln sich. Sie engagieren sich für eine gute Sache und stärken damit ihr Wohlbefinden und ihr Selbstwertempfinden. Motive für den ehrenamtlichen Einsatz sind sowohl eigennützige Gründe (individueller Nutzen, eigene Entwicklung) als auch das Engagement für einen guten Zweck.

3.2   Kinder- und Familienhilfe

Die Kinder- und Familienhilfe (Aide à l'Enfance et à la Famille, AEF) bietet im Interesse des Kindeswohls Unterstützungs- und Hilfemaßnahmen für Kinder, junge Erwachsene und Familien in Not. Zeigen Kinder und Jugendliche Schwierigkeiten in ihrer körperlichen, geistigen, psychischen oder sozialen Entwicklung oder sind sie Gefahren ausgesetzt, dann können sie Hilfeleistungen der Kinder- und Jugendhilfe in Anspruch nehmen. Das nationale Jugendamt (Office nationale de l'Enfance, ONE) ist zuständig für diese Hilfsmaßnahmen, die entweder auf freiwilliger Basis angefragt oder von den Justizbehörden verordnet werden. Die Kinder und Jugendlichen sowie ihre Familien können sich selbst an das nationale Jugendamt wenden oder aber über eine Vertrauensperson oder eine Fachkraft eines sozialen Dienstes um Hilfe oder Informationen anfragen. Nach Klärung der Hilfeanfrage wird diese vom ONE mit einem Maßnahmenpaket ausgestattet und an die zuständigen Hilfsdienstleister vermittelt. Öffentliche und private Träger können auf Grundlage dieser Leistungsbestimmung Maßnahmen umsetzen. Das nationale Jugendamt ONE untersteht dem Bildungsministerium (Ministère de l'Éducation nationale, de l'Enfance et de la Jeunesse, MENJE).

Jugendhilfemaßnahmen können innerhalb der Familien stattfinden oder bei Bedarf und in schwierigen Situationen auch außerhalb. Innerhalb der Familie findet Unterstützung statt durch Fallberater, Sozial- und Familienpfleger, durch psychischen, sozialen oder pädagogischen Beistand, durch psychotherapeutische Beratung, durch heilpädagogische Früherziehung, Psychomotorik, Ergotherapie oder Sprachtherapie. In schwierigen Situationen, bei akuten Krisen kann ein Jugendlicher befristet auch außerhalb der eigenen Familie unterstützt werden – in einer Pflegefamilie, bei Tageseltern, in einer Einrichtung des Betreuten Wohnens oder bei Adoptiveltern.

Damit unterscheidet sich dieser Ansatz klar vom Ansatz der non-formalen Bildung. Während ersterer die Gesamtheit aller Kinder und Jugendlichen fokussiert, wird hier klar ein verletzliches, von sozialer Ausgrenzung bedrohtes oder in Notlage geratenes Klientel anvisiert. Die Problemlagen sind klar in einem Leistungskatalog beschrieben. Der Fokus auf Transitionen und Entwicklungsaufgaben ist weniger ausgeprägt als in der non-formalen Bildung, die akuten oder latenten Beeinträchtigungen und Gefahren in ihrer Vielfalt sind Arbeitsschwerpunkte.

Die Kinder- und Familienhilfe fokussiert damit eindeutiger und direkter den physischen und psychischen Gesundheitszustand ihrer Klienten: Erfolgreiche Arbeit mündet in einen besseren Gesundheitszustand respektive führt bei Wiederaufnahme in die Herkunftsfamilie zu verbessertem Wohlbefinden. Man könnte sagen, dass die non-formale Bildung vornehmlich das Fundament einer gelingenden Jugendphase bildet, bei Bedarf auch spezifische Unterstützung in Form von Information und Beratung anbietet und somit indirekt einwirkt (langfristige Stärkung). Die Kinder- und Familienhilfe hingegen bietet spezialisierte Angebote für Jugendliche in bereits schwierigen Situationen an.

Dienste des Roten Kreuzes aus dem Bereich der Kinder- und Familienhilfe, die Einfluss auf Gesundheit und Wohlbefinden von Jugendlichen nehmen:

Der Auftrag des *Service Perspectives* ist es, junge Erwachsene zwischen 18 und 27 Jahren in psychosozialer Not für eine bestimmte Zeit und in einem definierten Raum zu begleiten, um ihre eigenen Ressourcen und Fähigkeiten zu entwickeln, so dass sie zum autonomen Akteur ihres eigenen Lebensprojekts werden. Im Kontext des Betreuten Wohnens unterstützen die MitarbeiterInnen die Klienten, einen Plan für ihre Zukunft zu entwickeln und umzusetzen. Je nach Autonomiegrad ist die Unterstützung bedarfsgerecht angepasst. Die Kosten für die Leistungen werden über das Office National de l'Enfance (ONE) abgerechnet.

Psy-Jeunes bietet Kindern, Jugendlichen und jungen Erwachsenen von 0 bis 27 Jahren, eine ambulante psychologische und psychotherapeutische Unterstützung und Beratung, damit diese nachhaltig ein Leben in psychischer

Gesundheit und Wohlbefinden führen können. Zielgruppe sind Kinder, Jugendliche und junge Erwachsene, die einen Punkt in ihrem Leben erreicht haben, der
ihnen und/oder ihren Mitmenschen (Eltern, Geschwister, Erzieher und Lehrer)
als Sackgasse erscheint. Dieser Leidensdruck kann sich auf unterschiedlichste
Weise zeigen: emotionale Auffälligkeiten, Ängste, Verlust von Selbstwertgefühl
und Selbstvertrauen, Zurückgezogenheit, Aufmerksamkeits- und Konzentrations-
probleme, starke Unruhezustände, Tics, Zwänge, Essstörungen, Schlafstörungen,
Alpträume, Dissoziationsphänomene und andere Belastungsreaktionen. Der
Dienst arbeitet im Kontext von Beratung und Therapie mit vielfältigen, den
individuellen Bedürfnissen angepassten Methoden.

Die Psychotherapeuten stellen für jeden Klienten einen Antrag beim ONE
(Jugendamt). Bei Bewilligung dieses Antrages wird die Therapie durch das ONE
finanziert. Eltern können zur Beteiligung an den Kosten herangezogen werden.
Die Bewilligung der Therapie wird alle 6 Monate mit entsprechenden Berichten
erneut angefragt.

Psy-Jeunes arbeitet eng mit den anderen Diensten der Kinder- und Familienhilfe des Roten Kreuzes zusammen. Die intraorganisationale Vernetzung führt
deutlich zu positiven Effekten für die Klienten.

Das *Centre d'Accueil Norbert Ensch* ist eine dezentrale Heimstruktur für
Kinder und Jugendliche zwischen 4 und 27 Jahren aus schwierigen Familienver-
hältnissen. Es gibt sieben unterschiedliche Gruppen mit unterschiedlichen Zielgruppen. So gibt es zum Beispiel eine Gruppe für minderjährige Mütter und
schwangere Minderjährige, eine Kindergruppe, eine Jugendgruppe und gemischte
Gruppen.

Allen Bewohnern wird ein stabiles Lebensumfeld mit Regeln zum respektvollen Umgang untereinander, aber auch ausreichend Freiraum zur Selbst-
entfaltung angeboten. Ziel ist die Reintegration in die Herkunftsfamilien und
die Unterstützung der Autonomieentwicklung bis hin zur Begleitung in Schul-
fragen und der Suche nach einem geeigneten Ausbildungsplatz. Eine Einweisung
erfolgt in der Regel über das Jugendgericht *(Tribunal de la Jeunesse),* welches in
der Regel durch SozialarbeiterInnen oder Dritte über eine schwierige Familiensituation informiert wurde. Gründe für eine Herausnahme aus der Familie sind
zum Beispiel Gewalt, Vernachlässigung oder Misshandlung. Auch freiwillige Ein-
weisungen auf Anfrage sind möglich. Die Eltern werden so gut wie möglich ins
tägliche Leben ihrer Kinder im Heim eingebunden, etwa bei Arztbesuchen oder
Versammlungen in der Schule.

3.3   Soziale Arbeit

Im Perimeter der Sozialen Arbeit finden Notfallhilfe und Prävention statt. Zielgruppe sind Menschen, die von sozialer Ausgrenzung betroffen sind, darunter auch sehr viele Jugendliche, teils stellen sie sogar den größten Teil der Klienten dar, beispielsweise im Flüchtlings- und Migrantendienst. In der Regel werden Angebote, Aktivitäten und Maßnahmen über Fehlbedarfskonventionen mit dem Familienministerium finanziert, viele Angebote werden auch aus Spendenmitteln bestritten. In Abgrenzung zur Kinder- und Familienhilfe streben die sozialen Dienste des Roten Kreuzes an, soziale Probleme praktisch zu lösen, zu lindern oder zu verhindern. Es wird in der Regel ein sehr niederschwelliger Ansatz verfolgt, oft ohne direkt Bildungs- und Erziehungsziele oder Therapie- und Beratungsziele zu verfolgen. Hilfe in einer akuten Notlage steht im Vordergrund. Das Ziel ist stets die soziale Inklusion benachteiligter Menschen. Neben den Werten des Roten Kreuzes sind Menschenrechte, soziale Gerechtigkeit und Vielfalt grundlegende Werte dieser Arbeit. Auch hier wird über die direkte und pragmatische Hilfe eine Beziehung zu den Klienten aufgebaut. Diese Beziehung zwischen MitarbeiterIn und KlientIn ist Grundlage für weiterführende Information und Beratung.

Einige Dienste des Roten Kreuzes aus dem Bereich der Sozialen Arbeit, die Einfluss auf Gesundheit und Wohlbefinden von Jugendlichen nehmen:

Der *Service Migrants et Réfugiés* (Migranten- und Flüchtlingsdienst) informiert und unterstützt Migranten, insbesondere Antragsteller auf internationalen Schutz, während ihres Aufenthalts in Luxemburg. In 12 Unterkünften ist Platz für maximal rund 1500 Bewohner (zurzeit wohnen rund 1200 Menschen in den Unterkünften) unterschiedlicher Herkunft, Ethnie, Religion und unterschiedlichen Alters. Frauen und Männer, Familien, Mütter mit Kindern und unbegleitete Minderjährige werden in unterschiedlichen Settings unterstützt und begleitet. Circa 65 % aller Klienten des Dienstes sind unter 30 Jahre alt und 35 % aller Bewohner haben die Volljährigkeit noch nicht erlangt. Die MitarbeiterInnen stellen den Bewohnern Informationen über das Asylverfahren zur Verfügung, garantieren die Versorgung mit allem Lebensnotwendigen, betreuen und beraten die Bewohner in allen Angelegenheiten, insbesondere zum Gesundheitswesen, Schulsystem, Wohnungsmarkt und zu Ausbildungsmöglichkeiten für Jugendliche und Erwachsene in Luxemburg. Außerdem werden Freizeitangebote organisiert.

LISKO (Lëtzebuerger Integratiouns- a Sozialkohäsiounszenter) stellt einen Anschlussdienst des Migranten- und Flüchtlingsdiensts dar. Zielgruppe sind anerkannte Schutzbedürftige. Auch hier sind die meisten Klienten unter 30 Jahre alt. Mit der Anerkennung des Flüchtlingsstatus beginnt in der Regel die eigentliche Integrationsarbeit. Die anerkannten Flüchtlinge müssen in einem ihnen völlig fremden Land mit anderer Kultur und Sprache, anderen Institutionen, Regeln und Verhaltensweisen leben. Arbeitssuche und Spracherwerb sind Gelingensfaktoren für eine erfolgreiche Integration.

Lisko wurde im April 2016 auf Veranlassung des Familienministeriums gegründet, nachdem die Zahl der Flüchtlingsankünfte Ende 2015 zugenommen hatte. Eines der Ziele des Dienstes ist es, die Sozialämter bei ihrer Arbeit zu unterstützen und zu entlasten. Ziel der Arbeit ist soziale Integration und Hilfe bei der Wohnungssuche. Die Fachkräfte des Lisko sind hauptsächlich SozialarbeiterInnen, die sich mit Gesetzen und Verordnungen auskennen. Es findet aber auch psychologische Beratung statt.

Auch die Dienste *DropIn* (Unterstützung von SexarbeiterInnen) und Abricouer (Streetwork, Notunterkünfte) bieten vielen Jugendlichen Unterstützung an. DropIn bietet SexarbeiterInnen psychosoziale Unterstützung und gesundheitliche Betreuung in einer neutralen und sicheren Umgebung, auf diskrete und nicht verurteilende Weise, um ihre Lebensbedingungen und ihr Wohlbefinden zu verbessern, soziale Ausgrenzung und Stigmatisierung zu verhindern und Autonomie und Gesundheit zu fördern. Dabei kommen soziale, erzieherische und gesundheitliche Maßnahmen zur Anwendung. DropIn verfügt über ein eigenes Beratungszimmer, in dem regelmäßig ein Arzt zur Verfügung steht. Außerdem werden Kondome und Hygieneartikel gratis verteilt.

Abricoeur bietet durch Streetwork Menschen, die obdachlos sind oder in prekären Wohn- und Lebenssituationen leben, eine niedrigschwellige Hilfe an, um ihre materielle, soziale und gesundheitliche Lebenssituation mit dem Ziel einer nachhaltigen und menschenwürdigen Lebensqualität schrittweise zu verbessern.

Beide Dienste streben nicht in erster Linie einen Ausstieg aus dem jeweiligen Lebenszustand an, sondern bieten niederschwellige Hilfe, um in Würde und Gesundheit sein Leben zu verbringen.

3.4 Medizinische Unterstützung

Das luxemburgische Rote Kreuz ist mit vielen Diensten im medizinischen und im Pflegebereich tätig. Jugendliche sind nicht speziell als Zielgruppe formuliert, jedoch sind besonders bei der *HIV Berodung* auch sehr viele Jugendliche unter den KlientInnen.

Die Aufgabe der *HIV Berodung* besteht darin, Neuinfektionen von Hepatitis, sexuell übertragbaren Infektionen und HIV zu verhindern und ein den Bedürfnissen der Betroffenen entsprechendes Lebensumfeld zu fördern. Der Dienst wurde 1988 zur Unterstützung von an AIDS erkrankten Menschen gegründet und ist derzeit ein nationaler Akteur im Bereich des öffentlichen Gesundheitswesens für die Prävention vor HIV, Hepatitis C und anderen sexuell übertragbaren Infektionen und die psychosoziale Betreuung Erkrankter.

Die *HIV Berodung* bietet eine Telefon-Helpline sowie persönliche Gespräche für Personen, die Fragen zu Safer Sex, Safer Use oder einer konkreten Risikosituation in Bezug auf eine mögliche Infektion haben.

Auf Anfrage werden maßgeschneiderte Präventionssitzungen in Gymnasien, Jugendzentren oder für andere Zielgruppen organisiert, ebenso wie Trainingskurse für das Personal von sozialen, medizinischen und pädagogischen Organisationen. 2019 haben 135 Jugendliche an vier dieser Präventionsworkshops teilgenommen. Das Parcours Roundabout AIDS (ein mobiles, dynamisches und interaktives Präventionsprogramm) wird in Sekundarschulen angeboten. Informations- und Sensibilisierungskampagnen und Veranstaltungen sollen die gesamte Bevölkerung daran erinnern, dass diese Themen nach wie vor aktuell sind. Im Jahr 2019 wurden über 3000 Jugendliche so an Schulen sensibilisiert. Die Sensibilisierung von Jugendlichen ist besonders wichtig. Viele von ihnen glauben, alles zu wissen oder dass sie nicht betroffen sind.

In den Räumlichkeiten des Dienstes werden schnelle, kostenlose und anonyme HIV-, Hepatitis-C- und Syphilis-Screening-Sitzungen organisiert. 2019 wurden über 800 Schnelltests durchgeführt. Die Kenntnis des eigenen serologischen Status ermöglicht es einer Person, ihr zukünftiges Verhalten in Bezug auf die einzugehenden Risiken zu beurteilen. Die Bekanntgabe des HIV-Status ist oft ein Schock, und viele Menschen erleben Momente der Entmutigung. Fragen stellen sich auf der Ebene der Umgebung (wem soll man es sagen?), des Familienlebens (Schuldgefühle, Sexualleben, Kinderwunsch, was soll man den Kindern sagen?), wenn man eine neue Beziehung eingehen will oder auf der Ebene der Arbeit.

Die SozialarbeiterInnen des Dienstes begleiten Menschen mit HIV und/oder Hepatitis C, die sich in Behandlung befinden, und bieten Unterstützung in verschiedenen Schritten an, die in erster Linie auf den Zugang zur Versorgung abzielen. Andererseits geht es darum, eine stabile soziale Situation zu erhalten oder wiederherzustellen, um dem Klienten zu ermöglichen, sich unter den besten Bedingungen um seine Gesundheit zu kümmern: Einkommensanträge, Wohnungssuche oder Schuldenmanagement. Der Dienst stellt auch Informationen über Menschenrechte zur Verfügung und verweist den Kunden bei Bedarf an andere spezialisierte Dienste.

Die *HIV Berodung* verfügt außerdem über spezialisierte Unterkünfte für KlientInnen in psychischer, sozialer und gesundheitlicher Notlage im Zusammenhang mit ihrer HIV-Infektion. Es handelt sich um Übergangsheime, in denen Menschen, die nicht in der Lage sind, ihre Infektion selbstständig zu bewältigen, einen Weg zur Autonomie finden können.

Zwischen den Diensten und den jeweiligen Direktionen findet ein strukturierter und kontinuierlicher Austausch statt. Nutznießer und KlientInnen profitieren dadurch von der Möglichkeit, bei Bedarf schnell Unterstützung anderer Art erhalten zu können.

4 Herausforderungen und Entwicklungen

Das stetige Wachstum des sozialen Sektors in Luxemburg führt zu einem Mangel an Fachpersonal. Vor allem ErzieherInnen, aber auch SozialpädagogInnen sind auf dem Arbeitsmarkt begehrt. Aktuell bilden die Schule für ErzieherInnen (LTPES) und die Universität Luxemburg nicht ausreichend Fachkräfte aus. Diese Entwicklung vollzieht sich ähnlich wie die des Pflegesektors, der durch die Einführung der Pflegeversicherung am 1. Januar 1999 einen rasanten Ausbau erlebte.

Der Bedarf an erschwinglichem Wohnraum für Jugendliche in Luxemburg ist sehr groß, das Angebot hingegen sehr gering. Leider liegen für den Jugendbereich keine verlässlichen Zahlen vor. In der Praxis und von der Trägerseite her wird ein großer Bedarf festgestellt. Die Preise für kleine Wohnungen und Studios in Luxemburg sind höher, als viele Jugendliche in Bildung, Ausbildung oder zu Beginn ihres Berufslebens es sich leisten können. Es gibt viele Single-Haushalte und der Bedarf an Studio-Wohnungen ist entsprechend hoch. Darüber hinaus sind die administrativen und reglementarischen Hürden zur Gründung von Wohngemeinschaften hoch.

Der rasante Ausbau der *Maisons Relais* zwischen 2005 und 2015 ist von einer gesetzlich verankerten Qualitätsentwicklung und -sicherung abgelöst worden. Der Aspekt der Bildung rückt hier immer mehr in den Vordergrund. Eine Emanzipation aus der „Betreuungsecke" hin ins Bildungssegment findet statt.

Die non-formale Bildung mit dem Ansatz der Unterstützung von Transitionen und Entwicklungsaufgaben gewinnt an gesellschaftlicher und politischer Bedeutung. Komplementär zur Wissensaneignung der formalen Bildung verschreibt sie sich der Kompetenzentwicklung in den Bereichen der persönlichen und sozialen Integration, der Partizipation, der Autonomie und Selbstständigkeit.

Die Methoden und die Programme mögen dabei unterschiedlich sein, die zentralen Ziele der formalen und non-formalen Bildung sind letztlich sehr eng beieinander: Die Kinder stark machen, sodass sie die Herausforderungen der Zukunft eigenständig bewältigen können.

Das nationale Angebot an Jugendhäusern ist nahezu komplett. Dennoch sind in den letzten Jahren immer wieder Gemeinden zu der Erkenntnis gelangt, dass ein Jugendhaus die lokale Sozialraumentwicklung positiv beeinflussen kann. Das Rote Kreuz hat seit 2017 zwei neue Jugendhäuser eröffnet und betreibt im Frühjahr 2021 insgesamt 11 Jugendhäuser.

Die Dienste der Kinder- und Familienhilfe haben sich in den letzten Jahren seit der Umstellung vor der Fehlbedarfsfinanzierung hin zur Leistungsfinanzierung über das ONE im Jahr 2008 erweitert und vergrößert. Es gibt im Prinzip keine Deckelung der Anzahl der Klienten. Wenn das ONE einen Handlungsbedarf bei einem Jugendlichen identifiziert und einen Auftrag erteilt, kann der Träger aktiv werden. Der rasante Ausbau der vergangenen Jahre hat sich im Budgetjahr 2020 stark verlangsamt, denn es wurden wenig zusätzliche Maßnahmen bewilligt.

Die Angebote des Jugendwohnens hingegen boomen im Gegensatz zum Betreuten Wohnen. Diese bei weitem weniger intensive (und damit kostengünstigere) Maßnahme kann tatsächlich eine gute Ergänzung sein. Jedoch ist genau zu beobachten, dass dort, wo Beratung und Begleitung notwendig sind, diese auch zur Anwendung kommen.

Die Dienste der Sozialen Arbeit haben sich seit Beginn der Flüchtlingskrise vervielfacht. Der Flüchtlings- und Migrantendienst ist von weniger als 10 MitarbeiterInnen auf über 70 MitarbeiterInnen angewachsen. Nach einer sehr fordernden Phase 2015 und 2016 ist der Dienst nun von organisatorischer Seite her in ruhigen Fahrgewässern. Jedoch kommen immer noch Monat für Monat viele Antragsteller auf internationalen Schutz nach Luxemburg. Die Situation in den Aufnahmezentren ist oft schwierig. Das Personal kommt häufig an seine Grenzen. Aktuell sind die Plätze/Betten oft belegt, rund 50 % der BewohnerInnen sind anerkannte Flüchtlinge, die keine Wohnung auf dem freien Markt finden.

Die dargestellten Dienste sind alle mehr oder weniger stark im Wachstum begriffen. Der Staat verfügte in den vergangenen Jahren über die notwendigen Ressourcen, sich den verändernden sozialen Bedarfen durch die Finanzierung angepasster Aktivitäten und Programme sowie deren Ausweitung zu stellen. Wie sich diese Entwicklung in der Nach-Corona-Zeit darstellen wird, bleibt abzuwarten. Anzunehmen ist eine gebremste Weiterführung der aktuellen Bildungs- und Sozialpolitik.

5   Fazit

In diesem Artikel wurden die vier zentralen Strategien und zahlreiche zugeordnete Dienste des luxemburgischen Roten Kreuzes dargestellt, bei denen Gesundheit und Wohlbefinden von Jugendlichen zu den zentralen Zielen zählen. Es wurde gezeigt, dass es viele unterschiedliche Situationen und Begründungen gibt, warum Jugendliche die typischen Transitionen und Entwicklungsaufgaben des Jugendalters nicht aus eigener Kraft durchlaufen können und wie spezialisierte Dienste mit unterschiedlichen Arbeitsansätzen sie bei diesen Herausforderungen unterstützen können. Das Rote Kreuz begleitet bedürftige Jugendliche ein Stück auf ihrem Weg zur Selbstständigkeit und trägt durch seine Aktivitäten zu deren Wohlbefinden und Gesundheit bei.

Deutlich wird die Vielfalt der Leistungen auf Trägerseite: Es gibt viele spezialisierte Dienste für unterschiedliche Angebote. Die Dienste werden je nach zuständigem Ministerium unterschiedlich finanziert und reguliert. Ein vernetzter Ansatz, bei dem der Jugendliche im Mittelpunkt steht, ist nicht einfach umzusetzen. Das Rote Kreuz kann aufgrund seiner Größe viele unterschiedliche Angebote aus einer Hand anbieten und in gewissem Maße von einer intraorganisationalen Zusammenarbeit profitieren.

Es ist eine gewisse Versäulung auf Basis von Problemlagen und Strukturen bei Trägern, den zuständigen Ministerien sowie Administrationen und in den Dachverbänden zu beobachten: Eine Abteilung organisiert die Jugendhilfe, eine andere die non-formale Bildung bis zum Grundschulalter, eine weitere die Jugendarbeit usw. Eine Abteilung unterliegt den Regeln des Erziehungsministeriums, eine andere denen des Familienministeriums und eine dritte denen des Gesundheitsministeriums. Sicherlich gibt es gute Gründe dafür, warum themenspezifischer Austausch und themenspezifische Organisation sinnvoll sind. Ergänzend dazu aber ist es wichtig, einen professionellen, problemlagenübergreifenden und organisationsübergreifenden Austausch zu unterstützen und zu entwickeln, bei dem der Jugendliche im Mittelpunkt steht.

Literatur

Croix-Rouge Luxembourgeoise (CRL) (2021a). Jungen Menschen und Familien. https://www.croix-rouge.lu/de/wir-helfen/jungen-menschen-und-familien/. Zugegriffen: 13.06.2021.
Croix-Rouge Luxembourgeoise (CRL) (2021b). Die 7 Prinzipien des Roten Kreuzes. https://www.croix-rouge.lu/de/uber-das-luxemburger-rote-kreuz/unsere-mission/. Zugegriffen: 13. Juni 2021.

Eurostat (2020). Pressemitteilung Euroindikatioren 21/2020. https://ec.europa.eu/eurostat/documents/2995521/10159300/3-30012020-AP-DE.pdf/. Zugegriffen: 16. Januar 2021.

Heinz, A., van Duin, C., Catunda, C., Kern, M.R., Residori, C. & Willems, H. (2018). Gesundheit und Wohlbefinden von Kindern und Jugendlichen in Luxemburg – Bericht zur HBSC-Befragung luxemburgischer Schülerinnen und Schüler in Jahr 2014. INSIDE Research Reports. Esch/Alzette. https://orbilu.uni. u/bitstream/10993/38226/1/Report%20HBSC%202014_Final_Web.pdf. Zugegriffen: 17. Januar 2021.

Chambre de Députés (1998). Loi du 8 septembre 1998 réglant les relations entre l'Etat et les organismes œuvrant dans les domaines social, familial et thérapeutique. Memorial A82. http://legi ux.public.lu/eli/etat/leg/loi/1998/09/08/n4/jo. Zugegriffen: 13 Juni 2021.

Chambre de Députés (2016). Loi du 24 avril 2016 portant modification de la loi modifiée du 4 juillet 2008 sur la jeunesse. Memorial A81. http://legilux.public.lu/eli/etat/leg/loi/2016/04/24/n3/jo. Zugegriffen: 13. Juni 2021.

Ministère de l'Éducation nationale, de l'Enfance et de la Jeunesse & Université du Luxembourg (MENJE & UL) (Hrsg.) (2015). Nationaler Bericht zur Situation der Jugend in Luxemburg 2015. Übergänge vom Jugend- ins Erwachsenenalter. Luxembourg.

Ministère de l'Éducation nationale, de l'Enfance et de la Jeunesse & Service National de la Jeunesse (MENJE & SNJ) (Hrsg.) (2018). *Nationaler Rahmenplan zur non-formalen Bildung im Kindes- und Jugendalter.* Luxembourg : Ministère de l'Éducation nationale, de l'Enfance et de la Jeunesse & Service National de la Jeunesse Luxembourg.

STATEC (2020). Indicateurs de risque de pauvreté (en %) 2003 – 2019. https://statistiques.public.lu/stat/TableViewer/tableViewHTML.aspx?ReportId=12957&IF_Language=fra&MainTheme=3&FldrName=1&RFPath=29. Zugegriffen: 17. Januar 2021.

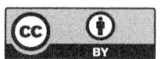

Trauererleben, Trauerbewältigung und die professionelle Unterstützung bei Kindern und Jugendlichen

Theoretische Konzepte und praktische Erfahrungen am Beispiel des „Kanner- a Jugendservice" von Omega 90

Jeanne Chomé, Martine Hentges, Andreas Hück, Solveig Nicolas, Gudrun Paulsen und Henri Grün

1 Trauer – zwischen Verlustbewältigung und Gesundheitsbeeinträchtigung

Trauer ist eine universell beobachtbare menschliche Reaktion auf den Verlust von wichtigen und geliebten Personen oder anderen Verlusterfahrungen. Sie zeichnet sich durch unterschiedlich lange Perioden von Trauererleben und

J. Chomé (✉) · M. Hentges · A. Hück · S. Nicolas · G. Paulsen · H. Grün
Omega 90, Luxemburg, Luxemburg
E-Mail: info@omega90.lu

M. Hentges
E-Mail: MartineHentges@omega90.lu

A. Hück
E-Mail: AndreasHueck@omega90.lu

S. Nicolas
E-Mail: SolveigNicolas@omega90.lu

G. Paulsen
E-Mail: GudrunPaulsen@omega90.lu

H. Grün
E-Mail: henri.gruen@pt.lu

© Der/die Autor(en) 2022
A. Heinen et al. (Hrsg.), *Wohlbefinden und Gesundheit im Jugendalter,*
https://doi.org/10.1007/978-3-658-35744-3_25

553

Trauerbewältigung aus, die mit Leiden einhergehen. Dieser Prozess wird von den meisten Menschen gut verarbeitet und integriert.

Die Trauer ist die unmittelbare Antwort auf diesen Verlust und geht einher mit Gefühlen wie intensive Traurigkeit, Schmerz und Wut. Der Trauerprozess hilft den Verlust zu begreifen, Abschied zu nehmen und sich dem Leben wieder zuwenden zu können. Somit ist der Trauerprozess ein gesunder Bewältigungsmechanismus in Bezug auf die veränderte Lebenssituation. Auch dieser Prozess wird von den meisten Menschen gut verarbeitet und integriert.

Eine Verlusterfahrung kann aber auch krisenhafte Ohnmachterfahrungen auslösen, die mit körperlichen und seelischen Gesundheitsbeeinträchtigungen verbunden sind. Dies gilt insbesondere dann, wenn Trauernde – wie etwa Kinder und Jugendliche – noch keine stabilen Bewältigungsmuster entwickelt haben und in ihrem Umgang mit Verlust und Trauer noch keine Erfahrungen haben. Hier ist die Gefahr dauerhafter psychischer und psychosomatischer Beeinträchtigungen aufgrund einer unzureichenden Bewältigung groß, mit langfristigen Folgen für Gesundheit und Wohlbefinden der Jugendlichen.

1.1   Einführung in theoretische Trauermodelle

Im Laufe der letzten Jahrzehnte wurde an Hand verschiedener Phasenmodelle versucht, den dynamischen und teilweise verwirrenden Ablauf der Trauer zeitlich zu strukturieren und Ähnlichkeiten im menschlichen Trauerprozess hervorzuheben. Dazu gehören:

- Das Phasenmodell nach Kübler-Ross (1969): Menschen durchleben 5 Phasen der Trauer: Verleugnung, Wut, Verhandlung, Depression und Akzeptanz; diese werden nacheinander und klar voneinander abgrenzbar durchlebt.
- Phasen nach Bowlby (1984): Der Autor geht davon aus, dass die von ihm beschriebenen Phasen (Phase der Betäubung, der Sehnsucht und Suche nach der verlorenen Bindung, der Desorganisation und Verzweiflung, der Reorganisation, der Verleugnung, der Wut und des Zorns, des Verhandelns, der Depression) mehrmals durchlebt werden können und von der Stärke der Bindung zum Verstorbenen abhängen. Demnach stellt Trauer den Versuch dar, die Bindung aufrechtzuerhalten.
- Traueraufgaben nach Worden (2002): Im Gegensatz zu einem „passiven" Erleben der Trauer schlägt er vier Aufgaben vor, die der Trauernde aktiv zu lösen hat: den Verlust als Realität/Wirklichkeit akzeptieren; den Trauerschmerz erfahren; sich anpassen an eine veränderte Umwelt, in der der

Verstorbene fehlt; dem Toten einen neuen Platz zuweisen und im Leben weitergehen.

- Trauerphasen nach Kast (2013): Nicht-Wahrhaben-Wollen; aufbrechende Emotionen; suchen, finden und sich trennen; neuer Selbst- und Weltbezug.
- Traueraufgaben nach Spierings (2006): In diesem Modell werden die Konzepte von Phasen der Trauer sowie Aufgaben der Trauer integriert: den Tod als Realität begreifen; den Trennungs- und Trauerschmerz durchleben; Erinnern und Wiedererleben der Beziehung zum Verstorbenen; Lösen der alten Bindung; sich anpassen an eine Welt ohne den Verstorbenen; neue Sinnfindung und Investition in das Leben.

1.2   Kritik an den Trauermodellen

Phasenmodelle versuchen zwar Ähnlichkeiten zwischen Trauernden hervorzuheben, vernachlässigen jedoch individuelle, soziale und kulturelle Unterschiede. Hinzu kommt oft eine mangelhafte empirische Überprüfung.

Trauernde unterscheiden sich in ihrem Erleben stark voneinander, was die Beurteilung „angemessene", „normaler" oder „abweichender" respektive „komplizierter" Trauerreaktionen erschwert. Phasenmodelle können missverstanden werden etwa als Zwang zum „richtigen" Trauern oder Verunsicherung und Stigmatisierungsängste bei Abweichungen vom vorgegebenen Schema auslösen.

In der praktischen Arbeit mit Trauernden zeigen sich die Trauerreaktionen auch häufig nicht linear, sondern verlaufen eher in Form einer Welle oder Spirale – eine Achterbahnfahrt der Gefühle, wie von Trauernden häufig berichtet wird.

Einem solchen flexiblen, dynamischen Prozess entspricht besser das duale Prozessmodell der Trauer nach Stroebe und Schut (1999). Dabei werden zwei Hauptarten der Bewältigung (Coping) des Verlustes unterschieden: die verlustorientierte und die wiederherstellungsorientierte. Erstere richtet sich auf die Verarbeitung verschiedener Aspekte des Verlustes selbst (Beziehung/Bindung zur verstorbenen Person, Gedanken, gemeinsame Erlebnisse, Grübeln, Weinen über den Tod). Die wiederherstellungsorientierte Bewältigung dagegen richtet sich auf die Folgen des Verlustes, wie z. B. Einsamkeit, und die Art der Bewältigung, wie z. B. neue Kontakte knüpfen mit ähnlich Betroffenen. Die Trauer bewegt sich zwischen diesen beiden Bewältigungsstrategien hin und her.

1.3   Multidimensionalität der Trauer

Die Trauerreaktionen, wie sie von Worden (1966) zusammengefasst und beschrieben werden, zeigen sich auf 4 Ebenen:

- Emotional (Traurigkeit, Angst, Wut, ….)
- Physiologisch (körperliche Reaktionen wie Schlafstörungen, Appetitverlust, Müdigkeit, Unruhe, ….)
- Kognitiv (Gedanken wie Selbstvorwürfe, Konzentrationsschwierigkeiten, Suizidgedanken, ….)
- Verhaltensbezogen (sozialer Rückzug, Aktivismus, Essstörungen,….)

Nach Spierings (2006) entwickelt sich normale Trauer in drei Beziehungs-dimensionen, verbunden mit entsprechenden Traueraufgaben:

- Eine neue Beziehung zu sich selbst, eine neue Identität finden
- Eine neue Beziehung zur Welt herstellen
- Eine neue Beziehung zum Verstorbenen entwickeln

1.4   Einfache und komplizierte Trauer

Trauernde unterscheiden sich in ihrem Erleben und dem Ausdruck von Trauer-gefühlen erheblich voneinander. Diese große Variabilität der Trauerreaktionen erschwert die Beurteilung „abweichender" und „komplizierter" Trauerreaktionen, zumal auch, wie bereits erwähnt, religiöse, soziale und kulturelle Aspekte zu berücksichtigen sind.

Folgende Aspekte können den Trauerprozess erschweren (nach Spierings 2006; Paul 2011):

- Verneinte Trauer: der Tod wird nicht anerkannt (kein Beginn der Trauer)
- Verzögerte Trauer: die Trauer kann nicht beginnen
- Chronische Trauer: die Trauer kann nicht beendet werden
- Verzerrte Trauer: der Zugang zu den Gefühlen ist erschwert
- Traumatische Trauer: zuerst muss das Trauma bewältigt werden
- Somatisierte Trauer: die Trauer drückt sich in körperlichen Symptomen aus

Paul (2011) nennt Risikofaktoren in vier Bereichen, die den Trauerprozess erschweren können:

- Begleitumstände des Todes/Todesart
- Beziehung zwischen Trauernden und Verstorbenen
- Lebensgeschichte und aktuelle Lebenssituation der Trauernden
- Soziale Faktoren

Spierings (2006) beschreibt konkret folgende Risikofaktoren (traumatische Verluste/Todesumstände), die die Notwendigkeit professioneller Unterstützung für die Betroffenen erhöhen:

- Plötzlicher, unerwarteter Verlust
- Suizid eines Angehörigen
- Verlust eines Kindes
- Tod wurde als vermeidbar angesehen
- Lang andauernder Krankheitsverlauf
- Ambivalente oder abhängige Beziehung zum Verstorbenen
- Mehrere Todesfälle gleichzeitig oder in kurzer Abfolge
- Fehlendes soziales Unterstützungssystem

1.5   Gesundheitsbeeinträchtigung durch anhaltende Trauerstörung

Die anhaltende Trauerstörung *(Prolonged Grief Disorder, PGD)* ist gekennzeichnet durch schwerwiegende, langanhaltende und beeinträchtigende Verlustreaktionen. 2019 wurde sie als Krankheitsbild in die internationale statistische Klassifikation (International Statistical Classification of Diseases, ICD-11) der Weltgesundheitsorganisation aufgenommen (WHO 2020). Diese soll 2022 offiziell in Kraft treten.

Eine vergleichbare Störung namens *Persistent Complex Bereavement Disorder (PCBD)* wurde zur weiteren Erforschung in das DSM-5 *(Diagnostic and Statistical Manual of Mental Disorders)* aufgenommen (Fleming & Drake 2020).

Es wird diskutiert, inwiefern die separate Kodierung einer Diagnose für „pathologische Trauer" zu einer Stigmatisierung der Betroffenen führen könnte.

2 Besonderheiten von Kinder- und Jugendtrauer als Grundlage für die Beratungspraxis

Der Verlust von engen Bezugspersonen ist für jeden Menschen, egal welchen Alters, von großer Bedeutung, da sich das Bindungsgefüge dadurch stark verändert. Kern et al. (2017) stellen in ihrem Buch „Wie Kinder trauern" fest, dass sich in den letzten drei Jahrzehnten die Sicht auf die kindliche Trauer verändert hat. Früher wurde angenommen, dass Kinder Verlust aufgrund fehlender emotionaler und geistiger Entwicklung nicht verstehen könnten und somit keine Trauer empfänden. Diese Meinungen sind heute revidiert.

Die Todesvorstellungen von Kindern sind schon früh vorhanden, unterscheiden sich jedoch von denen der Erwachsenen, weil die kindlichen Todeskonzepte von der jeweiligen Entwicklungsphase und der kognitiven Reife abhängig sind. Dabei prägen nicht nur elterliches Verhalten und deren Erklärungen über den Tod die Vorstellungen der Kinder, sondern auch die jeweilige religiöse und kulturelle Zugehörigkeit.

2.1 Verlustphänomene und Trauersymptome

Die Verlustphänomene und Trauersymptome zeigen sich auch bei Kindern und Jugendlichen auf verschiedenen Ebenen.

- Psychische, emotionale Ebene
- Physische, somatische Ebene; bei Kindern und Adoleszenten insbesondere durch somatoforme Schmerzen
- Wahrnehmungsebene (u. a. Verlangsamung, Zweifel, verminderter Selbstwert)
- Verhaltensebene (expressive Reaktionen wie: schreien, weinen, klagen; Imitieren der verstorbenen Person oder sprechen wie sie, Hyperaktivität, Verwahrlosung, Rückzug u. a.)

2.2   Entwicklung des Todeskonzeptes

Die Entwicklung des kindlichen Todeskonzeptes wird beeinflusst vom Entwicklungsalter, von vorherigen Erfahrungen sowie von Vorbildern im Umgang mit den Themen Sterben und Tod. Da die kindliche Entwicklung individuell sehr unterschiedlich verlaufen kann, sind die Altersangaben fluide und dienen der groben Orientierung; Abweichungen sind häufig festzustellen. Die folgende Beschreibung vom Verständnis des Todes bei Kindern orientiert sich an Webb (2010).

Das Kleinkind (0–2 Jahre)
Kinder ab etwa acht Monate zeigen Trauerreaktionen wie Ess- oder Schlafstörungen, Weinen, Unruhe, Angst, sich wegdrehen oder sich auf den Boden werfen.

Das Vorschulkind (2–7 Jahre)
Das Vorschulkind kann die Endgültigkeit des Todes noch nicht begreifen. Es geht davon aus, dass der Tod rückgängig gemacht werden kann.
  Ein Kind in diesem Alter hat meistens noch unrealistische Vorstellungen davon, wie lange man lebt, und es glaubt, dass auch nach dem Tod verschiedene Körperfunktionen weitergehen.
  Das Vorschulkind denkt magisch. So kann es glauben, es hätte den Tod selbst herbeigeführt oder verursacht.

Das Schulkind (7–11 Jahre)
Das Schulkind kann die Endgültigkeit und Unvermeidbarkeit des Todes begreifen. Es hat eine realistische Vorstellung davon, wie alt Menschen werden.
  Mit 7 Jahren gehen noch viele Kinder davon aus, dass der Tod nur alte und schwache Menschen trifft. Sie stellen sich den Tod als Person oder Skelett vor.

Das Grundschulkind (9–12 Jahre)
Das Grundschulkind ab 9/10 Jahren hat eine realistische Einschätzung folgender Subkonzepte des reifen Todeskonzeptes:

- Irreversibilität: Endgültigkeit des Todes
- Nonfunktionalität: Körperfunktionen sind stillgelegt beim Tod
- Universalität: Jeder stirbt früher oder später
- Kausalität: Es gibt immer eine Todesursache

Jugendliche

Im Jugendalter ist das Todeskonzept ausgereifter. Der Jugendliche befindet sich in einer Übergangsphase zum Erwachsenwerden. Findet zu diesem Zeitpunkt ein Todesfall statt, kann dies zu Schwierigkeiten in der Entwicklung führen. Es finden zahlreiche kognitive und körperliche Veränderungen statt. Viele Jugendliche sind unsicher und haben Probleme ihre Emotionen zuzulassen. Sie reden meist lieber mit Gleichaltrigen als mit Erwachsenen über den Tod. Jugendliche zeigen Verständnis und Interesse für Spirituelles und stellen philosophische Fragen.

2.3 Trauer und Trauerreaktionen bei Kindern und Jugendlichen

2.3.1 Unterschiede zu Erwachsenen

Weil bei Kindern und Jugendlichen die Fähigkeit der Affektregulation noch nicht voll entwickelt ist, sind schmerzhafte Emotionen für sie oft schwer auszuhalten. Auch ihre kognitive Entwicklung ist noch nicht ausgereift. Daher reagieren sie im Vergleich zu Erwachsenen stärker psychosomatisch. Meist leben sie eher im „Hier und Jetzt". Dennoch sind sie abhängig von Erwachsenen und sind an ihre Bezugspersonen gebunden. Sie brauchen Vorbilder in der Trauer. Erwachsene trauern oft kontinuierlicher, Kinder eher punktueller und manchmal verzögert. Ennulat (2013) findet hierfür ein eindrückliches Bild, in dem der Trauerprozess von Kindern mit dem Stolpern in und dem Herausspringen aus Pfützen verglichen wird.

2.3.2 Reaktionen Jugendlicher nach einem Todesfall – zwischen Ohnmacht und der Suche nach Bewältigung

Kinder und Jugendliche sind unterschiedlich und so zeigen sie auch ihre Trauer durch individuell ganz unterschiedliche Reaktionen. Die Reaktionen sollten nicht gewertet werden, sondern als normale Reaktion auf eine außergewöhnliche Situation angesehen werden. Die folgende Aufzählung von Trauerreaktionen bei Kindern und Jugendlichen erhebt keinen Anspruch auf Vollständigkeit, sondern gibt einen Ausschnitt aus unseren Beratungserfahrungen wieder. Mögliche Reaktionen auf einen Todesfall werden in den folgenden 4 Ebenen dargestellt:

Emotionale Ebene:	Verhaltensebene:
- Trauer: weinen, schreien - Aggressionen: Wut, andere schlagen, beschimpfen oder sich selbst verletzen - Angst: Sorgen um Familie, Freunde, sich selbst - Schuldgefühle (magisches Denken: „Weil ich nicht brav war, ist Papa gestorben.") - Schock, Erstaunen, Ohnmacht - Ungerechtigke tserleben - Verbundenheit, Liebe - Erleichterung - Einsamkeit - Vertrauensverlust - Sinnverlust	- Verändertes Schlafverhalten - Isolation und Rückzug - Nähe und Bindung suchen - Regressives Verhalten - Verhaltensunsicherheit - Weiterführen gewohnter Handlungen wie fernsehen, malen oder spielen - Konsum von Alkohol oder anderen Drogen - Veränderungen des Essverhaltens - Risikofreudigeres Verhalten - Reden, Fragen stellen - Abwechselnde Über- und Untererregungszustände - Vermeidungsverhalten
Somatische Ebene:	Kognitive Ebene:
- Schmerzen, Bauch- oder Kopfweh - Taubheitsgefühl - Erschöpfung - Zittern, Schwindel	- Unglauben, „Das ist nicht wahr!", Derealisation - Konzentrationsschwierigkeiten - Verminderter Selbstwert - Erinnerungslücken - Alpträume

(eigene Darstellung)

Allgemein sind Kinder und Jugendliche meist stärker und widerstandsfähiger, als von Erwachsenen angenommen wird. Bezüglich der Trauerverarbeitung und des Themas Tod sind jüngere Kinder im Kindergartenalter oft neugierig und unbefangen, denn sie kennen noch kein Tabu. Sie sind oftmals bereit, sich mit schwierigen Situationen auseinanderzusetzen.

Bei Jugendlichen stellt der Rückzug eine häufige Bewältigungsstrategie dar, mit manchmal unorthodoxen Reaktionen (scheinbar „coole" Reaktion z. B.: eine Bierflasche als Grabbeigabe). Familienmitglieder sind unterschiedlich resilient, dadurch sind sie auch nicht gleich betroffen.

2.4 Trauer und die Beeinträchtigung mentaler Gesundheit: zur Abgrenzung von Trauer zu Psychotrauma

Die Trauersituation kann, aber muss nicht zwangsläufig mit einem Psychotrauma einhergehen.

Zu Verlusten, die ein erhöhtes Risiko bergen, als traumatisch erlebt zu werden und in deren Folge sich traumabezogene Symptome entwickeln können, zählen u. a.

- Suizide
- der Verlust einer wichtigen Bindungsperson in Kindheit oder früher Jugend
- plötzliche, unerwartete Verluste, z. B. durch Unfall oder Herzinfarkt
- der Verlust nach langer chronischer Krankheit
- Verluste mit stark verändertem Aussehen des Verstorbenen
  - z. B. durch extreme Kachexie nach schweren Erkrankungen, etwa einer Krebserkrankung
  - durch livide Gesichtsverfärbung nach dem Tod (z. B. durch Ersticken)
  - oder auch durch die auftretenden Totenflecken und Verluste durch außergewöhnliche Todesarten wie Gewalt, Naturkatastrophen, Verbrennen, Flugzeugabsturz etc.

Solche Verluste können insbesondere bei Kindern traumatische Bilder und Flashbacks (Intrusionen) hervorrufen, falls sie unvorbereitet den Verstorbenen gefunden haben oder wenn sie sich genau vorstellen, wie der Verstorbene sein Leben verloren hat. Diese Bilder, auch wenn sie nur der eigenen Vorstellungskraft entspringen, können wiederum Hilflosigkeits- und Ohnmachtsgefühle hervorrufen und ein hohes Belastungspotential bergen.

Daher versuchen viele Betroffene diese Erinnerungen zu vermeiden und kapseln sich zum Beispiel ab. Eltern reden oft nicht mit Kindern über das Geschehene, sind selber sprachlos und verunsichert. Jugendliche und Kinder empfinden das als bedrückend und es verhindert, das Geschehene zu begreifen und zu verarbeiten. Oft unterdrücken sie dann ihre Gefühle. Oder sie entwickeln auch Minderwertigkeitsgefühle und/oder einen instabilen Selbstwert. Eine traumatische Trauerverarbeitung kann dann die Folge sein. In einem solchen Fall kann die Trauer erst dann verarbeitet werden, wenn das Trauma behandelt wurde. Bekannt ist ebenso die höhere, stressbedingte Krankheitsanfälligkeit bei Trauer und Trauma.

3 Der „Kanner- a Jugendservice" von Omega 90

3.1 Die Vereinigung Omega 90

Omega 90 ist eine gemeinnützige Vereinigung ohne Gewinnzweck (a.s.b.l.)[1], die 1990 mit der Aufgabe gegründet wurde, die Palliativpflege in Luxemburg zu verbreiten und zu fördern. Zu diesem Zweck werden Initiativen unterstützt, die sich mit der Begleitung von schwer bzw. unheilbar kranken und sterbenden Menschen und ihren Angehörigen beschäftigen sowie mit der Begleitung von trauernden Menschen. Unter einem erweiterten, gesellschaftlichen Blickwinkel möchte Omega 90 dazu beitragen, eine Kultur des Lebens zu entwickeln, die die Endlichkeit der menschlichen Existenz nicht verdrängt, sondern ins Leben integriert. Omega 90 ist nicht an eine bestimmte Ideologie oder Religion gebunden, sondern orientiert sich im Rahmen der geltenden gesetzlichen Regelungen an den Wertevorstellungen[2], wie sie in der Menschenrechtserklärung festgelegt sind. Die ethischen Richtlinien von Omega 90 sind im „Ethischen Orientierungsrahmen" der Gesellschaft beschrieben [3]

Um seine Ziele zu verwirklichen, hat Omega 90 unterschiedliche Angebote und Dienstleistungen entwickelt:

- *Haus Omega,* ein Zentrum für Palliativpflege in Luxemburg, mit 15 Betten für Menschen am Lebensende
- *Centre de Consultation,* eine psychologische Beratungsstelle für Menschen, die an einer unheilbaren Krankheit leiden, sich am Lebensende befinden oder nach einem Todesfall trauern; zur Beratungsstelle gehört auch der *Kanner- a Jugendservice*
- Fortbildungsprogramme in Palliativpflege für Ärzte, Pflegefachkräfte und Angehörige psychosozialer Berufe
- Ausbildung und Betreuung von ehrenamtlichen Mitarbeitern, die Menschen am Lebensende begleiten
- Sensibilisierungsaktionen für ein größeres Zielpublikum

---

[1] Folgende Vereinigungen sind Mitglieder von *Omega 90: Amiperas a.s.b.l., Croix-Rouge Luxembourgeoise, Doheem Versuergt, Fondation Cancer, Fondation Caritas Luxembourg, Stëftung Hëllef Doheem.*

[2] *Statuts modifiés adoptés par l'Assemblée générale de Omega 90 du 3 octobre 2012.*

[3] *Projet d'orientation de Omega 90 adopté par l'Assemblée générale de Omega 90 le 3 octobre 2012 point 2, page 4.*

3.2   Der „Kanner- a Jugendservice": Angebote, Methoden und Erfahrungen aus der Beratungspraxis

Der *Kanner- a Jugendservice* von Omega 90 besteht seit über 20 Jahren. Seine Hauptaufgabe besteht in der Begleitung von Trauer und traumatischen Verlusten bei Kindern und Jugendlichen. Er gehört zum Beratungsdienst *Consultation* von Omega 90, welcher auch Beratung, Begleitung und Psychotherapie für Erwachsene anbietet. In diesem Rahmen ist der *Kanner- a Jugendservice* eine teils eigenständige Abteilung. Die Arbeit mit trauernden Kindern und Jugendlichen unterscheidet sich von der Arbeit mit Erwachsenen, weil sie spezifische Anforderungen stellt und dementsprechende Kompetenzen verlangt. Im Jahr 2020 verfügte der *Kanner- a Jugendservice* über 1,75 Psychologenstellen (70 Wochenstunden).

3.2.1 Angebote des „Kanner- a Jugendservice"

Der *Kanner- a Jugendservice* bietet trauernden Kindern und Jugendlichen im Alter von 4 bis 18 Jahren – in Einzelfällen auch darüber hinaus – Begleitung in Form von Einzelgesprächen oder Gruppen an. Familiengespräche, Erziehungsberatung sowie Informationsvermittlung für Eltern, Angehörige und Professionelle im Umgang mit trauernden Kindern und Jugendlichen gehören ebenfalls zu den Angeboten.

Die Trauerbegleitung von Kindern, Jugendlichen und ihren Familien im *Kanner- a Jugendservice* kann aufgeteilt werden in:

- kurzfristige Beratung für Eltern, telefonisch oder im direkten Gespräch
- Kurzzeitbegleitungen für Kinder, Jugendliche und Eltern bei einfacher Trauer über einige Sitzungen (ca. 1–4 Termine)
- längerfristige Begleitungen für Kinder, Jugendliche und Eltern (meist bei komplexeren Situationen, Dauer länger als 5 Termine)
- Trauergruppen für Kinder und, je nach Anfrage, auch für Jugendliche

Trauergruppen

Der *Kanner- a Jugendservice* von Omega 90 bietet seit dem Jahr 2003 Trauergruppen für Kinder und für Jugendliche an. Diese Gruppen sollen eine gemeinsame Trauerarbeit und Austausch über die jeweiligen Lebenssituationen, Gedanken und Gefühle ermöglichen, wie z. B. Isolation (*„Meine Freunde verstehen mich nicht, die haben so etwas nicht erlebt."*). Das Gruppenangebot bietet

Unterstützung, um sich aus der erlebten Isolation zu befreien und neue Kontakte zu knüpfen. Kinder und Jugendliche können auf kreative und spielerische Art ihre Gefühle ausdrücken und lernen, mit dem Geschehenen umzugehen.

Die langjährige Erfahrung mit altersspezifischen Trauergruppen bei Omega 90 hat gezeigt, dass die Betroffenen erst psychisch stabil sein müssen und keine Intrusionen, Übererregungszustände o. Ä. mehr aufweisen sollten, wenn sie an einem Gruppenangebot teilnehmen möchten.

Fortbildungsangebote

Jedes Jahr bietet der *Kanner- a Jugendservice* verschiedene Fortbildungskurse zum Thema Krankheit, Tod und Trauer bei Kindern und Jugendlichen an. Teilnehmer an diesen Fortbildungen sind Professionelle aus sozio-edukativen oder Gesundheitsberufen. Für diese Berufsgruppen führen Mitarbeiter des Kanner- a Jugendservice auf Anfrage auch Supervisionen durch. Die Anfragen für Fort- und Weiterbildungen gehen mittlerweile über die Grenzen Luxemburgs hinaus.

Prävention: „Omega mécht Schoul", Beratung für Professionelle, „Trauerwallis"

Das präventive Projekt *Omega mécht Schoul* gehört seit der Durchführung des Pilotprojektes im Jahr 2011 ebenfalls zu den Angeboten des *Kanner- a Jugendservice.* Es wird im schulischen Umfeld durchgeführt, um Kindern einen angstfreien Umgang mit den Themen Krankheit, Tod und Sterben zu ermöglichen. An diesem Projekt nehmen auch speziell geschulte ehrenamtliche Mitarbeiter teil.

Bei schwerer Krankheit, nach einem Todesfall oder im Notfall können Lehrer, Schüler oder pädagogisches Fachpersonal Beratung in Anspruch nehmen.

2019 wurde im *Kanner- a Jugendservice* von Omega 90 die *„Trauerwallis"* als Instrument sowohl zur Krisenintervention als auch für die Präventions- und Trauerarbeit entwickelt. Sie kommt in Schulen und anderen Einrichtungen, die mit Kindern und Jugendlichen arbeiten, zum Einsatz, wenn ein Mitglied der Institution oder jemand aus dem Umfeld verstirbt. Der Koffer mit leicht anzuwendendem didaktischem Handbuch und pädagogischem Material mit konkreten Anleitungen für den Notfall soll Betroffenen in der Akutsituation helfen, ein Gefühl von Handlungsfähigkeit, Sicherheit und Kontrolle zu bewahren. Auch der auf einen Trauerfall folgende notwendige Prozess des Wahrhabens des Verlustes soll bei den Beteiligten mit Hilfe der *„Trauerwallis"* in Gang gebracht und gefördert werden.

3.2.2 Methoden und Ziele

Ziel der Trauerbegleitung bei Jugendlichen ist es, die akute Verlustbewältigung zu unterstützen und gesundheitliche Folgeerscheinungen nicht gelebter Trauer, wie psychosomatische Erkrankungen, soziale und emotionale Probleme und

Entwicklungsblockaden, zu vermeiden. Da Kinder in der Regel noch wenig Verlusterfahrungen verarbeiten mussten, haben sie meist noch keine entwickelten
Bewältigungsmuster und –routinen zur Verfügung, wie wir es von Erwachsenen
kennen. Von daher sind die Ziele der Trauerbegleitung von Jugendlichen nicht
nur auf die Vermeidung akuter physischer und psychischer Gesundheitsbeeinträchtigungen ausgerichtet, sondern zugleich immer auch auf die Entwicklung
von Bewältigungsmechanismen und nachhaltiger Resilienz.

Dabei ist es wichtig, dass die Entwicklungsphasen der Kinder und Jugendlichen auf der psychischen, emotionalen und sozialen Ebene beachtet werden. In
der Begleitung im *Kanner- a Jugendservice* orientieren wir uns unter anderem am
dualen Prozessmodell nach Stroebe und Schut (1999) sowie an den Traueraufga-
gaben nach Worden (2002).

Vor dem Hintergrund dieser Zielsetzungen finden im *Kanner- a Jugendservice*
finden folgende Methoden Anwendung: Systemische und analytische Therapie
für Kinder- und Jugendliche, traumazentrierte Therapie (z. B. EMDR, eine neuro-
psychologisch wirksame Behandlungsmethode, um Traumata zu verarbeiten),
Hypnotherapie, körperorientierte Psychotherapie, Tanztherapie, Sophrologie
und andere Entspannungsverfahren. Es wird integrativ gearbeitet. Die Sitzungen
werden den individuellen Bedürfnissen der Betroffenen angepasst und alters-
gerecht auf spielerische, kreative Art und Weise umgesetzt.

3.2.3 Erfahrungen aus der Beratungspraxis

Wer überweist Klienten an den „Kanner- a Jugendservice"?
Alle Mitarbeiterinnen des *Kanner- a Jugendservice* sind auf die Themen Krankheit, Sterben, Tod und Trauer spezialisiert und entsprechend in Trauerbegleitung
und Psychotherapie für Kinder und Jugendliche ausgebildet. Die Strukturen und
Institutionen, die deshalb Klienten an den Kanner- a Jugendservice überweisen,
sind breit gefächert: *Groupe de Support Psychologique* (GSP des CGDIS),
SePAS (Service Psycho-social et d'Accompagnement Scolaire), Professionelle im
schulischen Bereich, psychologische Dienste und Palliativstationen der Kliniken,
Haus Omega, Ärzte und Therapeuten in privater Praxis, *Fondation Cancer,*
Fondation Kriibskrank Kanner, ALAN, Famille plus, Office National de l'Enfance,
Familljen-Center, Familles Plus, Psy-Jeunes und Unterbringungsstrukturen.
Darüber hinaus verweisen Klienten, die bereits bei Omega 90 begleitet wurden,
auf uns. Andere Betroffene finden über die Internetseite von Omega 90 oder
durch Medienberichte den Weg zum *Kanner- a Jugendservice.*

Umgang mit trauernden Kindern und Jugendlichen
Die im Folgenden beschriebenen Richtlinien stellen in gewisser Weise die Essenz aus über 20 Jahren Trauerarbeit mit Kindern und Jugendlichen von Omega 90 dar. Es handelt sich um Erkenntnisse, Erfahrungen und Rückschlüsse aus unserer Praxis, die unterfüttert sind von theoretischer Auseinandersetzung mit und stetiger Weiterbildung in diesem Bereich.

Trauer ist eine normale Reaktion auf einen Verlust, ein persönliches Lebensgefühl, eine tiefgreifende und unausweichliche Erfahrung, die den ganzen Menschen erfasst (Hentges 2013). Sie beinhaltet eine Trennung die schmerzlich, aber notwendig ist. Unserer Erfahrung nach braucht es stabile Beziehungen, Orientierung, Halt und Sicherheit, um mit Trauer umzugehen. Das Durchleben der Trauer kann helfen, diese zu bewältigen und umzuwandeln. Dieser Prozess braucht in der Regel Gemeinschaft, Ausdruck, Raum und Zeit.

Ein Kind ist abhängig von seinen Eltern und Angehörigen, Jugendliche in der Regel auch von ihrer *Peergroup,* um sich schrittweise einem Leben anzupassen, in dem der Verstorbene fehlt. Kinder und Jugendliche brauchen Erwachsene, die für sie da sind, ohne sich aufzudrängen, die sie trösten und ihre manchmal widersprüchlichen Reaktionen aushalten. Darüber hinaus sollten Erwachsene ihnen den Ausdruck von Gefühlen ermöglichen und ein Vorbild sein für den Umgang mit und das Ausleben von Trauer.

Trauernde Kinder und Jugendliche brauchen klare Informationen über das Geschehen in ihrer Familie, sie sollten als vollwertige Mitglieder derselben behandelt werden. Es müssen nicht alle Details genannt werden, aber das, was einem Kind oder Jugendlichen mitgeteilt wird, sollte der Wahrheit entsprechen. Wird nichts erklärt, entstehen unter Umständen Phantasien, die schlimmer und ängstigender sein können, als es die verschwiegene Realität wäre.

Es gilt, betroffenen Kindern und Jugendlichen altersgerechte Antworten auf ihre Fragen zu geben, Unverständliches zu erklären und sie in die Rituale und das Geschehen rund um den Tod zu integrieren. Es braucht Erwachsene, die Betroffene nicht allein lassen, sondern sie trösten und bereit sind, auf ihre vielfältigen Gefühle und Gedanken einzugehen. Ein wichtiger Faktor ist die Wertschätzung der individuellen Fähigkeiten und Eigenheiten des Kindes oder des Jugendlichen. Durch diese wird das Selbstwertgefühl gestärkt und in der Folge kann die Trauer autonomer und dem individuellen psychischen Tempo entsprechend bewältigt werden. Im Idealfall findet ein Kind/Jugendlicher die genannten unterstützenden Faktoren in der eigenen Familie vor. Der Verlust einer engen Bezugsperson stellt für das trauernde Kind, den trauernden Jugendlichen, eine große Herausforderung dar, die sein Leben prägen wird. Es ist eine ganze Familie, die vom Tod betroffen ist. Die Trauer des einen beeinflusst die Trauer des anderen Familienmitgliedes, Rollen im Familiensystem verteilen sich neu, aus einem Geschwisterkind wird unter Umständen nun ein Einzelkind.

Unserer Erfahrung nach haben die Familienangehörigen der Kinder und Jugendlichen sowie ihre Begleitpersonen in der Schule oft nicht die nötigen Informationen, das Wissen oder die Zeit, um die Trauernden bestmöglich zu begleiten. Der Mangel an Informationen führt häufig zu der Angst, etwas Falsches zu sagen, was dann wiederum in Schweigen endet.

Des Weiteren erleben wir in unserer Arbeit Erwachsene, die das Thema meiden, weil sie Schwierigkeiten haben, mit ihrer eigenen Endlichkeit umzugehen. So fällt es jedoch schwer, den Kindern Zuversicht im Wissen um den Tod zu vermitteln.

Zusammenfassend kann man sagen, dass es eine Vielzahl von Gründen gibt, die es erschweren, trauernde Kinder und Jugendliche innerhalb ihres familiären und schulischen Umfeldes einfühlsam und ihrer Entwicklung entsprechend zu begleiten. Viele Familien greifen dann auf die fachliche Hilfe durch Begleitung und Therapie im *Kanner- a Jugendservice* von Omega 90 zurück.

Die Mitarbeiter von Omega 90 geben ratsuchenden Eltern und Professionellen häufig folgende Hinweise (die Aufzählung hat keinen Anspruch auf Vollständigkeit):

- Ehrlich und offen über den Tod reden
- Emotionen dürfen ausgedrückt und gezeigt werden
- Altersgerechte Ansprache und Erklärungen verwenden
- Möglichst zeitnah auf Fragen antworten
- Gespräch anbieten, aber nicht aufdrängen
- Sich und den anderen Trauernden Zeit lassen
- Aber auch schnell wieder gewohnte Abläufe in den Alltag einkehren lassen
- Mit Feingefühl die Bedürfnisse des Kindes/Jugendlichen erkennen
- Verhaltensänderungen beachten und ernst nehmen
- Wechsel zwischen Nähe und Distanz akzeptieren
- Das Kind oder den Jugendlichen nicht in eine (Erwachsenen-)Rolle drängen
- Kinder und Jugendliche in die unterschiedlichen Rituale rund um das Sterben und den Tod integrieren
- Selbstwirksamkeit fördern, Entscheidungen treffen lassen
- Wertschätzung zeigen und möglichst Ressourcen aktivieren

Trauer von Kindern und Jugendlichen
Insbesondere Kinder zeigen ihre Trauer über ihr Verhalten und über ihren Körper, jedes auf seine ganz persönliche Art und Weise. Kinder leben überwiegend in der Gegenwart und können schmerzliche und andere starke Gefühle nicht lange

aushalten. Anders als Erwachsene haben Kinder wenig Worte, um zu beschreiben, wie es ihnen geht. Sie zeigen ihre Trauer eher auf indirekte oder symbolische Art im Malen, im Spiel, in der Bewegung oder sonstigem kreativen Gestalten. Erwähnenswert ist in diesem Zusammenhang auch der Umgang mit kindlichen Schuldgefühlen. Kann ein Kind eine Situation nicht richtig einordnen oder verstehen, so glaubt es oft, es habe selbst etwas mit der Situation zu tun und trage Schuld z. B. an Krankheit und Tod. Kleine Kinder denken verstärkt magisch, d. h., sie meinen, ihre Gedanken können den Lauf der Dinge beeinflussen. Es ist wichtig, ihnen hierzu Erklärungen zu geben.

Jugendliche hingegen haben oft ein starkes Bedürfnis nach Autonomie. Wie bereits erwähnt, versuchen sie meist, Probleme eigenständig zu bewältigen, und wenden sich im Zweifelsfall eher an Gleichaltrige. Oft haben sie Schwierigkeiten, Affekte zuzulassen, auszudrücken und zu begreifen. So erleben sie ihre Gefühle als überwältigend, irritierend oder unkontrollierbar, was sie manchmal verunsichert und desorientiert zurücklässt. Inadäquate Bewältigungsstrategien wie Substanzmittelmissbrauch, Aggressivität oder soziale Isolation können die Problematik verstärken.

Eltern in Trauer, Trauerdynamik in der Familie, Prozess der Trauerberatung
Trauernde Eltern und Familienmitglieder sind oft so sehr von ihrem eigenen Leid überwältigt, dass sie selbst psychologische Hilfe benötigen, um ihr Leben wieder ins Gleichgewicht zu bringen. So kommt es oft vor, dass Erwachsene die Not der Kinder und Jugendlichen übersehen, besonders weil diese ihre Trauer anders erleben und zeigen als Erwachsene.

Wenn ein nahes Familienmitglied schwer erkrankt oder stirbt, benötigen Eltern oft fachliche Hilfe, um kurzfristige Entscheidungen für ihr Kind treffen zu können. Häufig werden folgende Fragen an die Mitarbeiterinnen des Kanner- a Jugendservice gestellt:

- *Unser Arzt hat mir eben mitgeteilt, dass meine Mutter in den nächsten Tagen sterben wird. Wie kann ich meinem fünfjährigen Jungen dies mitteilen? Welche Worte soll ich benutzen?*
- *Darf mein Kind die verstorbene Person sehen?*
- *Sollen Kinder an der Beerdigung teilnehmen und wie kann man sich in dieser Situation am besten als Familie organisieren und verhalten?*
- *Wie kann ich meinem Kind sagen, dass sein Vater lebensbedrohlich erkrankt ist?*
- *Mein Mann hat sich das Leben genommen. Was darf und was muss ich meinen Kindern sagen?*

- *Mein Kind fragt immer wieder, wann seine verstorbene Mutter zurückkommt. Was mache ich falsch?*
- *Mein Kind möchte nicht darüber reden. Ist das gut?*

Die Antworten auf diese Fragen sollten fachlich korrekt sowie verständlich formuliert sein und Orientierung bieten. Manchmal ist die Anfrage mit der Beratung über Telefon zufriedenstellend beantwortet. Oft ergibt sich später daraus eine Begleitung für das trauernde Kind.

Die Begleitung eines Kindes bei Omega 90 kann nur von seinen Eltern oder der Person, die das elterliche Sorgerecht innehat, angefragt werden. Die Bedingung für eine Trauerbegleitung ist die Einwilligung des Kindes oder Jugendlichen. Trauer kann erst bearbeitet werden, wenn der Betroffene bereit ist, sich mit seiner Trauer auseinanderzusetzen. Das Verdrängen der Trauergefühle kann für das Kind eine bestimmte Zeit lang eine normale Schutzreaktion sein. Für Eltern bedeutet die fachliche Begleitung ihres trauernden Kindes vor allem eine gewisse Entlastung in einer schwierigen Situation, mit der sie sich eventuell überfordert fühlen. In vielen Fällen wird die Begleiterin als fachliche Beraterin und als Vermittlerin zwischen den Welten der Kinder und Jugendlichen und denen der Erwachsenen angesehen.

Bei einem Erstgespräch mit den Eltern wird die familiäre Situation beschrieben und die Eltern erhalten unterschiedliche Informationen, wie z. B. häufige Reaktionen auf einen Todesfall oder den Verlauf von Trauer bei Kindern und Jugendlichen. Es wird geklärt, ob die Eltern ihr Kind selbst begleiten, ob es zu einer fachlichen Begleitung bei Omega 90 kommt oder ob eine andere Einrichtung empfohlen wird. Die Anfrage der Eltern an die Trauerbegleiterin erfolgt und eine Anfrage auf Kostenübernahme an das *Office National de l'Enfance (ONE)* wird formuliert. Drei oder vier Termine, meist in einem Intervall von jeweils zwei bis drei Wochen, werden anfänglich für das Kind vereinbart. Anschließend wird entschieden, welche weitere Begleitung das Kind benötigt. Ist es sinnvoll, das Kind weiter zu sehen? Ist wirklich Trauer das akut zu behandelnde Thema? Oder steht eventuell ein ganz anderes Thema als Trauer im Raum? Brauchen eher die Eltern weitere Unterstützung? Oder ist es angezeigt, das Kind in die Kindertrauergruppe aufzunehmen?

Trauer kann mit der Diagnose einer lebensbedrohlichen Krankheit beginnen. In manchen Fällen vertrauen uns erkrankte Väter oder Mütter ihr verunsichertes Kind an. Hier gilt es, sowohl den Eltern wie auch den Kindern und Jugendlichen Richtlinien zu geben, was in dieser schwierigen Zeit zwischen Leben und Tod für die Zukunft der Familie bedeutsam ist. In solchen Situationen möchte der schwerkranke Elternteil ebenfalls informiert werden, wie er das Kind oder den Jugendlichen auf den endgültigen Abschied vorbereiten und auf welche Art er ihm seine persönlichen Anliegen am besten mit auf den Lebensweg geben kann. Die Arbeit in solchen Situationen kann für die Mitarbeiterin des *Kanner- a Jugendservice* von Omega 90 einen zusätzlichen Auftrag darstellen.

Wenn die Therapeutin sowohl das Kind als auch den kranken/sterbenden Elternteil begleitet, ist dies oft sehr intensiv und eher längerfristig. Auch Geschwister von kranken Kindern oder Jugendlichen können bei Omega 90 begleitet werden. In manchen Fällen begleiten Eltern ihr Kind selbst und kommen regelmäßig in den *Kanner- a Jugendservice* bei Omega 90, um Rücksprache mit der Begleiterin zu halten. Auf diese Weise kann die Autonomie der Eltern gestärkt werden.

3.2.4 Zahlen zum Tätigkeitsbericht des „Kanner- a Jugendservice"

Im Jahr 2019 wurden insgesamt 313 Anfragen im *Kanner- a Jugendservice* durchgeführt, davon 218 (70 %) mit neuen Klienten. Der Auslöser für die Anfrage nach Beratung war in der Mehrzahl der Fälle ein Todesfall in der Familie oder im nahen Umfeld der Kinder oder Jugendlichen, in circa 10 % der Fälle eine lebensbedrohliche Erkrankung. In circa einem Drittel der Fälle wurde mit einer erwachsenen Bezugsperson gearbeitet, die Hilfe im Umgang mit Kindern und Jugendlichen in diesen Situationen suchte.

Die folgende Tab. 1 gibt Aufschluss über die Altersstruktur der Klienten im Jahr 2019. Es fanden insgesamt 910 Beratungs- und Therapiesitzungen statt, die 909 h reine Beratungszeit (ohne Vor- und Nachbereitungszeit, Fallgespräche,

Tab. 1 Altersstruktur der Klienten im Jahr 2019 (hier sind die Fälle nicht mitgezählt, bei denen erwachsene Bezugspersonen ohne die betroffenen Kinder oder Jugendlichen konsultierten). (eigene Darstellung)

Alter in Jahren	Anzahl	Anteil in Prozent
3–6	23	12,5
7–9	45	24
10–13	64	34,5
14–18	54	29
Total	186	100

Tab. 2 Dauer der Begleitungen von 2015 bis 2019. (eigene Darstellung)

Anzahl Sitzungen	Anzahl Klienten	Anteil in Prozent
1–2	597	56,1
3–5	250	23,5
6–10	147	13,8
>10	70	6,6
Total	**1064**	**100**

Kooperation, Bericht, …) in Anspruch nahmen. Hinzu kommen 194 h Psycho-
edukation, in denen Eltern in einem Beratungsgespräch Informationen bekamen,
wie sie mit ihren trauernden Kindern und Jugendlichen umgehen können.

Über die Dauer der Begleitungen, ermittelt für den Zeitraum von 2015 bis
2019, gibt Tab. 2 Auskunft.

Aus diesen Zahlen geht hervor, dass die Hälfte der Begleitungen nicht mehr
als zwei Sitzungen in Anspruch nahm, 80 % der Begleitungen nicht mehr als fünf
Sitzungen. Bei den Fällen, die mehr Sitzungen benötigten, handelte es sich um
komplexere Trauersituationen, wie sie in den vorherigen Kapiteln beschrieben
wurden.

4   Ausblick

Kinder sind verletzbar, doch zugleich sind sie resilient. Fachliche Begleitung
für trauernde Kinder und ihre Angehörigen ist eine wichtige und sehr nützliche
Dienstleistung von Omega 90. Durch relativ kurze, doch intensive Interventionen
können bei Kindern und Jugendlichen Blockaden verhindert oder aufgelöst
werden, und die Entwicklung von Bewältigungsmechanismen und Resilienz
unterstützt werden.

Ein sehr wichtiger Teil der Aufgaben des *Kanner- a Jugendservice* von
Omega 90 ist die Präventionsarbeit, zu der *„Omega mécht Schoul"* bereits einen
wichtigen Beitrag leistet.

Mit der *„Trauerwallis"* wurde die Präventionsarbeit um ein Projekt erweitert,
das gleichzeitig auch der Krisenintervention und Trauerarbeit dient. Wird eine
solche *„Trauerwallis"* von einer Institution erworben, die mit Kindern und
Jugendlichen arbeitet, müssen deren Mitarbeiter im Umgang mit dieser geschult

werden. Hierdurch hat sich die Aktivität des *Kanner- a Jugendservice* im Bereich Weiterbildung vergrößert. Sie wird in Zukunft noch weiter ausgebaut werden.

Darüber hinaus ist beabsichtigt, weitere Ausbildungen und Schulungen für die Öffentlichkeit anzubieten, um die Menschen für die Themen Tod und Trauer zu sensibilisieren und diese Themen weiter zu enttabuisieren. Menschen in ihrer Trauer zu informieren, zu beraten, zu orientieren, zu entlasten und zu unterstützen bleibt ein wichtiges Ziel.

Die 2019 etablierte Beratung für Kinder und Jugendliche in Ettelbrück ist ein geographisch erweitertes Beratungsangebot unseres Kanner- a Jugendservice, das sehr gut angenommen wird und in Zukunft personell erweitert werden sollte.

Neben der laufenden Trauergruppe „*Reebougrupp*" im *Kanner- a Jugend-service* wurde 2020 eine Trauergruppe für junge Eltern und Erwachsene angeboten, die zeitgleich stattfand. Dieses parallellaufende Angebot wird weiter ausgebaut.

Der Trauerprozess benötigt Zeit und Raum und sein Ausdruck in allen Aspekten findet in unserem Alltag meist wenig Anerkennung und Akzeptanz. Eine neue Trauerkultur zu finden, sprich neue Verhaltensformen, Rituale im Umgang mit unseren Verlusten, ist eine Herausforderung für unsere Gesellschaft.

Literatur

Bowlby, J. (1984). Attachment and Loss. New York: Penguin Books Ltd; 2nd Revised edition.
Ennulat, G. (2013). Kinder trauern anders. Freiburg: Herder.
Franz, M. (2008). Tabuthema Trauerarbeit. München: Don Bosco Verlag.
Hentges F. (2013) Kursunterlagen: Die Arbeit mit trauernden Kindern und ihren Angehörigen. Luxemburg: Kannerservice Omega 90.
Kast, V. (2013). Trauern: Phasen und Chancen des psychischen Prozesses. Stuttgart: Kreuz Verlag.
Kern, T., Rinder, N., & Rauch, F. (2017). Wie Kinder trauern. München: Kösel.
Kübler-Ross, E. (1969): On Death and Dying. New York: Scribner.
Paul, C. (2011). Trauerprozesse benennen, in. Paul C. (Hsg.) Neue Wege in der Trauer- und Sterbebegleitung: Hintergründe und Erfahrungsberichte für die Praxis. (S. 69–84). Gütersloher Verlagshaus.
Spiegel, Y. (1995). Der Prozess des Trauerns. Gütersloher Verlagshaus.
Spierings, J. (2006). EMDR und Trauer. Seminarmitschrift. Köln.
Stroebe, M., & Schut, H. (1999). The dual process model of coping with bereavement: rationale and description. Death Studies. Apr-May 1999; 23(3):197–224.
Fleming K., & Drake, M.E. (2020). Persistent Complex Bereavement Disorder DSM-5. https://www.theravive.com/therapedia/persistent-complex-bereavement-disorder-dsm--5.

World Health Organization (2020). International Classification of Diseases 11th Revision. https://icd.who.int/en.

Webb, N. (2010). Helping bereaved children. A handbook for practitioners. New York: Guilford Press.

Worden, W. J. (2002). Children and Grief. When a Parent dies. New York: Guilford Press.

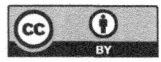

„Was wollt ihr von mir?" – Wohlbefinden und Gesundheit von Jugendlichen im stationären Kontext

Viviane Hansen, Nabila Özen und Claude Kohll

1 Einleitung

Ähnlich wie in den europäischen Nachbarländern erhöht sich auch in Luxemburg die Zahl der Kinder und Jugendlichen, die nicht in ihrer Herkunftsfamilie aufwachsen können. Diese Angebote von außer-familialer Erziehung werden überwiegend von Institutionen der Kinder- und Jugendhilfe vorgehalten. Die aktuellen Zahlen in Bezug auf stationäre Unterbringungen im Großherzogtum zeigen, dass über zwei Drittel der Heimplatzierungen im ersten Halbjahr 2020 durch die zuständigen Jugendgerichte angeordnet wurden und nur etwa 27 % auf freiwilliger Basis erfolgten (MENJE & ONE 2020).

Vor diesem Hintergrund haben Interventionsangebote in der stationären Kinder- und Jugendhilfe nur Aussicht auf Erfolg, wenn sie an das Lebensgefühl, die subjektive Wahrnehmung und den aktuellen Lebenskontext der Jugendlichen anknüpfen. Das subjektive Wohlbefinden von jungen Menschen in der Heimerziehung ist eine relevante Komponente in Bezug auf ihr eigenes Gesundheitsverhalten im Alltag.

In der pädagogischen Praxis stehen Erzieher und Erzieherinnen vermehrt unter dem Druck, eine Schutzfunktion gegenüber den ihnen anvertrauten Jugendlichen ausüben zu müssen, wenn sie den Eindruck haben, dass diese sich selbst oder

V. Hansen (✉) · N. Özen · C. Kohll
Arcus - Centre Formida pour jeunes, Esch-sur-Alzette, Luxemburg
E-Mail: viviane.hansen@arcus.lu

N. Özen
E-Mail: nabila.oezen@arcus.lu

C. Kohll
E-Mail: claude.kohll@arcus.lu

© Der/die Autor(en) 2022
A. Heinen et al. (Hrsg.), *Wohlbefinden und Gesundheit im Jugendalter,*
https://doi.org/10.1007/978-3-658-35744-3_26

auch anderen mit ihrem Verhalten schaden. Somit müssen die Fachkräfte davon überzeugt sein zu wissen, was „gut" und was „nicht gut" für die Jugendlichen ist. Die Frage (im Titel dieses Beitrags) „Was wollt ihr von mir?" gilt als beispielhaft für diese grundlegenden Situationen, in denen Jugendliche in der Kinder- und Jugendhilfe sich konfrontiert sehen mit Erziehungsauftrag und den Erziehungsvorstellungen der Professionellen, und sich dann oft missverstanden und bevormundet fühlen.

Im Folgenden soll dieses Spannungsfeld zwischen der Wahrnehmung der Jugendlichen und dem Verständnis bzw. der Resonanz der pädagogischen Fachkräfte auf die Handlungen der jungen Menschen beleuchtet werden.

Bevor wir uns mit dem Thema „Wohlbefinden und Gesundheit von Jugendlichen" auseinandersetzen, beschäftigen wir uns in einem ersten Schritt mit den Entwicklungsaufgaben und Grundbedürfnissen im Jugendalter (Abschn. 2.1). Parallel zum allgemeinen Entwicklungsprozess in dieser Altersphase kommen bei Jugendlichen im Heimkontext oft erschwerende Ausgangsbedingungen hinzu (Abschn. 2.2). Die Jugendlichen entwickeln im Umgang mit diesen, oft traumatischen Erlebnissen ganz unterschiedliche Resilienzfaktoren, die einen erheblichen Einfluss auf ihre Gesundheit und ihr Wohlbefinden haben (Abschn. 2.3).

Anschließend wird das Thema „Wohlbefinden und Gesundheit von Jugendlichen" anhand von drei Fallbeispielen aus der Kinder- und Jugendhilfe aus unterschiedlichen Perspektiven mit verschiedenen thematischen Schwerpunkten beleuchtet (Abschn. 3).

Bei der Entstehung dieses Buchbeitrags haben verschiedene MitarbeiterInnen[1] aus dem Erziehungshilfebereich von arcus mitgewirkt. Durch den Austausch von Praxisbeispielen aus internen Fallbesprechungen sowie die Auswertung von generalisierbaren Erfahrungswerten aus der Praxis wurden einrichtungsübergreifende Themen in Bezug zur Gesundheit von Jugendlichen im Heimkontext herausgefiltert. Dieses gemeinsam geteilte Erfahrungswissen findet sich sowohl innerhalb der alltagsnahen Beschreibung der drei konkreten Fallbeispiele wieder als auch im Ausblick auf eine Weiterentwicklung der Praxis zum Thema „Wohlbefinden und Gesundheit von Jugendlichen im stationären Kontext". Im letzten Abschnitt des Artikels werden die Ergebnisse unserer Überlegungen zusammengefasst. Wir hoffen, dadurch einige Hinweise zu Zielsetzungen, Aufgaben und

---

[1] Für eine gendergerechte Schreibweise werden in diesem Artikel stets beide Geschlechter genannt, wie beispielsweise MitarbeiterInnen oder SozialarbeiterInnen. Es sei denn, es wird sich explizit auf ein Geschlecht bezogen.

Handlungsstrategien geben zu können, die die Sensibilität für dieses Thema in der Praxis der Heimerziehung erhöhen und gleichzeitig dem Erleben und der Sichtweise von Jugendlichen mehr Gewicht verleihen.

Darüber hinaus konnten wir diesen Buchbeitrag nutzen, um einrichtungsinterne Lernprozesse anzustoßen. Durch die gemeinsame Arbeit an diesem Artikel ergaben sich viele Impulse und Denkanstöße, die eine differenziertere Auseinandersetzung mit dem Thema „Wohlbefinden und Gesundheit von Jugendlichen im stationären Kontext" voranbrachten.

Da das Thema „Wohlbefinden und Gesundheit von Jugendlichen im stationären Kontext" sehr viele Komponenten und eine große Komplexität aufweist, ist es uns wichtig, verschiedene Fragestellungen und Beobachtungen in ihrer Verbindung von Theorie und Praxis näher zu beleuchten.

2   Mehrfachproblematiken bei Jugendlichen in der stationären Jugendhilfe

Ausgehend von der Tatsache, dass Jugendliche mit vielen Entwicklungsschritten und mit der Befriedigung von ganz spezifischen Bedürfnissen konfrontiert sind, ist anzunehmen, dass es sich beim Jugendalter um eine sehr herausfordernde Phase handelt. Da die meisten Jugendlichen die Fremdunterbringung als zusätzliche Belastung erleben, zeigen sie oftmals Verhaltensweisen, welche für das erzieherische Personal besondere Herausforderungen im Alltag darstellen. Im folgenden Kapitel werden diese Mehrfachproblematiken bei Jugendlichen im stationären Kontext näher beleuchtet, indem die Entwicklungsschritte und die damit einhergehenden Grundbedürfnisse im Jugendalter sowie erschwerende Ausgangsbedingungen durch Biografie und Heimunterbringung vorgestellt werden. Außerdem werden die generellen Auswirkungen dieser Mehrfachproblematiken auf das Wohlbefinden und die Gesundheit bei Jugendlichen in der stationären Jugendhilfe kurz beschrieben.

2.1   Entwicklungsschritte und Grundbedürfnisse im Jugendalter

Basierend auf Theorien der Entwicklungspsychologie (Jean Piaget) und Soziologie (Robert Havighurst) werden wir uns im folgenden Kapitel mit den Veränderungsprozessen, den Entwicklungsaufgaben und den Bedürfnissen im Jugendalter beschäftigen. „Entwicklungsaufgaben beschreiben, welche Themen für ein bestimmtes Alter eine besondere Wichtigkeit haben und inwieweit deren Bewältigung zur erfolgreichen Entwicklung essenziell ist. Entwicklungsaufgaben entstehen durch das Zusammenspiel gesellschaftlicher Anforderungen und Erwartungen, wie zum Beispiel am Ende eines bestimmten Altersabschnittes aus dem Elternhaus ausgezogen zu sein, biologischer Entwicklungsveränderungen (z. B. Pubertät, Menopause) und der Persönlichkeit eines Individuums." (Schneider und Lindenberger 2018, S. 268).

Die körperlichen und hormonell bedingten Veränderungen während der Pubertät gehören zu den bedeutsamsten Entwicklungen in der frühen Adoleszenz, mit denen sich junge Heranwachsende auseinandersetzen müssen.

Der Wunsch nach dem Zusammensein mit Gleichaltrigen (Peergruppe) wächst aus dem Bedürfnis nach Zugehörigkeit und Sicherheit. In der Peergruppe finden Jugendliche andere Gleichaltrige, die sich innerhalb eines gemeinsamen sozialen Kontextes mit den gleichen Entwicklungsaufgaben beschäftigen. Dies begünstigt einen Prozess des besseren gegenseitigen „Verstehens". Als Folge des körperlichen Reifungsprozesses entwickeln Jugendliche sexuelle Bedürfnisse und den Wunsch nach Anerkennung und Zuwendung durch eine Partnerin oder einen Partner. Ebenso wie sie ihre Sozialbeziehungen zu Gleichaltrigen und Partnern weiterentwickeln, ändert sich auch die Beziehung zu den Eltern. In der Adoleszenz kommt es vermehrt zu Konflikten über alltägliche Probleme, aber auch zu Divergenzen über grundsätzliche Lebensthemen. Die Suche nach einer eigenen Identität, Individualität und der Wunsch nach Unabhängigkeit und Autonomie entstehen durch den Zuwachs an neuen Möglichkeiten und Herausforderungen (Schneider und Lindenberger 2018).

Die beschriebenen körperlichen Veränderungen in der Pubertät, die unterschiedlichen Entwicklungsaufgaben und die Bedürfnisse der Adoleszenz sind eng miteinander verknüpft. Körperliche sowie gesundheitliche Veränderungen und Probleme spielen während dieser Lebensphase genauso eine wichtige Rolle wie psychisches und soziales Wohlbefinden. Verhaltens- und Einstellungsänderungen ergeben sich aus der Reflexion über die körperlichen Veränderungen und lassen vielfach Konflikte mit der Umgebung entstehen oder führen nicht selten zu Pubertätskrisen (Remschmidt et al. 2005).

Jugendliche mit einer durchschnittlichen und relativ unproblematisch verlaufenden Entwicklung, welche unter allgemein guten Voraussetzungen aufwachsen und die notwendige soziale Unterstützung erfahren, sind in der Regel gut auf die beschriebenen Entwicklungsaufgaben vorbereitet. Vor diesem Hintergrund stellen diese Entwicklungsschritte positive und entwicklungsstimulierende Herausforderungen dar. Wenn Jugendliche allerdings durch mehrfach erschwerende Voraussetzungen, bedingt durch Heimunterbringung,

Traumatisierung oder Trennung der Eltern, nicht hinreichend bei der Auseinandersetzung mit den Anforderungen ihrer Lebensphase unterstützt werden,
kann dies zu erheblichen Entwicklungsproblemen führen (Remschmidt et al.
2005; Hurrelmann und Quenzel 2012).

Jugendliche der stationären Kinder- und Jugendhilfe zählen eher zur zweiten
Gruppe. Sie sind zusätzlich zu den typischen Herausforderungen, welche
die Pubertät und die damit zusammenhängenden Entwicklungsschritte und
Grundbedürfnisse mit sich bringen, weiteren Belastungen ausgesetzt. Diese
Belastungen sind häufig durch ihre Biografie und die Heimunterbringung selbst
begründet.

2.2 Erschwerende Ausgangsbedingungen durch Biografie und Heimunterbringung

Zu den allgemeinen Veränderungen und Herausforderungen, welche die Jugendphase mit sich bringt, kommt bei Jugendlichen, die stationär untergebracht sind,
hinzu, dass sie häufig bereits seit dem Kleinkindalter zusätzlichen Belastungen
verschiedenster Art ausgesetzt sind. Dazu gehören zerrüttete und konfliktreiche
Familienverhältnisse, welche heute zunehmend mit prekären Wohnverhältnissen
einhergehen. Zudem haben schwere traumatische Situationen in der Kindheit
häufig einen erheblichen Einfluss auf das Bindungsverhalten der Jugendlichen.

Es lässt sich beobachten, dass der Entwicklungsprozess der Identitätsfindung,
mit anschließendem Loslösungsprozess von erwachsenen Bezugspersonen, vermehrt durch viele Beziehungsabbrüche im Laufe ihrer Biografie gestört wird.
Um sich gesund loslösen zu können, sind positive Erfahrungen im Rahmen von
verbindlichen und tragfähigen Beziehungen mit erwachsenen Bezugspersonen
von großer Bedeutung. Meist haben die betroffenen Jugendlichen allerdings
nicht viele verlässliche Beziehungen in ihrer Biografie erlebt, verbrachten viele
Jahre ihrer Kindheit und frühen Jugend außerhalb ihres familiären Milieus und
haben schlimmstenfalls durch das Scheitern verschiedener Hilfesysteme auch
hier mehrere Beziehungsabbrüche erfahren müssen. Hinzu kommt, dass sie
durch häufiges Umziehen, sei es mit der Herkunftsfamilie oder aber bedingt
durch den Wechsel zwischen verschiedenen institutionellen Hilfemaßnahmen,
sich öfter als andere Jugendliche an ein fremdes schulisches und soziales Umfeld
anpassen müssen. Diese Diskontinuitäten erschweren wiederum den Anschluss
an eine feste Peergruppe und die Entwicklung eines Gefühls von Zugehörigkeit.
So kommt es, dass sich bei Jugendlichen aus der stationären Heimerziehung
die Frage stellt: Von welcher stabilen erwachsenen Bezugsperson soll oder kann

ein Ablösungsprozess stattfinden? Von ihren Eltern, mit denen das Zusammenleben oft von vielen unerfüllbaren Ansprüchen und unauflösbaren Ambivalenzen geprägt ist, was einen hohen Leidensdruck auf der Seite der Jugendlichen wie auch bei den Eltern erzeugt? Oder erfolgt der Loslösungsprozess eher von den ErzieherInnen, welche während einer bestimmten Zeit wichtige Ansprechpartner und Bezugspersonen darstellen? Durch die Diskrepanz zwischen ihrem eigenen Bedürfnis, Zeit mit ihrer Peergruppe zu verbringen, und dem Wunsch der Familie nach gemeinsamer Zeit mit ihren Kindern, sind Jugendliche aus der stationären Kinder- und Jugendhilfe in vielen Fällen zudem einem Loyalitätskonflikt ausgesetzt, der oftmals zu einem großen Unbehagen führt.

Außerdem steigt das Risiko von (internalisierenden und externalisierenden) Verhaltensauffälligkeiten bei sich kumulierenden Belastungsfaktoren gravierend. Dies hat zur Folge, dass viele Beziehungs- und Hilfeangebote der Kinder- und Jugendhilfe scheitern. Die vermehrten familiären und psychosozialen Risikofaktoren, welchen diese Jugendlichen ausgesetzt waren oder noch sind, gehen in vielen Fällen mit einer hohen Prävalenz von psychischen Störungen einher (Komorbidität). So stellte Marc Schmid (2007, S. 26) fest, dass „der Prozess der Hilfeplanung, die Trennung von den Bezugspersonen, familiengerichtliche Auseinandersetzungen, unklare Umgangsregelungen und vor allem das Scheitern von eingeleiteten Jugendhilfemaßnahmen und der damit verbundene erneute Wechsel der Bezugspersonen und die wiederholten Trennungserfahrungen etc. eine enorme Belastung für die Kinder darstellen." Die Studie basiert auf einer repräsentativen Stichprobe, die 20 deutsche Jugendhilfeeinrichtungen mit insgesamt 689 Kindern und Jugendlichen erfasst. Sie ergab, dass bei 60 % der Kinder und Jugendlichen „definierte klinische Diagnosen aus dem Gebiet der Kinder-und Jugendpsychiatrie (…)" festgestellt wurden (Schmid 2007, S. 13).

2.3   Auswirkungen auf Wohlbefinden und Gesundheit

Aufgrund der oben genannten Mehrfachbelastungen in der Herkunftsfamilie und traumatischen Erlebnissen auch in den institutionellen Hilfekontexten stehen die jungen Heranwachsenden vor der Herausforderung, neben den eigenen Entwicklungsaufgaben noch zusätzliche Problemlagen bewältigen zu müssen. Dabei fehlen ihnen häufig die dafür notwendigen Ressourcen und Schutzfaktoren, wie zum Beispiel eine sichere Bindungsrepräsentation, stärkende Vorerfahrungen oder ein unterstützendes soziales Umfeld. Dies hat zur Folge, dass die betroffenen

Jugendlichen vermehrt mit Rückschlägen und frustrierenden Situationen konfrontiert werden.

Aus internen Fallbesprechungen und Intervisionen geht hervor, dass die Kinder und Jugendlichen in Institutionen der Kinder- und Jugendhilfe unterschiedliche Verhaltensformen aufzeigen, die häufig mit einer Beeinträchtigung der Gesundheit und des Wohlbefindens einhergehen. In der Praxis beobachtete Verhaltensauffälligkeiten mit körperlichen Symptomen sind beispielsweise Essstörungen, Substanzmissbrauch (Tabak, Drogen), Schlafstörungen, selbstverletzendes und selbstgefährdendes Verhalten, Einnässen oder auch Störungen des Sexualverhaltens.

Zudem gilt es Entwicklungsstörungen, wie z. B. motorische Störungen, Sprachstörungen, Lernschwäche und kognitive Einschränkungen im Betreuungs- und Behandlungsalltagfrühzeitig zu erkennen, um gesundheitlichen Problemen von Kindern und Jugendlichen entgegenzuwirken.

Einige Jugendliche zeigen außerdem hohe Verhaltensauffälligkeiten. Auf der sozialen Ebene können sich diese sowohl in einem oppositionellen als auch in einem aggressiven Verhalten ausdrücken. Es fällt ihnen häufig schwer, sich auf verlässliche Beziehungen einzulassen.

Werden zentrale Grundbedürfnisse, wie das Bedürfnis nach Bindung, Kontrolle und Orientierung, Selbstwerterhöhung sowie positiver Lust auf lange Zeit nicht befriedigt, entwickeln Kinder und Jugendliche ihre eigenen Verhaltensmuster und Ich-Strukturen. So handelt es sich bei den als schwierig empfundenen Verhaltensweisen der Jugendlichen häufig um Schutzmechanismen, um sich vor weiteren verletzenden Erfahrungen zu schützen (Grawe 1999).

So können beispielsweise Essstörungen und oppositionelles Verhalten als Ausdruck für das Bedürfnis nach Kontrolle interpretiert werden. Aggressives und abweisendes Verhalten kann wiederum als emotionaler Schutz vor weiteren Abweisungen und Beziehungsabbrüchen erklärt werden.

Um das Verhalten der Jugendlichen im Heimalltag pädagogisch und therapeutisch adäquat auffangen zu können, gilt es die Hilfeleistung jeweils an die individuellen Bedürfnisse der Jugendlichen anzupassen.

Neue positive Erfahrungsmomente, partizipative Prozessgestaltungen, Erfolgserlebnisse und verlässliche Beziehungsangebote können einen großen Einfluss auf das Wohlbefinden der Jugendlichen haben (Wüsten und Pauls 2013; Pauls 2013). Die beschriebenen Auswirkungen auf Wohlbefinden und Gesundheit der Jugendlichen stellen also spezifische Anforderungen an das erzieherische Personal im Heimalltag.

3   Herausforderungen im Heimalltag – Fallbeispiele[2]

In den jetzt folgenden Fallbeispielen von Jugendlichen aus dem stationären Kontext der Kinder- und Jugendhilfe in Luxemburg handelt es sich um drei Jugendliche, bei denen die spezifischen Themen, Dynamiken und Problematiken, die wir beleuchten wollen, besonders deutlich werden.

Als Hintergrundinformation für die von uns ausgewählten Fallbeispiele wollen wir an dieser Stelle kurz die stationären Angebote von arcus beschreiben.[3]

In den geschlechtlich gemischten Lebensgruppen werden Kinder und Jugendliche von pädagogischen Fachkräften begleitet und betreut. Hierbei handelt es sich um junge Menschen, die sich in einer prekären Lebenssituation befinden, einem erhöhten Risiko von Gefährdungen ausgesetzt sind sowie eine befristete räumliche Trennung von ihren Eltern benötigen.

Die Lebensgruppen in den stationären Einrichtungen bieten den Kindern und Jugendlichen einen sicheren Ort des respektvollen Umgangs miteinander. Die Förderung der Gesundheit und der schulischen Entwicklung, der Aufbau familiärer und sozialer Beziehungen, die Befähigung zu einer eigenständigen Lebensgestaltung, die Bereitstellung eines strukturierten Alltags sowie die Aufarbeitung traumatischer Erlebnisse kennzeichnen das sozialpädagogische Arbeiten in unseren Lebensgruppen.

Neben der individuellen Förderung der Kinder und Jugendlichen erfährt die Unterstützung und Wertschätzung der leiblichen Eltern im Rahmen der stationären Unterbringung eine besondere Bedeutung. Eine größtmögliche Partizipation und Einbindung der Eltern in den Heimalltag wird von allen Lebensgruppen angestrebt. Die Stärkung der Familie sowie die Unterstützung der Erziehungsprozesse bilden grundlegende Schwerpunkte der pädagogischen Arbeit im Heimalltag.

Arcus bietet darüber hinaus für Kinder und Jugendliche, deren Wohl durch körperliche, psychische, sexuelle Misshandlung, Verwahrlosung oder andere traumatische Erlebnisse gefährdet wurde, eine intensivpädagogische stationäre Unterbringung an. Die intensivpädagogischen stationären Gruppen arbeiten in enger Kooperation mit Akteuren der Kinder- und Jugendpsychiatrie sowie für

---

[2] Die beschriebenen Fallbeispiele wurden so weit verfremdet, dass die Anonymität der Betroffenen gewahrt bleibt.

[3] https://www.arcus.lu/15/heimunterbringung. Zugegriffen: 04. März 2020.

die Umsetzung bedarfsorientierter Therapien mit dem „Berodungsdéngscht fir Kanner, Jugend a Famill" von arcus zusammen.

Die Förderung der Autonomiefähigkeit und der Selbstständigkeit ist zentrales Anliegen der stationären Unterbringung, dies besonders für die Lebensgruppen mit einem Aufnahmealter ab dem zwölften Lebensjahr. Die Umsetzung dieses Zieles findet sich in der pädagogischen Ausrichtung des Alltags wieder.

3.1 Jugendliche im Spannungsfeld zwischen selbst entscheiden (zu) dürfen und institutionellem Kontrollstreben

Der Fokus des ersten Fallbeispiels liegt auf der subjektiven Erlebnisdimension der eigenen Gesundheit und des Wohlbefindens eines Jugendlichen vor dem Hintergrund seiner biografischen Erlebnisse und seiner soziokulturellen Herkunft.

In der stationären Kinder- und Jugendhilfe gibt es oft eine noch stärkere Diskrepanz zwischen Selbsteinschätzung und Fremdeinschätzung der Gesundheit und des Wohlbefindens junger Menschen (zwischen externer Beobachtung/ Diagnose und Selbstwahrnehmung) im Vergleich zu Jugendlichen, die in ihrem Herkunftsmilieu aufwachsen.

Bezogen auf Gesundheitsthemen nehmen die pädagogischen MitarbeiterInnen oft eine eher kontrollierende Rolle und Haltung gegenüber den Jugendlichen und ihren Eltern ein. Sie fühlen sich stark verantwortlich, was sich dann im Alltag in einer Kommunikation mit sehr reglementierendem Aufforderungscharakter hinsichtlich der physischen und psychischen Selbstpflege der Jugendlichen widerspiegelt.

Für Jugendliche in der stationären Kinder- und Jugendhilfe ist Wohlbefinden eng mit der Mitbestimmung des eigenen Lebens verbunden. Die individuell entwickelten Alltagskonstruktionen der Jugendlichen in Bezug auf ihr Wohlbefinden und somit auch auf ihre Gesundheit sind oft schwer nachvollziehbar für die pädagogischen Fachkräfte.

Die alltagsbezogene Gesundheitsförderung kann nicht losgelöst von der Lebenswelt und den kognitiven, emotionalen sowie sozialen Ressourcen der Jugendlichen gesehen werden. Sie ist eng verbunden mit dem Hintergrund ihrer oft brüchigen Biografie. Zudem haben Jugendliche in der stationären Jugendhilfe und ihre Eltern kaum die Möglichkeit, sich im Alltag miteinander auseinanderzusetzen und hierdurch ihre Beziehung neu zu definieren. Ihre biografischen Verläufe erlauben es den Jugendlichen häufig nicht, sich eigene gesundheitsfördernde Handlungsfähigkeiten und -strategien anzueignen.

Tom

Tom ist 15 Jahre alt und lebt seit 3 Jahren in einer Jugendgruppe von arcus.

Als Tom 7 Jahre alt war, wurde bei ihm Diabetes diagnostiziert. Zu diesem Zeitpunkt lebte er bei seinen leiblichen Eltern. Als die Ehe 2014 geschieden wurde, wohnte Tom fortan bei seiner Mutter.

Der Mutter ging es nicht gut. Sie lebte selbst in einer für sie belastenden sozialen Situation. Vor allem die Verarbeitung einer Trennung, depressive Episoden und finanzielle Engpässe stellten für sie zeitweilig eine große Überforderung dar. Somit fiel es der Mutter in dieser Zeit sehr schwer, sich um Toms Gesundheit zu kümmern.

Entsprechend war bei den regelmäßigen Untersuchungen in der Kinderklinik Toms Zuckerspiegel oft zu hoch oder zu niedrig, sodass das Jugendgericht entschied, die Familie müsse eine ambulante Pflegekraft in Anspruch nehmen, um die Mutter zu unterstützen. Es kam jedoch sehr oft vor, dass Tom der Pflegekraft die Tür nicht aufmachte, wenn er allein zu Hause war und seine Mutter arbeitete. Sein Gesundheitszustand verschlechterte sich zunehmend. Nach einer erneuten Untersuchung in der Kinderklinik wurde Tom zuerst stationär in der Klinik und danach in einer Inobhutnahme-Struktur untergebracht. Die Mutter war teilweise präsent, jedoch weiterhin einer sehr instabilen Lebenssituation ausgesetzt, sodass keine Rückführung geplant werden konnte.

Mit 12 Jahren kam Tom in eine stationäre Lebensgruppe mit gleichaltrigen Jugendlichen.

Toms Gesundheitszustand, und vor allem der Umgang seiner Mutter mit der Krankheit, war einer der Hauptgründe für die Fremdunterbringung. Am Anfang des Aufenthaltes im Heim gab es nur wenig Kontakt zur Mutter. Sie wurde zu jedem schulischen und medizinischen Termin eingeladen, nahm diese Angebote jedoch meistens nicht wahr. Tom war ein etwas zurückhaltender Junge. Anfangs fiel es den ErzieherInnen sehr schwer einzuschätzen, wie autonom Tom mit seiner Krankheit umgehen konnte. Das zeigte sich in seinem heimlichen Essverhalten. Oft vergaß er seine Zuckerwerte einzugeben, sodass es ihm häufig schwindelig wurde und er sich insgesamt nicht gut fühlte.

Aufgrund kognitiver Defizite fiel es Tom schwer, eigene Entscheidungen mit Blick auf seine Gesundheit abzuwägen und kritisch reflektiert zu treffen. Der Jugendliche konnte den Sinn und Zweck eines gesundheitsförderlichen Verhaltens noch nicht erkennen. Gerade hohe Zuckerwerte verursachten bei den ErzieherInnen Alarmstimmung. Tom blieb dabei oftmals demonstrativ gelassen, da er die direkten Auswirkungen des hohen Zuckers nicht unbedingt zeitnah erlebte. Er zeigte sich dann aber im weiteren Verlauf solcher Situationen eher gestresst, da er z. B. nachts geweckt werden musste, um mehrmals Messungen der Blutzuckerwerte durchzuführen. Eine weitere Rolle spielte ein spezifischer Essensplan für Tom.

Er hatte große Schwierigkeiten, Anleitungen im Umgang mit seinem Diabetes zu verstehen und nachzuvollziehen, da sein Verhalten nicht zu sofortigen direkt wahrnehmbaren gesundheitlichen Krisen führte.

Anna Lena Rademaker (2018, S. 51) beschreibt in „Agency und Gesundheit in jugendlichen Lebenswelten", „dass zunächst einmal die Förderung von Wissen über verschiedene Gesundheitsaspekte" wichtig ist, „um vor diesem Hintergrund Entscheidungen mit Blick auf die eigene Gesundheit abwägen und kritisch-reflektiert treffen zu können. Es bedeutet die Stärkung von Selbstwirksamkeits-erfahrungen, damit junge Menschen sich als einflussmächtig mit Blick auf ihre Gesundheit erleben und die Förderung von Zukunftsoptimismus, um auch Sinn und Zweck in einem gesundheitsförderlichen Verhalten für sich finden zu können. Insbesondere ist dabei die Fähigkeit der selbstkritischen Reflexion eigener Ver-haltensweisen im Alltag mit Blick auf die Gesundheit zu bekräftigen."

In Bezug auf Toms Situation heißt das, wenn er etwas mit seiner Peergruppe unternehmen wollte, waren die ErzieherInnen sehr besorgt, da sie während mehrerer Stunden keine Handhabe über die notwendigen Vorkehrungen in Bezug auf den Diabetes hatten. Tom fühlte sich dadurch sehr eingeschränkt in seinem Alltag. Vieles musste für ihn vorab geplant werden. Für die ErzieherInnen stellte sich hier die Frage, wie sie die Spritz-, Kontroll- und Essenszeiten so gestalten konnten, dass die Zuckererkrankung nicht zu sehr die Alltagsabläufe bestimmte und Tom einen größtmöglichen Freiraum erleben konnte. Dabei standen die pädagogischen Fachkräfte unter einem diffusen Erwartungsdruck, da sie wussten, dass der nachlässige Umgang der Mutter mit der Erkrankung der zentrale Grund für die Fremdunterbringung war. Der unausgesprochene Auftrag an das Team lautete, dass in einem professionellen Kontext so etwas nicht passieren darf, was natürlich zu einer genaueren Ausweitung und weiteren Differenzierung der Kontrolle führte. Dies wiederum verstärkte tendenziell das Unwohlsein von Tom, da er nicht ausschließlich als „Diabetiker", sondern als eigenständige Person wahrgenommen werden wollte.

Toms eigener Umgang mit der Krankheit und sein Wohlbefinden hatten somit auch viel mit der Beziehung zu seiner Mutter zu tun. Funktionierte sein Alltag gut in der Lebensgruppe, empfand die Mutter dies als Kränkung, so als würde er ihr indirekt in den Rücken fallen. Wenn Toms Entwicklung in der Lebensgruppe stagnierte oder chaotisch verlief, war der Unterbringungsgrund aus ihrer Sicht hinfällig, da die ErzieherInnen es ja schließlich auch nicht besser hinbekamen als sie selbst.

Toms Mutter war am Anfang der Unterbringung sehr misstrauisch gegenüber der Einrichtung. Ihre Wahrnehmung war bestimmt vom Scheitern und von Schamgefühlen. Sie wollte nicht über das Thema „Diabetes" reden. Ihre subjektive Wahrnehmung, die sich in der Überzeugung „Mein Kind wurde mir weggenommen" ausdrückte, führte zu intensivem Stresserleben. So blendete sie das Thema „Diabetes" teilweise aus.

Häufig fühlen sich Eltern von Jugendlichen, die nicht mehr im Herkunftsmilieu leben, dadurch abgewertet, dass der Jugendliche in der Gruppe verschiedene Verhaltensweisen, welche von der Familie als auffällig erlebt wurden, im stationären Kontext zeitweise nicht mehr zeigt. Es musste also zuerst eine Vertrauensbasis zur Mutter aufgebaut werden. Erst dann konnte sie sich wieder schrittweise auf die angebotenen Unterstützungsmaßnahmen der ErzieheInnen einlassen.

Die Unterbringung in der stationären Kinder- und Jugendhilfe erfolgt selten auf freiwilliger Basis. Neben der Verlust- und Trennungserfahrung war es für Tom eher schwierig, sich in eine Peergruppe zu integrieren. Aufgrund seiner Erkrankung erfuhr er intensive Interventionen seitens der ErzieherInnen sowie Einschränkungen im Alltag (z. B. beim Ausgang mit seinen Freunden, Blutzucker messen und kurz danach Insulin spritzen zu müssen bei spontanen Snacks oder Unwohlsein). Dann gab es noch die regelmäßigen Aufenthalte am Wochenende bei seiner Familie, nach denen er mit sehr hohen Zuckerwerten zurück in die Einrichtung kam. Die Planung einer Rückführung war somit auch stets mit der Angst des Scheiterns bezüglich der Stabilisierung der gesundheitlichen Situation von Tom verbunden.

Tom war ständig hin- und hergerissen zwischen dem gesundheitsfördernden Umgang mit seiner Krankheit in dem für ihn schwierigen Kontext der Heimunterbringung und seinem Autonomiebestreben. Letzteres gestaltete sich oft schwierig, da seine selbstständigen Initiativen außerhalb des Betreuungskontextes stets mit Einschränkungen in Bezug auf seine Krankheit einhergingen. Diese Dynamik erschwerte Tom die allmähliche Loslösung von den erwachsenen Bezugspersonen, in seinem Fall von den Eltern und den ErzieherInnen, sowie eine stärkere Anbindung an seine Peergruppe.

Die generelle Schwierigkeit für Jugendliche in der Adoleszenz, eine Balance zwischen Autonomiebestrebungen, Bindungsbedürfnissen und Loyalitätsverpflichtungen zu finden, gestaltete sich für Tom als besondere Herausforderung, da er nicht zuhause lebte. Demnach war es für die pädagogische Begleitung wichtig, nicht ausschließlich Toms Krankheit im Blick zu haben, sondern auch die Faktoren, welche seine Gesundheit und sein Wohlbefinden positiv beeinflussen konnten.

In Toms Fall wurden im Verlauf der Hilfsmaßnahme gemeinsam mit der Familie wichtige Ressourcen herausgefiltert, welche es Tom zukünftig erlauben sollten, mehr Zeit mit seiner Familie zu verbringen. Eine weitere Intervention war, dass die Familienbesuche nicht sofort reduziert wurden, wenn der Jugendliche nach dem Wochenende bei einem Elternteil mit zu hohen Blutzuckerwerten in die Einrichtung zurückkehrte.

Zusammenfassend für diesen Fall bleibt aus unserer Sicht festzuhalten, dass es von großer Bedeutung im Sinne des Fallverstehens ist, die eigene Aufmerksamkeit sowohl auf das Autonomiebestreben der Jugendlichen, die Bedürfnisse und Wahrnehmung innerhalb der Familie als auch auf die mögliche Erwartung und die Ängste des Fachpersonals zu richten. Erst dieses mehrdimensionale Verstehen mit der Beteiligung der Adressaten erlaubte es den pädagogischen Fachkräften, zieldienliche und gesundheitsfördernde Interventionen für den Jugendlichen und seine Familie zu entwickeln.

3.2 Der Umgang mit Ambivalenzen als gemeinsamer Prozess zwischen Jugendlichen und Fachkräften

Das folgende Fallbeispiel setzt den Fokus auf das Wohlbefinden und die Gesundheit einer Jugendlichen in der Kinder- und Jugendhilfe und die damit verknüpften Entwicklungsschritte sowie Grundbedürfnisse des Jugendalters im Kontext einer psychopharmakologischen Behandlung.

Der Fakt, dass Jugendliche immer häufiger begleitend zu psychologischen und psychotherapeutischen Behandlungen auch einer psychiatrischen und medikamentösen Therapie unterzogen werden, bringt mit sich, dass sich diese Jugendlichen und ihr Umfeld mit unterschiedlichen Herausforderungen konfrontiert sehen, die direkte Auswirkungen auf ihr Wohlbefinden und die Gesundheit haben.

Julia

Julia ist 16 Jahre alt und lebt seit 10 Jahren getrennt von ihrer Familie in unterschiedlichen stationären Kontexten.

Ihre Familie wurde bereits vor ihrer Geburt durch diverse Erziehungshilfemaßnahmen unterstützt. Julia fiel schon als Kind im Kindergarten durch aggressive Verhaltensweisen auf. Schwere körperliche Misshandlungen vonseiten des leiblichen Vaters sowie der Fakt, dass die Mutter davon wusste, sie jedoch nicht schützte, sondern vielmehr Julia zu Falschaussagen ermutigte, führten dazu, dass die Jugendliche erstmalig fremdplatziert wurde. Dies war der Beginn einer Aneinanderreihung von sich wiederholenden Entlassungen und sich anschließenden Wiederaufnahmen in diversen stationären Fremdunterbringungsstrukturen. Während dieser Zeit verschlechterte sich Julias Verhalten zusehends. Zu dem bereits in der frühen Kindheit gezeigten aggressiven Verhalten gesellten sich impulsive Verhaltensweisen, Schwierigkeiten, mit Erwachsenen in Kontakt zu treten, sowie delinquentes Verhalten. Auch die schulische Betreuung gestaltete sich zusehends schwieriger. Vor diesem Hintergrund wurde ihr im Alter von 8 Jahren zum ersten Mal, durch den Neurologen der Mutter, Ritalin verschrieben.

Im beginnenden Jugendalter wurde Julia aufgrund sexueller Übergriffigkeiten gegenüber einem Mitbewohner aus ihrer damaligen stationären Struktur verwiesen und anschließend in der Kinder- und Jugendpsychiatrie untergebracht. Schlussendlich wurde die Jugendliche in einer neuen stationären Jugendwohngruppe aufgenommen.

Zu diesem Zeitpunkt wurde die Medikation von Julia nach 6 Jahren zum ersten Mal medizinisch überprüft. Bedenkt man, dass unter der kontinuierlichen Anwendung von Psychopharmaka regelmäßige Überprüfungen von Organfunktionen (z. B. Blutdruck und Puls) erforderlich sind und die Dosierung stets dem Gewicht, der Größe und dem Alter des Kindes oder Jugendlichen angepasst sein muss, ist es sehr bedenklich, dass die Medikation erst nach diesem langen Zeitraum zum ersten Mal überdacht wurde. Außerdem empfehlen Leitlinien für die Behandlung der meisten Störungsbilder im psychischen Bereich eine Kombination aus Psychotherapie und Medikamenten, was eine regelmäßige Überprüfung der Indikation für die Gabe von Medikamenten notwendig macht. Auch diese Empfehlung wurde also über mehrere Jahre hinweg im Fall von Julia nicht berücksichtigt.

Diese fast schon willkürliche Verschreibung des Medikamentes ist nicht zuletzt auch darauf zurückzuführen, dass eine kontinuierliche psychotherapeutische Betreuung durch die häufigen Wechsel der Strukturen nicht gegeben war. Julia musste also schon sehr früh erfahren, dass erwachsene Menschen, zu denen sie ohnehin einen schwierigen Zugang hatte, wichtige Themen über ihren Kopf hinweg entschieden. Sie musste unter der Anleitung von Erwachsenen dauerhaft ein Medikament einnehmen und erlebte dann im Nachhinein, dass sich niemand wirklich verantwortlich fühlte, die Indikation des Medikamentes im Laufe der Jahre zu evaluieren. Dass sich daraus ein Gefühl des Ausgeliefertseins und eine Abwehr gegen die Medikation entwickelte, scheint verständlich. Ihren Unmut äußerte Julia immer wieder deutlich und wehrte sich lauthals gegen das Einnehmen des Medikamentes. Dagegen bezogen sich die ErzieherInnen auf die Verschreibung des behandelnden Psychiaters und forderten das regelmäßige Einnehmen des Medikamentes ein. Allerdings ist zu beachten, dass die Evaluation der Medikation durch den Psychiater immer nur auf Basis der von den Fachkräften geschilderten Beobachtungen gemacht werden konnte. „Bei der Behandlung von Kindern im Rahmen institutioneller Betreuung ergeben sich für den verordnenden Arzt oft insofern Schwierigkeiten, dass eine kontinuierliche Beobachtung durch eine Bezugsperson meist nicht möglich ist (Schichtdienst o. ä.). Um Symptome adäquat und vergleichbar einschätzen zu können, ist eine intensive Kommunikation von wesentlicher Bedeutung: zwischen den Betreuern, aber auch zwischen den Betreuern und dem behandelnden Arzt." (Kämmerling und Linck, 2016, S. 38).

Im Laufe der Begleitung stellte sich heraus, dass es Julia gelungen war, während eines Zeitraums von 12 Monaten kein Medikament einzunehmen, ohne dass die pädagogischen Fachkräfte dies bemerkt hatten. Gleichzeitig pochten sie darauf, dass Julias Verhalten laut ihren Beobachtungen ohne Medikament nicht mehr tragbar sei. Dies bestärkte erneut Julias Unbehagen gegenüber Medikamenten und führte dazu, dass sich ihr Bedürfnis nach Unabhängigkeit und Autonomie immer weiter ausprägte, was Julia auch zum Ausdruck brachte. So wollte sie eigenständig, zusammen mit dem zuständigen Psychiater, Entscheidungen in Bezug auf ihre Medikation treffen. Schließlich würden die Betreuer sie eh nicht verstehen und sie brauche daher auch niemanden, der für sie entscheide, so Julia. Sie würde dies gerne selbst bestimmen. Der behandelnde Psychiater reagierte darauf mit einem Versuch, das Medikament langsam abzusetzen, damit die Jugendliche weiterhin mit ihm kooperierte. Das Verhalten verschlechterte sich kurzzeitig, wobei es sich nach einer wichtigen Gerichtsverhandlung, bei der grundlegende Entscheidungen in Bezug auf ihre Familiensituation getroffen wurden, wieder verbesserte. Eine spätere Rückführung in die Herkunftsfamilie funktionierte gut. Obwohl Julia weiterhin kein Medikament einnahm, blieb ihr Verhalten stabil.

Julias Beispiel zeigt deutlich, wie wichtig es ist, Jugendliche in die Entscheidung zur Medikamentengabe mit einzubinden und sie mitbestimmen zu lassen. Ihre Meinung und Wahrnehmung in Bezug auf ihr eigenes Wohlbefinden sind dabei von zentraler Bedeutung, nicht das Empfinden der ErzieherInnen, ob das Verhalten des Jugendlichen ohne Medikament tragbar ist oder nicht. Nur auf diese Weise wird dem Bedürfnis nach Unabhängigkeit, Autonomie und Selbstbestimmung Rechnung getragen.

Genauso wichtig sind die Berücksichtigung und das Anerkennen eines grundlegenden körperlichen Wohlbefindens des Jugendlichen. Julia beschwerte sich zum Beispiel immer wieder über starke Nebenwirkungen des Medikamentes, wie Schlafprobleme und verminderter Appetit. Zusammen mit dem Jugendlichen sollte abgewogen werden, inwieweit die auftretenden Nebenwirkungen den Alltag beeinflussen respektive ob die Wirkung des Medikamentes einen höheren Nutzen hat als das körperliche Wohlbefinden.

Zudem hat das Bedürfnis der Integration in die Gruppe von Gleichaltrigen eine wichtige Bedeutung. Julia fühlte sich stets stigmatisiert durch das Medikament. Sie hatte Angst, es könnte etwas mit ihr nicht stimmen, da sie auf ein bestimmtes Medikament angewiesen sei, um richtig funktionieren zu können. Sie dachte, dass Gleichaltrige dies genauso sehen würden und sie darum meiden könnten. Dies führte dazu, dass sie sich zum Schutz vor schmerzlichen Erfahrungen erst gar nicht auf Beziehungen zu Gleichaltrigen einließ. Sie äußerte, dass sie darunter leide, als krank angesehen zu werden, obwohl sie sich nicht als krank empfand.

Aus Sicht einer partizipativen Haltung zeigt Julias Beispiel, wie wichtig es ist, Jugendliche als Experten ihrer eigenen Lebenssituation anzuerkennen und somit, aus Sicht der pädagogischen Fachkräfte, gemeinsam mit ihnen alternative Lösungen, in diesem Fall in Bezug auf die Medikation, zu finden. Nur so können Fachkräfte im Umgang mit Jugendlichen, die ein herausforderndes Verhalten im Alltag zeigen, Sicherheit gewinnen und andere Lösungsstrategien zulassen. Hier gilt es stets die Bedürfnisse der Heranwachsenden im Auge zu behalten, um somit einer eventuell kontraproduktiven (medikamentösen) Behandlung vorzubeugen.

3.3 Problematisch erlebtes Verhalten als Ausdruck unerfüllter Bedürfnisse

Im abschließenden Fallbeispiel liegt der Fokus darauf, wie Jugendliche psychische Belastungen durch ein körperliches und soziales Verhalten zum Ausdruck bringen können, das häufig als problematisch erlebt wird. Zudem wird dargestellt, wie im Heimkontext darauf reagiert werden kann, um eine Verkörperung der „Symptome" zu verhindern.

Marie
Marie ist 16 Jahre alt und befindet sich seit ihrem 8. Lebensjahr in stationärer Unterbringung.

Im Verlauf ihrer Kindheit äußerte sich Maries Problematik in Einnässen, Albträumen, Schlafstörungen und auffälligem Sexualverhalten. Später im Jugendalter zeigten sich zudem aggressives und oppositionelles Verhalten, Drogenkonsum, Essstörungen und selbstverletzendes Verhalten.

Rückblickend auf Maries erste Lebensjahre in ihrer Herkunftsfamilie, könnte ihr distanzloses und von wenig Selbstwert zeugendes Verhalten auf die fehlenden Bezugspersonen, die keine stabile Bindungsentwicklung zuließen, zurückgeführt werden. Maries Vater verstarb an Krebs, als sie ein Säugling war. Ihre Mutter litt an Depressionen und konnte ihrer Rolle als wichtige Bindungsperson nicht gerecht werden. Der Kontakt zwischen Mutter und Tochter zeichnete sich seit der Unterbringung als sehr unregelmäßig und unverlässlich aus. Durch die Abwesenheit der Eltern fehlten Marie im frühen Kindheitsalter verlässliche, empathische Bezugspersonen, um eine sichere Bindung aufbauen zu können. Sie konnte daher wesentliche Schutzfaktoren im Leben nicht entwickeln. Ebenso fiel es ihr schwer, Emotionen zuzulassen, auszudrücken und zu regulieren. Da sie von Kindheit an sehr auf sich allein gestellt war und auch bereits früh ein großes Verantwortungsbewusstsein für das Wohlergehen ihrer psychisch stark belasteten Mutter entwickelte, konnte Marie außerdem keine Strategien zur Bewältigung von Herausforderungen und Konflikten erlernen und umsetzen.

Allgemein waren bei Marie bereits im frühen Jugendalter wenig Selbsteinschätzung hinsichtlich ihrer psychischen und physischen Gesundheit, keine Gefahreneinschätzung oder sexueller Schutz und eine gewisse Abgestumpftheit zu beobachten. Früh entwickelte sie außerdem ein aktives Sexualverhalten. Nach einer gynäkologischen Untersuchung wurde eine Geschlechtskrankheit bei der Jugendlichen diagnostiziert. Auf die Sorge der ErzieherInnen reagierte Marie mit Teilnahmslosigkeit.

Bezugnehmend auf Grawe (2004) könnte man annehmen, dass die Erfahrung von Vernachlässigung sowie geringe emotionale und liebevolle Kontakte zu ihren primären Bezugspersonen Marie daran gehindert haben, eine stabile psychische Struktur und Ressourcen zur Krisenbewältigung aufzubauen. Möglicherweise wurde der Aufbau einer sicheren Bindung dadurch erschwert, dass die Grundbedürfnisse im frühen Kindheitsalter nicht befriedigt wurden. Mit Blick auf die fehlenden positiven Beziehungserfahrungen in ihrer frühen Kindheit ließe sich auch Maries niedriges Selbstwertgefühl erklären.

Maries exzessives Weglaufen im Jugendalter und ihr Drang, sich gegen die Unterbringung im stationären Kontext zu wehren, könnten als Zeichen für ihr Bedürfnis nach Kontrolle und Orientierung interpretiert werden. So kamen die ErzieherInnen zur Hypothese, dass Marie durch das Weglaufen über ihre Perspektive und ihre Situation mitbestimmen konnte und gleichzeitig ihr im Jugendalter immer stärker werdendes Bedürfnis nach Unabhängigkeit erfüllt wurde.

Den Beobachtungen der pädagogischen Fachkräfte im Alltag zufolge fehlten Marie notwendige Ressourcen, Selbstwirksamkeitserfahrungen und die Fähigkeit, Konflikte zu lösen. Dies alles führte bei ihr zu großen Frustrationen. So richtete Marie in vielen Momenten erlebte Gewalt im familiären Kontext sowie tiefsitzende Verletzungen und Enttäuschungen in Form von Aggressionen gegen sich selbst. Die inneren Spannungszustände und Ambivalenzen zeigten sich auch in Form von distanzlosem sexuellem Verhalten, Drogen- und Alkoholkonsum sowie Suizidversuchen.

Marie hatte zudem seit ihrer Kindheit Übergewicht, verfügte aber abgesehen davon über einen guten Gesundheitszustand. Im Heimkontext war ihr Körpergewicht im Hinblick auf das gesundheitliche Wohlbefinden immer wieder Thema. So wurde sie durch die BetreuerInnen motiviert, sich in verschiedenen Sportvereinen zu integrieren. Die ErzieherInnen arbeiteten gemeinsam mit Marie an der Zielsetzung, mit Hilfe von gesunder und regelmäßiger Ernährung ihr Gewicht zu reduzieren. In vielen Austauschgesprächen wurde die Notwendigkeit von Diäten und einer Ernährungsberatung diskutiert. Hinzu kam, dass Marie große Schwierigkeiten hatte, soziale Kontakte zu knüpfen. Sie konnte sich nicht auf Beziehungen einlassen und schottete sich sehr von Gleichaltrigen ab. Die vermehrte Thematisierung ihrer körperlichen Erscheinung trug dazu bei, dass sie sich stets als minderwertig und nicht gut genug empfand. Sie konnte ihrem im Jugendalter zunehmenden Bedürfnis nach Zugehörigkeit und Zuneigung nicht gerecht werden.

Einerseits fühlten sich die ErzieherInnen dazu verpflichtet, Maries Körpergewicht als einen Gesundheitsfaktor zu betrachten, den es galt zu kontrollieren, um ihr Wohlbefinden zu gewährleisten. Andererseits schien die Jugendliche durch die körperliche Erfahrung des Essens lustvolle und erfreuliche Momente herbeizuführen. So galt es Maries Verlangen nach Essen nicht nur als defizitär anzusehen, sondern auch als Ressource und Ausgleich, um darauf aufzubauen. Ihre Leidenschaft wurde durch gemeinsames Kochen und Backen gefördert. So konnten ihre Fähigkeit und ihr Wunsch, sich selbst Gutes zu tun, gestärkt werden.

In Maries Fall stellte sich die Frage, welches Bedürfnis sich hinter ihren „Symptomen" versteckte. Mit Blick auf die Bedürfnisse im Jugendalter handelte es sich möglicherweise um eine Art der Selbstbestätigung, die sie woanders nicht bekam. Aber auch der Wunsch nach Sicherheit, Unabhängigkeit und Zugehörigkeit konnte in Maries Verhalten beobachtet werden. Daher war es aus professioneller Sicht wichtig, Maries Selbstbewusstsein zu stärken und ihr im Alltag die notwendige Zuneigung zu geben, wenn es ihr nicht gut ging. Dies bedeutete, ihr auch in schwierigen Situationen bedingungslose Wertschätzung entgegenzubringen. Durch das Angebot verlässlicher Beziehungen im stationären

Kontext konnte Marie mit der Zeit wieder Beziehungen zu anderen Menschen aufbauen. Die Anbindung an therapeutische Maßnahmen, sportliche Aktivitäten, viele Vieraugengespräche mit den ErzieherInnen und die Stärkung ihres Selbstbewusstseins halfen Marie ihren Körper zu akzeptieren. Sie entwickelte ihm gegenüber ein Gefühl der Sensibilität und Achtsamkeit.

In Bezug auf Maries Fall war es wichtig, die unerfüllten Bedürfnisse hinter ihrem Verhalten zu erfassen. Die intensive, beständige Beziehungsarbeit mit der Jugendlichen galt als Basis für ihre Stabilisierung. Im Heimkontext wurde ihr außerdem durch klare Regeln und Strukturen ein sicherer Rahmen geboten. Die durch die körperliche und seelische Reifung bedingten Veränderungen akzentuierten den Wunsch nach Sicherheit. Aber auch die Möglichkeit der Partizipation an wesentlichen Entscheidungsprozessen gab ihr ein Gefühl von Kontrolle und Orientierung. Durch Erfolgserlebnisse konnte sie Selbstwirksamkeit erfahren und in ihrem Selbstbewusstsein gestärkt werden. Durch eine enge, wertschätzende und akzeptierende Betreuung der ErzieherInnen konnte Marie im Alltag des stationären Kontextes neue Erfahrungen im Hinblick auf die Befriedigung ihrer Bedürfnisse nach Zugehörigkeit, Unabhängigkeit und Selbstentwicklung machen sowie vorhandene Ressourcen wiederentdecken und ausbauen.

4 Ausblick: Implikationen für präventive und gesundheitsfördernde Ansätze im stationären Kontext

Jugendliche befinden sich in einer Phase ihres Lebens, welche geprägt ist durch Veränderungen, neue Entwicklungsaufgaben und Unsicherheiten. Im stationären Heimkontext kommen häufig erschwerende Ausgangsbedingungen durch die Heimunterbringung selbst, zerrüttete Familienverhältnisse und traumatische Erlebnisse hinzu.

Rückblickend auf die oben beschriebenen Fallbeispiele zum Thema „Wohlbefinden und Gesundheit von Jugendlichen im stationären Kontext", haben sich folgende präventive und gesundheitsfördernde Ansätze in unserer Praxis sehr positiv bewährt.

a) Eine *mehrperspektivische* Sichtweise auf den gesamten Lebenskontext ist für die soziale Arbeit mit jungen und meist traumatisierten Menschen unentbehrlich. Auf Grundlage des bio-psycho-sozialen Modells können die wechselseitige Beeinflussung und die voneinander abhängigen Wirkungen auf der

Ebene von Person, Beziehung, Umfeld bzw. System betrachtet werden (Pauls 2013).

Es gilt die Multidimensionalität des auffälligen Verhaltens auf der körperlichen, psychischen und sozialen Ebene zu erfassen. Folgende Fragen können dabei hilfreich sein: Was sind die Hinweise auf das Problem? Welche Personen sind involviert, welche Faktoren rufen das als problemhaft empfundene Verhalten hervor und halten es aufrecht? Welche unerfüllten Bedürfnisse stecken hinter dem Verhalten? Über welche Ressourcen verfügen die Jugendlichen? Verfügen sie über ein soziales Netzwerk (ebd., S. 205ff.)? Fehlende persönliche und soziale Ressourcen, Entwicklungsanforderungen und Belastungen aus dem Umfeld sowie problematische Selbsteinschätzungen können hierdurch herauskristallisiert werden. Diese Faktoren blockieren eine positive Entwicklung der Jugendlichen und fördern häufig problematische Bewältigungsstrategien (ebd., S.117).

b) Des Weiteren spielt der, im Konzept der *Salutogenese* verankerte Begriff des *Kohärenzgefühls* eine sehr wichtige Rolle in der subjektiven Wahrnehmung der Gesundheit. Nach Antonovsky (1997) bestimmt diese Grundhaltung, wie gut Menschen ihre vorhandenen Ressourcen nutzen können. Sie wird im Laufe der Kindheit und Jugend von den jeweiligen Erfahrungen geprägt, die der Mensch in dieser Zeit macht. Was hält den Menschen gesund bzw. was hilft ihm, wieder gesund zu werden? Wie entwickelt er ein starkes Kohärenzgefühl? Das Konzept des Kohärenzgefühls beschreibt die Fähigkeit, angesichts vielfältiger gesellschaftlicher Optionen ein Gefühl von Verstehbarkeit, Sinnhaftigkeit und Handhabbarkeit (drei Grundkomponenten des Kohärenzgefühls) zu entwickeln. Nach Antonovsky (1997) entscheiden soziale Ressourcen und Belastungen mit darüber, in welchem Ausmaß das Kohärenzgefühl und die damit verbundene Fähigkeit, in Belastungssituationen über ein flexibles Bewältigungsinstrumentarium zu verfügen, entwickelt werden können. Antonovsky geht davon aus, dass das Kohärenzgefühl entscheidend für den Umgang mit Gesundheit und die Entwicklung von Resilienzfaktoren ist (Wydler et al. 2010). Für einen Jugendlichen, wie er im ersten Fallbeispiel beschrieben wird, ist es schwierig, ein solches Kohärenzgefühl zu entwickeln. In Toms Fall ist die „Verstehbarkeit" für ihn selbst nur begrenzt möglich, da verschiedene kognitive Prozesse in Bezug auf das Verständnis der Unterbringung wie auch im Hinblick auf das Verständnis im Umgang mit seiner Krankheit nicht umsetzbar sind. Somit wird auch die Handhabbarkeit seines Diabetes schwieriger. Diese Handhabbarkeit zeigt sich gerade in Situationen, in denen er einfach nur mit seiner Peergruppe etwas unternimmt, wo zum Beispiel spontanes Essen eine große Rolle spielt. Er will dann nur ein „ganz

normaler" Jugendlicher sein und nicht auffallen, indem er spezielle Essge-
wohnheiten zeigt und Messungen an seinem Körper durchführt. „Bedeutsamkeit": Für ihn steht der Diabetes in direktem Zusammenhang mit der
Unterbringung, also der Trennung von seiner Mutter. Gut mit der Krankheit
umzugehen, führt bei Tom zu ambivalenten Gefühlen wie zum Beispiel zu
dem Gefühl, seiner Mutter gegenüber nicht loyal zu sein. Zudem ist bei ihm
ständig eine gewisse Angst präsent, die Rückführung zur Mutter könnte nicht
realisierbar sein, wenn seine Werte nur bei den Aufenthalten zuhause schlecht
sind.

In Bezug auf Maries Situation wird die Entwicklung von Verstehbarkeit und
Achtsamkeit gegenüber sich selbst erst über das Anknüpfen der Fachkräfte an
wichtige Bedürfnisse und Themen der Jugendlichen möglich.

Eine salutogenetische Sichtweise mit Blick auf Ressourcen, positive
Erfahrungen und neue Bewältigungsmuster ist wichtig für eine positive Veränderung. Es gilt dabei den Fokus nicht zu sehr auf die „Thematisierung"
und „Aktivierung" der Symptomatik oder des Problems zu legen, sondern
vielmehr die Konflikte, Probleme und Schwierigkeiten hinter der nach außen
hin sichtbaren Symptomatik aufzudecken. Gesundheit, Krankheit und Beeinträchtigung können somit als biografisch und in sozialen Milieus verankert
gesehen werden. Erst bei der Betrachtung einer Person in ihrer Umgebung
kann ein Zusammenhang zwischen den Bedürfnissen nach Selbstwert, Selbstregulation, sozial-emotionalen Beziehungen und sozialer Unterstützung hergestellt und eine Intervention in die Wege geleitet werden (Gahleitner und
Pauls 2014).

c) Mit den wesentlichen Entwicklungsaufgaben der Adoleszenz gehen Grundbedürfnisse einher, auf welche bei Jugendlichen aus schwierigen Herkunfts-
verhältnissen häufig nicht adäquat reagiert werden kann. Umso wichtiger
erscheint es, dass *partizipative Strategien* in der Arbeit mit den Jugendlichen
und ihrem Umfeld im stationären Kontext verankert sind. Es ist notwendig,
die Jugendlichen und ihre Familie in alle Entscheidungsprozesse (Alltag,
Hilfeplan, Gesundheitsmaßnahmen) miteinzubeziehen. Dies kann zu einer
Förderung des Selbstwertgefühls und der Selbstwirksamkeit beitragen. Die
Jugendlichen und ihre Familie werden hierdurch als wichtig und kompetent
wahrgenommen. Durch transparentes Kommunizieren und Handeln können
Loyalitätskonflikte oder Machtgefälle vermieden werden. Die Partizipation
der Jugendlichen wird somit nicht allein durch vorstrukturierte Regel-
anwendungen erreicht, sondern benötigt eine gegenseitige Bereitschaft zur
Kooperation. Die ErzieherInnen und die Jugendlichen müssen sich einig
sein über das Ziel, das es zu erreichen gilt, und über den Weg, der dorthin

führt. Erziehung zur Selbstständigkeit und Selbstverantwortung heißt, die Jugendlichen ihrem Alter und Entwicklungsgrad entsprechend an allen sie betreffenden Entscheidungen zu beteiligen.

Es ist wichtig, dass die ErzieherInnen pädagogische Prozesse initiieren, in denen eine Balance gefunden wird zwischen dem altersangepassten Autonomiebestreben der Jugendlichen (sie wollen Freiheit, Unabhängigkeit und ein Recht auf Selbstbestimmung) und deren Einbindung in die Alltagsstrukturen der Lebensgruppe, was stärker ihrem Bedürfnis nach Zugehörigkeit entspricht. Für alle Jugendlichen sollte ein als positiv erlebtes Zusammenleben in der Lebensgruppe geschaffen werden, wo jedem Jugendlichen die Möglichkeit geboten wird, ein individuelles, auf den eigenen Ressourcen aufbauendes Lebensprojekt zu entwickeln und mitzubestimmen.

Es muss dabei gelingen, an die Wirklichkeitskonstruktionen der Jugendlichen (und ihrer Familien) anzuknüpfen, um gemeinsam Veränderungen in den Denk- und Handlungsmustern anzuregen. Es ist davon auszugehen, dass sowohl Jugendliche als auch Eltern versuchen, ihr bisheriges System und ihre Überzeugungen aufrechtzuerhalten. Genau hieran gilt es anzuknüpfen. Am Beispiel von Tom wird dies deutlich, indem die Loyalität in Bezug zu seiner Mutter von den ErzieherInnen gewürdigt und akzeptiert wird.

Es ist wichtig, als pädagogische Fachkraft mit einer systemischen Perspektive eigene Wirklichkeitskonstruktionen (z. B.: Was mir guttut, muss also auch dem anderen guttun) nicht auf die Jugendlichen zu übertragen. Die wertschätzende Kommunikation mit den Jugendlichen ist ein grundlegendes Element in der alltäglichen Zusammenarbeit und in der Erfassung ihrer Bedürfnisse.

d) Darüber hinaus sollten sich die Fachkräfte bewusst sein, dass ein partizipativer, ressourcenorientierter Ansatz zu einer *ambivalenten Rollenausgestaltung,* zwischen der Umsetzung des Schutzauftrags einerseits und der Wertschätzung gegenüber den Bedürfnissen der jungen Menschen andererseits, führen kann. Es gilt diese Ambivalenzen bewusst zu gestalten und konstruktiv sowie zieldienlich für den Hilfeprozess zu nutzen.

Anhand der drei Fallbeispiele wird klar, dass das sozialpädagogische Fachpersonal oft hin- und hergerissen ist zwischen protektiven Interventionen in Bezug auf die physische und psychische Gesundheit der Jugendlichen, und dem Wissen, dass eine Zusammenarbeit mit dem Jugendlichen nur dann funktioniert, wenn er sich in der Interaktion als selbstbestimmt erlebt. Wie das Fallbeispiel von Julia zeigt, wird die Einnahme von Medikamenten, welche dem Bereich der Neuroleptika zugeordnet werden, als besonders fremdbestimmt von ihr erfahren. Jugendliche, die sich in einer medikamentösen

Behandlung befinden, fühlen sich oft auch körperlich unwohl, da verschiedene Nebenwirkungen dieser Medikamente deutlich spürbar sind. Zusätzlich zum Schutzauftrag sehen sich die ErzieherInnen in der Verantwortung, für die Sicherheit der anderen Mitbewohner und Mitarbeiter zu sorgen. Wie im genannten Fallbeispiel erleben die ErzieherInnen die Jugendliche z. B. als aggressiv und unberechenbar, wogegen mit der Einnahme der Medikamente aus ihrer Sicht eine gewisse „Ruhe" eintritt. Somit spielt auch oft die Angst eine wesentliche Rolle, die Gruppendynamik wieder zu destabilisieren, sollten die Medikamente abgesetzt werden. Hier ist es sehr wichtig, mit dem Jugendlichen und seinem Umfeld zusammen alle möglichen Optionen in Bezug auf seine Gesundheit mit allen Vor- und Nachteilen zu besprechen, da eine medikamentöse Behandlung doch als sehr invasiv erlebt werden kann.

Eine ähnliche Ambivalenz in den erzieherischen Interventionen wird auch in den Fallbeispielen von Tom und Marie deutlich. Bei Tom ist es die Angst der Fachkräfte, dass die Symptome des Diabetes sich verschlimmern könnten, sollte keine genaue Kontrolle der Ernährung und der Regulierung seiner Insulingaben erfolgen. Die ErzieherInnen erleben jedoch parallel, dass Tom sich sehr unwohl fühlt, da er diese Begleitung als Einschränkung und Kontrolle in seinem Alltag erlebt.

Marie hat über Jahre immer mehr an Gewicht zugelegt. Die ErzieherInnen sorgen sich, dass eine weitere Zunahme zu schwerwiegenden Gesundheitsproblemen führen könnte und fühlen sich natürlich dazu verpflichtet, Marie täglich beim gemeinsamen Essen zu bremsen. Dies wiederum führt zu einer angespannten Situation.

e) Es stellt sich also die Frage, wie *günstige Rahmenbedingungen* geschaffen werden können, in denen sich der betroffene Jugendliche nach seinen eigenen Wünschen und Möglichkeiten verändern kann, dies immer im Hinblick auf Wohlbefinden und Gesundheit. Wie kann eine dynamische Interaktion zwischen belastenden und entlastenden sowie schützenden Rahmenbedingungen aufgebaut werden? Wie kann der Jugendliche in seiner Selbstwirksamkeit unterstützt werden, sodass er die Hilfemaßnahme der stationären Unterbringung akzeptieren und sie aktiv mitgestalten kann, um seine Gesundheit und sein Wohlbefinden zu fördern? Wichtig ist, dass alle Fachkräfte eine Neugier in die Gespräche einbringen, bewusst zuhören können und auch erfragen, was momentan beim jungen Menschen gut läuft. Was will der Jugendliche? Was kann der Jugendliche selbst tun? Welche Ressourcen und Kompetenzen hat er bereits? Welche Bedürfnisse liegen seinem Verhalten und seinen Schlussfolgerungen zugrunde?

Die praktische Arbeit in der stationären Jugendhilfe ist anspruchsvoll, da es gilt unterschiedlichen Anforderungen im Alltag gerecht zu werden und dabei stets die Notwendigkeit besteht, mehrere Perspektiven miteinzubeziehen. Die pädagogischen Fachkräfte brauchen also Handlungsstrategien und das notwendige Fachwissen, um auch schwieriges und sich wiederholendes symptomatisches Verhalten von Jugendlichen zu bewältigen und gegebenenfalls neu zu interpretieren. Dies setzt eine hohe Reflexionsfähigkeit und -bereitschaft voraus. Es ist wichtig, dass die pädagogischen Fachkräfte über konstruktive Strategien verfügen, die eigene Handlungsfähigkeit in schwierigen und herausfordernden Situationen aufrechtzuerhalten. Für diese Prozesse müssen ein spezifisches Bewusstsein und die notwendige Achtsamkeit in den jeweiligen Teams etabliert sein. Spezifische Fortbildung und Supervisionen helfen dieses Fachwissen und Bewusstsein aufzubauen. Darüber hinaus wird in unseren Strukturen das Vertrauen bei den Fachkräften gefördert, im Bedarfsfall Unterstützung und Hilfe im Teamzusammenhang zu suchen.

Um dieses Qualitätsniveau auf der Ebene des Fachpersonals mittelfristig zu garantieren, sind für uns Personalfürsorge sowie Entlastungs- und Schutzkonzepte in Bezug auf die psychische und emotionale Gesundheit der ErzieherInnen wichtige Bausteine in der Weiterentwicklung unserer Strukturen. Hierzu gehören z. B. Krisenverfahrenspläne, die die Begleitung von Jugendlichen als auch von betroffenen Fachkräften in sehr belastenden Situationen absichern, teaminterne Entlastungsstrategien und Verantwortungsaufteilung, aber auch regelmäßige Supervision und Fortbildung.

Somit kann ein günstiger Entwicklungsprozess für die Jugendlichen ermöglicht werden. Es ist wichtig, ihre individuellen Sichtweisen zu berücksichtigen und den Weg gemeinsam mit ihnen zu gehen. Erst wenn die Anforderungen es wert sind, sich dafür anzustrengen, und sie für die Jugendlichen einen subjektiven Sinn ergeben, kann ein gesunder Umgang mit ihrem Körper und der Befriedigung ihrer Bedürfnisse ermöglicht werden. Indem die individuellen Ressourcen stetig fokussiert und hervorgehoben werden, lässt sich bei den Jugendlichen ein Gefühl der Selbstwirksamkeit und Handlungsfähigkeit erreichen.

Literatur

Antonovsky, A. (1997). *Salutogenese. Zur Entmystizierung der Gesundheit.* Tübingen: Deutsche Gesellschaft für Verhaltenstherapie.

Arcus asbl. Elektronisches Dokument: https://www.arcus.lu/15/heimunterbringung. Zugegriffen: 4. März 2020.

Gahleitner, S. & Pauls, H. (2014). Biopsychosoziale Diagnostik als Voraussetzung für eine klinisch-sozialarbeiterische Interventionsgestaltung: Ein variables Grundmodell. In S. Gahleitner, G. Hahn, & Glemser R., *Psychosoziale Diagnostik: Klinische Sozialarbeit Band 5. (Klinische Sozialarbeit - Beiträge zur psychosozialen Praxis und Forschung.)* (S. 61–79). Köln Psychiatrie Verlag.

Grawe, K. (1999). Gründe und Vorschläge für eine allgemeine Psychotherapie. *Psychotherapeut* , S. 350–359.

Grawe, K. (2004). *Neuropsychoitherapie.* Göttingen: Hogrefe Verlag.

Kämmerling, L. & Linck, B. (2016). Heißes Eisen Psychopharmaka. *Jugendhilfe aktuell,* S. 37–39.

MENJE/ONE (2020). Aide et assistance - statistiques et études. Avril 2020. Elektronisches Dokument. https //men.public.lu/fr/publications/statistiques-etudes/aide-assistance/2004-aa-chiffres.html. Zugegriffen: 20.10.2020.

Pauls, H. (2013). *Klinische Sozialarbeit. Grundlagen und Methoden psychosozialer Behandlung (3. Auflage).* Weinheim und Basel: Beltz Juventa.

Quenzel, G. & Hurrelmann, K. (2012). *Lebensphase Jugend.* Weinheim und Basel: Beltz Juventa.

Rademaker, A. L. (2018). *Agency und Gesundheit in jugendlichen Lebenswelten - Herausforderungen für die Kinder- und Jugendhilfe. Mit einem Vorwort von Holger Ziegler (Prävention im Kindes- und Jugendalter).* Weinheim und Basel: Beltz Juventa.

Remschmidt, H., Quaschner, K., & Theisen, F. M. (2005). *Kinder- und Jugendpsychiatrie - Eine praktische Einführung.*

Schmid, M. (2007). *Psychische Gesundheit von Heimkindern: Eine Studie zur Prävalenz psychischer Störungen in der stationären Jugendhilfe.* Juventa.

Schneider, W. & Lindenberger U. (2018). *Entwicklungspsychologie.* 8., überarbeitete Auflage. Weinheim: Beltz.

Wüsten, G. & Pauls , H. (2013). In. H. Pauls, P. Stockmann , & M. Reicherts, *Beratungskompetenzen für die psychosoziale Fallarbeit - ein sozialtherapeutisches Profil* (p. 127 + 36). Freiburg: Lambertus Verlag.

Wydler, H., Kolip, P. & Abel, T. (2010) *Salutogenese und Kohärenzgefühl: Grundlagen, Empirie und Praxis eines gesundheitswissenschaftlichen Konzepts.* Weinheim und Basel: Juventa.

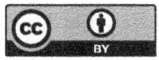

(Sucht)Prävention zwischen Restriktion, normativen Erwartungen und unterstützender Begleitung zur Gestaltung psychischer Gesundheit

Thérèse Michaelis, Jean-Paul Nilles und Uwe C. Fischer

1   Einleitung

„Bevor das Kind in den Brunnen fällt" ist nicht selten der Anspruch an Präventionsarbeit aus der Sicht der breiten Öffentlichkeit, aber auch von Geldgebern und Experten/innen. Der vorliegende Artikel versucht diesen Zugang kritisch zu hinterfragen, die Zielsetzungen an Präventionsarbeit differenzierter zu formulieren und vor allem von einem Verständnis einer möglichen Zauberformel für gefährdete, defizit- und problembehafteter Objekte zu „ent-führen". Mit dem Wissen um die praktische Umsetzung suchtpräventiver Arbeit wird im ersten Teil des Artikels der theoretische Unterbau für eine subjektorientierte Präventionsarbeit gelegt. Nachfolgend werden dann anhand der bisherigen Suchtpräventionsarbeit in Luxemburg am Beispiel des „CePT – Centre de Prévention des Toxicomanies" im Zeitraum 1995–2015 praktische Zugänge erörtert, um abschließend einen reflektierten Ausblick auf die Suchtprävention als emanzipative Bildungsarbeit und Förderung psychischer Gesundheit zu geben.

T. Michaelis
Rumelange, Luxemburg

J.-P. Nilles
Schifflange, Luxemburg

U. C. Fischer (✉)
Institut für Psychologie, Otto-Friedrich-Universität Bamberg, Bamberg, Deutschland
E-Mail: uwe.fischer@uni-bamberg.de

© Der/die Autor(en) 2022
A. Heinen et al. (Hrsg.), *Wohlbefinden und Gesundheit im Jugendalter,*
https://doi.org/10.1007/978-3-658-35744-3_27

2   Ein kritischer Blick auf die Zauberformel –
was soll, oder könnte (Sucht)Prävention sein?

Mit Prävention werden üblicherweise all jene Aktivitäten bezeichnet, die darauf abzielen, jemandem oder etwas zuvorzukommen (lat.: praevenire = zuvorkommen): vorbeugen, verhindern, vorbauen, verhüten, schützen, abwenden, sich versichern, zuvorkommen, abfangen, vereiteln, abwehren, ersparen, verunmöglichen, ablenken, nicht aufkommen oder entstehen lassen, unterbinden, abstellen, sich kümmern um, immunisieren und vieles andere mehr (vgl. Lüders 2011). Man tut etwas, *bevor* ein bestimmtes Ereignis oder ein bestimmter Zustand eintritt, damit dies nicht eintritt oder zumindest der Zeitpunkt des Eintretens hinausgeschoben wird oder die Folgen begrenzt werden. Alle Hoffnungen liegen demzufolge darin, dass per Präventionsmaßnahmen Schaden und Gefährdungen abgewendet oder verhindert werden können. Um dementsprechend gezielt zu intervenieren, so die Annahme und Vorgabe, löst die Prävention einen Ausschnitt aus der Wirklichkeit heraus, stellt Zusammenhänge zwischen gegenwärtigen Phänomenen und künftigen Ereignissen oder Zuständen her und konstruiert daraus ihr eigenes Aktionsfeld (Bröckling 2008, S. 39). So auch bei der Suchtprävention, wo das Phänomen Sucht, Abhängigkeit oder seit DSM 5 die Suchtmittelgebrauchsstörungen in den Mittelpunkt befürchteter Gefährdungen und demzufolge präventiver Maßnahmen gestellt werden. Während die fachliche Diagnose auf das Verhalten abzielt, wird von Außenstehenden zumeist nur die Substanz als sichtbare Gefahr gesehen. Eigentlich könnte deren Existenz niemanden stören, wären da nicht die Befürchtungen, dass diese Substanzen von Menschen konsumiert und die Einnahme eben bei diesen Menschen Störungen z. B. Suchtmittelgebrauchsstörungen auslösen würden.

Dass die „Droge" oder das damit verbundene Verhalten nur Mittel zum Zweck eines potenziell dysfunktionalen Umgangs mit der psychischen Gesundheit ist, wird häufig ignoriert. Die eigentlich „gebrauchende" Person wird in dem Moment zur von der Droge verführten passiven und damit hilfsbedürftigen abhängigen Person. Der hinter dem Substanzgebrauch stehende Mensch mit seinem Bedürfnis nach psychischem Wohlergehen im Kontext seines sozialen Umfelds erscheint zu komplex, nicht sichtbar und damit auch wenig greifbar. Die WHO-Definition zur Gesundheitsförderung (WHO 1986) mit ihren daraus ableitbaren Handlungsstrategien zur Unterstützung des Wohlergehens und ihres Setting Ansatzes, der auf das soziale Umfeld fokussiert, wird bei dieser Präventionssichtweise kaum in Betracht gezogen. Die Schuld auf eine „böse" Droge zu schieben, lenkt potenziell am besten von der eigenen Verantwortlichkeit ab.

Während die Kleinkinder meist noch in der Obhut der Eltern gesehen und von diesen beschützt werden (sollen) und die Erwachsenen sich selbst eher nicht als Zielgruppe suchtpräventiver Bemühungen verstehen, werden Kinder und insbesondere Jugendliche als „beliebteste" Zielgruppe suchtpräventiver Maßnahmen „erkoren". Wird doch die Phase Jugend als ein Werden verstanden, d. h. als ein noch nicht als [Erwachsen-]Sein definiert: „Hoffentlich übersteht sie/er das gut". Mit dem „Das" ist für viele die ganze Jugendzeit gemeint, ohne genau zu wissen wie lange diese gefährliche Zeit im Leben dauern mag. „Immer früher werden die Kinder zu Jugendlichen und immer später die Jugendlichen zu Erwachsenen. Die/der „junge Volljährige" gilt als noch nicht erwachsen, weil sie/er in den meisten Fällen keinen „tragfähigen gesellschaftlich anerkannten Grund unter den Füßen hat" (vgl. Kappeler 2007, S. 293). Die Altersspanne ‚Jugend' wird im alltäglichen Diskurs „[…] in erster Linie negativ als Defizit, als biopsychosozialer Mangel (an körperlicher und psychischer Reife, an sozialer Selbständigkeit etc…), als individuelle und gesellschaftliche Störung (individuell infolge psychischer Instabilität, gesellschaftlich infolge von Kriminalität und Gewalt), als Gefahr und Gefährdung oder neuerdings als Risiko (durch selbst- und/oder fremdgefährdendes Gesundheits-, Konsum-, Freizeit-Verhalten etc…) – in jedem Fall aber als ein soziales Problem gefasst" (Anhorn 2011, S. 24). Anhorn (2002) weist diese Negativität mit Einschränkungen auch für den wissenschaftlichen Diskurs im Bereich der (Drogenkonsum-)prävention nach, die selbst in der heutigen Zeit, wenn auch entdramatisiert und impliziter (z. B. entwicklungsbedingtes Risikoverhalten), noch präsent ist.

In einer solchen Diktion wird all zu leicht vergessen, dass es in dieser Altersphase vor allem darum geht, zu erfahren, wer man ist, sowie einen persönlichen Stil zu entwickeln und zum Ausdruck zu bringen. Es geht um Identitätssuche und -findung. Es geht dabei auch um Demonstration von Unabhängigkeit von Eltern, gar um bewusste Verletzung elterlicher Kontrolle, um gewollte Normverletzung und darum, ein eigenes Wertesystem und ein eigenes Normgefüge zu entwickeln. Auf diesem wichtigen und entwicklungsbedingt notwendigen Weg der Identitätsfindung und Individuation werden neue Freundschaften, intime Beziehungen etc. aufgebaut, zu denen auch Spaß haben und Genießen gehört (vgl. z. B. die funktionelle Rolle des Substanzkonsums bei den Entwicklungsaufgaben, Silbereisen und Reese 2001). Man könnte glauben, manche Erwachsene hätten ihr Langzeitgedächtnis verloren, sie könnten (oder wollten) sich nicht mehr erinnern, dass auch sie als Kinder und Jugendliche nicht nur „brav" waren und vor allem, wie wichtig diese eigenständigen Schritte der Aneignung der sie umgebenden Welt für ihre Persönlichkeit waren.

An dieser Stelle gilt es den Präventionsbegriff hinsichtlich seiner Funktionalität auf die Reproduktion sozialer und gesellschaftlicher Normalität hin zu denken, womit Strategien sozialer Kontrolle ins Blickfeld rücken. Es muss danach gefragt werden, ab wann und in welcher Weise gut gemeinte pädagogische Maßnahmen nicht auch in den Verdacht geraten, zu einer „Kolonialisierung der Lebenswelt" (Habermas), zu einer Entmündigungspädagogik, die auf Hilfsbedürftigkeit schließt und auf Beseitigung und Schutz vor Defiziten und möglichen Problemen schielt. Damit steht ebenso die Frage nach dem Menschenbild hinter den Präventionsgedanken, das es offenzulegen gilt.

Und, was wird von Prävention „von oben", d. h. von ihren Auftrags- und Geldgebenden erwartet? Dies führt uns nochmals an den Anfang des Artikels, wo Prävention zunächst als „Verhinderung von Nicht-Gewolltem" definiert wurde, oder mit Bröckling anders formuliert: „Vorausgesetzt ist dabei, dass sich erstens aus gegenwärtigen Indikatoren künftige unerwünschte Zustände prognostizieren lassen, dass sich zweitens Anzeichen von Fehlentwicklungen ohne Intervention verschlimmern, folglich drittens frühzeitige Eingriffe die größtmögliche Risikominimierung versprechen und sich die präventiven Interventionen viertens als Hilfe konzeptualisieren lassen" (Bröckling 2008, S. 38 f.). Der pathologische Blick, eine „negative Entwicklungslogik" steht hier Pate für die Legitimation von Präventionsmaßnahmen, wobei Prävention in diesem Kontext „die Magie einer Zauberformel" auferlegt wird. „Sie findet Anwendung in diversen Zusammenhängen und ist mit der Verheißung der Machbarkeit verbunden: Prävention und präventiven Maßnahmen wird ein massives Wirkpotential zugeschrieben. Dieses entfaltet sich vor dem Hintergrund von angenommenen Kausalitäten, so dass Prävention im sozialpolitischen Kontext ausschließlich in einem kausalen Sinne zu begreifen ist" (Wohlgemuth 2009, S. 258).

Am Beispiel Kinder- oder Jugendwohlgefährdungen werden mit Suchtprävention Maßnahmen zum Schutz der Zielgruppe ins Feld gerückt, die sich um das „gute" Aufwachsen und das Wohl von Kindern und Jugendlichen kümmern sollen. Was dabei „gutes Aufwachsen" sein soll, in wessen Ermessen diese Einschätzung liegt, bleibt nicht selten offen. Prävention folgt dem, was Otto et al. (2010, S. 142) über Soziale Arbeit geschrieben haben (vgl. Oelkers et al. 2008; Otto und Seelmeyer 2004), dass diese notwendigerweise von dem Problem der Normativität betroffen sei: „Sie ist auf gesellschaftspolitische Festlegungen und auf Resultate lebenspraktischer Entscheidungen bezogen, in die (explizite oder implizite) Annahmen über Anstrebenswertes und zu Vermeidendes, Achtenswertes und Verachtenswertes, Zulässiges und Unzulässiges, Zumutbares und Unzumutbares eingegangen sind. Sie kann also nicht darauf verzichten, zu lebenspraktischen Fragen wertend Stellung zu beziehen. So etwa zu den Fragen, was das Kindeswohl gefährdet oder welche Formen selbst- und fremdschädigenden Verhaltens hinzunehmen sind und welche Interventionen erforderlich werden lassen." Daraus lässt sich fragen, wessen Normvorstellungen Prävention folgt? Sind präventive Maßnahmen beliebig oder folgen sie denen, die das Sagen haben oder glauben es zu haben? „So wundert es nicht, dass Prävention immer wieder als Instrument hegemonialer Interessen gesehen wird, deren Hauptsäulen auf Kontrolle, Normalisierung und, soweit für notwendig erachtet, auch Disziplinierung menschlichen Verhaltens im Sinne der Verhinderung von Abweichung zielen. Damit stellt sich die Frage, wieweit sich und in welcher Weise Prävention in den Dienst einer Kolonialisierung von Lebenswelt stellt, die die Sicherung des Status quo anstrebt. Eine hegemoniale Indienstnahme der Präventionsarbeit steht somit im Raum" (vgl. Wohlgemuth 2009, S. 257). Was ist, wenn Prävention affirmativ (bzw. nicht-kritisch) ist, wenn sie sich den gesellschaftlich dominanten Deutungen und Bewertungen unterwirft? Was bleibt übrig, wenn Präventionsarbeit sich vor allem an normativen Maßstäben orientiert? (vgl. ad. Normative Sozialpolitik und Soziale Arbeit: Otto et al. 2010, S. 144).

Wenn Präventionsarbeit vor allem als Abwendung und Verhinderung von Schaden und Gefährdungen verstanden und gesehen wird, wird (Sozial) Politik wenig dagegen einzuwenden haben, markieren dabei doch „[…] Sicherheitsbedürfnisse den Antrieb und Sicherheitsfiktionen den Fluchtpunkt aller präventiven Anstrengungen. Das verleiht diesen den Charakter des Unabschließbaren: Vorbeugen kann man nie genug und nie früh genug. Prävention konstituiert damit eine Anthropologie im Gerundivum. Sie bestimmt „den Menschen" als ein zu schützendes und zu optimierendes Wesen. Sie sucht weder nach Universalien menschlicher Existenz, noch verwirft sie deren Möglichkeit, sondern übersetzt die Frage nach der conditio humana in die praktische Aufgabe, „Defizitmenschen" zu verhindern und „Voll- bzw. Normalmenschen" zu schaffen. Den an die Vorbeugungspraktiken geknüpften Sicherheitsversprechen liegt das Bild einer existentiell gefährdeten und gleichermaßen schutzbedürftigen wie zur vernunftmäßigen, d. h. risikominimierenden Lebensführung fähigen Spezies zugrunde" (Bröckling 2008, S. 42).

Wer würde sich schon gegen eine solch moralisch hohe Zielsetzung stellen? Prävention stößt in der Regel auf eine breite öffentliche Zustimmung, lässt sich gut legitimieren und findet so moralische Unterstützung seitens der Politik. Ja selbst als Instrument der Kostensenkung, lässt sich Prävention als betriebswirtschaftlicher Faktor argumentieren (Stichwort: Return on Investment). Hier klafft allerdings Anspruch/Wunsch und Realität auseinander, ein Dilemma nimmt Gestalt an, denn einerseits wird etwas befürwortet, was auf der anderen Seite nicht wirklich finanziert wird. Return on Investment bedeutet, dass man zuerst einmal investieren muss, bevor was zurückkommt. Die Praxis zeigt allerdings, dass suchtpräventiven Aktivitäten oft nur halbherzig und geringe finanzielle Mittel zur Verfügung gestellt werden. Während Polizei und Strafvollzug sowie Beratung und Therapie den „Präventionskuchen" zum größten Teil unter sich aufteilen, bleiben der eigentlichen Suchtprävention nur wenig Mittel. Ja, mehr noch, das was allgemein unter Suchtprävention verstanden wird, versuchen Suchthilfe und -beratung und auch Polizei als Teil ihrer Arbeit einzuverleiben, denn alles scheint Prävention zu sein bzw. jeder kann Prävention machen, man braucht nur alles Verhindern von Nicht-Gewolltem als Prävention zu definieren. Damit wird das Betätigungsfeld der Präventionsarbeit zu einem offenen Buch. Problemzentrierte Negativdiagnosen sind allgegenwärtig und Helfende, mit und ohne Hochschulabschluss, bieten ihre Dienste zuhauf an. Was ist mit dem Anspruch, dass „gute" pädagogische Arbeit das Ziel verfolgen muss, Kindern und Jugendlichen ein selbstbestimmtes und zufriedenes Leben zu ermöglichen, und dies über allen anderen, kleinschrittig formulierten Zielen stehen müsse? Prävention kann nicht nur als „Hüterin von Bestehendem" gesehen werden, das einer „Abwesenheitsdoktrin" (Abstinenz) folgt: Gesundheit als Abwesenheit von Krankheit oder Sicherheit als Ausbleiben von Verbrechen/Kriminalität etc. definiert. Prävention muss mehr sein als Sicherung eines vermeintlichen „positiven Status quo", „Hilfe in", „Schutz vor" oder „Verhinderung von".

Prävention ist nicht nur als „erzieherische" pädagogische Maßnahme zu verstehen, sondern impliziert auch die gesundheitliche Zielsetzung. Wie eingangs bereits eingeführt, verleitet die Kombination aus Prävention und Gesundheit zur einfachen Schlussfolgerung, dass die Verhinderung von Krankheit, also Prävention automatisch einen Gesundheitszustand herbeiführen könne. Diese Konstruktion von Gesundheit als Abwesenheit von Krankheit hält der Realität, dem überwiegenden Laienverständnis (s. Faltermeier 2005) und der fachlichen Orientierung (vgl. WHO-Definition) nicht Stand.

Gesundheit wird eher ganzheitlich verstanden und bezieht neben der somatischen Gesundheit v. a. die psychische Gesundheit ein. Die WHO (2001) formuliert das wie folgt:

„Psychische Gesundheit ist ein Zustand des Wohlbefindens, in dem der Einzelne seine eigenen Fähigkeiten ausschöpfen, die normalen Lebensbelastungen bewältigen, produktiv und fruchtbar arbeiten kann und imstande ist, etwas zu seiner Gemeinschaft beizutragen".

In dieser Formulierung taucht kein „Verhindern" oder „Schützen vor" auf. Im Gegenteil betont es die Fähigkeit Lebensbelastungen zu bewältigen. Entsprechend gilt es Ressourcen und Fertigkeiten aufzubauen. Mit Gesundheitsförderung meint die WHO (1986):

„[…] ein Prozess, der Menschen dazu in die Lage versetzen soll, mehr Einfluss auf ihren Gesundheitszustand zu entwickeln und ihre Gesundheit aktiv zu verbessern. Ziel ist die Erreichung eines Zustandes vollständigen körperlichen, geistigen und sozialen Wohlbefindens, der dadurch erreicht werden soll, dass Individuen und Gruppen unterstützt werden, eigene Wünsche wahrzunehmen und zu realisieren, Bedürfnisse zu befriedigen, sowie die Umgebung zu verändern oder sich an diese anzupassen. Gesundheit ist ein positives Konzept, das sowohl soziale und individuelle Ressourcen als auch körperliche Fähigkeiten betont. Aus diesem Grund ist Gesundheitsförderung nicht nur im Kompetenzbereich des Gesundheitssektors anzusiedeln, sondern Gesundheitsförderung geht weiter als ein gesunder Lebensstil zum Wohlbefinden" (S. 1).

Geht es tatsächlich um dasselbe gesundheitliche Ziel bei der Prävention und Gesundheitsförderung, sollen diese kompatibel in einem Konzept integriert werden. Die praktizierte Prävention geht allerdings häufig nicht mit dieser Gesundheitsüberzeugung einher. Suchtverhalten ist kein delinquentes Verhalten (mehr), das erzieherisch sanktioniert werden soll, sondern stellt, wenn die fachlichen Kriterien insgesamt auf einen Leidensdruck hinweisen, eine Beeinträchtigung der psychischen Gesundheit dar. Selbstverständlich gilt es auch hier kritisch auf der Hut zu sein, wer den Gesundheitsbegriff für sich definitorisch bemächtigt, um möglicherweise hegemonial Normen zu bestimmen, die wiederum eine Kontrollinstanz legitimieren könnten. Dabei sind auch Macht- und ökonomische Interessen ersichtlich, die ein zumeist unerreichbares Selbstoptimierungs-Ideal zur allgemeinen objektivierenden Norm bestimmt. Die WHO-Definition gibt bewusst keine normierende objektivierende Gesundheitsweise vor, sondern betont die Unterstützung der individuellen und gruppenbezogenen Bedürfnisse sowie die eigenständige selbstwirksame Einflussnahme auf die eigene Gesundheit.

Angesichts des vorab kritischen Verständnisses von Präventionsarbeit, gilt es nachfolgend einen Blick auf die praktische Suchtpräventionsarbeit in Luxemburg im Zeitraum 1995 bis 2015 zu wagen, um ihre Identität zwischen von außen häufig geforderter Restriktion und Normierung und der modernen Auffassung von psychischer Gesundheit und Bildungsarbeit zu finden.

3   Suchtprävention in Luxemburg am Beispiel „CePT – Centre de Prévention des Toxicomanies" im Zeitraum 1995 bis 2015

Seit seiner Gründung, als Stiftung, durch Parlament und Regierung 1995 orientierte sich das CePT – Centre de Prévention des Toxicomanies (Zentrum für Suchtprävention) an der Formulierung der „Ottawa Charta" (WHO 1986): „Gesundheit wird von den Menschen in ihrer alltäglichen Umwelt geschaffen und gelebt, dort, wo sie spielen, lernen, arbeiten und lieben. Gesundheit entsteht dadurch, dass man sich um sich selbst und für andere sorgt, dass man in der Lage ist, selber Entscheidungen zu fällen und Kontrolle über die eigenen Lebensumstände auszuüben sowie dadurch, dass die Gesellschaft, in der man lebt, Bedingungen herstellt, die allen ihren Bürgern Gesundheit ermöglichen." Daraus hatte das CePT für seinen Präventionsansatz abgeleitet: „Der Mensch steht im Mittelpunkt, nicht die Droge". Dieses Menschenbild steht für ein suchtpräventives Handeln, bei dem der Mensch und insbesondere sein psychisches Wohlbefinden erste Priorität haben. Der Mensch wird dabei im Kontext seines sozialen, gesellschaftlichen und materiellen Umfeldes betrachtet (Michaelis 2009; Michaelis und Fischer 2009). Prävention geht einher mit dem Konzept der Gesundheitsförderung.

Das grundlegende Ziel des CePT war es, Sucht zu verhindern, Missbrauch zu vermindern und den Beginn des Konsums hinauszuzögern. Daher wurde dem entwicklungsgerechten Schutz von Kindern und Jugendlichen vor Drogen besondere Beachtung geschenkt. Die Verantwortung für diesen Schutz wurde in erster Linie bei den Erwachsenen gesehen. Die Suchtprävention bezog sich daher nicht schwerpunktmäßig auf Jugendliche und Kinder, sondern hatte als Hauptansprechpartner die Erwachsenen. Die Stärkung von Schutzfaktoren, in Form von persönlichen und sozialen Kompetenzen sowie der Aufbau sozialer Ressourcen waren Schwerpunkte der Zielsetzung. Der Aufbau suchtpräventiver Netzwerke, die Förderung der Kommunikation und das soziale Miteinander sowie die Verbesserung der strukturellen Bedingungen stellten langfristige Ziele dar. Insbesondere sollte die Entwicklung gesellschaftlicher Rahmenbedingungen, die einen suchtpräventiven Lebensstil ermöglichen, unterstützt werden. Als Hauptzielgruppe wurden Multiplikatoren/innen angesprochen, die das suchtpräventive Denken und Handeln an die intermediären Zielgruppen Kinder, Jugendliche und Erwachsene vermitteln und umsetzen. Die allgemeinen Aufgabenfelder mit denen die Zielsetzungen verknüpft wurden, bestanden in der Aufklärung und Sensibilisierung; Fort- und Weiterbildung sowie der Betreuung eines Suchttelefons. Daneben wurde eine Bibliothek aufgebaut und unterhalten, Studien initiiert sowie kontinuierlich eine interne Qualitätssicherung durchgeführt.

3.1 Ausgangssituation bei der Gründung

Während in den 1970er Jahren auch in Luxemburg noch Aufklärungs- und Abschreckungskampagnen im Vordergrund standen, richtete sich zu Beginn der 1980er Jahre der Blick stärker auf die Ursachen von Suchtgefahren. Im Laufe der 1990er Jahre vollzog sich ein grundlegender Paradigmenwechsel: Die Suchtprävention des CePT entwickelte sich schrittweise von einer vorgefundenen defizitorientierten hin zu einer neu zu gestaltender gesundheitsfördernden (salutogenetischen) Perspektive. Dies führte zur Etablierung so genannter Life-Skills-Ansätze (Botvin und Tortu 1988; WHO 1999), die Ressourcen und Kompetenzen mehr und mehr in den Vordergrund rückten und die substanzunspezifische Basis des suchtpräventiven Ansatzes des CePT bildeten. Die Bedeutung der Ressourcen tritt vor allem dann hervor, wenn sie dazu beitragen, bei vorhandenen Risikofaktoren die Widerstandsfähigkeit (Antonovsky 1987, 1997) zu erhöhen. Auf der Grundlage sozialer und persönlicher Lebenskompetenzen können dann konkrete Informationen zu Substanzen und suchtgefährdenden Verhaltensweisen vermittelt werden. Dabei ist es wichtig, an die Erfahrungswelt der Menschen anzuknüpfen, Raum für Austausch und Dialog zu schaffen, bei dem die unterschiedlichen Aspekte ihres Lebens – so auch des Konsums psychoaktiver Substanzen (vulgo Drogenkonsum) – thematisiert werden können (Erlebnisräume, Gefühlszustände, Gruppenintegration, Ritualisierungen, Verlockungen und Gefahren, ...).

Daneben stand die Beschäftigung mit der Drogenkultur unserer Gesellschaft, ein konkretes Wissen über Drogen, eine Auseinandersetzung mit dem kulturellen und sozialen Status von Rausch und Sucht (Freitag und Hurrelmann 1999), sowie die Thematisierung von gesundheitlichen Schäden oder Verstößen gegen geltende Gesetze oder Jugendschutzbestimmungen im Blickfeld suchtpräventiver Arbeit. Dabei wurde nicht außer Acht gelassen, dass der Verzicht auf den Konsum psychoaktiver Substanzen ebenfalls eine Option darstellt oder in manchen Fällen gar gefordert wird.

Bleiben wir einmal dabei, dass Suchtprävention als gesamtgesellschaftliche Querschnittsaufgabe ihre Daseinsberichtigung hat, dann gilt es die Rahmenbedingungen zu klären, unter denen sie dies leisten kann, dies vor allem, wenn sich Prävention nicht als Gehilfin einer Etablierung und Begründung normativer

Maßstäbe, als funktionalistische Ausrichtung im Sinne eines pädagogischen Sicherheits-Denkens verstehen bzw. vereinnahmen lassen will.

3.2 Aufbauphase 1995–2010 mit dem Fokus auf Settingansatz und Verhältnisprävention

Seit Mitte der 1990iger Jahre hatte das CePT als gemeinnützige Privatstiftung die Suchtprävention in Luxemburg kontinuierlich ausgebaut, so etwa in unterschiedlichen Settings (Gemeinde, Schule) wie auch in vielen Organisationen der Jugend- und Sozialarbeit, in denen Fachkräfte des CePT intervenierten. Das CePT als Fachstelle für Suchtprävention entwickelte im Laufe der Jahre eine eigenständige fachliche Identität, losgelöst vom individuumsbezogenen Beratungsdruck (klientenzentrierte Beratungsarbeit), jedoch in direktem Kontakt mit den Szenen (Stichwort: Partyszene und „Freizeitkonsum" bis hin zu konkreten Risikogruppen). Im Vordergrund stand die Vernetzungsarbeit mit offiziellen aber auch inoffiziellen Gruppen und Organisationen um möglichst viele Personen zu erreichen und zu involvieren.

Dieses Handlungswissen, das sich sowohl aus der oben beschriebenen Kooperation mit den nationalen Beratungsstellen, aus Erkenntnissen aus dem Alltag, als auch im Austausch mit internationalen Präventionsstellen sowie aus der Präventionsforschung entwickelte, bildete eine wichtige Ressource für die Entwicklung praxisnaher Präventionskonzepte in unterschiedlichen Settings.

Das CePT hatte über die Jahre unterschiedlichste Formen der Vermittlung suchtpräventiver Botschaften eingesetzt, etwa über Kampagnen, Broschüren, Flyer etc., durch Trainings, praktische und interaktive Übungen oder Diskussionen. Im Rahmen von Seminaren, Schulstunden, Projekten oder durch Ansätze wie Theater-, Erlebnis-, Abenteuer- oder Wildnispädagogik und mithilfe anderer „kreativer Methoden" wurde dies umgesetzt.

Menschen wurden in ihren Lebensweltbereichen wie Familie, Schule, Jugendarbeit, Gemeinde, Betriebe, Freizeit, Partyszene etc. angesprochen. Innerhalb dieser Systeme wiederum in unterschiedlicher Weise partizipativ beteiligt, so etwa im System Schule Schüler/-innen, Lehrpersonal, Eltern, Schulleitung, Schulpersonal etc. Dies führte u. a. dazu, dass die Suchtprävention neben individuellen, verhaltenspräventiven Maßnahmen auch strukturelle Veränderungen im Sinne einer nachhaltigen Verhältnisprävention initiierte.

Grundlegend für die Vorgehensweise des CePT in dieser Phase war eine systemische Sichtweise, die vor allem von innen heraus, also gemeinschaftlich, partizipativ und auf Diskurse aufbauend, am System und den gegebenen

Verhältnissen ansetzte. Daher lässt sich das Vorgehen in der Anfangsphase schwerpunktmäßig als Verhältnisprävention einordnen, bei der kooperativ Strukturen entwickelt wurden, um verschiedene betroffene Gruppen zu beteiligen, die dann mit fachlicher Unterstützung idealerweise aus sich heraus, im Sinne des Empowerments (Rappaport 1987), aktiv für die Suchtprävention wurden. Dies zeigte sich u. a. deutlich in den ersten gemeindebasierten Suchtpräventionsprogrammen (Fischer et al. 2002). Es wurde eine Pilotgruppe aus vielschichtigen Vertretern/-innen der Gemeinde gebildet, die von dem jeweiligen Gemeinderat überparteilich unterstützt wurde und erste Informations- und Diskussionsrunden für die Gemeindemitglieder veranstaltete. Dies ermöglichte den Diskurs um die Prävention innerhalb der Gemeinde und der Herausbildung einer Freiwilligengruppe, die vom Gemeinderat legitimiert Setting-spezifische Angebote offerierte, Ressourcen aufbaute und auch strukturelle Veränderungen initiierte. Angesprochen wurden vor allem Personen und Institutionen, die mit der eigentlichen Zielgruppe zu tun haben bzw. in Verantwortung stehen, also Eltern, Lehrende, Erziehende, Personen im Freizeit-, Vereins- und Sportbereich, Verkaufspersonal etc. Dieses Prinzip des strukturellen Aufbaus von Präventionsgruppen aus dem Setting heraus, dem Ressourcenaufbau und der Vernetzung verschiedener involvierter Gruppen konnte, je nach Gegebenheit, auf andere Settings, wie Schule, Betrieb, Partyszene etc. angepasst und übertragen werden.

3.3 Weiterentwicklung 2010–2015 mit dem Fokus auf emanzipatorische pädagogische Identitätsarbeit

Die Präventionsarbeit des CePT stellte die vielfältigen Suchbewegungen, die individuellen und kollektiven Praktiken der Identitätsarbeit in der weiteren Phase noch stärker in den Mittelpunkt und half dabei, Lebensbedingungen mit den Jugendlichen immer wieder neu zu definieren. Ein daraus abgeleitetes Handeln ging von den Problemen, Bedürfnissen, Potentialen, Fähigkeiten und Interessen Jugendlicher aus.

In zunehmendem Maße fand auch das Thema Risikominimierung stärker Eingang in die Präventionsarbeit des CePT. Dies liegt u. a. daran, dass einerseits das Dogma Abstinenz in der Öffentlichkeit an Bedeutung verloren hat und andererseits die gesellschaftliche Realität tagein, tagaus bestätigt, dass Konsum (illegalisierter) Substanzen trotz Verbote stattfindet und damit auch die jahrzehntelange Maxime „Krieg gegen die Drogen" nicht zu halten ist und dass nicht jeder Konsum direkt zu Sucht führt (wenn auch durchaus verbunden mit unterschiedlichsten Risiken und Problemlagen – die man nicht bagatellisieren darf).

Den sogenannten „Freizeitkonsum" ins Blickfeld der Präventionsarbeit des CePT zu nehmen, schien umso wichtiger, da die Anzahl jener Personen, die Konsumerfahrungen mit psychoaktiven Substanzen (legale wie illegalisierte Substanzen) haben – bis hin zu Risikogruppen – hoch ist und diese vor allem in den entsprechenden Settings (Party-Szene, Festivals, öffentlicher Raum, ...) erreicht werden sollten.

Wenn es darum geht, wie oben beschrieben, Jugendliche nicht als Objekte zu degradieren oder defizitär zu definieren und zu behandeln, war und ist es notwendig danach zu trachten, wie Jugendlichen Chancen der Entwicklung autonomer Entscheidungs- und Handlungsfähigkeit zugänglich gemacht werden können. Unter einer solcherart verstandenen Jugendarbeit versteht Scherr (1997, 2002, 2008a, 2008b) eine „Praxis der Subjekt-Bildung" und schlägt vor, (offene) Kinder- und Jugendarbeit theoretisch und konzeptuell als subjektorientierte Bildungspraxis zu modellieren (vgl. Scherr 2008a, S. 167).

Präventionsarbeit, in diesem Sinne, zielte darauf ab, Individuen dazu zu befähigen, sich mit sich selbst sowie den gesellschaftlichen Lebensbedingungen auseinanderzusetzen und diese zu begreifen. Daraus sind Angebote der Prävention als Bildungsgelegenheiten zur Lebens- resp. Welterfahrung zu verstehen, die die Bildung mündiger und selbstbewusster Individuen fördern und unterstützen. Der Gebrauchswert der Präventionsarbeit leitet sich ab aus der Aufgabe Bildungsprozesse anzuregen, durch die eine Distanzierung von Ritualen, Routinen, Gewohnheiten („Alltagsbewusstsein") ermöglicht wird, damit andere Erfahrungen und neue Anfänge sich entwickeln können. „... jede Selbstbildung erfolgt durch ständige Irritation der eigenen Erfahrungen. Ihr kommt es nicht auf die schnellen Antworten an, sondern auf die Arbeit an den Antworten" (Lindner 2009, S. 36). Bildungsprozesse sind „sozial, zeitlich und räumlich nicht eingrenzbar, sondern geschehen der Möglichkeit nach immer dann, wenn Individuen an Kommunikations- und Handlungszusammenhängen teilnehmen, die dazu geeignet sind, Veränderungen im Individuum anzuregen" (Scherr 2008b, S. 140).

Hilfreich war daher ebenfalls die Vermittlung von Informationen und Hilfsangeboten, wie auch Angebote zur Selbstreflexion mit Elementen zum Umgang mit dem eigenen Körper, zum Wohlbefinden und zum Substanzkonsum sowie eine kritische Reflexion über Gefahren, Risiken und gesundheitliche Schäden (Schadens- und Risikominimierung) bzw. die Schärfung des Risikobewusstseins für substanzbedingte Problematiken.

Um dies realisieren zu können, brauchte es einen umfassenden pädagogischen Zugang, der auf die Selbstbestimmung und Selbsttätigkeit der Beteiligten setzt und ein auf die Selbstbildung beruhendes Bildungskonzept. Suchtprävention muss durch das Aktivieren selbstreflexiver Prozesse – der Reflexion des eigenen oder subkulturellen Lebensstils, der Auseinandersetzung mit den subjektiven Entwicklungspotenzialen und Lebensperspektiven – zur individuellen Bildungsbiographie in Beziehung gesetzt werden. Ausgangspunkt einer solchen präventiven Herangehensweise war stets die Frage nach den vorherrschenden Bedürfnissen nach Rausch und die Suche nach Grenzerfahrungen, sprich die Frage nach den Konsummotiven und möglicher weniger schädigenden Alternativen.

3.4   Nachhaltige Kontinuität u. a. durch den Einbezug von Multiplikatoren/-innen in der Gesamtphase

In den unterschiedlichsten Handlungsfeldern/Settings waren für das CePT die haupt- wie ehrenamtlich Tätigen – die Multiplikatoren/-innen – in Schule, Aus- und Weiterbildung, Sozial- und Jugendarbeit, Verantwortliche in Vereinen usw. die erste Zielgruppe suchtpräventiver Maßnahmen. Mit diesen Multiplikatoren/-innen wurde in Fortbildungen und Schulungen, in Beratungen und in Kooperationen die präventive Funktion ihres professionellen Handelns im Berufsalltag thematisiert sowie Konzepte und Maßnahmen entwickelt (Nilles et al. 2005). In ihren jeweiligen Berufs- bzw. Tätigkeitsfeldern sind sie aufgrund ihrer unmittelbaren und mittelbaren Bedeutung für die Sozialisation von Kindern und Jugendlichen, ihrer gesellschaftlichen Integration und persönlicher Individuation die eigentlichen „Agenten" der Präventionsarbeit. Durch die möglichst wertschätzende Bindung, die die Multiplikatoren/-innen zu den Personen haben, wirken sie als Vorbilder, deren Verhalten im positiven, wie im negativen Sinne nachgeahmt wird. Dies gilt auch für die pädagogischen Interventionen, die im Falle von Auffälligkeiten (z. B. in Zusammenhang mit Drogenkonsum) zu planen und durchzuführen sind. Die Handlungskompetenzen dieser Multiplikatoren/-innen (einschließlich Eltern) werden gestärkt, so dass sie über die konkrete Kooperation hinaus selbstwirksam in der Lage sind, ein Stück am Aufbau und Stärkung der psychischen Gesundheit mitzuwirken. Dies gilt auch bei der Einbeziehung von jugendlichen Multiplikatoren/-innen (Peers) in spezifische Projekte.

Die Projekte von und mit Multiplikatoren/-innen zeigten auch auf, dass präventive Maßnahmen sich letztendlich nur wirksam realisieren lassen konnten, wenn verschiedene Institutionen daran beteiligt wurden. Suchtprävention ist somit zu verstehen, als eine integrative Kooperationsdisziplin unter Einbeziehung betroffener und interessierter Akteure/-innen (Personen und Institutionen) und als eine Gemeinschaftsaufgabe in den unterschiedlichen Settings.

Weitere kontinuierliche Maßnahmen betrafen u. a. das Suchttelefon und die Qualitätssicherung. Das CePT hatte im Laufe seines Bestehens die universelle Präventionsarbeit bei der Primärprävention in den Vordergrund gestellt, ohne dabei die Bereiche der selektiven oder indizierten Prävention auszublenden. So wurde über zehn Jahre im Rahmen des CePT das so genannte „Suchttelefon" angeboten, ein Beratungsdienst von ehrenamtlichen Mitarbeitern/-innen, die Ratsuchenden und Konsumierenden zur Seite standen. Das Suchttelefon wurde 2007 im CePT durch den Service-Bereich FroNo ersetzt. Im Jahr 2014 wurde das Pilotprojekt „Drugchecking" (Kürzel: DUCK) vom CePT ins Leben gerufen.

Die Umsetzung der verschiedenen Maßnahmen wurde stets reflexiv und evaluativ begleitet, um den Prozess und die Ergebnisse hinsichtlich ihrer Akzeptanz, Verbreitung und Wirkung kritisch und empirisch im Sinne der Qualitätssicherung zu hinterfragen. Neben qualitativen Methoden konnten in manchen Fällen auch umfangreiche quantitative Evaluationsstudien initiiert werden (z. B. Fischer et al. 2002; Grimm et al. 2013).

Zusammenfassend lassen sich in Bezug auf die eingangs eingeführten Kritikpunkte folgende Besonderheiten festhalten: Die Prävention setzte nicht bei der Droge, sondern zuerst beim Menschen mit seinen Bedürfnissen und seinen sozialen Bezügen an. Hauptzielgruppe des CePT waren die Erwachsenen, die in ihrem Setting als Multiplikatoren/-innen eine wesentliche Verantwortung gegenüber ihren Bezugspersonen haben und denen ihre Rolle möglichst bewusst gemacht wurde. Die Bedürfnisse und Identitätsansprüche der verschiedenen Jugend- und Freizeitkulturen wurden akzeptierend aufgegriffen und partizipativ im Setting mit dem Aufbau von Ressourcen, Alternativen und Kompetenzen zu einem gesundheitlich kohärenten Lebensstil entwickelt. Dies stand im Gegensatz zu Maßnahmen, die auf externe soziale Kontrolle der etablierten Norm, „sichernde" Restriktionen und sozialer Degradierung selbstständiger Heranwachsender zu Hilfsbedürftigen basierten. Der gesundheitliche Paradigmenwechsel im 20. Jahrhundert hin zu einer ressourcenorientierten Gesundheitsförderung im Sinne der WHO findet sich hier deutlich wieder.

4   Gemeinsame Wege der Gesundheitsförderung und der emanzipatorischen Jugendarbeit – ein Ausblick

Angesichts der kritischen Betrachtung der Prävention und der Dokumentation der praktischen Präventionsarbeit am Beispiel des CePT, das einen konstruktiven Weg im Umgang mit den potenziellen Stolpersteinen der Prävention aufwies, gilt es die gemeinsamen gestalterischen Möglichkeiten der Prävention aus der Sicht der Pädagogik und aus der Sicht der Gesundheitsförderung im Ausblick darzustellen.

Suchtprävention ist darauf angewiesen sich vom worst case Szenario: Sucht zu befreien, bei dem man leicht den Eindruck gewinnen kann, es gäbe nur die Zustände Abstinenz und Sucht. Oder wie Quensel formuliert: „Die Sucht-Prävention begreift Drogen, Drogenkonsum und Drogen-Konsument vom negativen Ende her" (2010, S. 106 ff.). Ein am Genuss orientierter Konsum von Alkohol und anderen Drogen gibt es quasi nicht, dies, obwohl alltäglicher Praxis und besseren Wissens. Damit man dies glauben kann, werden Menschen für unmündig erklärt.

Bevormundende und entmündigende politische und juristische Behinderungen stehen einer emanzipatorischen Erziehung zum mündigen Drogengebrauch (Stichwort: Drogenmündigkeit) im Wege. Hierzu ließe sich auf Theodor W. Adorno und sein Essay „Erziehung zur Mündigkeit" (1972) oder Horkheimer und Adorno (1969) „Dialektik der Aufklärung" verweisen, die Kappeler (2007) in diesem Kontext auf die Kurzformel gebracht hat: „Erst, wenn keine Illegalisierungs- beziehungsweise Kriminalisierungsdrohung mehr besteht und wenn die wirtschaftlichen Voraussetzungen geschaffen sind, kann ein primär am Genuss orientierter Konsum von Drogen entwickelt werden. Solange die Gesellschaft nichts Anderes zulässt ist für die große Mehrheit ihrer Mitglieder eine Vorstellung von unmittelbar genießendem Umgang mit Drogen vergeblich" (S. 301). Die/der mündige Bürger/-in ist gefordert mit all ihrer/seiner „Wissens-, Urteils- und Handlungskompetenz" (vgl. Widmaier 2012, S. 14) aber auch ihrer/seiner sozialen Kompetenz (vgl. auch Soziabilität bei Barsch 2008).

Eine derartige emanzipatorische Suchtprävention braucht einen umfassenden pädagogischen Zugang, der sich nicht in Stoffkunde oder Geboten und Verboten erschöpfen kann, sondern sie setzt sich in Beziehung zur individuellen Bildungsbiographie durch das Aktivieren selbstreflexiver Prozesse, der Reflexion des eigenen oder subkulturellen Lebensstils, der Auseinandersetzung mit den subjektiven Entwicklungspotenzialen und Lebensperspektiven. Ausgangspunkt einer solchen pädagogischen/präventiven Herangehensweise könnte die Frage nach den vorherrschenden Bedürfnissen nach Rausch und die Suche nach Grenzerfahrungen, sprich den Konsummotiven sein.

Wie bereits dargelegt, ist Identität nicht einfach gegeben und garantiert, sondern ein Prozess, der in Auseinandersetzung mit den vorgefundenen, dynamischen und widersprüchlichen Alltagsroutinen erfolgt. Es gilt Menschen jeden Alters, hier insbesondere Heranwachsende, im Prozess ihrer Subjektwerdung zu unterstützen, d. h. ihnen dabei zu helfen, ein selbstbewusstes und selbstbestimmtes Leben führen zu können. Bildung fungiert dabei als Teil, Unterstützung und Bedingtheit von Lebensbewältigung (Lindner 2009).

In Anbetracht diverser individueller und gesellschaftlicher Herausforderungen ist es wichtig, bei Jugendlichen ein „offensives Nachdenken über Möglichkeiten der Lebensgestaltung und des sozialen Zusammenlebens anzuregen sowie ihre biografischen, kulturellen und politischen Suchprozesse nicht still zu stellen, sondern zu begleiten und zu unterstützen" (Scherr 2006, S. 101).

Eine solche Identitätsarbeit stellt einen prozessualen und ständigen Balanceakt dar. „Diese Balance entspricht auf der Seite des Individuums der Struktur von Prozessen kommunikativen Handelns, an denen das Individuum teilnimmt. Interaktionsprozesse in einer Gesellschaft mit divergierenden Normen und getragen von Individuen mit unterschiedlichen Biographien können nur fortdauern, wenn die Beteiligten ihre Ich-Identität zu erkennen geben. Für jedes Individuum ist seine balancierende Ich-Identität ein ständiger Versuch, sich gegen Nicht-Identität zu behaupten, weil diese den Interaktionsprozess überhaupt oder jedenfalls die eigene Mitwirkung daran gefährden würde" (Krappmann 2005, S. 79).

Es geht in dieser Konzeption darum, dass jede/jeder Einzelne in ihrem/seinem Wesen Anerkennung findet, d. h. auch Jugendliche nicht als Objekte irgendwelcher, wie auch immer gearteter pädagogischer Interessen/Zwecksetzungen (manchmal in Form gut gemeinter Ratschläge oder Bevormundung) verstanden werden. Es geht um das Spannungsverhältnis von selbstbestimmter Lebensführung, um die Realisierung von eigenverantwortlichen Lebensentwürfen und um den Beitrag, den Präventionsarbeit leisten kann, um die Jugendlichen zu einer aktiven und bewussten Auseinandersetzung mit den ihnen auferlegten Lebensbedingungen zu stärken.

In Anlehnung an den von Bock und Otto (2007, S. 208) verwendeten Bildungsbegriff, ließe sich Präventionsarbeit verstehen „als ‚kritisches Konzept' zwischen derzeit bestehenden Lebensverhältnissen und ökonomischen Zumutungen, in denen die eigene Biographie immer wieder neu hergestellt werden muss, inmitten irrationaler und zum Teil vollkommen widersprüchlicher Angebote, Gestaltungsaufgaben und Zumutungen, die zwischen äußeren Vorgaben und eigenen Optionen zu bewältigen sind" (vgl. Thiersch 2002; Bock et al. 2006).

Dieser Anspruch der emanzipatorischen Bildungsarbeit an die Prävention lässt sich sehr gut in Einklang bringen und ergänzen mit der von der WHO geforderten Ausrichtung der Prävention an die Förderung der psychischen Gesundheit.

Die beiden Disziplinen erscheinen sich manchmal wie „Fremde" (vgl. Keupp 2010) und doch ermöglicht ihre inter- oder besser noch transdisziplinäre Zusammenarbeit konstruktiv den Zielen der WHO näher zu bringen. Dies kristallisiert sich vor allem in den allgemeinen Zielen zur Entwicklung von Lebenskompetenzen (WHO 1999) auf der Ebene der Individuen und dem Aufbau von Kapazitäten (capacity building) und „Ermöglichungsräumen" (Capability-Ansatz) auf der gemeinschaftlichen organisatorischen Ebene. Unter den wesentlichen Kompetenzen der Life-Skills werden u. a. vom Schwerpunkt her (Mischformen einbezogen) kognitive (Entscheidungsfindung, Problemlösung, kreatives Denken, kritisches Denken), emotionale (Emotions- und Stressbewältigung) und soziale Kompetenzen (Empathie, Selbst-Wahrnehmung, effektive Kommunikation, Beziehungsfähigkeit) benannt. Etwas unter gehen dabei allerdings die Selbstmanagement-Kompetenzen (Bergo et al. 2008), also Planungs- und Umsetzungsfertigkeiten, die es erst ermöglichen die anderen Kompetenzen selbstwirksam in einer Handlung zu realisieren. Die Entwicklung von solchen Fertigkeiten stehen im Einklang mit der Konzeption von Gesundheitsförderung, wie es die WHO (1999) formuliert: Es gilt Ressourcen aufzubauen, die es letztendlich verhindern, dass das Gleichgewicht der eigenen Gesundheit sich kontinuierlich in ein Unwohlsein bis hin zu einem Krankheitsstadium verlagert und diese auch in belastenden Situationen unterstützen im Sinne einer Resilienz (Fröhlich-Gildhoff und Rönnau-Böse 2019). Solche „Widerstandsressourcen" gehören vor allem zum Kernkonzept der Salutogenese von Antonovsky (1987, 1997) und tragen mit zum generalisierten Kohärenzgefühl bei. Herausfordernde Situationen werden dadurch verstehbarer, handhabbarer und bedeutsamer in der aktiven Auseinandersetzung damit. Auf die Prävention bezogen könnte man vereinfacht die Rolle von Droge und Konsumierenden so ausdrücken: Nicht die ‚Droge' sucht ihre Konsumierenden, um diese süchtig zu machen, sondern die Konsumierenden entscheiden sich in belastenden Situationen auf der Basis ihrer jeweiligen Ressourcen, welche Mittel zur kurz- oder langfristigen Wiederherstellung des psychischen Wohlbefindens beitragen. Je mehr eigene und äußere Ressourcen zur Verfügung stehen, desto selbstwirksamer, konstruktiver und nachhaltiger wird die Person damit umgehen können; je weniger davor vorhanden ist, desto eher wird auf kurzfristige vermeintliche Verbesserungen des Wohlbefindens zurückgegriffen, die bei andauernden Belastungen zu krankmachenden Verhaltensweisen (u. a. Sucht, Gewalt, Passivität, ...) oder Zuständen führen können, die langfristig die psychische Gesundheit gefährden.

Antonovsky bezieht in seinem Konzept auch die äußeren Verhältnisse (ökonomische, materielle und gesellschaftliche) als wichtige Ressourcen mit ein. Gesundheit kann nicht allein auf das individuelle Handeln zurückgeführt werden. Gesundheit, insbesondere psychische Gesundheit, und gesundheitliches Handeln vollzieht sich in der Interaktion mit seiner (sozialen) Umwelt. Der Setting-

Ansatz der WHO bettet das individuelle Handeln in lebensalltägliche, zumeist räumlich verortete, gemeinschaftliche Organisationen ein. Damit bieten sich konkrete Ansatzpunkte für die sonst so klassisch benannte Verhältnisprävention in Familien, Schulen, Betrieben, Gemeinden etc. Der Ansatz setzt da an, wo die Menschen in ihrer alltäglichen Lebensumwelt „[…] spielen, lernen, arbeiten und lieben. Gesundheit entsteht dadurch, dass man um sich selbst und um andere kümmert, dass man in die Lage versetzt wird, selbst Entscheidungen zu treffen und Kontrolle über die eigenen Lebensumstände auszuüben" (WHO 1986, S. 4).

Die daraus abgeleiteten grundlegenden Strategien betonen die aktive Beteiligung der Betroffenen (Partizipation) am gesamten Planungs-, Umsetzungs- und Entscheidungsprozess sowie das Empowerment-Konzept, zur Vermittlung von Kompetenzen, die zum selbstbestimmten und eigenverantwortlichen Handeln in einer Gemeinschaft befähigen. Darüber hinaus werden Strategien zur Strukturentwicklung von „gesunden" Organisationen benannt (vgl. Engelmann und Halkow 2008). Auch hier sollte der Fokus nicht auf Hilfe und Dienstleistung liegen, sondern den Aufbau von Kapazitäten im Sinne von „Verwirklichungschancen" (capabilities), Befähigung und Ermöglichungsräume (Grundmann 2008; Sen 2000) strukturell fördern. Dies vereint zudem die beiden Interessen der emanzipatorischen Bildungsarbeit und nachhaltigen Gesundheitsförderung.

Die Zauberformel muss letztendlich jede Person selbst und autonom für sich entwickeln, jeweils den eigenen Bedürfnissen im sozialen Kontext angemessen. Wir, als Präventionsarbeitende, können Ihnen nur die Ressourcen und Möglichkeitsräume bieten, im Sinne einer unterstützenden Bildungsarbeit und einer psychischen Gesundheitsförderung, die eine selbstreflexive Erarbeitung eines nachhaltigen kohärenten Gleichgewichts des eigenen psychischen Wohlergehens im jeweiligen Setting ermöglicht.

Literatur

Adorno, T.W. (1972). *Erziehung zur Mündigkeit*. Frankfurt am Main: Suhrkamp.
Anhorn, R. (2002). Jugend - Abweichung - Drogen: Zur Konstruktion eines sozialen Problems. In F. Bettinger, C. Mansfeld, & M. M. Jansen (Hrsg.), *Gefährdete Jugendliche? – Jugend, Kriminalität und der Ruf nach Strafe* (S. 47–74). Opladen: Leske u. Budrich.
Anhorn, R. (2011). Von der Gefährlichkeit zum Risiko – Zur Genealogie der Lebensphase „Jugend" als soziales Problem. In B. Dollinger, & H. Schmidt-Semisch (Hrsg.), *Handbuch Jugendkriminalität. Kriminologie und Sozialpädagogik im Dialog* (S. 23–42). Wiesbaden: Springer VS.
Antonovsky, A. (1987). *Unravelling the mystery of health*. San Francisco: Jossey-Bass.

Antonovsky A. (1997). *Salutogenese. Zur Entmystifizierung der Gesundheit.* Tübingen: dgvt.

Barsch, G. (2008). *Lehrbuch Suchtprävention. Von der Drogennaivität zur Drogenmündigkeit.* Geesthacht: Neuland.

Bergo, C., Jung, C., Fischer, U.C., Bogdáni, I., Gombkötö, E.H., Kosir, M, Morand-Aymon, B., Nägele, D., Passa, A., Paulos, C., Ries, J., Salovaara, A., & Michaelis, T. (2008). *Förderung von sozialen und personalen Kompetenzen bei sozial Benachteiligten als Voraussetzung für Lebenslanges Lernen. Trainingskonzept.* Luxemburg: CePT.

Bock, K., Andresen, S., & Otto, H.-U. (2006). Zeitgemäße Bildungstheorie und zukunftsfähige Bildungspolitik. Ein „Netzwerk Bildung" als Antwort der Kinder- und Jugendhilfe. In H.-U. Otto, & J. Oelkers (Hrsg.), *Zeitgemäße Bildung. Herausforderung für Wissenschaft und Bildungspolitik* (S. 332–347). München: reinhardt.

Bock, K., & Otto, H.-U. (2007). Die Kinder- und Jugendhilfe als Ort flexibler Bildung. In M. Harring, C. Rohlfs, & C. Palentien (Hrsg.), *Perspektiven der Bildung. Kinder und Jugendliche in formellen, nicht-formellen und informellen Bildungsprozessen* (S. 203–217). Wiesbaden: Springer VS.

Botvin, G.J., & Tortu, S. (1988). Preventing adolescent substance abuse through life skills training. In R.H. Price, E.L. Cowen, R.P. Lorion, & J. Ramos-McKay (Eds.), *Fourteen ounces of prevention* (p. 98-110). Washington: American Psychological Association.

Bröckling, U. (2008). Vorbeugen ist besser. Zur Soziologie der Prävention. *Behemoth. A Journal on Civilisation, 1*, S. 35–48. http://www.zeithistorische-forschungen.de/sites/default/files/medien/material/2013-3/Broeckling_2008.pdf. Zugegriffen: 29.06.2013.

Engelmann, F., & Halkow, A. (2008). *Der Setting-Ansatz in der Gesundheitsförderung: Genealogie, Konzeption, Praxis, Evidenzbasierung. Discussion Papers/Wissenschaftszentrum Berlin für Sozialforschung, Forschungsschwerpunkt Bildung, Arbeit und Lebenschancen, Forschungsgruppe Public Health, 2008-302.* Berlin: Wissenschaftszentrum Berlin für Sozialforschung gGmbH. https://nbn-resolving.org/urn:nbn:de:0168-ssoar-294064.

Faltermaier, T. (2005). Subjektive Konzepte und Theorien von Gesundheit und Krankheit. In R. Schwarzer (Hrsg.), *Gesundheitspsychologie. Enzyklopädie der Psychologie C/X/1* (S. 31–53). Göttingen: Hogrefe.

Fischer, U.C., Michaelis,T., & Krieger,W. (2002). Gemeindenahe primäre Prävention von Drogenmissbrauch und Sucht. In B. Röhrle (Hrsg), *Prävention und Gesundheitsförderung Bd. II* (S. 285–325). Tübingen: dgvt.

Freitag, M. & Hurrelmann, K. (1999). *Illegale Alltagsdrogen. Cannabis, Ecstasy, Speed und LSD im Jugendalter.* Weinheim Juventa.

Fröhlich-Gildhoff, K., & Rönnau-Böse, M. (2019). *Resilienz.* München: Ernst Reinhardt Verlag.

Grimm, S., Residori C., Joachim, P., Décieux, J P., & Willems, H (2013). *Lokale Netzwerkbildung als strategisches Konzept in der Prävention.* Wiesbaden: Springer VS.

Grundmann, M. (2008). Handlungsbefähigung – Eine sozialisationstheoretische Perspektive. In H.-U. Otto, & H. Ziegler (Hrsg.), *Capabilities* (S. 131-142). Wiesbaden: Springer VS.

Horkheimer, M., & Adorno, T.W. (1969). *Dialektik der Aufklärung.* Frankfurt am Main: Suhrkamp.

Kappeler, M. (2007). Du sollst selbständig werden! – aber bitte so, wie es sich gehört. Prävention als pädagogischer Imperativ und als Dauerstress für Erziehende und Zu-Erziehende. In B. Dollinger, & H. Schmidt-Semisch (Hrsg.), *Sozialwissenschaftliche Suchtforschung* (S. 289–307). Wiesbaden: Springer VS.

Keupp, H. (2010). Gesundheitsförderung durch Kinder- und Jugendhilfe – zwischen Hilfe und Kontrolle. In Sozialpädagogisches Institut des SOS-Kinderdorf e.V. (Hrsg.), *Gesundheitsförderung in der Kinder- und Jugendhilfe* (S. 7–34). München: Eigenverlag.

Krappmann, L. (2005). *Soziologische Dimensionen der Identität. Strukturelle Bedingungen für die Teilnahme an Interaktionsprozessen*. Stuttgart: Klett-Cotta.

Lindner, W. (2009). Bildungsverständnis der Jugendsozialarbeit. Sozialpädagogische Bildung und Lebensbewältigung. *Sozial Extra, 9/10*, S. 35–37.

Lüders, C. (2011). Von der scheinbaren Selbstverständlichkeit präventiven Denkens. *DJI Impulse, 2*, S. 4-6.

Michaelis, T. (2009). Suchtprävention - eine Alltagssache! In Ministère de la Famille et de l'Intégration, Entente des Foyers de Jour, Syndicat des Villes et Communes Luxembourgeoises, & Université du Luxembourg (Hrsg.), *Maisons relais pour enfants: le manuel - das Handbuch* (S. 202–204). Luxemburg: Editions le Phare.

Michaelis, T., & Fischer, U.C. (2009). Suchtprävention. In H. Willems G. Rotink, & D. Ferring (Hrsg.), *Handbuch der sozialen und erzieherischen Arbeit in Luxemburg. Band 2* (S. 1249–1257). Luxemburg: Éditions Saint-Paul.

Nilles, J.P., Krieger, W., & Michaelis, T. (Hrsg.) (2005). *Multiplikatoren in der Primären Suchtprävention. Ein Handbuch*. Luxemburg: CePT.

Oelkers, N., Steckmann, U., & Ziegler, H. (2008). Normativität in der Sozialen Arbeit. In J. Ahrens, R. Beer, U.H. Bittlingmayer, & J. Gerdes (Hrsg.), *Beschreiben und/oder Bewerten I. Normativität in sozialwissenschaftlichen Forschungsfeldern. Münsteraner Schriften zur Soziologie Bd. 1* (S. 231–256). Münster: LIT.

Otto, H-U., Scherr, A., & Ziegler, H. (2010). Wieviel und welche Normativität benötigt die Soziale Arbeit? Befähigungsgerechtigkeit als Maßstab sozialarbeiterischer Kritik. *neue praxis, 2*, S. 137–163.

Otto, H-U., & Seelmeyer, U. (2004). Soziale Arbeit und Gesellschaft – Anstöße zu einer Neuorientierung der Debatte um Normativität und Normalität. In S. Hering, S., & U. Urban (Hrsg.), *„Liebe allein genügt nicht". Historische und systematische Dimensionen der Sozialpädagogik* (S. 45–63). Opladen: Leske + Budrich.

Quensel, S. (2010). *Das Elend der Suchtprävention. Analyse - Kritik – Alternative*. Wiesbaden: Springer VS.

Rappaport, J. (1987). Terms of empowerment/exemplars of prevention: Toward a theory for communitiy psychology. *American Journal of Community Psychology, 15*, 121-148.

Scherr, A. (1997). *Subjektorientierte Jugendarbeit*. Weinheim: Juventa.

Scherr, A. (2002). Subjektbildung in Anerkennungsverhältnissen. Über „soziale Subjektivität" und „gegenseitige Anerkennung" als pädagogische Grundbegriffe. In B. Hafeneger, P. Henkenborg, & A. Scherr (Hrsg.), *Pädagogik der Anerkennung: Grundlagen, Konzepte, Praxisfelder* (S. 26–44). Schwalbach: Wochenschau.

Scherr, A. (2006). Mündigkeit als Grundprinzip einer pädagogischen Theorie der Jugendarbeit? Anmerkungen zu Klaus Mollenhauers „Versuch 3": In W. Lindner (Hrsg.), *1964 – 2004: Vierzig Jahre Kinder- und Jugendarbeit in Deutschland* (S. 95-102). Wiesbaden: Springer VS.

Scherr, A. (2008a). Gesellschaftspolitische Bildung – Kernaufgabe oder Zusatzleistung der Jugendarbeit? In H.-U. Otto, & T. Rauschenbach (Hrsg.), *Die andere Seite der Bildung. Zum Verhältnis von formellen und informellen Bildungsprozessen* (S. 167–180). Wiesbaden: Springer VS.

Scherr, A. (2008b). Subjekt- und Identitätsbildung. In T. Coelen, & H.-U. Otto (Hrsg.), *Grundbegriffe Ganztagsbildung. Das Handbuch* (S. 137–145). Wiesbaden: Springer VS.

Sen, A. (2000). *Ökonomie für den Menschen*. München: Hanser

Silbereisen, R.K., & Reese, A. (2001). Substanzgebrauch Jugendlicher: illegale Drogen und Alkohol. In J. Raithel (Hrsg.), *Risikoverhaltensweisen Jugendlicher. Formen, Erklärung und Prävention* (S. 131–153). Opladen: Leske + Budrich.

Thiersch, H. (2002). Bildung – alte und neue Aufgaben der Sozialen Arbeit. In R. Münchmeier, H.-U. Otto, & U. Rabe-Kleberg (Hrsg.), *Bildung und Lebenskompetenz. Kinder- und Jugendhilfe vor neuen Aufgaben* (S. 57–71). Opladen: Leske + Budrich.

WHO (1986). Ottawa Charter for Health Promotion. https://www.euro.who.int/de/publications/policy-documents/ottawa-charter-for-health-promotion,-1986. Zugegriffen: 11.06.2020.

WHO (1999). *Partners in Life Skills Education*. Genf: WHO.

WHO (2001). Strengthening mental health promotion. *Fact sheet no. 220*. Genf: WHO.

Widmaier, B. (2012). Außerschulische politische Bildung nach 1945 – Eine Erfolgsgeschichte? *Aus Politik und Zeitgeschichte, 62,* Bd. 46–47, S. 9–16.

Wohlgemuth, K. (2009). *Prävention in der Kinder- und Jugendhilfe. Annäherung an eine Zauberformel*. Wiesbaden: Springer VS.

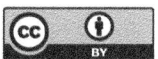

Gesundheitliche Probleme und Beeinträchtigungen des Wohlbefindens bei Jugendlichen – eine Analyse auf Basis der Arbeitsdokumentation des Service Psy-Jeunes Luxemburg

Christiane Weintzen, Manuela Woll, Malou Zeyen
und Dina Dias

> *„Zwei Dinge sollten Kinder von ihren Eltern bekommen:*
> *Wurzeln und Flügel. "*
>
> *Johann Wolfgang Goethe*

1   Ziel des Beitrages

Wohlbefinden ist ein sehr komplexes multidimensionales Konstrukt, welches nicht mit Glück oder der Abwesenheit von Leid und Störungen gleichzusetzen ist. Subjektives Wohlbefinden wird definiert als die subjektive, affektive und kognitive Bewertung des eigenen Lebens. Es besteht aus drei Komponenten: der Lebenszufriedenheit (kognitive Bewertung), dem Vorhandensein positiver Emotionen/Stimmungen und der Abwesenheit negativer Emotionen/Stimmungen (Diener 1984). Grundsätzlich ist davon auszugehen, dass der Mensch im

C. Weintzen (✉) · M. Woll · M. Zeyen · D. Dias
Psy-Jeunes, Croix-Rouge luxembourgeoise, Luxemburg, Luxemburg
E-Mail: Christiane.weintzen@croix-rouge.lu

M. Woll
E-Mail: Manuela.woll@croix-rouge.lu

M. Zeyen
E-Mail: Malou.zeyen@croix-rouge.lu

D. Dias
E-Mail: Dina.dias@croix-rouge.lu

Allgemeinen nach einer Maximierung von Zufriedenheit, Freude und Glück im Leben strebt und Schmerzen und Leid zu vermeiden sucht. (Bundeszentrale für gesundheitliche Aufklärung 2018)

Aus psychologischer Sicht liegt beim Wohlbefinden der Fokus auf dem persönlichen Wachstum und der Selbstrealisierung. Ein hohes psychologisches Wohlbefinden ist dann gegeben, wenn man in seinem Leben autonom handeln kann, Umweltanforderungen meistern kann, persönliches Wachstum erlebt, positive Beziehungen mit anderen Personen pflegt, Sinn im Leben erkennt und sich selbst akzeptiert (Ryff und Keyes 1995).

Keyes' (2002) Theorie zu psychischer Gesundheit (mental health) erweitert das Konzept des subjektiven und psychologischen Wohlbefindens um den sozialen Aspekt. Individuen funktionieren gemäß Keyes dann gut, wenn sie die Gesellschaft verstehen und sie als sinnvoll erleben, in ihr die Möglichkeit sehen, persönlich zu wachsen, sich der Gesellschaft zugehörig und akzeptiert fühlen, sie größtenteils akzeptieren und das Gefühl haben, selbst etwas zur Gesellschaft beizutragen.

Eingebettet in diesen theoretischen Rahmen soll der Beitrag durch konkrete Fallbeispiele einen Einblick geben in die Belastungen, aufgrund derer Kinder, Jugendliche, Eltern und andere Bezugspersonen sich an einen Psychologen des Service Psy-Jeunes in Luxemburg wenden. Hierbei ist es wichtig hervorzuheben, dass aufgrund der Spezifizität der Beratungs- und Betreuungsangebote des Service Psy-jeunes hier nur ein Teilbereich der möglichen psychischen Probleme und Belastungen aufgezeigt werden kann. Die spezifische Problematik der Suchterkrankungen etwa oder das Mobbing z. B. werden hier nicht berücksichtigt.

Mit unserem Beitrag möchten wir den Blick der Leser dafür schärfen, dass verhaltenskreative Kinder und Jugendliche häufig keinen anderen Ausweg sehen, als sich so zu verhalten, wie sie es tun. Dabei wünschen sie sich nichts mehr, als gesund und glücklich zu sein.

2 Aufgaben und Ziele des Psy-Jeunes

Der Service Psy-Jeunes wurde am 1. Oktober 1993 gegründet mit dem Ziel, für Jugendliche im Alter zwischen 12 und 24 Jahren mit belastenden Lebensereignissen eine therapeutische Begleitung anzubieten.

In den vergangenen Jahren hat sich der Service für eine breitere Population geöffnet. Kinder, Jugendliche und junge Erwachsene, die sich freiwillig melden, können eine ambulante, psychologische und psychotherapeutische Hilfe und Unterstützung bekommen, damit sie nachhaltig ein Leben in psychischer Gesundheit und Wohlbefinden führen können.

Das Angebot richtet sich sowohl an den Jugendlichen bzw. das Kind selbst wie auch an sein Umfeld: seine Eltern, Geschwister sowie Erzieher und Lehrer.

Oft haben Jugendliche und junge Erwachsene, die die Hilfe des Service Psy-Jeunes in Anspruch nehmen, einen Punkt im Leben erreicht, wo es in ihren Augen und/oder in den Augen ihrer Familienmitglieder/Freunde nicht mehr weitergeht. Dieser belastende Lebensmoment kann sich in folgenden Verhaltensauffälligkeiten zeigen:

- Affektive Störungen: anhaltende leichte bis starke Schwankungen im Stimmungs-, Antriebs- und Aktivitätsbereich
- Neurotische Belastungs- und somatoforme Störungen: Reaktionen auf schwere Belastungen und Anpassungsstörungen, Angst- und Zwangsstörungen, somatoforme Störungen
- Verhaltens- und emotionale Störungen mit Beginn in Kindheit- und Jugend: hyperkinetische Störungen, Störung des Sozialverhaltens, Störung der Emotionen, Ticstörungen
- Verhaltensauffälligkeiten mit körperlichen Störungen und Faktoren: z. B. Essstörungen und Schlafstörungen

Die Erfahrungen aus der therapeutischen Praxis des Service Psy-Jeunes haben gezeigt, dass Verhaltensauffälligkeiten oftmals Folgen von nicht verarbeiteten belastenden und/oder traumatischen Ereignissen sind, die das Kind oder den Jugendlichen an Leib und Leben oder massiv in seinem Selbstwert bedroht haben. Das kann z. B. geschehen, wenn sich Eltern voneinander trennen; wenn ein Elternteil oder naher Angehöriger verstirbt oder von schwerer Krankheit bedroht ist; wenn dem Jugendlichen respektive jungen Erwachsenen seelische, körperliche und sexuelle Misshandlungen im außer- oder innerfamiliären Umfeld widerfahren; wenn er einen schweren Unfall überlebt hat oder auch Zeuge davon wird; oder, wenn er in der Schule ausgegrenzt oder gemobbt wird oder sich aufgrund von schlechten Leistungen als Versager fühlt. Gefühle, die durch solche Ereignisse ausgelöst werden, sind u. a. Scham- und Schuldgefühle, Ängste vor Kontrollverlust und/oder Versagensängste, Gefühle von Hilflosigkeit, Hoffnungslosigkeit, Einsamkeit oder innere Leere. Die Jugendlichen entwickeln daraufhin oft eigene Strategien, um mit diesen Gefühlen umzugehen. In vielen Fällen führen diese Strategien zu Verhaltensauffälligkeiten.

Diese Kinder, Jugendlichen und jungen Erwachsenen brauchen Hilfe und Unterstützung, um neue Ziele für sich zu finden. Dabei ist es wichtig, ihnen zu helfen, Sicherheit nach innen und außen herzustellen, damit sie in ihrer Situation die notwendige psychische Stabilität finden können. Diese beiden Faktoren sind ausschlaggebend dafür, belastende Erfahrungen verarbeiten zu können, damit ein Leben in psychischer Gesundheit und Wohlbefinden möglich wird.

Verhaltenstherapie, systemische Therapie, Gesprächspsychotherapie, Hypnotherapie, Traumatherapie und EMDR. Durch häufige Fort- und Weiterbildungen wird der Pool der therapeutischen Möglichkeiten ständig erweitert. Ebenfalls sind Intervision und Supervision wichtige Bestandteile des Arbeitsalltags. Sie unterliegen laut Psychotherapeutengesetz vom 14.07.2015 Art.7 der Schweigepflicht.

3 Methoden und Hilfsangebote

In einem psychotherapeutischen Prozess werden häufig verschiedene Phasen durchlaufen. Obwohl dies meist ein sehr individueller Prozess ist und es kein festes Ablaufschema gibt, können die wichtigen Momente einer Psychotherapie wie folgt festgehalten werden:

- sich finden und Vertrauen fassen
- zu schwierigen Themen vorstoßen
- eigene Ressourcen neu entdecken
- alte Konfliktmuster aufbrechen und verstehen und Probleme bearbeiten
- sich neu erfahren und kennen lernen
- Konflikte austragen lernen und durcharbeiten
- neue Handlungs- und Erlebnismöglichkeiten entdecken

Auch die Schwerpunkte und Inhalte der Psychotherapie sind individuell sehr verschieden, je nachdem was die Person erlebt hat, welche Lösungsstrategien sie bisher entwickelt hat, welche Fähigkeiten und Ressourcen sie mitbringt und welche Herangehensweise ihr am besten entspricht. Im Folgenden sollen die wichtigsten therapeutischen Ansätze und Konzepte des Service Psy-Jeunes kurz dargestellt werden. Ein besonderer Schwerpunkt des Service ist die Arbeit mit Traumata und EMDR.

Ein Trauma ist „[...] ein belastendes Ereignis oder eine Situation kürzerer oder längerer Dauer, mit außergewöhnlicher Bedrohung oder katastrophenartigem Ausmaß, die bei fast jedem eine tiefe Verzweiflung hervorrufen würde." (Dilling und Freyberger 2010, S. 174) (Beispielsweise: Naturkatastrophe oder menschlich verursachtes schweres Unheil, ein sogenanntes „man-made disaster", ein Kampfeinsatz, ein schwerer Unfall, eine Beobachtung des gewaltsamen Todes anderer oder Opfersein von Folter, Terrorismus, Vergewaltigung oder anderen Verbrechen.)

Die Reaktionen auf ein Trauma können unmittelbar nach dem Ereignis auftreten oder aber erst Wochen. Monate oder Jahre danach. Manchmal kann es sein, dass die Betroffenen zwischen ihren Symptomen und dem Trauma überhaupt keinen Zusammenhang mehr herstellen können. Mögliche Reaktionen sind:

- Symptome des Wiedererlebens: sich aufdrängende, belastende Erinnerungen an das Trauma, Flashbacks, Alpträume
- Vermeidungssymptome: emotionale Stumpfheit, Gleichgültigkeit und Teilnahmslosigkeit der Umgebung und anderen Menschen gegenüber, aktive Vermeidung von Aktivitäten und Situationen, die Erinnerungen an das Trauma wachrufen könnten. Manchmal können wichtige Aspekte des traumatischen Erlebnisses nicht mehr (vollständig) erinnert werden
- Vegetative Übererregtheit: Schlafstörungen, Reizbarkeit, Konzentrationsschwierigkeiten, erhöhte Wachsamkeit, übermäßige Schreckhaftigkeit, erhöhte Ängstlichkeit, Panikattacken

EMDR steht für „Eye Movement Desensitization and Reprocessing" (zu Deutsch: Desensibilisierung und Verarbeitung durch Augenbewegung). Dies ist eine Methode zur Trauma-Integration, also der Verarbeitung traumatischer Erlebnisse. Die Methode wurde von Francine Shapiro entwickelt. Inzwischen wird diese Methode nicht nur bei Traumata, sondern auch bei anderen Diagnosen angewendet und ist mehrfach wissenschaftlich validiert worden. Studien haben gezeigt, dass nach der Behandlung einer einfachen posttraumatischen Belastungsstörung mit EMDR sich 80 % der Patientinnen und Patienten deutlich entlastet spüren – und das bereits nach wenigen Sitzungen.[1] Weitere Verfahren zur Verarbeitung von Traumata sind z. B. narrative Techniken, Ego-States-Therapie, imaginative Verfahren, Bildschirmtechnik.
    Weitere im Service Psy-Jeunes angewandte Methoden sind:

- **Klinische Hypnose (MEG)**
    Klinische Hypnose/Hypnotherapie gilt als ressourcenorientierter Ansatz, der es Patienten erlaubt, körperlichen Symptomen und psychischen Problemen mit positiven Erfahrungen und eigenen Bewältigungskompetenzen zu begegnen (MEG, Milton Erickson Gesellschaft).

---

[1] http://www.emdria.de/emdr/was-ist-emdr/.

- **Klientenzentrierte Psychotherapie**
  Ist eine Therapieform der humanistischen Psychologie. Sie geht auf ihren Begründer Carl R. Rogers zurück.
- **Psychologische Schmerztherapie**
  Schmerzen haben erheblichen Einfluss auf die Psyche des Menschen. Oft sind psychologische Verfahren der einzige Weg, chronische Schmerzen zu lindern. Psychologische Methoden versuchen am affektiven, kognitiven und sozialen Aspekt chronischer Schmerzen anzusetzen. Es werden spezifische Verfahren zur Veränderung ungünstiger Verhaltens- und Empfindungsgewohn-heiten vermittelt und in den Alltag des Patienten transferiert. Es können auf-arbeitende (Konflikt-, Gedanken- und Beziehungsanalyse) oder vorwiegend modifikatorische (Aktivitätsänderung, Verhaltenslenkung, Entspannungs- und Visualisierungstechniken, Hypnotherapie) zur Anwendung kommen.
- **Verhaltenstherapie**
  Die Verhaltenstherapie versucht für gegenwärtige Probleme individuelle, maßgeschneiderte Interventionen zu bieten. Sie setzt an den prä-disponierenden, auslösenden und aufrechterhaltenden Bedingungen an und ist zielorientiert. Der Patient ist aktiv beteiligt. Es geht nicht nur um Reflexion und Gewinnung von Einsicht, sondern um praktisches Handeln und aktives Erproben neuer Verhaltens- und Erlebnisweisen. Der Therapeut bietet dem Patienten „Hilfe zur Selbsthilfe" und ist dabei transparent.
  Zu den verhaltenstherapeutischen Methoden, die im Service Psy-Jeunes angewendet werden, gehören u. a.: Desensibilisierungs- und Konfrontations-methoden, Rollenspielmethoden, Entspannungsverfahren, soziales Kompetenztraining, Stressbewältigungstraining und Elterntraining.
- **Entwicklungspsychologische Beratung (EPB)**
  Die EPB ist ein Angebot zur Förderung der elterlichen Feinfühligkeit in der frühen Kindheit. Sie dient dem Aufbau einer gelingenden Eltern-Kind-Beziehung und einer sicheren emotionalen Bindung beim Kind.
- **Schematherapie**
  Die Schematherapie ist eine Form der Psychotherapie. Sie zählt zur sogenannten dritten Welle der kognitiv-verhaltenstherapeutischen Therapien und erweitert die Methoden der kognitiven Therapie um Elemente psycho-dynamischer Konzepte und anderer etablierter psychologischer Theorien und Therapieverfahren wie der Objektbeziehungstheorie, der Transaktionsanalyse, der Hypnotherapie und der Gestalttherapie. Sie wurde von Jeffrey E. Young entwickelt (Young 2005).

4   Gesundheitliche Probleme und Beeinträchtigungen des Wohlbefindens bei jugendlichen Klienten des Psy-Jeunes

„Ich will mich entfalten. Nirgends will ich gebogen bleiben, denn dort bin ich gelogen, wo ich gebogen bin." Rainer Maria Rilke.

Die psychische Entwicklung eines jeden Menschen wird von mehreren Faktoren beeinflusst. Sowohl genetische Prädispositionen und Temperament auf der einen Seite, aber auch unsere Erfahrungen und unser soziales Umfeld (Familie, Schule, Freizeit, Freunde) bestimmen, wie wir uns entwickeln.

Im Folgenden werden einige Lebensgeschichten vorgestellt und deren Einfluss auf die Entwicklung des jeweiligen Kindes und auf die Beeinträchtigung seines Wohlbefindens.

Klientin 1 (16 Jahre)

Zum Zeitpunkt der Anmeldung lebte die Klientin seit 6 Wochen im Heim. Sie wurde aufgrund ihres aggressiven Verhaltens und der vielen Konflikte in der Schule vorgestellt. Im Erstgespräch zeigte sich die Klientin abweisend. Alles sei gut, es habe sich viel verändert, seitdem sie im Heim sei; sie brauche keine Hilfe. Nur sehr vorsichtig ließ sie sich auf die Fragen der Therapeutin ein. Sie berichtete, dass sie sich sehr schnell angegriffen/bedroht fühle und dann zuschlage. Sie sei dadurch auch bereits stationär und teilstationär in Behandlung gewesen. Wenn ihre Gefühle unerträglich werden, ritze sie sich. Im Laufe der Therapie zeigte sich, dass die Klientin die Menschen von sich wegstieß, die sie mochte. Sie fühlte sich ungeliebt. Sie hatte das Gefühl, immer alles falsch zu machen und von anderen nur negativ bewertet zu werden. Was auch tatsächlich der Fall war. Jeder sah in ihr nur „die Aggressive". Die Klientin hatte verlernt auf ihre eigenen Bedürfnisse zu hören, ihren Gefühlen zu vertrauen. In ihr waren tief verwurzelt Gefühle von Verzweiflung, Traurigkeit und Selbsthass.

Zur Geschichte: Die Klientin war das älteste von 5 Geschwistern. Ihre Mutter war sehr jung, als sie schwanger wurde. Als die Klientin auf der Welt war, konnte die Mutter nicht auf die Bedürfnisse des Babys eingehen. Sie fühlte sich überfordert und gab das Kind zur Großmutter in ein anderes Land. Dort wuchs die Klientin auf, bis sie 3 Jahre alt war. Dann wollte die Mutter ihr Kind zurück. Sie hatte immer noch Schwierigkeiten, auf die Emotionen ihres Kindes zu reagieren. Die Klientin beschreibt die Mutter als kühl und distanziert. Den Vater beschreibt sie als liebevoll. Sie hätten regelmäßig Sachen unternommen, viel gespielt. Als sie ca. 7 Jahre alt war, hatte der Vater einen Verkehrsunfall, wodurch sich seine Persönlichkeit stark veränderte. Aus dem liebevollen Vater wurde ein Vater, der sie immer häufiger schlug und misshandelte. Nach einiger Zeit fing er an sie zu missbrauchen. Sie erzählte es ihrer Mutter, doch diese glaubte ihr nicht. Als sie 12 Jahre war, trennten sich ihre Eltern und der Missbrauch hörte auf.

Analyse: In einer Lebensphase, in der der Aufbau einer sicheren Bindung von höchster Bedeutung für ein Baby ist, wurde die Klientin von ihrer leiblichen Mutter getrennt, um in ein völlig fremdes Umfeld gesetzt zu werden. Bereits im Mutterleib beginnt der Aufbau einer Bindung zur Mutter. Das Ungeborene hat Kontakt zu seiner Außenwelt. Es hört die Stimmen seines Umfeldes; Geräusche, die es sich bereits einprägt. Kurz nach der Geburt ist ein Baby fähig, die Stimme seiner Mutter von anderen Frauenstimmen zu unterscheiden. Die Trennung eines Säuglings von seiner Mutter, ist für nahezu jedes Kind ein traumatisches Erlebnis.

Die Bindungstheorie gilt als eine der weltweit wichtigsten Theorien zur Erklärung der sozial-emotionalen Entwicklung von der Geburt bis ins hohe Alter. Bowlby beschreibt Bindung als ein emotionales Band zwischen einem Kind und einer oder mehreren vertrauten Bezugspersonen. Laut Bowlby existiert ein biologisch festgelegtes Bindungsverhaltenssystem, das das Überleben und die psychische Gesundheit des Kindes garantiert (Cierpka 2014).

Ein weiteres Mal wird das Kind mit 3 Jahren aus seinem gewohnten Umfeld gerissen. Zu diesem Zeitpunkt ist die Bindung gefestigt. Das Kind entwickelt in diesem Alter eine innere Repräsentation davon, wer es ist und wo es hingehört. Es fühlt sich sicher und geborgen. Das Kind hat erste soziale Kontakte außerhalb der Familie, die wichtig für seine Entwicklung sind. Es hat ein Zugehörigkeitsgefühl entwickelt. Aus diesem Umfeld wird es rausgenommen, um in ein neues Umfeld gesetzt zu werden, zwar mit seinen leiblichen Eltern, die es aber bis dahin kaum kennen lernen durfte, doch in ein fremdes Land, mit einer fremden Sprache und neuen Gesichtern – alles Bekannte und Vertraute ist weg. Hier kann man von Bindungstraumata sprechen.

Als die Klientin 7 Jahre alt war, veränderte sich die Persönlichkeit des Vaters. Dies war für das Kind mit massiven Ängsten verbunden. Neben der Gewalt erfuhr das Kind eine tiefe Verletzung seiner körperlichen und seelischen Integrität. Zu diesem Entwicklungszeitpunkt ist das Kind zwar fähig das Verhalten des Vaters als falsch zu empfinden, jedoch nicht seinen Vater infrage zu stellen. Da das Kind danach strebt, die Welt zu verstehen und zu erklären, gibt es sich selbst die Schuld am Verhalten des Vaters.

Die Aggressionen des Kindes sind zum einen als Ventil aller Emotionen zu verstehen, zum anderen befindet sich das Kind in einem Zustand ständiger Wachsamkeit und Kampfbereitschaft.

Klient 2 (15 Jahre)

Anmeldegründe dieses Klienten waren Zwangsgedanken und Zwangshandlungen, starke innere Anspannung, Selbstverletzung, sowie Impulskontrollstörungen. Zum Zeitpunkt der Anmeldung lebte der Klient mit seiner älteren Schwester und den leiblichen Eltern in einem Haushalt.

Im Erstgespräch zeigte der Klient eine depressive Stimmung und äußerte Schlafstörungen zu haben. Dies hatte zur Folge, dass sich der Klient in der Schule schlecht konzentrieren konnte und sich selbst sehr unter Druck setzte, um seinen Ansprüchen gegenüber den schulischen Leistungen gerecht zu werden. Des Weiteren hatte der Klient aufgrund des selbstverletzenden und impulsiven Verhaltens ein sehr negatives Selbstbild entwickelt. Dies führte zur Vermeidung sozialer Kontakte und sozialem Rückzug.

Zur Geschichte: Der Vater des Klienten litt unter einer chronifizierten posttraumatischen Belastungsstörung aufgrund eigener traumatischer Erfahrungen in Kindheit und Jugend. Er bestimmte den Alltag der Familie, indem er eigene Bedürfnisse in den Vordergrund stellte. Sein starkes Kontrollverhalten ließ es nicht zu, dass die Mutter oder die Kinder eigene Wünsche, Bedürfnisse oder Ideen einbringen konnten. Der Alltag der ganzen Familie wurde von ihm durchstrukturiert. Freundschaften waren nur bedingt erlaubt, da der Vater sie als Verrat ihm gegenüber empfand. Der Klient hatte nie gelernt spontan zu sein oder auf die eigenen Bedürfnisse zu hören. Er musste sich anpassen und eigene Bedürfnisse zurückstellen.

Analyse: Die Traumafolgestörung des Vaters machte es ihm nicht möglich, auf die Bedürfnisse oder Wünsche seiner Familienmitglieder einzugehen. Aufgrund der Vernachlässigung der Grundbedürfnisse nach Autonomie, Anerkennung, sich mitzuteilen und Spontaneität konnte beim Klienten keine gesunde psychische Entwicklung stattfinden. Die rigiden Forderungen des Vaters machten es dem Klienten unmöglich, eigene Bedürfnisse zu zeigen. Durch die ständige Unterdrückung der eigenen Gefühlswelt und die dauerhafte Anpassung an ein erkranktes Familiensystem verlor das Kind mit der Zeit das Gespür für sich selber. Das hochbeängstigende Verhalten des Vaters führte auf Seiten des Klienten zur Entwicklung von Zwangsgedanken und Zwangshandlungen im Sinne einer Kompensationsstrategie. Dies, um in überfordernden Situationen ein Mindestmaß an Kontrolle zurückzugewinnen. Der daraus resultierenden hohen inneren Anspannung steuerte der Klient mit Hilfe von Selbstverletzung entgegen.

Die Selbstbestimmungstheorie (Ryan und Deci 2000) postuliert drei psychologische Grundbedürfnisse – Autonomie, Kompetenz und soziale Eingebundenheit –, deren Befriedigung zu psychologischem Wachstum, Integrität und Wohlbefinden sowie zu Vitalität und Selbst-Kongruenz führt. Maslow definierte die Grund-

bedürfnisse Sicherheit, Geborgenheit, Autonomie/Selbstständigkeit, Anerkennung/
Akzeptanz, Freiheit, sich mitzuteilen, realistische Grenzen, Liebe und Aufmerk-
samkeit, Spontaneität und Spiel (Schneider und Margraf 2009*)*.

Klient 3 (11 Jahre)

Anmeldegründe dieses Klienten waren Konzentrationsschwierigkeiten, emotionale Instabilität, Dissoziationen, Ängste (vor allem Verlustängste) und Schlafstörungen. Zum Zeitpunkt der Aufnahme lebte der Klient seit 3 Monaten in Fremdunterbringung.

Im Erstgespräch wurde der Klient von seiner Erzieherin begleitet. Die Äußerungen des Klienten ließen auf ein vermindertes Selbstwertgefühl und eine geringe Frustrationstoleranz schließen. Schulisch fiel es dem Klienten schwer mitzukommen, auch weil er sehr langsam in seinen Denkprozessen war. Aufgrund der Ängste war der Klient wenig selbstständig und skeptisch gegenüber anderen Menschen. Er hatte Schwierigkeiten, soziale Kontakte aufzubauen und aufrechtzuerhalten.

Zur Geschichte: Der Klient wuchs bis zu seinem 11. Lebensjahr mit seiner alleinerziehenden psychisch erkrankten Mutter (Alkoholabhängigkeit und Depressionen) auf. Der Alltag war unstrukturiert und chaotisch. Die Mutter war in ihrem Verhalten unberechenbar. Sie konnte sehr liebevoll sein, war aber häufig auch emotional abwesend. Bereits sehr früh musste der Klient Verantwortung übernehmen, morgens selber aufstehen, sich fertig machen und die Mutter wecken. Häufig musste er die Verantwortung für die Mutter übernehmen, versteckte den Alkohol oder entsorgte diesen. Er brachte die Mutter häufig ins Bett, wenn sie betrunken auf dem Fußboden lag. Bereits mit 5 Jahren konnte er sich selbst versorgen. Wegen der Alkoholerkrankung der Mutter machte er sich sehr oft Sorgen um sie. Angst war sein ständiger Begleiter: Angst um die Mutter, Überforderung im Alltag, Angst, wie es weitergehen sollte. Die Fremdunterbringung wurde veranlasst, als das Kind die Mutter nach einem Selbstmordversuch bewusstlos in der Wohnung auffand.

Analyse: Psychische Erkrankungen eines Elternteils wirken sich massiv auf die Entwicklung von Kindern aus. Wenn das andere Elternteil die Bedürfnisse des Kindes ebenfalls nicht beantworten kann, wirkt sich dies verstärkend auf die Belastung aus. Die frühkindlichen Erfahrungen in der Interaktion machen es dem Kind unmöglich, eine sichere Bindung aufzubauen. Im beschriebenen Fall wechselten sich liebevolles und vernachlässigendes Verhalten ab, was sich in einem desorganisierten Bindungsstil zeigen kann. Das Kind entwickelte daraufhin Bewältigungs- und Schutzstrategien für das erkrankte Elternteil und Überlebensstrategien für sich selbst. Es übernahm die Ver-

antwortung für die Mutter (Parentifizierung). Dadurch konnte es sich häufig nicht auf die Schule konzentrieren, hatte Schlafstörungen. Gleichzeitig konnte es nicht mehr Kind sein. Soziale Interaktionen fielen ihm schwer, weil es so viel anderes „Wichtigeres" im Kopf hatte. Soziale Ausgrenzung war die Folge. Wenn die Gefühle übermächtig werden, schaltet das Gehirn auf Dissoziation um, die der emotionalen Distanzierung dienen soll. In diesen Moment wirkt das Kind auf andere abwesend, verträumt. Häufig resultiert aus dieser ständigen Überforderung ein sehr hohes Ausmaß an innerer Anspannung und Angst. Hyperarousal und permanente Wachsamkeit sind die Folgen. Ebenso sind heftige Wutausbrüche und starke Impulskontrolldurchbrüche möglich.

Der Selbstmordversuch eines Elternteils verunsichert das Kind in seinem Urvertrauen und entzieht im „den Boden unter den Füßen". Massive Verlustängste sind die logische Folge. Das Kind reagiert mit heftigen Schuldgefühlen einerseits, weil es nicht da war, um das zu verhindern. Gleichzeitig ist dieser Akt für das Kind ein Zeichen, der Bezugsperson nicht wichtig und bedeutend genug zu sein.

Grossmann und Grossmann (2003) konnten nachweisen, dass die Bindungserfahrungen von Kindern mit den wichtigen Bindungspersonen die Grundlage für das (Ur-)Vertrauen in sich, in andere und die Welt darstellen. Die Wertschätzung von Gefühlen, die Bedeutung von Beziehungserfahrungen und das tiefere Verständnis für die Folgen solcher Erfahrungen verpflichten die Fachleute zu einem biografisch orientierten Vorgehen, gerade bei den besonders unsicheren und durch die Bindungspersonen selbst belasteten Kindern in Heimen und Pflegefamilien. Ohne die Bindungsforschung und den Blick auf die Bindungsgeschichte von Menschen könnten wir ihr auffälliges Verhalten und die Sehnsucht nach Nähe dahinter viel weniger verstehen.

Klient 4 (8 Jahre)
Der Klient wurde aufgrund von Konzentrationsproblemen in der Schule vorgestellt. Er sei für sein Alter nicht aufmerksam genug, er „träume" sich weg, müsse immer wieder ans Arbeiten erinnert werden. Zum Zeitpunkt der Anmeldung lebte der Klient mit seiner Mutter und den 2 jüngeren Brüdern in einem Haushalt.

Zur Geschichte: In der Anamnese des Jungen zeigten sich Gewalterfahrungen in der Familie. Immer wieder erlebte er, wie sein Vater seine Mutter schlug. Der Klient stellte sich häufig zwischen beide, weil der Vater dann von der Mutter abließ. Die Situation eskalierte, als der Junge seine Mutter bewusstlos auffand und Hilfe holte, da er dachte, sie sei tot. Daraufhin schaffte es die Mutter, sich von ihrem Partner zu trennen. Der Vater übte weiterhin Druck auf die Familie aus.

Immer wieder tauchte er auf, verhielt sich aggressiv gegenüber der Mutter und zeigte impulsives Verhalten gegenüber den Kindern. *Laut Lutz Ulrich Bessser, Facharzt für Psychiatrie und Psychotherapie, Kinder- und Jugendpsychiatrie und psychotherapeutischer Medizin, konnten wissenschaftliche Studien inzwischen belegen, dass es für das Belastungserleben irrelevant ist, ob das Kind die Gewalt am eigenen Körper erlebt oder nur beobachtet. Die Auswirkungen auf das Gehirn seien die gleichen (Besser 2013). Das Kind entwickelt eine ständige Wachsamkeit, im Sinne einer Handlungsbereitschaft im Falle eines Vorfalls. Kinder übernehmen häufig eine Schutzrolle gegenüber dem Partner, der die Gewalt erfährt. Sie fühlen sich verantwortlich dafür, dass dem Opfer und den Geschwistern nichts passiert. Ist das Gehirn des Kindes im Zustand der Wachsamkeit und Angst, ist es ihm nicht möglich, Denkprozesse oder konzentrierte Arbeiten zu leisten.*

Klientin 5 (21 Jahre)

Anmeldegrund waren wechselnde Stimmungen sowie Angstanfälle. Die Klientin sagte, sie sei schnell wegen Kleinigkeiten gereizt beziehungsweise verärgert. Daraufhin werde sie wütend, beleidige und werfe mit Gegenständen. Anschließend fühle sie sich schuldig, werte sich ab und fühle sich unwichtig. Sie fühle sich ihren Gefühlszuständen machtlos ausgeliefert. Sie fügte sich selbst verschiedene Verletzungen zu (Ritzen, in die Wand schlagen, sich selbst blutig schlagen). Zum Zeitpunkt der Aufnahme lebte sie mit ihrem Freund zusammen. Frühere pädagogische, psychologische ambulante sowie stationäre Hilfsmaßnahmen waren bereits erfolglos. Nach einer etwas turbulenten Schullaufbahn hatte sie dennoch die Sekundarstufe geschafft.

Zur Geschichte: Die Klientin wuchs als Einzelkind mit ihren leiblichen Eltern auf. Sie erlitt Gewalt von Seiten der Mutter. Der Vater stand dem Verhalten seiner Partnerin hilflos gegenüber. Er selber sei körperlich krank. Häufig bangte die Klientin um sein Leben. Die Klientin erlebte die Mutter als unberechenbar. Sie rastete nicht nur tagsüber aus, sondern riss die Klientin nicht selten auch nachts aus dem Bett, um sie zu beschimpfen und zu schlagen. Die Mutter gab ihr das Gefühl unerwünscht zu sein und äußerte immer wieder, die Klientin habe ihr Leben zerstört. Finanzielle Ressourcen nutzte die Mutter für sich selbst. Hierbei stellte sie ihre eigenen Bedürfnisse vor die Wünsche der Klientin, ignorierte zum Beispiel ihren Wunsch nach einem Hobby. In der Schule zeigte die Klientin auffälliges Verhalten; sie schwänzte immer wieder, ihre Leistungen fielen drastisch ab. Eine stationäre Aufnahme war die Folge, brachte aber keine Entlastung. Belastend hinzu kamen häufige Wohnungs- und Ortswechsel.

Analyse: Gewalterfahrungen durch die Mutter führten beim Kind zu massiven Ängsten. Neben den Schlägen und Abwertungen verletzte der Satz „Du bist nicht gewollt" das Kind in seinem tiefsten Inneren. Das Kind fragte sich, wenn meine Eltern mich nicht wollen, wer soll mich dann wollen? Da diese Erfahrungen tagtäglich stattfanden und der Vater keinerlei Schutz gewährleisten konnte, musste das Kind allein Bewältigungsstrategien finden. In diesem Fall passte es sein Weltbild derart an, dass Aggressivität als normal empfunden wurde. Das Kind zeigte Beschwichtigungsversuche, indem es sich dem Alltag anpasste, sehr ruhig wirkte und bestmögliche Leistungen in der Schule brachte (überangepasstes Verhalten). Diese Strategien funktionierten jedoch nur zeitbegrenzt, bis sich die erlebten Aggressionen im Kind re-inszenierten. Das Gefühl von Wertlosigkeit durch die erlebten Erfahrungen unterstützte die Selbstaggressionen. Die Oma konnte in diesem Fall dem Kind zwar Halt geben, die Situation aber nicht unterbinden, da ihr das Kind nie etwas erzählt hat. Die Klientin hatte Angst, es werde schlimmer, bzw. sie befürchtete, die Oma unternehme tatsächlich etwas dagegen und die Eltern könnten ihr daraufhin den Kontakt verbieten. Ihre eigenen Aggressionen waren ein Hilferuf.

Klientin 6 (16 Jahre)
Die Anmeldung erfolgte aufgrund von Angstzuständen und Panikattacken. Die Klientin gab an, sie empfinde eine unspezifische Traurigkeit sowie ein Gefühl des Kontrollverlustes. Ihr Angstzustand war von Sorgen über verschiedene Lebensbereiche (Schule, Familie, Wohnung) beeinflusst. Sie beschrieb sich selbst als eine ängstliche Person, welche sich schnell Sorgen macht. Die geschilderten Symptome haben sich seit einiger Zeit noch verschlimmert.

Zur Geschichte: Die junge Frau war 16 Jahre alt und lebte zusammen mit ihrer Mutter und ihren zwei älteren Geschwistern. Die Eltern hatten sich getrennt, als die Klientin 9 Jahre alt war, und standen seitdem in Konflikt. Die Beziehung zum Vater, welche bisher aufrechterhalten wurde, war seit kurzem eher distanziert, weil sie sich von ihm manipuliert fühlte. Der Vater war seit der Trennung von ihrer Mutter nur selten anwesend. Die Mutter hatte nach der Trennung eine weitere Partnerschaft, die aber nach zwei Jahren auseinanderging. Der Partner gab damals den Kindern die Schuld für die Trennung. Zeitnah musste sich die Klientin in der Schule für eine schulfachbezogene Sektion entscheiden. Ihre Entscheidung bereute sie schnell, ihr wurde ein Wechsel nicht gewährt. Aufgrund der schlechteren Leistungen warfen die Mutter und ihre Schwestern ihr vor, sich nicht genug Mühe zu geben, nicht hart genug für die Schule zu arbeiten. Im Zuge dieser Situationen begannen sich die Symptome zu zeigen.

Die Klientin war sich zum Zeitpunkt des Therapiebeginns der elterlichen Konflikte vor nicht allzu langer Zeit erst wirklich bewusst geworden. Im Laufe des Jahres hatte sie mehrere schwierige Ereignisse erlebt (Einbruch, Übergriff auf ein Familienmitglied, Verschärfung der Konflikte zwischen den Eltern).

Analyse: Bei der Trennung der leiblichen Eltern mit den daraus resultierenden Konflikten übernahm die Klientin einen Teil der Verantwortung. Sie bekam viele indirekte Konflikte mit und fühlte sich gezwungen Lösungen zu finden. Zu diesem Zeitpunkt entwickelte die Klientin keinerlei störungsrelevante Symptome. Es zeigt also, dass Kinder durchaus in der Lage sind, belastende Lebensereignisse durchzustehen, wenn sie genug Ressourcen und Unterstützung zur Verfügung haben. Die anhaltenden Konflikte zwischen den leiblichen Eltern, die erneute Trennung von Mutter und Partner sowie der schulische Leistungsdruck führten jedoch dazu, dass die Ressourcen der Klientin erschöpft waren. Da die Klientin bereits vom Temperament her eher ängstlich war und sich viele Sorgen machte, führten diese belastenden Situationen zu einer Verstärkung der Angst. Sie versuchte die Dinge so gut es ging nach ihren Möglichkeiten zu bewältigen, erlebte aber immer wieder Kontrollverlust: die erneute Trennung, schulische Überforderung, den Einbruch. Aus diesen wiederholten Situationen der Macht- und Hilflosigkeit resultierte die unspezifische Trauer. Sie wusste eigentlich sehr genau, was sie brauchte. Die Klientin hatte eigentlich immer einen guten Zugang zu ihrem inneren Gespür und zu ihren Bedürfnissen. Ihr Umfeld hatte nicht immer ein Gehör dafür.

Resilienzfaktoren sind „Eigenschaften, die das Kind in der Interaktion mit der Umwelt sowie durch die erfolgreiche Bewältigung von altersspezifischen Entwicklungsaufgaben im Verlauf erwirbt; die Faktoren haben bei der Bewältigung von Lebensaufgaben eine besondere Rolle" (Wustmann 2004, S. 46).

Klientin 7 (3 Jahre)

Die Eltern stellten die Klientin aufgrund von folgender Problematik vor: Sie habe sich in den letzten Monaten im Verhalten geändert. Sie sage zu allem nein, zeige sich teilweise aggressiv gegenüber ihren Spielkameraden. Derzeit gäbe es viele Konflikte bezüglich der Sauberkeitserziehung. Sie weigere sich, aufs Klo zu gehen. Stuhlgang sei kein Problem. Konflikte seien vorwiegend mit dem Vater. Zum Zeitpunkt der Anmeldung lebte die Klientin mit ihrem jüngeren Bruder und der Mutter in einem Haushalt. Die Eltern hatten sich vor einigen Monaten getrennt. Am Anfang sah der Vater die Kinder jedes Wochenende, inzwischen waren die Kinder abwechselnd bei beiden Elternteilen. Die Eltern gaben an sich gut zu verstehen. Die Mutter habe an einer postnatalen Depression gelitten.

Analyse: Das problemindzuierende Verhalten zeigte sich stärker beim Vater als bei der Mutter. Die Mutter ging gelassener mit der Sauberkeitserziehung um, der Vater stellte höhere Erwartungen an sein Kind. Insgesamt seien Vater und Tochter im Charakter sehr ähnlich. Mit ihren 3 Jahren musste die Klientin bereits einige Hürden überwinden. Die postnatale Depression macht es Müttern nicht möglich, feinfühlig und für das Neugeborene emotional verfügbar zu sein. Das kompetente Baby kann diese schwierige Situation jedoch gut bewältigen, wenn andere Bezugspersonen es auffangen und ihm Halt geben. Die Geburt eines jüngeren Geschwisterchens stellt häufig eine weitere Herausforderung dar. Das ältere Kind muss lernen seine Eltern zu teilen. Auch dies braucht einen Anpassungsmoment für alle Beteiligten. Die Trennung der Eltern, selbst wenn sie noch so „gut" verläuft, ist für Kinder ein sehr einschneidendes Erlebnis. Alles, was sie bisher gekannt haben, alles Gewohnte, die Rituale, ihr Zuhause, die Familie, wird entzweit. Kinder reagieren darauf teils mit sehr unterschiedlichen Emotionen. Eine Möglichkeit zeigt sich hier: Das Kind versuchte die Aufmerksamkeit seiner Eltern auf sich selbst zu lenken. Dies machen Kinder teils unbewusst. Sie versuchen so ein Stück Sicherheit und Halt zurückzugewinnen. Egal ob wir positive Gefühle mit unseren Kindern teilen oder wir mit ihnen schimpfen, wir teilen einen Moment mit dem Kind, sind präsent, fokussiert und konzentriert auf das Kind. Häufig in solchen unsicheren Lebensmomenten ist es diese Aufmerksamkeit, ob positiv oder negativ, die Kinder brauchen und einfordern.

Jedes Kind wird mit einer unverwechselbaren Identität und Individualität geboren. Die Kinderpsychiater Stella Chess und Alexander Thomas haben den Ausdruck „goodness of fit" eingeführt, der besagt, dass ein Kind sich dann optimal entwickelt, wenn eine Übereinstimmung zwischen seinem Temperament und seiner Motivation einerseits und den Erwartungen, Anforderungen und Möglichkeiten andererseits besteht (Chess und Thomas 1984).

Klientin 8 (10 Jahre)

Die Eltern stellten die Klientin aufgrund folgender Problematik vor: Das Kind zeige eine große Sensibilität und lasse sich leicht aus dem Gleichgewicht bringen. Sie sei übertrieben perfektionistisch, habe eine niedrige Frustrationstoleranz und könne nicht mit Niederlagen umgehen. Sie sei in mehreren Bereichen stark verunsichert und zeige diverse unspezifische und objektgebundene Ängste. Sie habe Schwierigkeiten, sich an neue Situationen anzupassen. Außerdem leide sie unter Schlafstörungen. Ihr Verhalten sei zeitweise aufmüpfig und wenig respektvoll. Auch gebe es häufig Konflikte mit ihrer Schwester. Zum Zeitpunkt der Anmeldung lebte die Klientin gemeinsam mit der jüngeren Schwester und den Eltern in einem Haushalt. Die Familie war in der Vergangenheit aus beruf-

C. Weintzen et al.

lichen Gründen sehr häufig umgezogen. Der Vater war aus denselben beruflichen Gründen ein ganzes Jahr von der Familie getrennt.

Analyse: Die häufigen Länderwechsel erforderten von der Klientin ein Höchstmaß an Anpassung. Nicht nur dass Kultur und Sprache immer wieder wechselten, die Klientin musste sich bei jedem Umzug ein neues soziales Umfeld aufbauen und das Gewohnte hinter sich lassen. Es kam also immer wieder zu Beziehungsabbrüchen. Die Folge können eine allgemeine Verunsicherung und hohe innere Anspannung sein. Der Perfektionismus entwickelt sich im Sinne einer kompensatorischen Strategie. Niederlagen werden dadurch nur sehr schwer akzeptiert. Durch die allgemeine innere Unruhe und Anspannung kann das Kind nachts nicht zur Ruhe kommen. Mit dem Eintritt in die Schule werden Freunde für die Entwicklung des Kindes immer bedeutungsvoller. In einer Freundschaft gewinnen Kinder nicht nur Spielgefährten. Freunde teilen die gleichen Interessen, geben sich gegenseitig Unterstützung. Die Klientin musste sich ständig neue Freunde suchen, was mit zunehmendem Alter schwieriger wird, da sich bereits im Kindergarten Freundschaften formen und „die Neue" häufig erst einmal einen schwierigen Standpunkt hat. Die einzige Konstante im Leben des Kindes war die Mutter. Sie war liebevoller Wegbegleiter. Es war für sie sicher nicht immer leicht, da auch sie sich immer wieder den neuen Gegebenheiten anpassen und ein soziales Umfeld für sich selbst und die Familie aufbauen musste; häufig allein, da der Vater abwesend war. Sie selbst war vom Temperament her ähnlich wie die Klientin eher unsicher. Sie stellte hohe Erwartungen an sich selbst, welche von Selbstzweifeln begleitet waren. Es ist davon auszugehen, dass die Mutter ihrer Tochter trotz aller Liebe nicht genügend Halt, Ruhe und Gelassenheit vermitteln konnte. Ihre eigenen Sorgen färbten auf das Kind ab.

Klientin 9 (16 Jahre)

Die Klientin kam im Alter von 16 Jahren in unseren Service zur Psychotherapie. Sie nannte als Anmeldegründe ausgeprägte Stimmungsschwankungen und Panikgefühle sowie den Drang, sich selbst zu verletzen in Form von Schneiden (bereits mit 12 Jahren). Auch habe sie wiederkehrende Suizidgedanken, konnte sich jedoch zum Zeitpunkt des Therapiebeginns von akuter Suizidalität glaubhaft distanzieren. Die Klientin hatte bereits drei Suizidversuche in der Vergangenheit unternommen. Im therapeutischen Kontakt zeigte die Klientin zu Beginn ein hohes Maß an Misstrauen und Vorsicht. Es fiel ihr sehr schwer, über Erlebtes zu sprechen. Sie gab an, sie habe große Schwierigkeiten, sich emotional zu öffnen oder Gefühle zu zeigen. Immer wieder betonte sie im Kontakt, sie habe Angst, in Tränen auszubrechen und beim Weinen gesehen zu werden. Die Klientin gab an, sie fühle sich häufig körperlich und emotional total erschöpft. Vertrauensvolle

Beziehungen einzugehen gelinge ihr kaum. In ihrem Alltag meide sie Kontakte möglichst und gehe nur in guten Phasen „unter die Leute". Zum Zeitpunkt der Therapie lebte die Klientin mit der leiblichen Mutter und deren Partner in einem Haushalt.

Zur Geschichte: In der biografischen Anamnese beschrieb die Klientin eine von emotionaler Vernachlässigung geprägte Entwicklung sowie erlebte Gewalt durch den alkoholkranken Vater. Sie könne sich an längere Phasen ihrer Kindheit kaum oder nicht erinnern. Manche verfügbaren Erinnerungen erlebe sie in Gedanken und Gefühlen ungewollt immer wieder: So beschrieb sie z. B. eine Situation, in der sie der alkoholisierte Vater zur Strafe mit einem Strick ans Auto gebunden und hinter dem fahrenden Auto hergezogen habe. Die Erinnerungen an diese Gewalterlebnisse drängten sich der Klientin wiederkehrend und unaufhaltsam auf in Form von Bildern und Filmen. Ebenfalls beschrieb sie körperliche Intrusionen wie Herzklopfen und Schmerzen. Zum Zeitpunkt des Therapiebeginns waren die Eltern bereits geschieden und es bestand kein Kontakt mehr zum Vater, was die Klientin als stark entlastend erlebte. Die psychische Erkrankung der Mutter äußere sich in Alkoholmissbrauch und unberechenbarem Verhalten. Sie sei häufig ausgerastet, manipuliere und drohe mit Suizidalität. Sie habe häufig wechselnde Partner, deren Meinungen sie über die ihre stelle.

Analyse: Gewalterfahrungen durch wichtige Bindungspersonen stellen für die psychische Entwicklung des Kindes eine existentielle Bedrohung dar. Es fehlt eine gesunde Vorbildfunktion, die Halt und Sicherheit gibt. Gleichzeitig erlebt das Kind Vernachlässigung und weitere massive Formen von Gewalt, die zerstörerisch wirken. Das Kind entwickelt Überlebensstrategien, um in diesem erkrankten System funktionieren zu können. Genetisch kann auf der Ebene der Chromosomen bereits ein Einfluss dieser hoch stressrelevanten Erfahrungen nachgewiesen werden. Kinder, die solche traumatischen Lebensbedingungen durchlaufen, können schnellere Reifungsprozesse zeigen. Auf andere wirken sie frühreif und selbstständig in alltäglichen Situationen. Emotional hingegen sind diese Kinder in ihrer Entwicklung verzögert, sie zeigen häufig schnell wechselnde Gefühle, die für ihr Umfeld nur schwer nachvollziehbar sind, da sie nicht den typischen Entwicklungsphasen zugeordnet werden können (wie z. B. einer Trotzphase). Durch die Gewalt und die Vernachlässigung erlebt das Kind ständigen Kontrollverlust, der sich in Ohnmachtsgefühlen und Hoffnungslosigkeit zeigt. Das Kind in seiner Natur versucht die Welt um sich herum zu verstehen, um sich in ihr zurechtzufinden. In solch kranken Systemen bleibt dem Kind häufig nur die Erklärung, nicht in Ordnung zu sein, und somit die Ablehnung der Eltern als gerechtfertigt zu übernehmen und zu reinszinieren. Dies zeigt sich dann in Form von Selbsthass, Selbstverletzung und Suizidalität.

Klient 10 (19 Jahre)

Der Klient hatte sich im Alter von 19 Jahren wegen schon länger bestehender Zwangsgedanken und -handlungen in unserem Service angemeldet. Er berichtete über die zwanghafte Vorstellung, ihn eigentlich abstoßende sexuelle Handlungen begehen zu müssen. Da der Klient den starken Drang verspürte, diese der Partnerin zu „beichten", war die Beziehung des Paares zu diesem Zeitpunkt stark belastet. Die Zwangssymptomatik führte dazu, dass er, wenn er für sein Studium etwas verschriftlichen sollte, immer wieder von vorn beginnen musste, sobald ein „unreiner Gedanke" auftrat. Die Zwangsgedanken und Zwangshandlungen waren insgesamt mit starker Angst verbunden. Wenn er sie nicht durchführe, war er überzeugt, dass der Freundin „etwas Schlimmes zustoßen" werde. Durch den Zwang, das schon Geschriebene zu löschen und wieder von vorn anfangen zu müssen, wurden schriftliche Arbeiten für ihn zu einer Herkulesaufgabe. Auch berichtete er über einen Ordnungszwang und Rituale nahmen irgendwann mehrere Stunden in Anspruch. Im Verlauf der Erkrankung sah der Klient sich für eine Weile gezwungen, sein Studium zu unterbrechen, da er den Anforderungen nicht mehr in ausreichendem Maße nachkommen konnte. Ihm war die Unsinnigkeit seiner Gedanken zu jedem Zeitpunkt bewusst, jedoch schämte er sich sehr dafür bis hin zu starken Zweifeln am eigenen Charakter. Er versuchte, sein zwanghaftes Verhalten immer mehr zu verstecken, und isolierte sich vom Freundeskreis zunehmend.

Zur Geschichte: Der Klient berichtete, ein eher ängstliches Kind gewesen zu sein, das von Mutter und Großmutter stark behütet worden sei. Mutter und Großmutter waren beide stark depressiv. Jedoch sei es während seiner Entwicklung durch einen älteren und verhaltensauffälligen Bruder zunehmend häufiger zu gewaltsamen Auseinandersetzungen zwischen dem Vater und diesem Bruder gekommen. Zum Zeitpunkt des ersten Auftretens der Symptome habe der Klient sich aufgefordert gefühlt, in die körperlichen Auseinandersetzungen zwischen Vater und Bruder beschwichtigend einzugreifen; jedoch meist erfolglos.

Analyse: Depressionen von Bindungspersonen wirken sich auf das Bindungsverhalten der Kinder aus, da sie die Feinfühligkeit sowie die Interaktion direkt beeinflussen. Der Bindungsperson fällt es schwer, auf die Kontaktversuche des Kindes einzugehen, sie ist emotional erstarrt, wertet Signale des Kindes zu schnell als Ablehnung. Das Kind braucht die emotionale Nähe, um ein Gefühl der Geborgenheit und Sicherheit zu entwickeln. Einer sich im Säuglingsalter entwickelnden sicheren Bindung wird eine protektive Funktion für den Entwicklungsverlauf des Kindes zugeschrieben. Längsschnittstudien haben gezeigt, dass dadurch prosoziale Verhaltensweisen gefördert werden und eine gewisse belastbare psychische Stabilität im Sinne von „Resilienz" (Brisch 2010).

Spiegelneurone im Gehirn führen dazu, dass das Kind bestimmte emotionale Zustände des Gegenübers übernimmt. Hinzu kommen die Auseinandersetzungen des Bruders mit dem Vater, was eine zusätzliche Belastung in Form von Verunsicherung darstellt. Dies kann bei Kindern Gefühle von Hilflosigkeit, von Verantwortungsübernahme, aber auch Angst auslösen. Das starke Stressempfinden seitens des Kindes kann dazu führen, dass es Zwangsgedanken- und handlungen im Sinne einer Kompensationsstrategie entwickelt.

Diese einzelnen Falldarstellungen haben einen Einblick in die unterschiedlichen Ursachen für die Entwicklung psychischer Beeinträchtigungen und Belastungen von Kindern und Jugendlichen gegeben und die biografischen Hintergünde ausgeleuchtet. Das familiäre Umfeld und die Bindungen zu den Eltern sind dabei die zentralen Faktoren. Die Fallbeispiele haben gezeigt, wie wichtig es ist, die Bedürfnisse der Kinder wahrzunehmen und wie bedeutsam die Verantwortung der Erwachsene (insbesondere der Eltern) gegenüber Kindern ist. Gleichzeitig wurde auch deutlich, dass erforderliche Interventionen durch Hilfs- und Unterstützungsangebote häufig erst zu spät erfolgen.

5 Herausforderungen und Entwicklung

Kinder kommen mit einer angeborenen Fähigkeit auf die Welt, ihre Umgebung verstehen zu wollen und lernen zu wollen. Wenn das System, in welches sie hineingeboren werden, nicht mit dem angeboreren Verhaltensrepertoire übereinstimmt, werden die bestehenden Verhaltensprogramme verändert und angepasst, damit sich das Kind in seiner Welt zurechtfinden kann. Dies entspricht einem unbewussten Lernvorgang. Symptome entwickeln sich als ein Anpassungsvorgang an äußere Gegebenheiten, welche die Bedürfnisse des Kindes nicht oder ungünstig beantworten. Das Kind selbst ist lange Zeit nicht in der Lage, ein krankes System als solches infrage zu stellen. Zum einen weil es kein anderes System als Vergleichsmodell hat. Zum anderen weil seine kognitiven Kompetenzen ein solches Hinterfragen bis zu einem gewissen Alter nicht zulassen. Hinzu kommt, dass es in einer absoluten Abhängigkeit zu seinen Bezugspersonen steht, die vermeintlich als einzige Personen sein Überleben garantieren können. Das Kind hat also keine anderen Möglichkeiten, als sich anzupassen. Bis zu einem gewissen Alter wird es nicht um Hilfe bitten oder bitten können. Aber es wird aufgrund seiner Ausdrucks- und Verhaltensweisen, seiner Interaktionen mit Erwachsenen und Gleichaltrigen zeigen, dass es ihm nicht gut geht. Diese Hilferufe sind für sein Umfeld jedoch nicht immer zu erkennen. Ab einem gewissen Alter, etwa im Jugendalter, sind Kinder in der Lage, selbst um Hilfe zu bitten. Allerdings versuchen sie i. d. R. „allein klarzukommen" und melden sich häufig erst dann, wenn sie den Eindruck haben, dass nichts mehr geht. Symptome können sich zu diesem Zeitpunkt bereits chronifiziert oder schon zu schwerwiegenden Konsequenzen geführt haben, wie z. B. ungünstige Schullaufbahn, Schulabbruch, Suchterkrankungen, Verlust des Freundeskreises. Präventionsmaßnahmen – wie zum Beispiel die Eingliederung bestimmter Themen wie Emotionsregulation, Achtsamkeit und soziales Kompetenztraining in den Schulstoff – können den Kindern und Jugendlichen bereits erste alternative Handlungsstrategien im Umgang mit schwierigen Gefühlen zeigen.

Eine Herausforderung ist es, die Belastungen der Kinder frühzeitig zu erkennen. Verhaltensauffälligkeiten wie starker Rückzug, Weinerlichkeit und Aggressionen sind Ausdrucksversuche des Kindes, seinem Gegenüber eine Botschaft zu senden. Es braucht hier Unterstützung und Hilfe von geschulten Fachkräften, die die Botschaften des Kindes sehen, verstehen und als Hilferufe ernst nehmen.

Ebenso muss der Zugang zu entsprechenden Hilfen gewährleistet sein. Es braucht Fachkräfte, die dem Kind und seiner Familie unterstützend zur Seite stehen, ihnen helfen Lösungen zu finden und das Kind dabei unterstützen, alternative Handlungsstrategien zu entwickeln. Diese pädagogischen, psychologischen/psychotherapeutischen und medizinischen Hilfen müssen zeitnah installiert werden. Lange Wartezeiten, Aufnahmestopps sowie ein Mangel an Fachkräften sollten nicht nicht im Wege stehen. Hierzu braucht es deshalb ein politisches Gehör. Wenn Familien und Fachkräfte um die Kinder herum ein System als belastend für die psychische Entwicklung der Kinder einstufen, braucht es die Möglichkeiten sowie Ressourcen, dieses System kindgerechter zu gestalten. Wir müssen die Welt mit den Augen der Kinder sehen, aus dem Denken der Kinder verstehen und mit dem Herzen der Kinder fühlen lernen.

Literatur

Besser, L. U. (2013). Wenn die Vergangenheit Gegenwart und Zukunft bestimmt. Wie Erfahrungen und traumatische Ereignisse Spuren in unserem Kopf hinterlassen, Gehirn und Persönlichkeit strukturieren und Lebensläufe determinieren. In. Jacob Bausum, Lutz Ulrich Besser, Martin Kühn und Wilma Weiß (Hrsg.). Traumapädagogik. Grundlagen, Arbeitsfelder und Methoden für die pädagogische Praxis. Weinheim, Basel: Beltz Juventa, S. 38–55.
Bundeszentrale für gesundheitliche Aufklärung (2018). Wohlbefinden/Well-Being. https://www.leitbegriffe.bzga.de/alphabetisches-verzeichnis/wohlbefinden-well-being/.

Brisch, K.-H. (2010). Der Säugling – Bindung, Neurobiologie und Gene. Stuttgart: Klett Cotta Verlag Stuttgart.

Brisch, K.-H. (2011). Bindungsstörungen. Stuttgart: Klett Cotta Verlag Stuttgart.

Cierpka, M. (2014). Frühe Kindheit 0-3 Jahre. Heidelberg: Springer Verlag.

Chess, St. & Thomas, A. (1984). Origins an evolution of behavior disorders. New York: Bruner und Maze .

Diener, E. (1984). Subjective well-being. *Psychological Bulletin, 95*(3), 542–575.

Dilling, H, & Freyberger, H. J. (2010) (Hrsg.). Taschenführer zur ICD–10–Klassifikation psychischer Störungen. Bern: Verlag Hans Huber.

Grossmann, K.E. & Grossmann, K. (Hrsg.) (2003). Bindung und menschliche Entwicklung. John Bowlby, Mary Ainsworth und die Grundlagen der Bindungstheorie und Forschung. Stuttgart: Klett-Cotta Verlag.

Huber, M. (2009). Trauma und die Folgen. Paderborn: Junfermann Verlag.

Keyes, C. (2002). The Mental Health Continuum: From Languishing to Flourishing in Life. Journal of health and social behavior. 43. 207–22.

Petermann, F. (2008). Lehrbuch der klinischen Kinderpsychologie. Göttingen: Hogrefe Verlag.

Ryan, R. M. & Deci, E. L. (2000). Self-determination theory and the facilitation of intrinsic motivation, social development, and well-being. *American Psychologist, 55*(1), 68–78.

Ryff, C. D. & Keyes, C. L. M. (1995). The structure of psychological well-being revisited. *Journal of Personality and Social Psychology*, 69(4), 719–727.

Schneider, W. & Lindenberg, U. (2012). Entwicklungspsychologie. Weinheim: Beltz Verlag.

Schneider, S. & Margraf, J. (2009). Lehrbuch der Verhaltenstherapie. Band 3. Heidelberg: Springer Verlag.

Wustmann, C. (2004). Resilienz: Widerstandsfähigkeit von Kindern in Tageseinrichtungen fördern. Weinheim und Basel: Beltz Verlag.

Young, J.E. (2005). La thérapie des schémas. Brüssel: De Boeck.

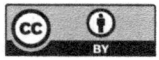

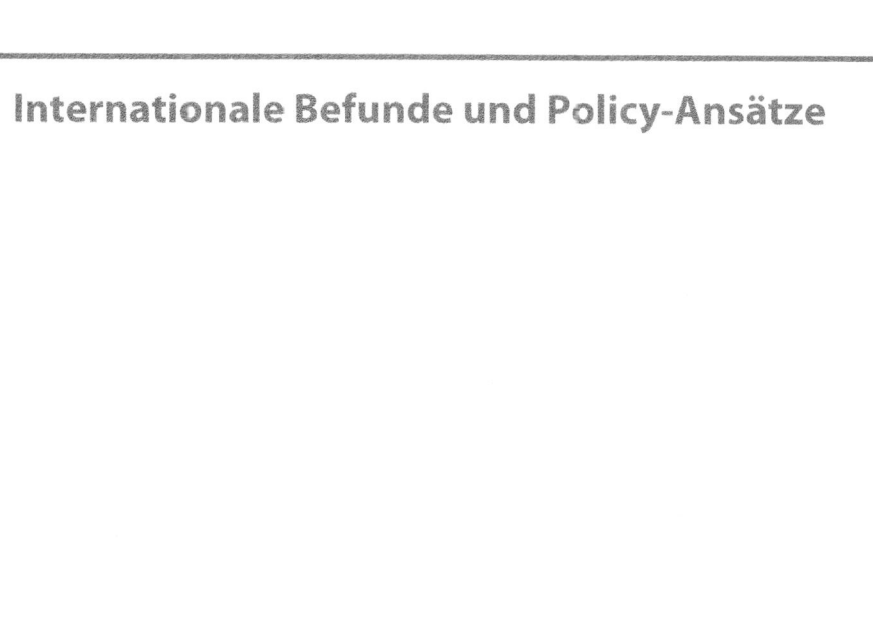

Internationale Befunde und Policy-Ansätze

Adolescent Health and Wellbeing in the UK

Yvonne Kelly

1   Introduction

The UK population is relatively 'young' and has high rates of fertility compared with most European countries, for instance 17.8 % of the total population are under 15 years of age, compared with the average for the European Union at 15.6 % (OECD 2014a), and this is mirrored by the fertility rate which in 2017 was 1.74 in the UK compared with the EU average of 1.60 (OECD 2014b). On a global footing the UK fares well along with other high income country settings on broad indicators of adolescent wellbeing, such as the WHO and UNICEF 'flourishing index' which includes markers of growth and nutrition, educational attainments, reproductive freedom, exposure to violence and mortality. In a recent report, using this measure of flourishing, the UK was ranked tenth behind Norway, South Korea, Netherlands, France, Eire, Denmark, Japan, Belgium, Iceland and on an equal footing with Germany, Switzerland, Singapore, Luxembourg and Sweden (Clark et al. 2020). Adolescent health has long term consequences for wellbeing and functioning throughout the lifecourse, for instance, the bulk of mental health conditions emerge during this time, and obesity along with certain habits and health behaviours tend to track from adolescence into the adult years. Today's young people are tomorrow's workforce and parents, and this, taken together with lifecourse implications, highlights the

Y. Kelly (✉)
ESRC International Centre for Lifecourse Studies in Society and Health (ICLS),
University College London, London, UK
E-Mail: y.kelly@ucl.ac.uk

© Der/die Autor(en) 2022
A. Heinen et al. (Hrsg.), *Wohlbefinden und Gesundheit im Jugendalter,*
https://doi.org/10.1007/978-3-658-35744-3_29

importance of supporting the development and maintenance of health during this phase of life.

Overarching influences on young people's health include the social determinants and the forces of commercial marketing, both of which pose major challenges for societies. The last decade of austerity measures in the UK has seen sweeping cuts to youth services and support for educational provision. These cuts have been accompanied by widening inequalities in poor health outcomes and increases in youth violence. Two recent high profile reports (Royal College of Paediatrics and Child Health 2020; Marmot et al. (2020)) have called for the social determinants of health to feature centre stage in all government policy, arguing that health should be positioned alongside economic productivity to reflect societal success. Young people are exposed as never before to commercial marketing pressures from corporate powers including for tobacco, alcohol, sugar sweetened beverages, gambling and social media, and there is widespread inappropriate use of personal data. Clearly, governments need to protect children from harmful commercial behaviour, but this requires agile regulation which is often opposed by powerful lobby groups and well-resourced lawyers. Currently, in the UK, legislation on protecting children from commercial harms is largely absent (Clark et al. 2020).

While the picture described in this chapter is of a pre-Covid19 context, it is conceivable that aspects of health such as mental health and health behaviours will be adversely affected in the short term and beyond by the current pandemic. Furthermore, there are likely wide ranging implications for the development and implementation of policies aimed at improving and supporting young people's health and wellbeing. For instance, it seems likely that the period of austerity experienced over the last decade will deepen even further. This chapter describes patterns of health conceptualised broadly in line with the WHO definition, as a state of physical, mental and social wellbeing and not merely the absence of disease or illness, (WHO 1946) including mental health, overweight and obesity, health behaviours and aspects of social relationships.

2   Mental Health and Wellbeing

Youth mental health is a major public health concern, which poses substantial societal and economic burdens globally (WHO 2013). Decades of underfunding in research, prevention strategies and effective treatment have resulted in unprecedented unmet need among young people in the UK (House of Commons Education and Health and Social Care Committees 2018). The UK does not compare well with other countries when considering young people's mental health and wellbeing, for instance recent Programme for International Student Assessment (PISA) survey findings show that the UK was ranked relatively low among Organisation for Economic Co-operation and Development (OECD) countries on feelings of sadness, fearfulness, and joyfulness (OECD 2019). According to the most recent figures for England, one in eight children and young people age 5 to 19 have mental health problems including anxiety, depression, conduct and hyperactivity disorders (NHS Digital 2018a), and it is estimated that about one in four girls and one in ten boys aged 14 have clinically relevant depressive symptoms (Kelly et al. 2018). Adolescence is widely regarded as a particularly vulnerable time for the development of poor mental health with 50 % of problems emerging by age 14 (WHO 2013). Alongside this, a general deterioration in mental health and wellbeing has been observed over the adolescent period for both young women and young men (Department of Education 2019), and it is estimated that 75 % of lifetime mental health problems develop before the transition from adolescence into adulthood (McLaughlin and King 2015; Kessler et al. 2007).

There have been significant changes over time, with secular trends since the late 1990s suggesting a worsening in mental health among British youth (NHS Digital 2018a; Collishaw et al. 2004; Ross et al. 2017). A recent paper compared mental health problems in two birth cohorts born a decade apart, in the early 1990s and 2000s and suggested that clinically relevant depressive symptoms in 14–15 year olds had doubled for girls (12.4–24.0 %), increased by more than half for boys (5.7–9.2), and the proportion experiencing self-harm had increased by a third for girls (16.9–22.8) and by a quarter for boys (6.9–8.5) (Patalay and Gage 2019). The burden of poor mental health is unequally distributed and this begins early in life (Kelly et al. 2011): data from the UK Millennium Cohort Study show that young people from economically disadvantaged groups tend to be worse off compared with their more affluent peers. For instance, Figure 1 shows that approximately 20 % of girls in the richest income group have clinically relevant depressive symptoms compared with 25–30 % of those in the poorest groups, and although levels of depressive symptoms are lower in boys, similar socioeconomic patterns are observed.

Many factors have been proposed to influence young people's mental health including the importance of school, friends, family, appearance and use of leisure time (Department of Education 2019). However, the underlying reasons for observed inequalities, and overall worsening in mental health among British youth are not well understood, nevertheless, a range of explanations have been proffered relating to changes in the contexts of young people's lives, including

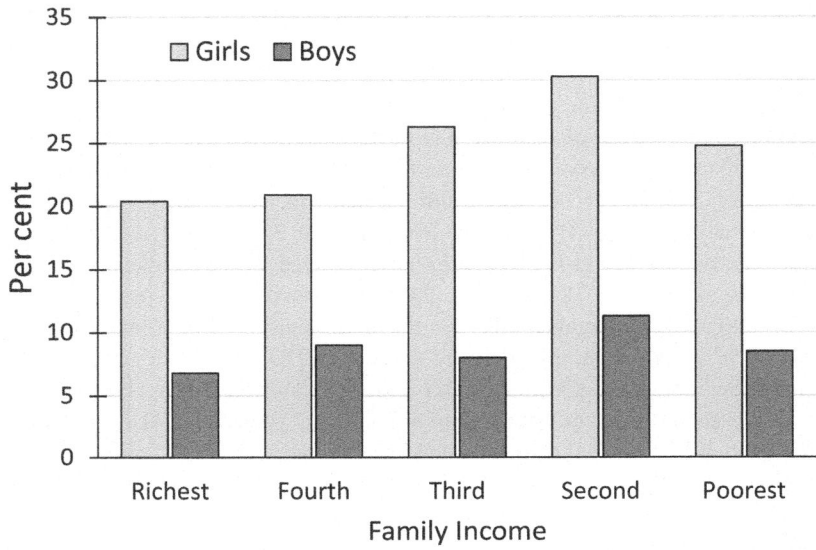

Fig. 1 Prevalence of clinically relevant depressive symptoms (age 14) by family income (own illustration)

more time spent engaging with digital technologies, increased exam pressures and educational expectations, uncertainty about future employment and housing prospects, climate change and given the current pandemic the prospect of new emerging infections may become important. The contribution of these in relation to young people's mental health and wellbeing are supported to varying degrees by extant research.

Young people are growing up in a rapidly changing digital age characterised by seamless transitions across multiple forms of media including TV and movies, social networking and gaming sites. Undoubtedly the benefits of digital technology use are wide ranging, for example, improved knowledge acquisition and social connectedness with geographically dispersed support networks. On the other hand, the observed decline in mental health has coincided with ubiquitous digital technology use and has led to growing concerns about the potential pitfalls of how, where, when and why people engage in digital activities. This has led to a flurry of research but questions remain, for instance about the directionality of observed associations (is it poor mental health that leads to problematic use, or vice-versa?), and about the potential for vulnerability of young people from marginalised groups (Kelly et al. 2018; Booker et al 2018; Odgers 2018). Social relationships are important throughout the lifecourse, and in the transition between childhood and adolescence friends and peer groups become more important influences on individual behaviours and experiences. A recent report indicated that young people's levels of happiness with their friendships has dropped over the last decade (The Children's Society 2019), and studies suggest that loneliness and social isolation are becoming more common in young people (Lasgaard et al. 2016). The ways in which use of digital technologies, on and off line relationships and experiences, and school engagement combine to influence young people's mental health are currently a major focus for research.

Mental health policy

There is a substantial unmet need for mental health provision across the UK with only one third of young people who need it receiving treatment (NHS Digital 2018a). The most recent policy developments laid out in *Transforming children and young people's mental health provision* position educational establishments in the front line role of promoting and protecting children and young people's mental health and wellbeing (House of Commons Education and Health and Social Care Committees 2018). This policy initiative proposes to improve the timeliness and quality of care by having a designated member of staff who has a lead role for mental health in every school and college, by having mental health support teams linked to groups of schools and colleges, and by trialling reduced waiting times for specialist care services. It is envisaged that initiatives will be rolled out in Trailblazer projects with 20–25 % coverage by 2022/2023. However, the policy has attracted a significant amount of criticism on several fronts, including for failing to recognise the extent of fragmentation in service provision, a lack of joined up thinking and effective coordination across Government Departments such as Health, Education, Justice and Culture (House of Commons Education and Health and Social Care Committees 2018). Specifically the Government's current stance fails to look at contributory factors for poor mental health and preventive strategies, it does not take account of marginalised groups, it puts pressure on already overburdened teaching professionals without appropriate allocation of resources, it fails to invest in the health professional workforce that is needed and it does not address the transition into adult care (Care Quality Commission 2017).

3   Obesity and Overweight

Overweight is associated with poor health and lost productivity throughout life and is currently estimated to cost 3 % of UK GDP, equivalent to £60B in 2018 (McKinsey Global Institute 2014; The Chief Medical Officer 2019). The public health importance of overweight is substantial, being predictive of poor physical and mental health at all life stages, including early puberty (Kelly et al. 2016a), poor psychosocial wellbeing in adolescence (Kelly et al. 2016b), non-communicable disease risk and early death (Di Angelantonio et al. 2016). The most recent data for England commissioned by the Department for Health and Social Care show that over a third of 11–15 year olds are classified as overweight including obese (NHS Digital 2018b, 2018c), important to note here is that national level data collections classify overweight and obesity according to British growth curves derived in 1990. More recent and globally comparable reference values generated by the International Obesity Task Force (IOTF) (Cole and Lobstein 2012) provide more conservative estimates of the proportion of children and young people classified as overweight or obese. Applying IOTF cut-points to nationally representative data from the UK Millennium Cohort Study shows that over a quarter of 14 year olds are overweight (including obese) and approximately one in twelve are obese (Table 1). Recent decades have seen increasing rates of overweight and obesity and this has largely been attributed to environmental changes over the same period often referred to as the obesogenic environment which fosters conditions in which people consume more and move less than we did before. The obesogenic environment exerts its influence via multiple aspects of people's lives from structuring individual behaviours including what and how much we eat and drink, and the amount of exercise we get through to broader determinants such as the communities in which people live—their proximity to food outlets and recreational facilities, and commercial sector regulation. These influences are not evenly distributed, for example, poor diet and low levels of physical activity are more common among families living in disadvantaged circumstances (Goisis et al. 2016). Perhaps unsurprisingly then, stark inequalities in obesity are evident, these start early in childhood, and continue to widen, for instance, data from the Millennium Cohort Study show at the start of adolescence a three-fold difference in the prevalence of obesity for those in the poorest income quintile versus the richest, and by age 14 the gap has widened further to a four-fold difference (Goisis et al. 2016 and Fig. 2). Moreover, inequalities are worsening over time, the gap for young people living in the least and most deprived areas of England having widened by a further 50 % over the last decade (NHS Digital 2018b).

Table 1 Markers of health among 14 year olds from the UK Millennium Cohort Study (own illustration)

	All	Girls	Boys
Clinically relevant depressive symptoms	16.33	23.83	9.26
Self-harmed in last 12 months	15.46	22.88	8.51
Happy with ...			
School	74.78	71.76	77.63
Family	84.89	81.67	87.94
Friends	86.97	84.57	89.23
The way they look	60.70	47.55	73.13
Life as a whole	78.32	71.21	85.03
Overweight or obese	27.16	28.70	25.79
Obese	8.01	8.27	7.78
Ever had an alcoholic drink	48.26	47.62	48.85
Binge drank (5 + drinks per occasion) in last 12 months	9.78	10.44	9.16
Smoking			
Ever smoked	16.91	18.49	15.41
Current occasional smoker	2.11	2.64	1.61
Current regular smoker	2.71	3.32	2.13
E-cigarettes			
Ever used e-cigarettes	17.61	16.44	18.72
Occasional e-cigarette user	3.04	3.22	2.87
Regular e-cigarette user	0.48	0.38	0.58
Any illicit drug use	5.66	5.56	5.75
Moderate to vigorous physical exercise every day	37.71	28.43	46.24
Breakfast every day	50.02	41.77	59.56
Short sleep ($\leq$7 h)	13.37	14.48	12.33
Disrupted sleep (difficulties staying asleep)	21.09	25.60	19.60
TV use for 3 + hours per day	44.24	46.23	42.41
Gaming for 3 + hours per day	29.41	11.97	45.50
Social media use for 3 + hours per day	34.69	46.19	24.09

(continued)

Table 1   (continued)

	All	Girls	Boys
Intimate partnered activities			
None	31.56	32.35	30.83
Light	57.52	58.49	56.60
Moderate	7.55	5.96	9.05
Heavy	3.37	3.20	3.52
Any gambling (last 4 weeks)	12.33	7.40	16.97
Physical fighting	31.65	21.25	41.44
Ever carried a weapon	2.82	1.85	3.73
Ever been a in a street gang	4.00	4.53	3.51

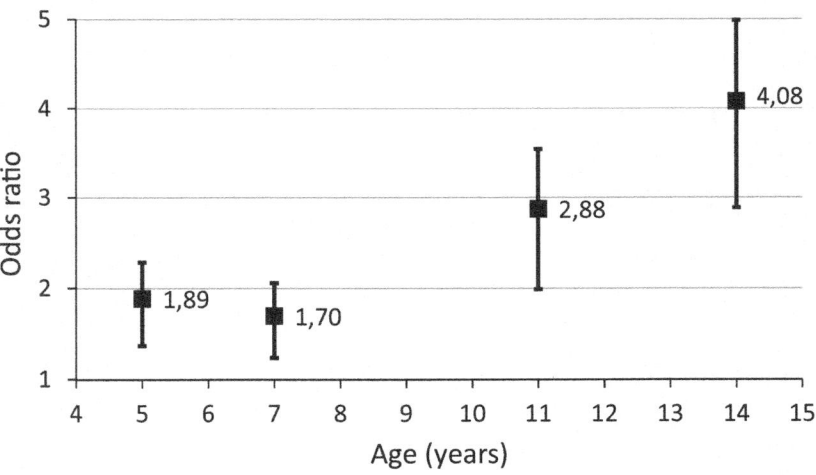

Fig. 2 Obesity (odds ratios) by family income quintiles, poorest vs. richest (own illustration)

Obesity policy

The British Government's ambition is to halve obesity rates by 2030, however, given their current action plan, this stated desire has been roundly criticised as unachievable, most notably by the Chief Medical Officer for England

(The Chief Medical Officer 2019; HM Government 2018; NHS 2019). Rising rates of obesity and socioeconomic inequalities in obesity over recent decades has coincided with an increasingly obesogenic environment in which opportunities for burning energy have diminished, whilst those for consuming energy dense food and drink have skyrocketed. Inequalities are perpetuated at least in part by the substantial price gap between more and less healthy foods, with healthy foods costing 3 times as much as less healthy foods per 1000 kcal, and evidence suggesting that healthy foods are becoming more expensive over time (Jones et al. 2014).

The fact that obesity levels show little sign of reducing has led some to assume the epidemic is a somewhat intractable problem. However, the challenge has been created by societies themselves, influenced by powerful commercial interests at the cost of public health. There is widespread suspicion of a lack of political appetite for high level interventions requiring increased regulation and the potential to harm commercial interests (Adams et al. 2016; Vallgårda 2018). A major problem many societies, including the UK, face is one of identifying where changes need to be made and taking steps to affect change, and unfortunately, the British Government has historically aimed the bulk of its interventions at low level downstream factors. Currently in the UK, with the exception of the sweetened drinks levy, there is an absence of high level 'upstream' interventions aimed at reducing obesity and associated socioeconomic inequalities. Instead policies focus on individual 'downstream' behaviours and firmly place responsibility for changing behaviours with young people themselves, their parents and carers (Vallgårda 2018; Hillier-Brown et al. 2014). This approach is problematic and has not worked to reduce levels of obesity or inequalities. The central challenge here is that behaviour change typically requires high levels of agency, as the amount of agency and resources that individuals possess influences how well they benefit from interventions aimed at changing behaviours. What makes high level upstream interventions such as reversing the erosion of safe public spaces and limiting the availability of low cost energy dense foods more attractive is that they are examples of changes that require low levels of individual agency, and it is these sorts of interventions that could be the most effective and potentially most equitable (Adams et al. 2016). Interestingly, a recent opinion poll suggested that an overwhelming majority of the British public would support upstream initiatives aimed at reducing obesity, with three quarters of people agreeing that healthy food should be cheaper than unhealthy options, that there should be reduced exposure to marketing of unhealthy foods, that the sugar content of food should be reduced, and that there should be reduced concentration of fast food outlets near to schools (Savanta ComRes 2015). This evidence of the public's enthusiasm for change highlights a clear disconnect between public opinion and action from decision makers at national and local government levels and underscores the fact that considerable political resolve will be required if we are to be successful in tackling the current epidemic.

Achieving the Government's stated target will require wide ranging action from multiple stakeholders, including physical, commercial and environmental interventions such as the creation of safe public spaces, limits on the availability of low priced calorie dense foods, and making 'healthy' food options more affordable (The Chief Medical Officer 2019). One initiative being piloted in selected London Boroughs is the formation of 'School Super-zones' which have a mix of upstream and downstream level interventions, including: the ending of child poverty; the creation of more active, playful streets and public spaces—making it safe to walk or cycle to school, along with making free London water available; stopping the marketing and incentivising of unhealthy food and drink; and the transformation of fast-food businesses by rebalancing of food and drink sold making healthy options more attractive. At the time of writing this initiative remains in its infancy and implementation will be at the local level rather than the rolling out of a 'one size fits all' scheme. Consequently, the evaluation of School Super-zones will be highly complex and multi-faceted, and it is likely that there will be lengthy delays before any potential benefits are revealed.

4   Health Behaviours and Activities

In tandem with the myriad developmental changes occurring during adolescence, are an increased sense of autonomy, agency and the formation of various aspects of identity. In keeping with this perspective, adolescence is widely viewed in the 'western tradition' as a time of experimentation particularly in relation to various health behaviours such as alcohol consumption, smoking and drug use in addition to the exploration of intimate relationships and changes in social networks more broadly. It is also a time of profound change in aspects of physical activity, sleeping patterns, leisure time activities, and digital technology use.

4.1   Drinking, Smoking and Drug Use

In the UK over recent decades there have been dramatic reductions in the proportions of young people who drink alcohol, smoke and take illegal drugs, for example in the late 1990s just under half of 11–15 year olds had ever smoked and this had fallen to 16 % by 2018 (NHS Digital 2019). Table 1 shows percentages of 14 year olds from the Millennium Cohort Study who reported to smoke, drink alcohol and use drugs. Approximately one in six had ever smoked cigarettes or had ever vaped, and there was some evidence of gender patterning with girls more likely than boys to have smoked (18.5 vs. 15.4 %), but interestingly, girls were less likely to have vaped (16.4 vs. 18.7 %). The most recent SDD survey figures suggest that about 5 % of 11–15 year olds are current smokers, and that 6 % can be classified as current vapers (NHS Digital 2019). Data from the Millennium Cohort Study suggest no clear gender differences for drinking or for drug use, about a half of 14 year olds had drank alcohol and approximately one in ten had experienced binge drinking—having had 5 or more drinks on a single occasion, and approximately one in twenty reported having taken illegal drugs (Table 1). There are, in the main, similarities with recent estimates of drinking, smoking and drug use from other contemporary national level surveys, where there are variations this is likely due to differences in phrasing of questions asked and the age ranges surveyed (for examples see NHS Digital 2019; Inchley et al. 2020; Brooks et al. 2020).

4.2 Physical Activity, Sleep and Digital Technology Use

Physical activity has many benefits for health not least in helping to prevent overweight and obesity and is widely thought to boost mental health and wellbeing. The current WHO guidelines recommend that young people get 60 min per day of moderate to vigorous physical activity (World Health Organization 2010). Over the last two decades a WHO initiative has been tracking population level physical activity on a global scale with the aim of improving levels of 'sufficient' physical activity. Against these targets, a recent report showed that the UK was falling well short of sufficient activity levels for adolescents, and importantly, there had been no improvement in the 20 years since the initiative began. It was found that only one in five young people took sufficient exercise on a daily basis, and gender inequalities were apparent too with just 15 % of girls versus 25 % of boys with sufficient activity levels (Guthold et al. 2020). In the Millennium Cohort Study, just under two out of five 14 year olds report engaging in moderate/vigorous activity on a daily basis, and boys are more likely to report doing so compared with girls (46.2 vs. 28.4 %— see Table 1). Examination of objective accelerometery data from a sub-sample of approximately 3500 MCS participants revealed that overall 40 % did 60 min or more of moderate to vigorous activity per day (Pearson et al. 2019).

Whilst there are no official UK Government guidelines on the amount of sleep adolescents should get, the importance of sleep for healthy development is becoming increasingly recognised. Sleep quantity and quality are thought to be influential across a range of developmental domains including BMI (Kelly et al. 2016b), mental health (Kelly et al. 2013a), and cognitive performance (Kelly et al. 2013b). About one in eight 14 year olds in the MCS reported short sleep duration (7 h or less per night, Table 1). A higher proportion reported having difficulties with disrupted sleep and this was more common for girls than boys (25.6 vs. 19.6 %).

The question of whether the use of digital technologies is causally linked to poor health (as already discussed in relation to mental health) is not clear cut. Sleep has been put forward as one of the potential pathways via which use of screens might impact on health (Kelly et al. 2018) and this has been recognised in a recent Chief Medical Officers' report which includes guidelines on use of screens and getting enough sleep (Davies et al. 2019). Digital technology use is almost universal and many country settings, including the UK (Davies et al. 2019) endorse daily limits of around 2 h. These limits are exceeded by substantial proportions of young people, as detailed in Table 1, about two in five 14 year olds watch TV for 3 or more hours per day. Gaming is overall less prevalent but is heavily gendered, it is more common in boys than girls 45.5 vs. 12.0 %, whilst social media use is oppositely gendered, being more common among girls than boys, 46.2 vs. 24.1 % for 3 or more hours daily.

4.3   Intimate Partnered Relationships

Partnered intimate activity in adolescence is increasingly considered a normative part of development (Halpern 2010; Van de Bongardt et al. 2015). Much of the prior work on intimate activity in adolescence has had a narrow focus on the timing and circumstances of sexual debut, usually referring to first vaginal intercourse. Younger age at sexual debut correlates with unplanned teenage pregnancy and is associated negatively with sexually transmitted infections, mental health and educational attainment. Moreover, good sexual health in youth is associated with better sexual health and relationships throughout the lifecourse. In the UK, the legal age of consent is 16 and early sexual debut generally refers to having had sex prior to this age. In the UK there have been dramatic drops in teenage pregnancy rates over the last two decades from 43.9/1000 in 2000 to 16.8/1000 in 2018 (Office for National Statistics 2018). Alongside this, recent British prevalence estimates suggest that early sexual debut is becoming less common.

For example, among young people born in the 1980s and 1990s, approximately 30 and 20 % respectively, report having had sex before age 16 (Mercer et al. 2013; Heron et al. 2015). Table 1 shows rates of partnered intimate activities among MCS participants aged 14. Activities are grouped into three categories: 'light' (handholding, kissing and cuddling); 'moderate' (touching and fondling under clothes); and 'heavy' (oral sex and sexual intercourse) (Mawditt et al. 2019). The majority of 14 year olds report some sort of partnered intimacy and only about one in thirty report having had intercourse/oral sex (Table 1).

4.4   Gambling and Violence

Gambling is increasingly recognised as a public health challenge in the UK, with problem gambling often going hand-in-hand with mental health problems and substance misuse. Commercial harms to health are clearly relevant here, with gambling companies spending billions of pounds marketing and advertising their products, targeting children and young people (Clark et al. 2020). It is estimated that some 55,000 adolescents (aged 11–16) are problem gamblers and about twice this number are at risk of becoming problem gamblers (Gambling Commission 2019). In an attempt to treat the complex health problems co-occurring with problem gambling, in 2019 the UK NHS announced the launch of gambling addiction clinics for 13–25 year olds. There is an important lifecourse dimension to gambling behaviours, and current estimates suggest that in the UK there are 300,000 adult problem gamblers with a further 1.7 million at risk (Conolly et al. 2018). Government policy on age restrictions vary depending on the type of gambling, for example, age 16 for the National Lottery, and age 18 for online betting and casinos as well as high street gambling outlets, whilst there are no age restrictions on the use of low stakes slot machines, and gambling products with virtual currency are freely available (Wardle 2018). In 14 year olds from the MCS about one in eight reported some form of gambling in the prior month (Table 1), and this was markedly more common for boys compared with girls. These figures are similar to other UK studies, for example the Gambling Commission's annual survey reveals similar proportions of 11–16 year olds reporting gambling, including on slot machines and private bets (Gambling Commission 2019).

Youth violence has implications for mental health, substance use, social relationships, educational engagement and interactions with the criminal justice system. Paralleling wide ranging cuts, over the last decade, in youth services, and the removal of financial assistance for young people from economically disadvantaged families to stay in education, rates of youth violence have increased markedly (Marmot et al. 2020). About one third of 14 year olds from the MCS reported getting into physical fights and this was twice as common for boys than girls (41.4 vs. 21.3 %, Table 1), as was carrying a weapon (boys 3.7 vs. girls 1.9 %) on the other hand, street gang membership, although relatively rare being reported by one in twenty five, was slightly more common among girls than boys (4.5 vs. 3.5 %).

5 Conclusion

Over the last two decades there have been substantial changes in adolescent health in the UK. Overweight and obesity and poor mental health have become more common, and socioeconomic inequalities have widened. Conversely, there have been dramatic falls in the uptake of potential health damaging behaviours such as drinking and smoking, and declining rates of teenage pregnancy. Globally, technological changes mean that our worlds are highly interconnected and online communications are almost universal with young people typically spending several hours per day engaging in activities via social media and gaming platforms. The social determinants of health are increasingly acknowledged as important influences in young people's lives, and the potential for commercial harms are unprecedented. Historically, UK public health policy has tended to concentrate on 'downstream' factors such as behaviours of young people themselves and their carers. Future policy developments aimed at improving health will require high level political buy-in to intervene on 'upstream' factors including commercial and broader social environments.

References

Adams, J., Mytton, O., White, M. & Monsivais, P. (2016). Why Are Some Population Interventions for Diet and Obesity More Equitable and Effective Than Others? The Role of Individual Agency. PLoS Med.; 13(4):e1001990. doi: https://doi.org/10.1371/journal.pmed.1001990.

Booker, CL., Kelly, YJ. & Sacker, A. (2018). Gender differences in the associations between age trends of social media interaction and well-being among 10–15 year olds in the UK. BMC Public Health; 18(1):321. doi: https://doi.org/10.1186/s12889-018-5220-4.

Brooks, F., Klemera, E., Chester, K., Magnusson, J. & Spencer, N. (2020). HBSC England National Report: Findings from the 2018. HBSC study for England. Hatfield, England: University of Hertfordshire.

Care Quality Commission (2017). Review of children and young people's mental health services.

Clark, H., Coll-Seck, AM., Banerjee, A., Peterson, S., Dalglish SL., Ameratunga, S. et al. (2020). A future for the world's children? A WHO-UNICEF-Lancet Commission. The Lancet. doi: https://doi.org/10.1016/S0140-6736(19)32540-1.

Cole, TJ. & Lobstein, T. (2012). Extended international (IOTF) body mass index cut-offs for thinness, overweight and obesity. Pediatric obesity; 7(4):284–94.

Collishaw, S., Maughan, B., Goodman, R. & Pickles, A. (2004). Time trends in adolescent mental health.

Conolly, A., Davies, B., Fuller, E., Heinze, N. & Wardle, H. (2018). Gambling behaviour in Great Britain in 2016 Evidence from England, Scotland and Wales. Journal of Child Psychology and Psychiatry;45(8):1350–62. doi: https://doi.org/10.1111/j.1469-7610.2004.00335.x.

Davies, SC., Atherton, F., Calderwood, C. & McBride, M. (2019). United Kingdom Chief Medical Officers' commentary on 'Screen-based activities and children and young people's mental health and psychosocial wellbeing: a systematic map of reviews'. Department of Health and Social Care; 2019.

Department of Education (2019). State of the nation 2019: children and young people's wellbeing. Education and Health and Social Care Committees (2018). The Government's Green Paper on mental health: failing a generation.

Di Angelantonio, E., Bhupathiraju, SN., Wormser, D., Gao, P., Kaptoge, S., de Gonzalez, AB. et al. (2016). Body-mass index and all-cause mortality: individual-participant-data meta-analysis of 239 prospective studies in four continents. The Lancet; 388(10046):776–86. doi: https://doi.org/10.1016/S0140-6736(16)30175-1.

NHS Digital (2019). Smoking, Drinking and Drug Use among Young People in England 2018.

Gambling Commission (2019). Young People and Gambling Survey 2019. A research study among 11–16 year olds in Great Britain.

Goisis, A., Sacker, A. & Kelly, Y. (2016). Why are poorer children at higher risk of obesity and overweight? A UK cohort study. Eur J Public Health; 26(1):7–13. doi: https://doi.org/10.1093/eurpub/ckv219

Guthold, R., Stevens, GA., Riley, LM. & Bull, FC. (2020). Global trends in insufficient physical activity among adolescents: a pooled analysis of 298 population-based surveys with 1·6 million participants. The Lancet Child & Adolescent Health; 4(1):23–35. doi: https://doi.org/10.1016/S2352-4642(19)30323-2.

Halpern, CT. (2010). Reframing research on adolescent sexuality: healthy sexual development as part of the life course. Perspect Sex Reprod Health; 42(1):6–7. doi: https://doi.org/10.1363/4200610.

Heron, J., Low, N., Lewis, G., Macleod, J., Ness, A. & Waylen, A. (2015). Social factors associated with readiness for sexual activity in adolescents: a population-based cohort study. Arch Sex Behav; 44(3):669–78. doi: https://doi.org/10.1007/s10508-013-0162-5

Hillier-Brown, FC., Bambra, CL., Cairns, J-M., Kasim, A., Moore, HJ. & Summerbell, CD. (2014). A systematic review of the effectiveness of individual, community and societal level interventions at reducing socioeconomic inequalities in obesity amongst children. BMC Public Health;14(1):834.

HM Government (2018). Childhood obesity: a plan for action, chapter 2

House of Commons Education and Health and Social Care Committees (2018). The Government's Green Paper on mental health: failing a generation.

Inchley, J., Mokogwu, D., Mabelis, J. & Currie, D. (2020). Health Behaviour in School-aged Children (HBSC) 2018 Survey in Scotland: National Report. MRC/CSO Social and Public Health Sciences Unit: University of Glasgow.

Jones, NR., Conklin, AI., Suhrcke, M. & Monsivais, P. (2014). The growing price gap between more and less healthy foods: analysis of a novel longitudinal UK dataset. PLoS ONE; 9(10):e109343.

Kessler, RC., Amminger, GP., Aguilar-Gaxiola, S., Alonso, J., Lee, S. & Üstün, T. (2007). Age of onset of mental disorders: a review of recent literature. Curr Opin Psychiatry; 20(4):359–64. doi: https://doi.org/10.1097/YCO.0b013e32816ebc8c.

Kelly, Y., Sacker, A., Del Bono, E., Francesconi, M. & Marmot, M. (2011). What role for the home learning environment and parenting in reducing the socioeconomic gradient in child development? Findings from the Millennium Cohort Study. Archives of disease in childhood; 96(9):832–7. doi: https://doi.org/10.1136/adc.2010.195917.

Kelly, Y., Kelly, J. & Sacker, A. (2013a). Changes in bedtime schedules and behavioral difficulties in 7 year old children. Pediatrics; 132(5):e1184–93. doi: https://doi.org/10.1542/peds.2013-1906.

Kelly, Y., Kelly, J. & Sacker, A. (2013b). Time for bed: associations with cognitive performance in 7-year-old children: a longitudinal population-based study. Journal of epidemiology and community health; DOI:https://doi.org/10.1136/jech-2012-202024. doi: https://doi.org/10.1136/jech-2012-202024.

Kelly, Y., Zilanawala, A., Sacker, A., Hiatt, R. & Viner, R. (2016a). Early puberty in 11-year-old girls: Millennium Cohort Study findings. Arch Dis Child. doi: https://doi.org/10.1136/archdischild-2016-310475.

Kelly, Y., Patalay, P., Montgomery, S. & Sacker, A. (2016b). BMI Development and Early Adolescent Psychosocial Well-Being: UK Millennium Cohort Study. Pediatrics; 138(6). doi: https://doi.org/10.1542/peds.2016-0967.

Kelly, Y., Zilanawala, A., Booker, C. & Sacker, A. (2018). Social Media Use and Adolescent Mental Health: Findings From the UK Millennium Cohort Study. EClinicalMedicine; 6:59–68. doi: https://doi.org/10.1016/j.eclinm.2018.12.005.

Lasgaard, M., Friis, K. & Shevlin, M. (2016). "Where are all the lonely people?" A population-based study of high-risk groups across the life span. Soc Psychiatry Psychiatr Epidemiol; 51(10):1373–84. doi: https://doi.org/10.1007/s00127-016-1279-3.

Marmot, M., Allen, J., Boyce, T., Goldblatt, P. & Morrison, J., (2020). Health equity in England: The Marmot Review 10 years on.

Mawditt, C., Sacker, A., Britton, A., Kelly, Y. & Cable, N. (2019). The stability of health-related behaviour clustering during mid-adulthood and the influence of social circumstances on health-related behaviour change. Prev Med; 121:141–8. doi: https://doi.org/10.1016/j.ypmed.2019.02.009.

McKinsey Global Institute (2014). Overcoming obesity: an initial economic analysis.

McLaughlin, KA. & King, K. (2015). Developmental trajectories of anxiety and depression in early adolescence. J Abnorm Child Psychol;43(2):311–23. doi: https://doi.org/10.1007/s10802-014-9898-1.

Mercer, CH., Tanton, C., Prah, P., Erens, B., Sonnenberg, P., Clifton, S. et al. (2013). Changes in sexual attitudes and lifestyles in Britain through the life course and over time: findings from the National Surveys of Sexual Attitudes and Lifestyles (Natsal). Lancet; 382(9907):1781–94. doi: https://doi.org/10.1016/S0140-6736(13)62035-8.

NHS Digital (2018a) Mental Health of Children and Young People in England, 2017.

NHS Digital (2018b). Health Survey for England 2017, Adult and child overweight and obesity

NHS Digital (2018c). National Child Measurement Programme: England, 2017/18 school year

NHS (2019). The NHS Long Term Plan.

Odgers, C. (2018). Smartphones are bad for some teens, not all. Nature.. 554(7693):432–4. doi: https://doi.org/10.1038/d41586-018-02109-8.

OECD (2014a). Young population 2014 https://www.oecd-ilibrary.org/content/data/3d774f19-en.

OECD (2014b) Fertility rates. https://www.oecd-ilibrary.org/content/data/8272fb01-en

OECD (2019). PISA 2018 Results (Volume III).

Office for National Statistics (2018). Conceptions in England and Wales: Statistical bulletin 2020.

Patalay, P. & Gage, SH. (2019). Changes in millennial adolescent mental health and health-related behaviours over 10 years: a population cohort comparison study. Int J Epidemiol; 48(5):1650–64. doi: https://doi.org/10.1093/ije/dyz006.

Pearson, N., Sherar, LB. & Hamer, M. (2019). Prevalence and Correlates of Meeting Sleep, Screen-Time, and Physical Activity Guidelines Among Adolescents in the United Kingdom. JAMA Pediatrics; 173(10):993–4. doi: https://doi.org/10.1001/jamapediatrics.2019.2822.

Ross, A., Kelly, Y. & Sacker, A. (2017). Time trends in mental well-being: the polarisation of young people's psychological distress. Soc Psychiatry Psychiatr Epidemiol; 52(9):1147–58. doi: https://doi.org/10.1007/s00127-017-1419-4.

Royal College of Paediatrics and Child Health (2020). State of Child Health 2020.

Savanta ComRes (2015). Fat chance? The challenge of tackling obesit.

The Children's Society (2019). The Good Childhood Report 2019.

The Chief Medical Officer (2019). Time to Solve Childhood Obesity.

Vallgårda, S. (2018). Childhood obesity policies–mighty concerns, meek reactions. Obes Rev.;19(3):295–301.

Van de Bongardt, D., Yu, R., Deković, M. & Meeus, WHJ. (2015). Romantic relationships and sexuality in adolescence and young adulthood: The role of parents, peers, and partners. European Journal of Developmental Psychology; 12(5):497–515. doi: https://doi.org/10.1080/_7405629.2015.1068689

Wardle, H. (2018). Trends in children's gambling 2011–2017.

World Health Organization (WHO) (1946). Constitution of the World Health Organization. International Health Conference.

World Health Organization (WHO) (2010). Global recommendations on physical activity for health. Geneva World Heal Organ; 60.

World Health Organization (WHO) (2013). Mental Health Action Plan 2013–2020 House of Commons.

Risk Behaviours: Tracking Youth Health and Well-Being in Bulgaria 2006–2018

Tatyana Kotzeva und Elitsa Dimitrova

1 Introduction

The health and health status of children and young people is a foundational element of the quality of life and future generations' wellbeing (UNICEF 2011). Today's young people may expect to live longer than ever before, the prevalence of chronic illnesses in the 16–29 age group is lower than those in older groups with a higher self-rated health perception of youngsters: 91 % of the EU-28 young people at age 15–24 years reported that they were in good or very good health in 2016 (Eurostat 2017). However, the conceptualization of health not merely as a lack of illness but as physical, psychological, and social wellbeing assumes that youth's health behaviours and health outcomes have to be seen in a broader social context of young people's lifestyles. Prevention of diseases and promotion of healthy lifestyles and healthy environments are stated as key objectives in the EC strategic documents: EU public strategy 'Health Programme' (Multi-annual programme of EU action in the field of health for the period 2014–2020 (Regulation EU N 282/2014))[1] and the European Commission Youth—Discover EU's Role—EU Youth

---

[1] https://ec.europa.eu/health/funding/programme_en (Accessed 24.09.2021).

T. Kotzeva (✉) · E. Dimitrova
Institute for Population and Human Studies, Bulgarian Academy of Sciences,
Sofia, Bulgaria
E-Mail: t.kotzeva@iphs.eu

E. Dimitrova
E-Mail: e.dimitrova@iphs.eu

© Der/die Autor(en) 2022
A. Heinen et al. (Hrsg.), *Wohlbefinden und Gesundheit im Jugendalter*,
https://doi.org/10.1007/978-3-658-35744-3_30

Strategy—Health and Wellbeing website[2]. Recognizing the unique psycho-social conditions of adolescence, the recent WHO documents 'Investing in Children: the European Child and Adolescent Health Strategy' (WHO 2014a), 'Health for the World's Adolescents: A Second Chance in the Second Decade' (WHO 2014b) and 'Global Strategy for Women's, Children's and Adolescents' Health' (WHO 2015) direct public attention and policy actions to this specific age group. Issues of health inequalities, mainly based on socioeconomic circumstances, have also been a focal point in public policies in order to facilitate better health and secure wellbeing for young people.

Among factors related to socioeconomic circumstances, tobacco and drug use, alcohol consumption, reduced physical activity, unhealthy eating habits, involvement in violence resulted in physical injuries, and early start of sexual activity[3] are of special importance for providing safe and healthy lifestyles for young people. From an individual perspective, the regularity of risky behaviours during adolescent age could impede physical, social, and emotional wellbeing later in young adults' lives (Kann et al. 2018).

Adolescence has been recognized as a 'second birth,' a period when young people gain new experiences and social relations. Increased emotional intensity, social engagement, novelty-seeking, and creative explorations are key features of adolescents' perceptions of the world, which implicates both mental excitement and mental confusion (Siegel 2014). Embedded in physiological changes in the brain around puberty (Steinberg 2008), sometimes adolescents' risk-taking behaviours lead to long-standing habits resulting in nicotine, alcohol, and drug addictions. On the other hand, despite the adverse health effects, adolescents develop risky behaviours as a coping mechanism to reduce school stress and boredom, make contacts with the opposite gender and peers, boost their self-esteem, and get accepted as mature and self-reliant companions.

Recent studies on adolescent health apply a socio-ecological model through which an interaction of factors explains risky behaviours at five levels: individual, interpersonal, institutional/organizational, community and public policy (McLeroy et al. 1988; McLaren and Hawe 2005). Individual-level factors

---

[2] https://ec.europa.eu/youth/policy/youth-strategy/health-wellbeing_en (Accessed 24.09.2021).

[3] The Centre for Disease Control (CDC) has suggested six primary domains of risk among youth and young adults: tobacco use, alcohol and illicit substance use, sexual behaviour related to unintended pregnancy and sexually transmitted infections, injury-prone and violent behaviour, unhealthy dietary patterns, and physical inactivity (Kann et al. 2018).

(for example, gender, age, life satisfaction, etc.) are related to adolescents' developmental, psychological and behavioural characteristics. At the inter-personal level, adolescent health and health behaviours are influenced by relation-ships with family members, classmates, peers, and other regular social contacts. The institutional/organizational level involves factors within an institution/ organization that impact on adolescent health. Findings from previous HBSC studies have shown that school policies regarding nutrition, physical activity, prevention of violence, use of harmful substances, etc. significantly impact students' healthy and risky behaviours (Currie et al. 2008). The community-level involves the relationships between organizations, social networks, norms, and practices related to promoting healthy behaviours, e.g., the availability of sport and recreation venues such as sports clubs, parks, sports grounds, etc. to stimulate physical activity of the young people. The most general level of public policies concerns the policies, regulations, and laws aiming to create and support healthy environments (Subramanian et al. 2003), e.g., existing national policies to imple-ment dietary food at school canteens and programs to increase sports activities.

The main objectives of this paper are:

- To describe and evaluate the prevalence and trends of adolescents' risky behaviours[4] in Bulgaria over a 13 year period (2006–2018);
- To estimate the relationships between health risk behaviours, individual-level factors (gender, age) and some interpersonal level factors, mainly from the family domain (family structure and family affluence);
- To present the country-level policies and some strategic programs that aim to improve young people's health in Bulgaria.

The analysis is based mainly on the data from the Bulgarian samples of the Health Behaviour among School-aged Children (HBSC) study. HBSC is a large-scale international study conducted under the World Health Organization aegis every four years since the start of the 1980s in multiple European and North American countries. Students aged 11, 13, and 15 years fill out self-assessing questionnaires at school (with parents' consent) and provide information on different aspects of health and health behaviours and their family, school, and peers. The HBSC study assets provide a broad set of representative data for the

---

[4]We refer to a scope of risky behaviours as they are defined according to the HBSC methodology (Inchley et al. 2013a).

target population with an internationally standardized and validated questionnaire that makes possible cross-national comparative analyses. Despite the collection of large cross-national data over a 30 year period, the HBSC study faces methodological limitations concerning the self-reported data that may imply overreporting or underreporting on some sensitive topics at the adolescent age and cross-sectional type of the data that impedes a causality analysis.

In Bulgaria, the HBSC study was conducted three times in the following waves: 2005/2006, 2013/2014, and 2017/2018[5]. Although the waves do not cover three successive surveys, the time period covers a ten-plus-year period that allows monitoring and evaluating trends of adolescent health and health behaviours. The same sampling procedure (based on a random sampling of schools and classes in the 28 country's regions), as well as the use of identical questions and responses/ categories across survey years, provide the data quality for sufficient trend analysis (Schnohr et al. 2015).

HBSC indicators on risk behaviours and statistical analysis
For this analysis, we use questions on current cigarette smoking, current alcohol consumption, lifetime drunkenness, participation in physical fights and bullying perpetration at school, cannabis use during the last 30 days, and early start of sexual life.

The HBSC study involves the question of current smoking *"How often do you smoke tobacco at present?"* with four categories *'every day'*, *'less than once a week,'* *'at least once a week but not every day,'* *'don't smoke.'* Weekly smoking combines the first two answers.

The question used for risky alcohol consumption concerns beverage-specific use: *"At present, how often do you drink anything alcoholic, such as beer, wine, spirits (like rakia, vodka, whisky, tequila), alcopops, any other drink that contains alcohol?"* with five options: *'every day,'* *'every week,'* *'every month,'* *'rarely,'* *'never.'* The weekly alcohol use combines the two answers: 'everyday' and 'every week.' The second indicator used for alcohol misuse is drunkenness in a lifetime *"Have you ever had so much alcohol that you were really drunk in your lifetime?"* with the categories *'no, never',* *'yes, once,'* *'yes, 2–3 times',* *'yes, 4–10 times',* *'yes, more than 10 times'.*

---

[5] The sample size of the HBSC respondents is 4854 in 2005/2006, 4796 in 2013/2014 and 4548 in 2017/2018. In the last wave of the survey the response rate for the three age groups is 60.3 % for 11-year olds, 68.1 % for 13-year olds, and 65.1 % for 15-year olds.

We use current (last 30 days) prevalence for cannabis use as one of the most spread illicit substance in adolescent age *"Have you ever taken cannabis?"* with the scope of frequency: *'never,' '1–2 days', '3–5 days', '6–9 days','10–19 days', '20–29 days'* and *'30 days or more'*. Only 15-year old students answer this question.

An indicator for the students' sexual initiation is the question, *"Have you ever had sexual intercourse?"* with two options: *'yes'* and *'no.'* The question is asked only to 15-year old participants.

Two questions are used for youth violence and bullying. The first question indicates the prevalence of the students' participation in a physical fight *"During the past 12 months, how many times were you in a physical fight?"* with answers *'I have not been in a physical fight in the past 12 months', '1 time', '2 times', '3 times'* and *'4 times or more'*. The presented proportions of the students who have participated in a physical fight at least 3 times include the last two responses. The frequency of bullying perpetration (bullying others) at school is measured by the question *"How often have you taken part in bullying another student(s) at school in the past couple of months?"* with the options: *'I have not bullied another student(s) at school in the past couple of months,' 'It has only happened once or twice,' '2 or 3 times a month', 'About once a week,' 'Several times a week.'* The presented proportions of the students who have bullied 2–3 times a month comprise the last three responses.

We apply logistic regression models to test the difference between the waves in the prevalence of risky behaviours. In these models, we test the effect of the time when the survey was conducted, and we also control for gender, age, family structure, and family affluence. Family structure is created as a composite measure and includes the following categories: students who live with two parents, students who live with one parent, and students who live with other relatives or in a child home/foster care. Family affluence is assessed through the Family Affluence Scale (FAS III)—a brief assets-based measure including 4 items: number of computers owned by the family, number of cars, number of travels/holidays abroad, having an own bedroom. The total scale score ranges from 0 to 9, with scores 0–3 representing the category of families with low affluence, the scores 4–6—the families with medium affluence, and the scores 7–9—the families with high affluence.

2   Findings

2.1   Prevalence of Risky Behaviours Across the Survey Waves, by Age and Gender

Current tobacco smoking
Findings in Fig. 1 demonstrate a steep growth of the proportion of weekly smokers by age with a crucial transition between the ages of 13 and 15 when their share increases three-four times. A positive statistically significant trend has been observed for a decline of the share of regular smokers among 15-years olds between the three waves, especially for girls, while for the boys, the percentage remains almost the same between 2014 and 2018. Gender differences present a higher prevalence in girls' weekly smoking, and this trend remains across the three HBSC waves.

Current alcohol consumption and excessive drinking
Findings in Fig. 2 show that the prevalence of weekly alcohol consumption increases with age, particularly for boys between ages 13 and 15. Overall, weekly drinking is more typical for boys with gender differences greater than ten percentage points for all ages. Alcohol prevalence among Bulgarian boys and girls (significant for both genders at $p < = 0.001$) increases significantly in 2018 with clearly indicated growth for girls.

Data presented in Fig. 3 shows that the prevalence of getting drunk in a lifetime (on two or more occasions) increases with age, particularly between 13 and 15 years. Boys report having been drunk more often than girls. However, gender difference diminishes over the years as the proportions of boys who report

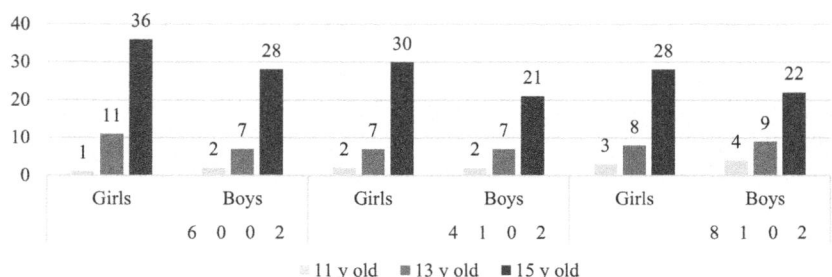

Fig. 1 Adolescents who reported smoking at least once a week, by age and gender (%). (Source: HBSC-BG 2006, 2014, 2018. Own calculations)

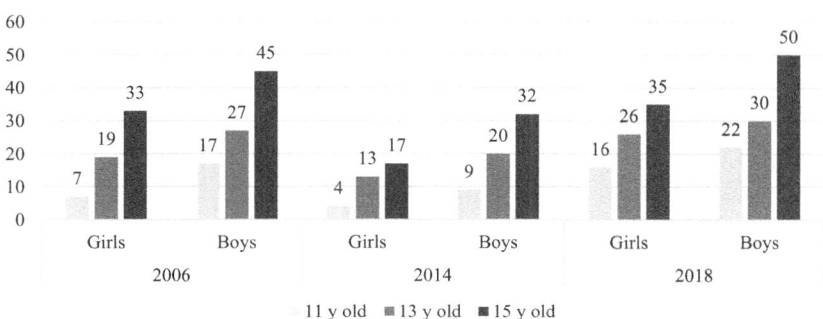

Fig. 2 Adolescents who reported drinking alcohol at least once a week, by age and gender (%). (Source: HBSC-BG 2006, 2014, 2018. Own calculations)

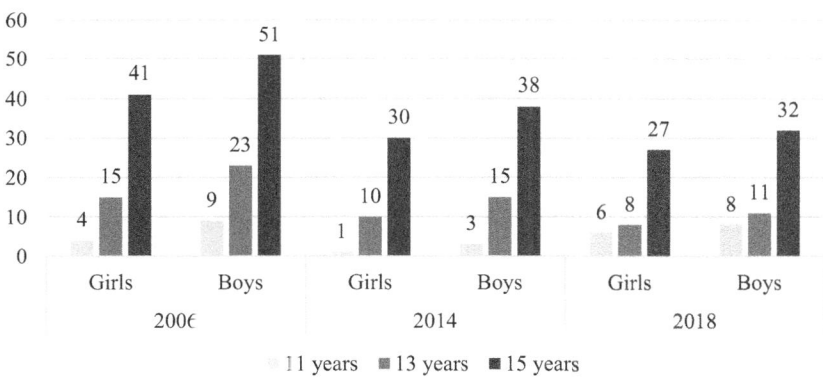

Fig. 3 Adolescents who reported to have been drunk on two or more occasions, by age and gender (%). (Source: HBSC-BG, 2006, 2014, 2018. Own calculations)

excessive drinking decrease significantly, unlike the increasing proportion of girls who experiment with excessive alcohol consumption. There is a time trend of a decrease in alcohol abuse among 13- and 15-year olds and a slight increase among 11-year old students.

Current cannabis use
Findings presented in Fig. 4 show the proportions of Bulgarian adolescents at the age 15 who had used cannabis on at least one day during the last 30 days (current

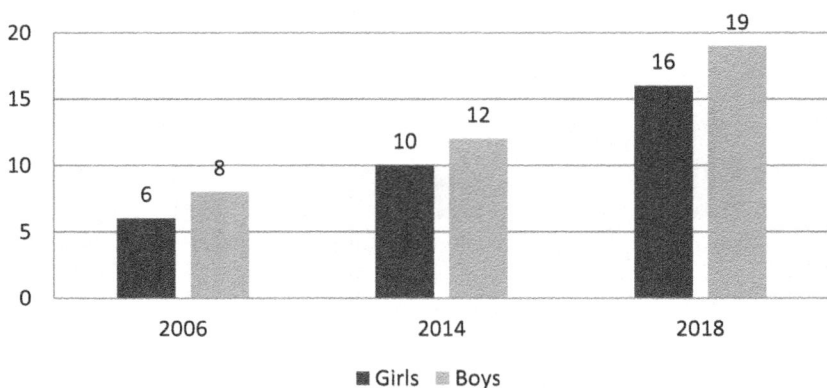

Fig. 4 15-year old adolescents who reported using cannabis in the last 30 days, by gender (%). (Source: HBSC-BG, 2006, 2014, 2018. Own calculations)

use). There is a steep increase in current cannabis use over the survey years, which is significant for both genders.

Age of initiation of risky behaviours—first cigarette, first alcohol drink and first drunkenness
The age of initiation of risky behaviours is of crucial importance for the design of intervention programs that should approach adolescents. Data presented in Figs. 5 and 6 show that the key age for the beginning of the most prevalent risky behaviours—smoking tobacco and alcohol consumption is 14 years for both boys and girls. For girls, there is a second peak at the age of 15.

Sexual initiation
Data in Fig. 7 shows that boys are more likely to report having had sexual intercourse. Gender disparities remain across the survey waves. A significant decrease in the reported sexual onset is observed between 2006 and 2018 for both genders and a slight increase for girls between 2014 and 2018.

Youth Violence
Findings in Fig. 8 show the proportions of those who reported physical fighting involvement three times and more for the last 12 months. The proportions tend to decline significantly with age and over time, particularly for boys. However, for girls who have been less involved in physical aggression, there is a significant increase in the proportions in 2018.

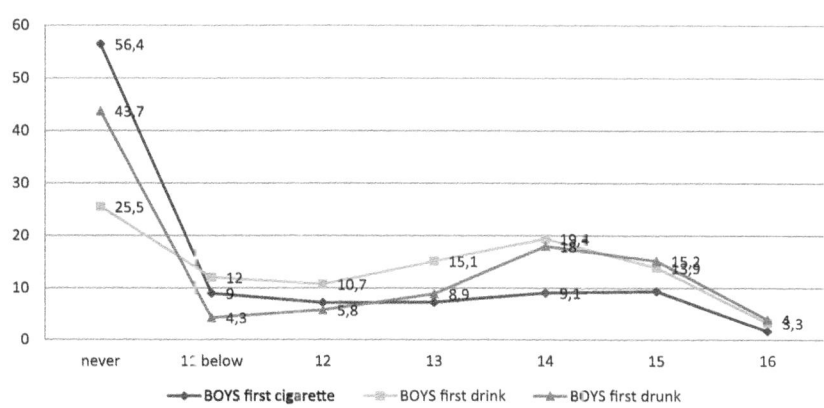

Fig. 5 Initiation of risky behaviours for boys (%). (Source: HBSC-BG, 2006, 2014. No data available for 2018. Own calculations)

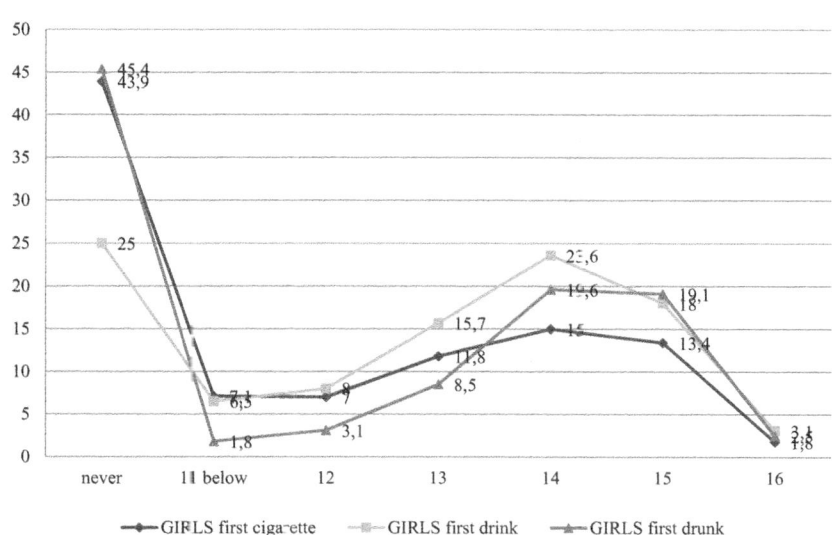

Fig. 6 Initiation of risky behaviours for girls (%). (Source: HBSC-BG, 2006, 2014. No data available for 2018. Own calculations)

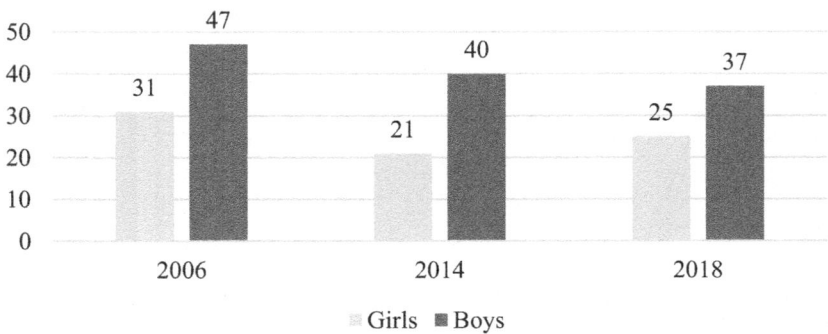

Fig. 7 15-year old students who responded "yes" to having had sexual intercourse, by gender (%). (Source: HBSC-BG, 2006, 2014, 2018. Own calculations)

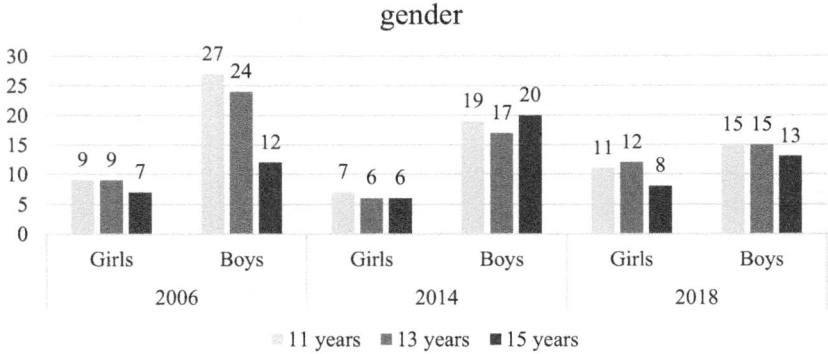

Fig. 8 Adolescents who have been involved in a physical fight at least 3 times in the last 12 months, by age and gender. (Source: HBSC-BG, 2006, 2014, 2018. Own calculations)

Bullying perpetration

Data presented in Fig. 9 show that the proportions of students who have bullied other(s) at school at least 2–3 times a month increase over time. Changes across survey waves are observed with the highest prevalence at the age of 13 for boys and girls. Generally, bullying perpetration is significantly higher for boys, but girls' participation in bullying has increased across survey waves.

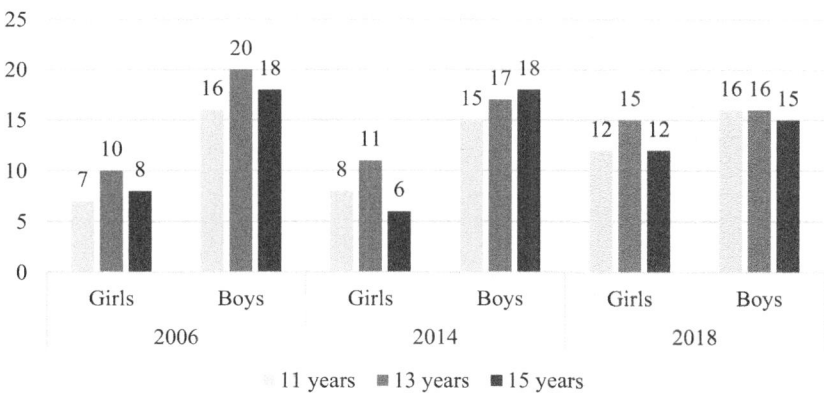

Fig. 9 Adolescents who have bullied other(s) at school at least 2–3 times in the past couple of months, by age and gender. (Source: HBSC-BG, 2006, 2014, 2018. Own calculations)

2.2   Multivariate trend analysis of risky behaviours

On Table 1 we present the results from logistic regression analysis of the time trends in young people's risky behaviours. Apart from the study's wave, in the models, we control for age, gender, and family structure, and family affluence.

The models' results reveal significant changes over time in the prevalence of certain risky behaviours among young people in Bulgaria. There is a statistically significant decrease in smoking tobacco, excessive alcohol consumption (getting drunk), involvement in a physical fight and the early start of sexual life compared to the first wave of HBSC in 2006 (reference year). Trends of a significant increase in regular alcohol consumption and cannabis use in a lifetime have also been observed.

Gender differences are statistically significant for five of the studied risky behaviours. The multivariate analysis results reveal that the odds of regular alcohol consumption, alcohol abuse (getting drunk), early start of sexual life, physical fight and bullying perpetration is significantly lower for girls than boys (reference category). The likelihood of smoking tobacco is significantly higher for girls. In the case of current cannabis use, gender differences are not statistically significant.

Table 1. Logistic regressions of Bulgarian adolescents' risky behaviours

	Current cigarette smoking		Current alcohol consumption		Getting drunk—lifetime		Early start of sexual life		Cannabis use—last 30 days		Bulling perpetration		Physical fights	
	OR	Sig	OR	Sig	OR	Sig	OR	Sig	OR	Sig	OR	Sig	OR	Sig
Wave														
2006 (ref.)	1		1		1		1		1		1		1	
2014	0.71	***	0.53	***	0.62	***	0.63	***	1.10		1.03		0.76	***
2018	0.88	**	1.22	***	0.60	***	0.66	***	1.49	**	1.02		0.72	***
Gender														
Boy (ref.)	1		1		1		1		1		1		1	
Girl	1.35	***	0.58	***	0.92	*	0.51	***	1.02		0.57	***	0.40	***
Age														
11 y.o. (ref.)	1		1		1						1		1	
13 y.o	3.53	***	1.99	***	2.15	***					1.42	***	0.98	
15 y.o	13.47	***	3.94	***	5.02	***					1.18	***	0.79	***
Family structure														
Two parents (ref.)	1		1		1		1		1		1		1	
One parent	1.83	***	1.30	***	1.20	**	1.35	***	1.84	***	1.30	***	1.23	***

(continued)

Table 1. (continued)

	Current cigarette smoking		Current alcohol consumption		Getting drunk—lifetime		Early start of sexual life		Cannabis use—last 30 days		Bulling perpetration		Physical fights	
	OR	Sig	OR	Sig	OR	Sig	OR	Sig	OR	Sig	OR	Sig	OR	Sig
Other relative/ foster care/ children's home	2.03	***	1.48	***	1.29	**	1.94	***	1.79	**	1.44	***	1.52	***
Family affluence scale														
FAS—low (ref.)	1		1		1		1		1		1		1	
FAS—medium	0.92		1.17	**	0.99		1.03		1.00		1.02	5	1.02	
FAS—high	1.10		1.44	***	1.08	***	1.62	***	1.90	***	1.24	***	1.26	***
Constant	0.03	***	0.16	***	0.13	***	0.72	***	0.03	***	0.45	***	1.02	***
N. of observations	13,877		13,772		11,119		4613		4354		13,755		13,798	
Log likelihood	−5212.7		−6881.7		−4870.4		−2820.55		−843.5		−8447.0		−8654.1	

Source: HBSC-BG, 2006, 2014, 2018. Own calculations
Notes: 1) *** $p \leq 0.01$; ** $0.01 < p \leq 0.05$; * $0.05 < p \leq 0.10$
2) The analysis of early start of sexual life and cannabis use in the last 30 days includes only 15-years old students

T. Kotzeva und E. Dimitrova

The effect of age reveals that the prevalence of cigarette smoking, regular alcohol consumption, getting drunk and bullying perpetration significantly increases with age. The effect is negative only in the case of physical fights.

There is a statistically significant relationship between the studied risky behaviours and family structure. The students who live in a one-parent family and a family of their relatives or in foster care are more likely to report that they smoke cigarettes, regularly drink alcohol, get drunk, have risky sexual behaviour and are aggressive towards others in school compared to those who live with both parents (reference category).

Family affluence is also significantly associated with some of the adolescents' risky behaviours. The students from high FAS families are more likely to report that they regularly drink alcohol, have an early start of sexual life, use cannabis and show aggressiveness at school (bullying perpetration and participation in physical fights) compared to young people from low FAS families (reference category).

3   Discussion

The frequency of risky behaviours in Bulgarian adolescence over 13-years period of time indicates a chronic prevalence of unhealthy activities. Between one-third and one-fourth of schoolchildren aged 11–15 years report having been involved in tobacco smoking, alcohol use and abuse, cannabis use, early unsafe sexual experience, participating in physical fights and bullying others at school. From a cross-national perspective, the Bulgarian adolescents outnumber most of their peers in the other countries participating in HBSC and typically occupy the first ten risky behaviours (Inchley et al. 2016; Inchley et al. 2020b).

Over the years, trend analysis demonstrates a significant decrease in adolescents' current cigarette smoking, excessive alcohol use, involvement in a physical fight, and sexual activity before age 15 and an upward trend of adolescents' regular alcohol consumption and drug use.

From a cross-national perspective, despite the substantial decline of adolescent smoking for the last 30 years in the European countries, the prevalence of regular smokers among 15-years old Bulgarians is very high. Bulgaria leads the ranking out of 44 countries in cigarette smoking in the last 30 days—38 % of Bulgarian girls and 26 % of Bulgarian boys at the age of 15 report weekly smoking in 2018 (Inchley et al. 2020b, p. 92). According to the European Health Interview

Survey (2014), 36 % of men and 21 % of women in Bulgaria are daily smokers, representing along with Cyprus (38 %) and Latvia (37 %) the largest proportion of regular smokers among the EU countries (National Statistical Institute 2019, p. 99). The Eurostat data reveal a high prevalence of daily smoking among Bulgarian men aged 15–24 (Eurostat 2017). These data confirm that adolescence is a crucial time for tobacco initiation and nicotine addiction that may be difficult to quit in adult life (WHO 1996).

Although HBSC survey waves reveal a trend of decline of regular drinking among boys and girls in the European region (Inchley et al. 2018b), drinking, including binge drinking, is still widespread among Bulgarian adolescents. Bulgarian 11- and 13-years olds report the highest share of current (last 30 days) alcohol consumption and 15-olds occupy the 6th position by this indicator in the international ranking (Inchley et al. 2020b, p. 82–83). Although Eurostat data show that in later age 15–24 years olds Bulgarians are not among the leaders in alcohol consumption (Eurostat 2017), Bulgarian adolescents rank on some of the first places by the prevalence of drunkenness at least twice in a lifetime. The frequent and excessive use of alcohol in adolescence may have adverse effects on young people's physical and mental health and is associated with low academic achievements, more aggression, deviant behaviours at school, drug use (Kuntsche et al. 2012; Kuntsche and Gmel 2013) and unplanned and risky sex (Cooper 2002).

Cannabis, as the most frequently used drug by young people in Europe, is a risk factor for behaviour problems and mental disorders at this age (Inchley et al. 2018a). Trend analysis displays an expansion of the current use (last 30 days) of cannabis with a statistically significant increase between 2014 and 2018. Bulgarian students top rank the countries by this indicator (Inchley et al. 2020b, p. 95). Cannabis initiation and its regular use in adolescence is associated with dropouts and low school performance, unsafe sex, aggression and delinquency, anxiety and depression, cognitive disorders and brain deterioration (Kokkevi et al. 2006; Volkov et al. 2014). However, Eurostat data for cannabis use at the next age group (15–24 years) places Bulgaria among the countries with a low prevalence (Eurostat 2017).

Sexual health is part of adolescents' social and personal wellbeing. The analysis across years presents a statistically significant downward trend of adolescent sexual activity. However, the Bulgarian 15-year old boys outnumber their coevals in most countries participating in the last wave of HBSC by this indicator (Inchley et al. 2020b, p. 76). We may consider that boys' data on reported sexual onset is partially biased due to the adolescents' aspirations to be perceived as mature men. On the other hand, Eurostat data reveal one of the highest proportions of abortions and births at the under the age of 20 years in Bulgaria (Eurostat online database. Section "Abortion indicators"[6]). Early unprotected sex has its potential risks on adolescent physical and mental health: its effects are related not only to the risk of unintended pregnancy and induced abortion but as well as to sexually transmitted infections with a long term effect on reproductive health, emotional wellbeing, self-perception and social status of young people (Spriggs Madkour et al. 2010). Bacalso and Mihajlović (2018) draw the conclusion relevant to Bulgaria's case that the high age barriers in accessing sexual and reproductive health services are contrary to the often lower age of consent to sexual relationships and even marriage at younger ages.

Physical fighting is the most vivid display of youth aggression and is considered an indicator of multiple risk behaviours (Sosin et al. 1995). Trend analysis for adolescents' participation in physical fights reveals a statistically significant decrease in Bulgaria's youth violence over the 13 years. In 2018 Bulgarian 15- and 13-year olds rank in the 9th position and 11-year olds⁻in the 14th position by involvement in a physical fight at least three times in the past 12 months (Inchley et al. 2020b, p. 106–107).

Trend analysis for bullying perpetration does not present substantial changes over the survey years. In a cross-national comparison, 11-year olds occupy the 3rd rank, 13-year olds⁻the 4th rank, and 15-year olds⁻the 5th rank by bullying others at least twice in the past couple of months (Inchley et al. 2020b, p.100–101). The high prevalence of bullying at school among Bulgarian adolescents is a major concern for public health as young people's aggression is associated with other risky behaviours such as alcohol and drug use, alienation from school life, and lower overall life satisfaction, etc. (Walsh et al. 2013).

Gender differences are a substantial gradient for risky behaviours, with boys outnumbering girls in all risky behaviours, except cigarette smoking. There is a pattern of increasing the share of girls' unhealthy behaviours over the years, especially in alcohol and drug consumption and aggression at school. The age of 14 is crucial for the onset of risky behaviours for both genders.

Cross-comparative data from Eurostat on the proportions of regular smoking, alcohol consumption, and drug use at the age of 15–24 show that Bulgarian young people continue unhealthy activities initiated during adolescent years. This effect is especially true for smoking tobacco that started in adolescent years and

---

[6] https://ec.europa.eu/eurostat/databrowser/view/demo_fabortind/default/table?lang=en (Accessed—24.09.2021).

became a daily habit for 26 % of Bulgarian males aged 15–24. By this indicator, Bulgaria ranks among the countries with the highest proportion of male daily smokers.

The HBSC study applies a socio-ecological model where health behaviours and health outcomes are influenced by social, psychological, and ecological factors. Macro-level influences, including economic, political, cultural and environmental factors, are essential gradients of the socio-ecological model of understanding adolescents' health and wellbeing. At the micro-level, the main determinants of adolescents' health are delineated through social settings/contexts approach, including the effects of family, peers, and school.

Family structure and family affluence turn to be strongly associated with schoolchildren's risky behaviours. Adolescents living in one-parent families or in families with relatives have higher odds of risky behaviours. Our previous studies (Dimitrova and Kotzeva 2009) prove that social support, close relations with the parents and high satisfaction with family life have a preventive effect on schoolchildren's risky behaviours.

Family affluence is another significant gradient in defining the prevalence of risk behaviours. The multivariate statistical analysis shows that young people from high FAS families in Bulgaria are more likely to report that they regularly drink alcohol, have an early start of sexual life, use cannabis and show aggressiveness at school (bullying perpetration and physical fights) compared to young people from low FAS families. These results correspond to our previous findings (Dimitrova and Kotzeva 2019), which reveal that young people from high-status families are more likely to report certain types of risky behaviours. An association between the prevalence of risky behaviours and high affluence families is mostly found for the Baltic countries (Zaboriskis et al. 2006), unlike most West European countries where risky behaviours are more associated with lower socioeconomic status (Currie et al. 2012).

4 Youth Policy and Intervention Strategies in Bulgaria

Survey data, including HBSC data, have served as a valuable source for setting up policy agendas and developing evidence-based strategies and programs directed towards improving adolescents' health and wellbeing in Bulgaria. The National

Health Strategy (2014–2020)[7], esp. policy direction 7 "Effective functioning of maternal, child and school healthcare" and the auxiliary National Program for the Improvement of Maternal and Child Health (2014)[8] are the main policy-driven documents based on the European framework "Investing in Children: the European Child and Adolescent Health Strategy 2015–2022 (The WHO Regional Office for Europe)" and on the UN Convention on the Rights of the Child (General comment N 20 (2016) on the implementation of the rights of the child during adolescence).

Based on evidence-informed and rights-based principles the country-level health documents are directed to supporting growth during adolescence, reducing exposure to violence and risk, achieving a tobacco-free millennial generation, promoting healthy nutrition and physical activity, tackling depression and other mental problems in adolescence, addressing the unfinished agenda of preventable death and infectious diseases (Dimova et al. 2018).

The key areas for improving health literacy and health promotion for young people are risky behaviours, obesity, sexual and reproductive health, aggression and violence and mental health, with a special focus on at-risk groups, including the Roma community. In Bulgaria, state-run institutions and NGOs support policies and enhance programs responsive to adolescents' needs and capacities and enable effective participation of young people in policy implementation. Among such programs is the national student contest 'Missioners of health' launched in 2018 by the Ministry of Health in partnership with other governmental and non-governmental organizations such as WHO's office for Bulgaria and the Bulgarian Red Cross Youth. The contest aims at encouraging more schools to be involved in the initiative to raise schoolchildren's health literacy concerning tobacco and alcohol abuse, unhealthy eating, and reduced physical activity.

The reduction of risk factors such as tobacco smoking and alcohol abuse is a priority of health promotion and health education programs in Bulgaria. Although smoking is banned in public spaces by the Health Act, tobacco advertising is prohibited, alcohol and cigarettes are not sold to people under the age of 18, the restrictions are often violated, and smoking is highly tolerated in public,

---

[7] https://www.mh.government.bg/media/filer_public/2015/04/08/nacionalna-zdravna-strategia_2014-2020.pdf (Accessed—24.09.2021).

[8] https://srzi.bg/uploads//pages/Stolichna_RZI/1.Organizacionna_struktura/org_struktura/Programi/Majchino%20i%20detsko%20zdrave/National_Programme_for_Improveme.pdf (Accessed 24.09.2021).

including the increasing habits of smoking water pipes, which are equally toxic as smoking regular cigarettes. The effective intervention programs against drug abuse and addictions should be based not only on information campaigns but on improving coordination between school authorities and police to stop the illegal spread of drugs near schoolyards.

Sexual and reproductive health education exists as an option in a few schools in Bulgaria. Adolescents, especially from marginalized social groups, face barriers to access medical advice on contraception and abortion. At the EU baseline, the country has a high rate of abortions and births under the age of 18, making programs to reduce inequalities and transform gender violence between adolescent boys and girls crucial. The National Centre for Public Health and Analyses (NCPHA) promotes youth empowerment through sexual and reproductive health and rights, gender equality, and peacebuilding programs. In partnership with the International Institute for Youth Development PETRI, UNFPA, and Youth Peer Education Network (Y-PEER), PETRI-Sofia Center[9] provides peer-to-peer education using alternative education methods (theatre-based techniques, role games, simulations), organizes meetings, and builds an international network of young volunteers and experts.

The NCPHA completed the project "Improved mental health services" with the sponsorship of EEA grants[10]. The project activities comprise training and online educational programs for general practitioners, psychologists, and social workers in primary care to detect anxiety and depression and suicidal symptoms. Other activities include organizing public campaigns to increase people's sensitivity to mental health issues and media specialists' training on how to cover the topic.

Another important area for policy interventions is combatting violence in adolescent age. 'Childhood without violence' Coalition[11] comprises 20 NGOs and academic representatives aiming to build up public intolerance and change attitudes toward violence. In cooperation with parents and children and professionals working with children, the NGOs activists work on creating sustainable public services and measures to protect children against violence,

---

[9] http://petri-sofia.org/en/homepage/ (Accessed 24.09.2021).
[10] http://bgmental.ncpha.government.bg/bg (Accessed 24.09.2021).
[11] http://endviolence.bg/ (Accessed 24.09.2021).

developing of instruments for detection and reporting about children at risk, providing advocacy for changes in legislation and policies, organizing information and awareness campaigns and mapping the situation through research studies.

5   Conclusion

The surveys' findings show that some of the risk-taking behaviours started during adolescence as part of youth culture of experimentation, mood improvement and peers' appreciation, relevant for 'fruit-bearing age,' but they may lead to substance addiction and chronic physical, social and psychological problems in adult life. Additionally, risky and unhealthy behaviours are observed simultaneously, producing multiple risk-taking. The policy agenda of national programs should address the health risk multiplicity and involve teachers, parents, NGOs, and young people to coordinate and unify different stakeholders' efforts to encourage healthy lifestyles for young people.

The school environment is of paramount importance to health promotion and building up healthy habits among schoolchildren, but health education is not a substantial gradient of school curricula in Bulgaria. There is a considerable need for an increase of social workers, psychologists, and special needs assistants at schools as a strategy to tackle aggression and bullying and as a way to monitor students' mental health and personal development. Providing more opportunities for extracurricular activities for sports, art, social volunteering, and school community building are tools to achieve resilience to unhealthy behaviours and stimulate young people's capacities to establish rewarding relationships with others and develop pro-social lifestyles.

References

Bacalso, C. & Mihajlović, D. (2018). *Age Matters! Understanding age-related barriers to service access and the realization of rights of children, adolescents and youth.* Final Synthesis Report. UNICEF: Youth Policy Labs.

Cooper, ML. (2002). Alcohol use and risky sexual behavior among college students and youth: Evaluating the evidence. *Journal of Studies on Alcohol,* Suppl. 14: 101–117.

Currie, C., Nic Gabhainn, S., Godeau, E., Roberts, C., Smith, R., Currie, D., Pickett, W., Richter, M., Morgan, A. & Barnekow, V (Eds.) (2008). *Inequalities in young people's health: HBSC international report from the 2005/06 Survey. Health Policy for Children and Adolescents,* No. 5. Copenhagen: WHO Regional Office for Europe.

Currie, C. et al. (Eds.) (2012). *Social determinants of health and wellbeing among young people. Health Behaviour in School-aged Children (HBSC) study: international report from the 2009/2010 survey.* Copenhagen: WHO Regional Office for Europe; 2012 (Health Policy for Children and Adolescents, No. 6).

Dimitrova, E. & Kotzeva, T. (2009). Risk behaviors of the Bulgarian school-aged children: family predictors and determinants. In: *Bulgarian Journal of Psychology. The South-East Regional Conference of Psychology "South Eastern Europe Looking Ahead: Paradigms, Schools, Needs and Achievements of Psychology in the Region.* Sofia, Bulgaria, 30–1 Nov 2009, Is.3–4, pp. 43–55.

Dimitrova, E. & Kotzeva, T. (2019) Socio-economic Inequalities and Risk Behaviors among School-aged Children in Bulgaria: Results of the HBSC. *Sociological Problems.* Special Issue "How We Live Together: Communities, Institutions, Networks, 51, 2019, ISSN:0324-1572, 102–124.

Dimova, A., Rohova, M., Koeva, S., Atanasova, E., Koeva-Dimitrova, L., Kostadinova. T. & Spranger, A. (2018). Bulgaria: Health system review. 2018. *Health Systems in Transition*, 20(4): 1–256.

European Commission. *EU Health Programme (Multi-annual programme of EU action in the field of health for the period 2014–2020 (Regulation EU N 282/2014)).* https://ec.europa.eu/health/funding/programme_en (Accessed 24.09 2020).

European Commission. *Youth—Discover EU's Role—EU Youth Strategy—Health and Well-being website.* https://ec.europa.eu/youth/policy/youth-strategy/health-wellbeing_en, (Accessed 24.09.2020).

Eurostat (2017). Being Young in Europe Today—Health. Data extracted in December 2017. https://ec.europa.eu/eurostat/statistics explained/index.php?title=Being_young_in_Europe_today_-_health#Health_status, (Accessed 24.09.2020).

Inchley, J., Currie, D., Budisavljevic, S., Torsheim, T., Jåstad, A., Cosma, A. et al. (Eds.) (2020a). *Spotlight on adolescent health and wellbeing. Findings from the 2017/2018 Health Behaviour in School-aged Children (HBSC) survey in Europe and Canada. International report.* Volume 1. Key findings. Copenhagen: WHO Regional Office for Europe. Licence: CC BY-NC-SA 3.0 IGO.

Inchley, J., Currie, D., Budisavljevic, S., Torsheim, T., Jåstad, A., Cosma, A. et al. (Eds.) (2020b). *Spotlight on adolescent health and wellbeing. Findings from the 2017/2018 Health Behaviour in School-aged Children (HBSC) survey in Europe and Canada.* International report. Volume 2. Key data. Copenhagen: WHO Regional Office for Europe. Licence: CC BY-NC-SA 3.0 IGO.

Inchley, J., Currie, D., Cosma, A. & Samdal, O. (Eds.). (2018a) Health Behaviour in School-aged Children (HBSC). *Study Protocol: background, methodology and mandatory items for the 2017/18 survey.* St Andrews: CAHRU.

Inchley, J., Currie, D., Vieno, A., Torsheim, T., Ferreira-Borges, C., Weber, M., Barnekow, V. & Breda, J. (Eds.). (2018b). *Adolescent alcohol-related behaviours: trends and inequalities in the WHO European Region, 2002–2014.* Observations from the Health Behaviour in School-aged Children (HBSC) WHO collaborative cross-national study.

Inchley, J., Currie, D., Young, T. et al. (Eds.). (2016). Growing up unequal: gender and socioeconomic differences in young people's health and wellbeing. Health Behaviour in School-aged Children (HBSC) study: international report from the 2013/2014 survey.

Health Policy for Children and Adolescents, No. 7. Copenhagen: WHO Regional Office for Europe.

Kann, L., McManus, T., Harris, W.A., Shanklin, S.L., Flint, K.H., Queen, B., Lowry, R., Chyeu, D., Whittle, L., Thornton, J., Lim, C., Bradford, D., Yamakawa, Y., Leon, M., Brener, N. & Ethier, K.(2018). Youth risk behavior surveillance—United States, 2017. *Morbidity and Mortality weekly Report—Surveillance Summaries*. 67(8): 1–114. Published online 2018 Jun 15. doi: https://doi.org/10.15585/mmwr.ss6708a1, (Accessed 24.09.2020).

Kokkevi, A., Nic Gabhainn, S., Spyropoulou, M. & the Risk Behaviour Focus Group of the HBSC. (2006). Early initiation of cannabis use: A cross-national European perspective. *Journal of Adolescent Health*, 39(5): 712–719.

Kuntsche, E., Rossow, I., Simons-Morton, B., ter Bogt, T., Kokkevi, A. & Godeau, E. (2012). Not early drinking but early drunkenness is a risk factor for problem behaviors among adolescents from 38 European and North American countries. *Alcoholism: Clinical and Experimental Research*, Volume first published online 2012.

Kuntsche, E. & Gmel, G. (2013). Alcohol consumption in late adolescence and early adulthood—Where is the problem? *Swiss Medical Weekly*, 143, p. w13826 https://doi.org/10.4414/smw.2013.13826, (Accessed 24.09.2020).

McLaren, L. & Hawe, P. (2005). Ecological perspectives in health research. *Journal of Epidemiology & Community Health*, 59 (1): 6–14. doi: https://doi.org/10.1136/jech.2003.018044.

McLeroy, KR., Bibeau, D., Steckler, A. & Glanz, K. (1988). An ecological perspective on health promotion programs. *Health Education Quarterly* 15: 351–377. doi: https://doi.org/10.1177/109019818801500401.

Marmot, M. (2009). Social determinants and adolescent health. *International Journal of Public Health*, 54(2): 125–127.

National Statistical Institute. (2019). *Sustainable Development in Bulgaria 2005–2016*. Sofia: NSI.

Schnohr, W., Molcho, M., Rasmussen, M., Samdal, O. et al. (2015).Trend analyses in the health behaviour in school-aged children study: methodological considerations and recommendations. *European Journal of Public Health*, vol.25, Supplement 2: 7–12.

Siegel, D. (2014). *Brainstorm. The Power and Purpose of the Teenage Brain*. Tarcher Perigee.

Sosin, DM., Koepsell, TD., Rivara, FP. & Mercy, JA. (1995). Fighting as a marker for multiple problem behaviors in adolescents. *Journal of Adolescent Health*, Mar:16(3):209–15.

Spriggs Madkour, A., Farhat, T., Halpern, CT., Godeau, E. & Nic Gabhainn, S. (2010). Early adolescent sexual initiation and physical/psychological symptoms: a comparative analysis of five nations. *Journal of Youth and Adolescence*, 39(10): 1211–1225.

Subramanian, SV., Jones, K. & Duncan, C. (2003) Multilevel methods for public health research. Kawachi I, Berkman LF, (Eds.). *Neighborhoods and Health* [Internet]. Oxford: Oxford University Press: 65–111.

Steinberg, L. (2008). A social neuroscience perspective on adolescent risk-taking. *Developmental Review* 28: 78–106.

UNICEF. (2011). *The State of the World's Children. Adolescence: an age of opportunity*. New York, United Nations Children's Fund. https://www.unicef.org/publications/index_57468.html, (Accessed 24.09.2020).

Volkow, ND., Baler, RD., Compton, WM. & Weiss, SR. (2014). Adverse health effects of marijuana use. *New England Journal of Medicine*, 370(23): 2219–2227.

Walsh, SD., Molcho, M., Craig, W., Harel-Fisch, Y., Huynh, Q., Kukaswadia, A. et al. (2013). Physical and emotional health problems experienced by youth engaged in physical fighting and weapon carrying. *PLoS One*. Feb 21; 8(2):e56403.

World Health Organization (1995). *Tobacco, alcohol and illicit drugs. WHO Fact Sheet No. 127*.

World Health Organization (2014a). *Investing in children: the European child and adolescent health strategy 2015–2020*. Copenhagen: WHO Regional Office for Europe. http://www.euro.who.int/en/health-topics/Life-stages/child-and-adolescent-health/policy/investing-in-children-the-european-child-and-adolescent-health-strategy-20152020, (Accessed 24.09.2020).

World Health Organization (2014b). *Health for the World's Adolescents: A second chance in the second decade*. Geneva, World Health Organization. https://www.who.int/maternal_child_adolescent/documents/second-decade/en/, (Accessed 24.09.2020).

World Health Organization (2015). *The Global Strategy for Women's, Children's and Adolescents' Health (2016–2030)*. Geneva: World Health Organization. https://www.who.int/life-course/publications/global-strategy-2016-2030/en/, (Accessed 24.09.2020).

Zaboriskis, A., Sumskas, L., Maser, M. & Pudule, I. (2006). Trends in drinking habits among adolescents in the Baltic countries over the period of transition: HBSC survey results 1993–002. *BMC Public Health* 6:67 doi:https://doi.org/10.1186/1471-2458-6-67.

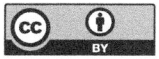

Current Findings and Policy Concepts Concerning School-Related Health and Well-Being in Finland – School Burnout and Engagement

Katariina Salmela-Aro

1 Introduction

Finland is a country in which students have been successful in the OECD's PISA comparison studies. However, student wellbeing is an issue. Finland was ranked almost last in the OECD comparisons in terms of student happiness in school. In addition, there is a widening achievement gap, and some signs of segregation in the metropolitan area of Helsinki. Moreover, according to the OECD PISA study, the largest gap in achievement nationally is between native-born Finns and immigrants. Gendered wellbeing and achievement gaps are also present. Boys are more likely to be underachievers, whereas girls suffer from mental-health issues.

In the present paper I first describe the context of Finland, then I focus in particular on school-related health and wellbeing. I present the key models on which I base the results: the modern expectancy-value-cost theory and the related stage-environment fit theory, as well as the demands-resources model in the school context. I present results showing how school wellbeing (burnout and engagement in particular) changes during middle school and transitions to educational tracks, later in high school and gap years, and during third decade of life in tertiary education and the transition to working life. I also show how school wellbeing can spill over to other life domains, negatively and positively, through depression, excessive Internet use and life satisfaction, for example. The social context of parents, peers, and teachers plays a key role in the health and well-being of

K. Salmela-Aro (✉)
Departement of Educational Sciences, University of Helsinki, Helsinki, Finland
E-Mail: katariina.salmela-aro@helsinki.fi

© Der/die Autor(en) 2022
A. Heinen et al. (Hrsg.), *Wohlbefinden und Gesundheit im Jugendalter*,
https://doi.org/10.1007/978-3-658-35744-3_31

689

adolescents, too, and I focus on peer selection and influence effects, for example. Finally, I discuss some recent policy issues in Finland concerning the promotion of student engagement and wellbeing.

2   School Burnout in Research

Burnout has attracted the interest not only of the scientific community but also of the general public in the last few decades. Given the rationale that school is a place in which students work (Salmela-Aro and Tynkkynen 2012, p. 929), the three-component construct of burnout has recently been applied to the context of formal education (Salmela-Aro et al. 2009a; Salmela-Aro 2017; Walburg 2014): exhaustion due to school demands, a cynical and detached attitude towards school, and feelings of inadequacy as a student (Salmela-Aro et al. 2009a). Exhaustion refers to being tired, ruminating on school-related issues and experiencing sleep problems; cynicism implies an indifferent or distal attitude towards studying in general, a loss of interest in studying and not seeing it as meaningful; and a sense of inadequacy as a student refers to a diminished feeling of academic competence, achievement and accomplishment. It is possible to study these three dimensions of school burnout from the perspective of modern expectancy-value-cost theory (Eccles and Roesner 2009). Within this framework, the feeling of inadequacy as a student refers to having low expectations; having a cynical attitude towards school refers to the value component of the expectancy-value-cost model, which includes values such as attainment, utility, and interest; and exhaustion refers to the high emotional costs of studying (Salmela-Aro 2017).

Although a relatively new research topic, school burnout has rapidly captured international attention, a fact that reflects its perceived relevance in many countries (e.g., May et al. 2015; Meylan et al. 2015; Yang and Chen 2016; Herrmann et al. 2019). The phenomenon has been observed among students in countries with different educational systems and academic policies, thus indicating that it is neither culturally nor geographically restricted (Walburg 2014). Although this paper focuses on Finland, the results are largely generalizable to other countries. According to PISA surveys, 15-year-old students in Finland outperform their peers in other countries. However, there is a large gap between native Finns and immigrants, and between boys and girls. In this paper, I present recent findings on school burnout and engagement in the context of the new challenges of digitalization and diversity that schools are facing. Today's teenagers outperform all previous generations in terms of Internet use, and ethnic diversity has become the rule rather than the exception in most European countries, including Finland.

According to the OECD, the definitive test of how effectively immigrants integrate into their receiving societies is how well their children are doing. Positive school adaptation is a precursor of future adaptation among young people, hence school burnout may have negative, possibly cascading, future consequences. The promotion of positive school engagement is thus of paramount importance for the future success and wellbeing of young people and society.

The demands-resources model adapted for use in the school context (Salmela-Aro and Upadyaya 2014) and the stage-environment fit theory (Eccles and Midgley 1989; Salmela-Aro and Tynkkynen 2012) could help to explain school burnout and engagement. The two theories approach school burnout as a mismatch between individual needs and the demands imposed by the school context, causing students to experience energy depletion without gaining appropriate returns, and engagement as a match between these needs and demands. The key psychological needs are competence, autonomy, and relatedness (see also self-determination theory, Deci and Ryan 2000). According to the adapted demands-resources model, the more school-related demands that students experience, the higher their level of school burnout, whereas the more resources they possess, the stronger their engagement. Consequently, two processes can be identified: a motivational process according to which resources lead to increased motivation, and a health-impairment process during which demands lead to strain and impaired health. In support of the model, longitudinal research results show that school burnout and engagement also spill over from the domain-specific school context to general ill- and wellbeing (Salmela-Aro and Upadyaya 2014): burnout predicts later depressive symptoms, whereas engagement predicts later life satisfaction. Moreover, the spillover is not restricted to wellbeing, and also extends to further educational choices, achievements and pathways. Findings from longitudinal studies indicate that school engagement predicts higher grades, successful transition from high school to tertiary studies, and later satisfaction with chosen educational pathways. School burnout, in turn, predicts involuntary gap years after high school, lowered educational aspirations, and a fourfold greater likelihood of dropping out. In line with the stage-environment fit theory, the risk of school burnout is greater when the school context does not support the psychological needs of students.

Longitudinal studies conducted in the school context show that when students are autonomously motivated to pursue their educational goals, they invest more effort in them and thereby achieve high levels of progress. High goal progression, in turn, is related to high levels of school engagement and success in future educational transitions, whereas low progress is associated with drop-out intentions and school burnout (Vasalampi et al. 2009).

3   Students at Elementary School: Growing Up in the Digital Era

Members of the current generation of young people are often described as digital natives (Prensky 2001). Most adolescents use mobile devices and social media for maintaining constant connections and hanging out with an extended network of peers. Patterns of socio-digital participation are nevertheless heterogeneous in that only some young people cultivate advanced computer and media skills, and pursue their interests by actively joining various network communities (Gee and Hayes 2011). Some investigators express concern that adolescents who are accustomed to dealing with intensive flows of information through working simultaneously with multiple media (i.e., media multitasking, Veen and Vrakking 2008), and navigating through relatively short fragments of text, may develop "grasshopper minds" (Carr 2010), rendering them unable and unwilling to embark on disciplined intellectual activity. It is also suggested that some young people are driven by harmonious passions in their engagement in intensive socio-digital participation (Vallerand et al. 2007), which enable them to develop their skills and competences, and to engage in increasingly more complex activities (Ito et al. 2010). Others, however, may develop obsessive passions (Vallerand et al. 2007) or even addictions that involve repeated participation in compulsive, monotonous activities related to computer gaming or surfing the Internet, for instance. Adopting (Bergman and Andersson's (2010) person-oriented approach to examining homogeneous subgroups of students with varying initial levels and developmental trends of engagement and burnout, we identified four profiles (Salmela-Aro et al. 2016a) among students at elementary school: engaged, stressed, cynical, and burned out. The engaged students formed the largest group (50 % of the sample), with moderate scores on school engagement and relatively low scores on all three dimensions of school burnout. Students in the stressed group comprised 4 % of the sample, expressing very high levels of exhaustion and inadequacy, whereas those at risk of burnout (5 %) were characterized by high levels of all three components of school burnout. Finally, those in the cynical group (41 %) showed highly cynical attitudes towards school. The results further revealed that the cynical students were more likely to be males, whereas those who were stressed and burned out were more likely to be females. Those in the cynical group also reported that they would be more engaged at school if they could use digital devices in the classroom. Although the incorporation into formal education of socio-digital technologies to support pedagogical transformations such as inquiry-, phenomenon-, and game-based study practices might enhance student engagement, digitalization remains a double-edged sword.

Experiencing a high level of school engagement is beneficial for students in terms of academic performance and well-being (Salmela-Aro and Upadyaya 2012; Upadyaya and Salmela-Aro 2013a), and this should therefore be among the main goals of modern pedagogies. However, although Finnish students show high mean levels of school engagement overall, we identified subgroups struggling with disengagement and cynicism. It has been suggested that the ways in which students use digital technologies out of school are out of sync with the presumably more traditional pedagogical practices of formal education. This phenomenon is known as the *gap hypothesis* (see e.g., Prensky 2001; Salmela-Aro et al. 2016b), as it concerns the gap between digital engagement and school-related engagement among adolescents. The hypothesis is that students who are engaged in learning via digital technologies out of school do not find traditional educational practices similarly engaging. This is in line with the above-mentioned findings that students who report more cynicism towards schoolwork also report that they would be more engaged in their schoolwork if they were able to make extensive use of digital technologies in doing it (Salmela-Aro et al. 2016b). Digitalization presents a new challenge to young people generally and in the school context. Our cross-lagged path models showed further that a cynical attitude towards school predicted later excessive Internet use after controlling for the previous level. Moreover, sleep problems mediated school burnout and excessive internet use.

4 Students at Middle School: Growing Up in Diversity

A further new challenge for today's educational system, alongside digitalization, is increasing student diversity. For example, Finland has the widest gap between immigrants and natives in terms of academic achievement. Our results revealed an increase in school burnout during middle school (grades 7 to 9), and the burnout pattern was gendered.

Among girls the increase was in feelings of inadequacy as a student, whereas the boys, particularly recent immigrants, had an increasingly cynical and negative attitude towards school. One reason for this is the high demands on these students: Finnish schools do not provide enough support to help them to overcome language barriers and thereby to promote learning. However, burnout was lower among immigrant girls than among native Finns, a finding that could reflect the immigrant paradox among girls (see the special issue, Motti-Stefanidi and Salmela-Aro 2018). As posited in the demands–resources model, their resources for academic adaptation and resilience may stem from their personal and social resources (Salmela-Aro and Upadyaya 2014). Cynicism, which as already stated is increasingly prevalent among recent immigrant boys, has been shown to increase the risk of dropping out fourfold (Bask and Salmela-Aro 2013). The proneness of immigrant boys to displaying an increasingly cynical attitude towards school, and thus possibly to being at risk of dropping out, makes the process of integrating them into Finnish society even more demanding. At worst, these children disengage first from school, and then from society. Programs are needed that allow immigrant youth to experience school as a safe haven, support their learning and engagement, and combat discrimination. How well these young people perform in school is a major test for the receiving society and its educational system. It seems that Finland faces many challenges in this respect. Diversity should be understood as a resource rather than a risk for society as a whole.

5   Beyond High School

Finnish adolescents in post-compulsory academic education have been compared to those in vocational education for signs of school burnout and engagement (Salmela-Aro et al. 2008). According to the results, feelings of inadequacy are more likely to be experienced by students on an academic as opposed to a vocational track. The nature of the Finnish academic and vocational educational environments, and of the transition itself, strongly affects any changes in how students think and feel about their education (stage-environment fit, Wigfield et al. 1996). Eccles and Midgley (1989) suggested that negative developmental changes could ensue if young people were not provided with developmentally appropriate educational environments. A negative developmental fit may lead to school burnout if the educational context does not support the students' psychological needs. It has been shown that the transition to high school is particularly stressful in view of the increased academic demands and changes in the sources of social support it involves. A recent study reported a 30-percent increase in school burnout among Finnish girls at high school over the previous two years. It also seems that school burnout increases across the years at high school (Sorkkila et al. 2018).

Tuominen-Soini and Salmela-Aro (2014) identified four profiles among a cohort of high school students: engaged (44 %), engaged-exhausted (28 %), cynical (14 %), and burned-out (14 %). High-school engagement may also be associated with burnout in that some students who experienced high engagement simultaneously reported high levels of exhaustion and low educational achievement. Students who simultaneously experienced high levels of both engagement and exhaustion felt more exhausted and stressed because of their high educational aspirations than those who only experienced engagement, who were more worried about possible failure and more readily gave up when faced with academic challenges. Nevertheless, most students experienced high levels of engagement and well-being, and only a small proportion reported low engagement and adjustment problems However, findings from the new millennium cohort indicated that the proportion of engaged students had fallen to 37 %, compared to rises to 45 % among the engaged-exhausted students and 18 % among the burned-out students.

It was reported in a recent study that the proportion of students suffering from school burnout is even higher among aspiring athletes at high school. Although the health benefits of practicing sport are widely acknowledged, increasing concern has been expressed about student-athletes who combine academic pursuits with high-level competitive sports, in that success in one domain often comes at the cost of failure in the other (Sorkkila et al. 2018). The European Commission (2012) acknowledges that high-achievement sport should be organized in a socially responsible manner to avoid school dropout among elite-level athletes. It was found that student-athletes were at risk of sport- and school-related burnout even at the beginning of upper secondary school, almost half of them risking burnout. Furthermore, symptoms of sport and school burnout increased and became more generalized over time, and school-related exhaustion spilled over to the sports domain. High individual and parental expectations at the beginning of upper secondary school were negatively related to burnout in the same domain, but positively related to burnout in the other one. Furthermore, mastery goals related to sport- and school-related achievement buffered against cynicism and feelings of inadequacy in the same domain, whereas school-related performance goals predicted school-related cynicism.

6 Study Burnout Increases During Higher Education

We adopted a person-oriented approach to identify the profiles of study engagement and burnout in higher education in a representative sample of 12,394 higher-education students at different phases of their studies in universities and polytechnics in Finland. Again, we identified four profiles: engaged (44 %), engaged-exhausted (30 %), inefficacious (19 %), and burned-out (7 %) (Salmela-Aro and Read 2017). The engaged students tended to be in the earlier stages of their studies, whereas the burned-out and the inefficacious had been studying the longest. This pattern indicates that students start out being highly engaged, and burnout becomes more common later in their academic career. In support of the demands-resources model, the covariates reflecting demands were higher, and those reflecting resources were lower, among the burned-out and inefficacious students than among the engaged. Some students who experience difficulties in graduating from higher education and thus prolong their studies are at an elevated risk of burnout: prolonging one's studies is assumed to be stressful and to lead to cynicism concerning the meaningfulness of studying as well as feelings of inadequacy as a student. As a consequence, burnout also presents a risk of later dropout (Bask and Salmela-Aro 2013) and depression (Salmela-Aro and Upadyaya 2014). Further in line with the demands-resources model, the inefficacious and burned-out students reported more depressive symptoms than their engaged counterparts.

Our new analyses during the COVID-19 showed that remote learning increased university students' burnout dramatically. Among a sample of 1500 university students from the University of Helsinki, 18 % suffered from severe burnout, whereas 29 % was engaged during remote learning. Moreover, 24 % was in risk of burnout and 29 % engaged-exhausted. These results need to be taken seriously.

Analyses of individual differences in the development of study engagement showed an increase in engagement among some students (14 %) following the transition to higher education or to working life (Salmela-Aro 2009; Upadyaya and Salmela-Aro, 2013b, 2017), possibly reflecting the better person-environment fit of the new study or work environment (Eccles and Midgley 1989; Eccles and Roeser 2009). Other studies have also shown that high engagement in school facilitates career choices, whereas many students who disengage from school feel that their studies are less significant and experience more insecurity concerning their career choices (Ketonen et al. 2016). Many young people starting out on their higher-education studies or their career may perceive the new environment as better suited to their future goals, thereby providing a better person-environment fit (Eccles and Midgley 1989; Eccles and Roeser 2009) and offering opportunities for change in engagement.

7 Social Context: Sharing Burnout and Engagement

Adolescents typically do not face challenging educational transitions alone but seek advice from and discuss opportunities with their significant others. This behavior is also posited in the life-span model of motivation (Salmela-Aro 2009). More specifically, it is argued that the goals of individuals going through critical transitions are influenced not only by their own beliefs and motivation but also by the perceptions, attitudes and expectations of significant others. Thus, affective support from their interpersonal environment during challenging educational transitions may be a critical resource for adolescents (Gniewosz et al. 2012). The influence of parents and peers on student choices has been particularly emphasized (Nurmi 2004). School- and work-related engagement and burnout always occur in a larger social context, which includes family, peers/coworkers, principals/management, and the school/work environment (Eccles and Roeser 2009). These contexts, together with the individual's stage-environment fit, serve as a framework for understanding student engagement and burnout (Upadyaya and Salmela-Aro 2013b). Mutual interaction between members of these different contexts serves as an ecological asset that promotes wellbeing.

With regard to family characteristics, several studies have shown that parental involvement, affection, monitoring, and support all promote engagement with school/work (Englund et al. 2008; Upadyaya and Salmela-Aro 2013b; Wang and Eccles 2012). Close and supportive relationships, including parental affection in general (i.e., affective support and warmth from one's parents), typically increase adolescents' engagement in their studies during educational transitions (Upadyaya and Salmela-Aro 2013b), and help them to attain their educational goals (Melby et al. 2008). Likewise, supportive relationships with peers have proved to be beneficial. Having friends and feeling accepted at school appear to support involvement and engagement in school-related activities (Wentzel et al. 2010, 2017), as well as fostering positive feelings about school (Estell and Perdue 2013) and good school performance (Ladd et al. 1997): all these things increase the likelihood of graduating from school (Véronneau and Vitaro 2007).

Parents, teachers, peers, coworkers, and supervisors serve as sources of support for students/young adults in promoting high engagement, adjustment to transitions, and educational and vocational success (Englund et al. 2008; Upadyaya and Salmela-Aro 2013b). In the school context, teacher autonomy, support, and enthusiasm tend to have positive effects on student engagement (Watt et al. 2017). Parental autonomy and social support may serve as an environmental protective factor, and the more sources of social support one has, the higher one's levels of positive outcomes and engagement (Duineveld et al. 2017; Rosenfeld et al. 2000). Multiple sources of support may serve as ecological assets among adolescent students, which together with strong high-school engagement promote positive youth development (Lerner et al. 2012) and a successful school-to-work transition: this, in turn, is a precursor of successful career development (Pinquart et al. 2003). Educational and occupational transitions are also optimal periods in which to make interventions designed to prevent the possible weakening of engagement. This, in turn, supports positive youth development and the overall adjustment of students and young adults to their new educational and vocational environments.

Moreover, recent research also attests to an increase in school burnout and related disengagement (Salmela-Aro et al. 2016b), and that some students who experience high levels of engagement simultaneously report high exhaustion and reduced well-being (Tuominen-Soini and Salmela-Aro 2014). Thus, it would be useful to examine student engagement and burnout conjointly (Salmela-Aro 2015, 2017). Similarly, there is a need for future studies to better identify the processes leading to disengagement, and to plan interventions that could prevent low and diminishing engagement trajectories among students and young adults (Symonds et al. 2016). Changes in engagement are especially prevalent during educational and vocational transitions, for example, which offer students and workers opportunities to make positive changes (Li and Lerner 2011; Upadyaya and Salmela-Aro 2013b).

8   Outlook

As a new policy, one way of facilitating continuing engagement among adolescent students and young adults would be to develop innovative transition programs designed to give them a deeper understanding of their study and career possibilities (Vinson et al. 2010), and to enhance their career exploration (Perry 2008). Such programs could feature a wide range of novel, innovative, and traditional activities (e.g., tutoring in small groups, undertaking research projects, Google mapping) with an emphasis on clarifying future possibilities and the purposes of student courses and activities (for more examples, see Vinson et al. 2010). Moreover, helping students to identify their intrinsic career values prior to the transition to higher education/work may also enhance engagement in school/ work (Sortheix et al. 2013). Teachers and educators could incorporate such programs into their own teaching and thus support successful transition to higher education/work among students.

References

Bask, M., & Salmela-Aro, K. (2013). Burned out to drop out: Exploring the relationship between school burnout and school dropout. *European Journal of Psychology of Education*, *28*, 511–528.

Bergman, L. R., & Andersson, H. (2010). The person and the variable in developmental psychology. *Journal of Psychology, 218*, 155–165.

Carr, N. (2010). *The shallows: How the Internet is changing the way we think, read, and remember.* London: Atlantic.

Deci, E. L., & Ryan, R. M. (2000). The „what" and „why" of goal pursuits: Human needs and the self-determination of behavior. *Psychological Inquiry, 11*(4), 227–268.

Duineveld, J., Parker, P., Ryan, R., Ciarrochi, J., & Salmela-Aro, K. (2017). The link between perceived maternal and paternal autonomy support and adolescent well-being across three major educational transitions. *Developmental Psychology, 53*, 1–17.

Dweck, C. (2017). *Mindset-updated edition: Changing the way you think to fulfil your potential.* Hachette UK.

Eccles, J. S., & Midgley, C. (1989). Stage-environment fit: Developmentally appropriate classrooms for young adolescents. In R. Ames & C. Ames (Eds.), *Research on motivation and education: Goals and cognitions* (vol. 3. pp. 139–186). New York: NY, Academic Press.

Eccles, J. S., & Roeser, R.W. (2009). Schools, academic motivation, and stage-environment fit. In R. M. Lerner and L. Steinber (Eds.) *Handbook of adolescent psychology* (3rd ed.) (pp. 404–434). Hoboken, N.J.: John Wiley & Sons.

Englund, M. M., Egeland, B., & Collins, W. A. (2008). Exceptions to high school dropout predictions in a low-income sample: Do adults make a difference? *Journal of Social Issues, 64*, 77–93

Estell, D. B., & Percue, N. H. (2013). Social support and behavioral and affective school engagement: The effects of peers, parents, and teachers. *Psychology in the Schools, 50*(4), 325–339.

Gee, J. P., & Hayes, E. R. (2011). *Language and learning in the digital age.* Routledge.

Gniewosz, B., Eccles, J. S., & Noack, P. (2012). Secondary school transition and the use of different sources of information for the construction of the academic self-concept. *Social Development, 21*(3), 537–557.

Herrmann, J., Koeppen, K., & Kessels, U. (2019). Do girls take school too seriously? Investigating gender differences in school burnout from a self-worth perspective. *Learning and Individual Differences, 69*, 150–161.

Ito, M., Baumer, S., Bittanti, M., Cody, R., Herr-Stephenson, B., Horst, H. A., Lange, P., Mahendran, D., Martínez, K. Z., Pascoe, C. J., Perkel, D., Robinson, L., Sims, C., & Tripp, L. (2010). *Hanging out, messing around, and geeking out.* The MIT Press.

Ketonen, E. E., Haarala-Muhonen, A., Hirsto, L., Hänninen, J. J., Wähälä, K., & Lonka, K. (2016). Am I in the right place? Academic engagement and study success during the first years at university. *Learning and Individual Differences, 51*, 141–148.

Ladd, G. W. (1990). Having friends, keeping friends, making friends, and being liked by peers in the classroom: Predictors of children's early school adjustment?. *Child Development, 61*(4), 1081–1100.

Ladd, G. W., Kochenderfer, B J., & Coleman, C. C. (1997). Classroom peer acceptance, friendship, and victimization: Destinct relation systems that contribute uniquely to children's school adjustment?. *Child Development, 68*(6), 1181–1197.

Lerner, R. M., Bowers, E. P., Geldhof, G. J., Gestsdóttir, S., & DeSouza, L. (2012). Promoting positive youth development in the face of contextual changes and challenges: The roles of individual strengths and ecological assets. *New Directions for Youth Development, 2012*(135), 119–128.

Li, Y., & Lerner, R. M. (2011). Trajectories of school engagement during adolescence: Implications for grades, depression, delinquency, and substance use. *Developmental Psychology, 47*, 233–247.

May, R. W., Bauer, K. N., & Fincham, F. D. (2015). School burnout: Diminished academic and cognitive performance. *Learning and Individual Differences, 42*, 126–131.

Melby, J. N., Conger, R. D., Fang, S. A., Wickrama, K. A. S., & Conger, K. J. (2008). Adolescent family experiences and educational attainment during early adult-hood. *Developmental Psychology, 44*, 1519–1536.

Meylan, N., Doudin, P. A., Curchod-Ruedi, D., & Stephan, P. (2015). School burnout and social support: The importance of parent and teacher support. *Psychologie Française, 60*, 1–15.

Motti-Stefanidi, F. & Salmela-Aro, K. (toim). (2018). Youth and Migration: What promotes and what challenges their integration? *European Psychologist: Special issue, Vol. 23*.

Nurmi, J. E. (2004). Socialization and self-development. *Handbook of Adolescent Psychology*, 2, 85–124.

Perry, J. C. (2008). School engagement among urban youth of color: Criterion pattern effects of vocational exploration and racial identity. *Journal of Career Development, 34*, 397–422.

Pinquart, M., Juang, L. P., & Silbereisen, R. K. (2003). Self-efficacy and successful school-to-work transition: A longitudinal study. *Journal of Vocational Behavior, 63*, 329–346.

Prensky, M. (2001). Digital natives, digital immigrants. *On the New Horizon, 9*, 1–6.

Rosenfeld, L. B., Richman, J. M., & Bowen, G. L. (2000). Social support networks and school outcomes: The centrality of the teacher. *Child and Adolescent Social Work Journal, 17*, 205–226.

Salmela-Aro, K. & Upadyaya, K. (2012). The Schoolwork Engagement Inventory: Energy, Dedication and Absorption (EDA). *European Journal of Psychological Assessment, 28*, 60–67.

Salmela-Aro, K. & Upadyaya, K. (2014). School Burnout and Engagement in the Context of the Demands-Resources Model. *British Journal of Educational Psychology, 84*, 137–151.

Salmela-Aro, K. (2009). Personal goals and well-being during critical life transitions: The four C's—Channelling, choice, co-agency and compensation. *Advances in Life Course Research, 14*, 63–73.

Salmela-Aro, K. (2015). Toward a new science of academic engagement. *Research in Human Development, 12*, 304–311.

Salmela-Aro, K. (2017). Dark and bright sides of thriving–school burnout and engagement in the Finnish context. *European Journal of Developmental Psychology, 14*, 337–349.

Salmela-Aro, K., & Tynkkynen, L. (2012). Gendered pathways in school burnout among adolescents. *Journal of adolescence, 35*(4), 929–939.

Salmela-Aro, K., Kiuru, N., & Nurmi, J. E. (2008). The role of educational track in adolescents' school burnout: A longitudinal study. *British Journal of Educational Psychology, 78*(4), 663–689.

Salmela-Aro, K., Kiuru, N., Leskinen, E., & Nurmi, J. E. (2009a). School burnout inventory (SBI) reliability and validity. *European Journal of Psychological Assessment, 25*(1), 48–57.

Salmela-Aro, K., Moeller, J., Schneider, B., Spicer, J., & Lavonen, J. (2016a). Integrating the light and dark sides of student engagement using person-oriented and situation-specific approaches. *Learning and Instruction*, *43*, 61–70.

Salmela-Aro, K., Muotka, J., Alho, K., Hakkarainen, K., & Lonka, K. (2016b). School burnout and engagement profiles among digital natives in Finland: A person-oriented approach. *European Journal of Developmental Psychology*, *13*, 704–718.

Salmela-Aro, K. & Read, S. (2017). Study engagement and burnout profile among Finnish higher education students. *Burnout Research, 7, 21–28.*

Sorkkila, M., Aunola, K., Salmela-Aro, K., Tolvanen, A., & Ryba, T. V. (2018). The co-developmental dynamic of sport and school burnout among student-athletes: The role of achievement goals. *Scandinavian Journal of Medicine & Science in Sports, 28(6)*, 1731–1742.

Sortheix, F. M., Dietrich, J., Chow, A., & Salmela-Aro, K. (2013). The role of career values for work engagement during the transition to working life. *Journal of Vocational Behavior*, *83*, 466–475.

Symonds, J., Schoon, I., & Salmela-Aro, K. (2016). Developmental trajectories of emotional disengagement from schoolwork and their longitudinal associations in England. *British Educational Research Journal*, *42*, 993–1022.

Tuominen-Soini, H., & Salmela-Aro, K. (2014). Schoolwork engagement and burnout among Finnish high school students and young adults: Profiles, progressions, and educational outcomes. *Developmental Psychology*, *50*, 649–662.

Upadyaya, K., & Salmela-Aro, K. (2013a). Development of school engagement in association with academic success and well-being in varying social contexts: A review of empirical research. *European Psychologist, 18*, 136–147.

Upadyaya, K., & Salmela-Aro, K. (2013b). Engagement with studies and work: Trajectories from post-comprehensive school education to higher education and work. *Emerging Adulthood, 1*, 247–257.

Upadyaya, K., & Salmela-Aro, K. (2017). Developmental dynamics between young adults' life satisfaction and engagement with studies and work. *Longitudinal and Life Course Studies, 8(1)*, 20–34.

Vallerand, R. J., Salvy, S. J., Mageau, G. A., Elliot, A. J., Denis, P. L., Grouzet, F. M., & Blanchard, C. (2007). On the role of passion in performance. *Journal of Personality, 75(3)*, 505–534.

Vasalampi, K., Salmela-Aro, K., & Nurmi, J.-E. (2009). Adolescents' self-concordance, school engagement, and burnout predict their educational trajectories. *European Psychologist, 14*, 1–11.

Veen, W., & Vrakking, B. (2008). Homo Zappiens and his consequences for learning, working and social life. *Trend Study within the BMBF Project "International Monitoring"*.

Véronneau, M. H., & Vitaro, F. (2007). Social experiences with peers and high school graduation: A review of theoretical and empirical research. *Educational Psychology, 27(3)*, 419–445.

Vinson, D., Nixon, S., Walsh, B., Walker, C., Mitchell, E., & Zaitseva, E. (2010). Investigating the relationship between student engagement and transition. *Active Learning in Higher Education, 11*, 131–143.

Walburg, V. (2014). Burnout among high school students: A literature review. *Children and Youth Services Review, 42*, 28–33.

Wang, M.-T. & Eccles, J. S. (2012). Social support matters: Longitudinal effects of social support on three dimensions of school engagement from middle to high school. *Child Development, 83*, 877–895.

Watt, H. M., Carmichael, C., & Callingham, R. (2017). Students' engagement profiles in mathematics according to learning environment dimensions: Developing an evidence base for best practice in mathematics education. *School Psychology International, 38*, 166–183.

Wentzel, K. R., Battle, A., Russell, S. L., & Looney, L. B. (2010). Social supports from teachers and peers as predictors of academic and social motivation. *Contemporary Educational Psychology, 35*(3), 193–202.

Wentzel, K. R., Muenks, K., McNeish, D., & Russell, S. (2017). Peer and teacher supports in relation to motivation and effort: A multi-level study. *Contemporary Educational Psychology, 49*, 32–45.

Wigfield, A., Eccles, J. S., & Pintrich, P. R. (1996). Development between the ages of ll and 25. *Handbook of educational psychology, 148*.

Yang, H., & Chen, J. (2016). Learning perfectionism and learning burnout in a primary school student sample: A test of a learning-stress mediation model. *Journal of Child and Family Studies, 25(1)*, 345–355.

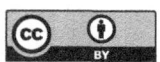

Adolescent Health in the European Region: Policy Development and the Role of WHO

Ross Whitehead, Eileen Scott, Aixa Aleman-Diaz, Susanne Carai and Martin W. Weber

1   Introduction

Adolescents within the WHO European Region are generally the healthiest in the world. However, we can still do more to improve their health and wellbeing and ultimately their prospects of a long, healthy life. Adolescence represents a unique developmental window in which action to improve physical, mental and social welfare can have life-long consequences.

The rapid physical and psychological development that occurs in adolescence accompanies a significant shift in social and cultural roles and relationships in preparation for adulthood. As part of this transition, young people may experiment with many of the behaviours that can lead to poor health outcomes in adulthood. Unfortunately, this can also mean that adolescents have greater expo-

R. Whitehead (✉) · E. Scott
Public Health Scotland, Edinburgh, Scotland
E-Mail: ross.whitehead1@phs.scot

E. Scott
E-Mail: eileen.scott1@phs.scot

A. Aleman-Diaz
Copenhagen Business School, Copenhagen, Denmark

S. Carai · M. W. Weber
WHO Regional Office for Europe, Copenhagen, Denmark
E-Mail: carais@who.int

M. W. Weber
E-Mail: weberm@who.int

© Der/die Autor(en) 2022
A. Heinen et al. (Hrsg.), *Wohlbefinden und Gesundheit im Jugendalter*,
https://doi.org/10.1007/978-3-658-35744-3_32

sure to risk factors to their immediate health, whilst having fewer resources to deal with these risks.

Investment in adolescent health is vital in achieving the United Nations Sustainable Development Goals. The 17 goals, adopted in 2015 by the UN General Assembly, set out a series of ambitious targets relating to poverty, inequality, climate change, the environment, peace and justice for global governments to achieve by 2030 (UN 2015). Action to promote the health and wellbeing of today's adolescents will help to underpin the ultimate success of these.

In 2014, *"Investing in children: the child and adolescent health strategy for Europe 2015–2020"* (WHO 2014) was unanimously endorsed by the 53 member states of the region. The strategy prioritises investment in protecting adolescents, promoting their health and well-being, and preventing disease. Tackling depression and other mental health problems in adolescence was recognized as a specific priority in addressing adolescent health in the European Region.

To help countries around the globe respond to the unique challenges to adolescent health, the WHO in 2017 in conjunction with UNAIDS, UNESCO, UNFPA, UNICEF, UN Women and the World Bank published *"Global Accelerated Action for the Health of Adolescents (AA-HA!): Guidance to support country implementation"* (WHO 2017a). Alongside this publication, WHO produced a suite of associated resources including case studies, youth-friendly materials and infographics on morbidity and mortality. In 2019 a European adaptation of this guidance was created by the WHO regional office for Europe to suit the specific needs of adolescents in the European regions and to help governments address their needs (Scott et al. 2019).

Consistent with these aims, in February 2020, in collaboration with UNICEF, WHO published "A future for the world's children? A WHO-UNICEF-Lancet commission" (Clark et al. 2020), which highlights the long-term benefits of improving young people's health (with a particular focus on climate change), outlines the proper role of government, and describes the need for multisectoral approaches to health.

Since March 2020, normal adolescent behaviour, and school-related activities have been seriously disrupted owing to the COVID-19 pandemic, which caused widespread closures of schools in April 2020 across Europe, and prevented adolescents from undertaking their normal activities and socializing. Health service access and delivery has also been impacted. At the time of writing (the end of 2020), there is still no prospect of normal activities being completely reinstated, with countries facing significant challenges in keeping schools open and returning to normal levels of health service delivery.

2 Adolescent Health in Europe: The Current Situation

Adolescent mortality in the European Region has declined substantially in recent decades. Annual deaths of 10–19-year-olds are estimated to have fallen from over 70,000 in 1990 (representing an all-cause rate of 53 per 100,000) to 31,617 in 2017 (30 per 100,000). Nevertheless, the remaining deaths are largely due to causes that are either preventable (e.g. road injuries) or receptive to high-quality health care (e.g. cancer and respiratory infections). The majority (over 60 %) of 10–19 year-olds' deaths in 2017 were attributable to the following six cause-groupings (IHME 2020):

- Road injuries—5810 deaths (5.5 per 100,000)
- Cancer—4623 deaths (4.4 per 100,000)
- Self-harm—4374 deaths (4.2 per 100,000)
- Drowning—1790 deaths (1.7 per 100,000)
- Lower respiratory infections—1260 deaths (1.2 per 100,000)
- Interpersonal violence—1232 deaths (1.2 per 100,000)

The non-fatal burden of illness during adolescence also remains mostly preventable, with significant scope for reductions in the number of years of healthy life lost. Preventable or treatable mental health problems, including anxiety, conduct and depressive disorders, self-harm, bipolar disorders and eating disorders are responsible for over 20 % of adolescents' total morbidity burden.

Aggregate statistics such as these, however, mask significant inequalities within and between countries in the region. There is substantial variation in mortality between sub-regions with an especially large gap in 10–19-year olds' death rate between Commonwealth of Independent States (CIS) and Western European (EU-15) nations (46.6 per 100,000 versus 15.5 per 100,000, respectively). The specific causes of death that account for the majority of this difference are especially receptive to high-quality clinical care and environmental safety measures (liver diseases, lower respiratory infections and drowning). There also exist significant gender differences in the adolescent mortality rate. The rate amongst males is approximately double that for females (39 per 100,000 versus 20 per 100,000, respectively), which is largely attributable to higher injury mortality in males.

Socioeconomic status is a strong predictor of health status within and across the WHO European region, with those from more affluent families tending to experience lower rates of death and disease. Developmental changes are moulded by the social and environmental circumstances that adolescents are growing up in, providing access to resources like money, education and social relationships which drive future life opportunities and health outcomes.

The HBSC survey (described in more detail below, and in other chapters of this book) highlights the socioeconomic patterning of health-promoting behaviours. Those from more affluent families tend to exhibit increased engagement in health-promoting behaviours (such as physical activity, tooth brushing and consumption of fruit and vegetables) and reduced participation in harmful activities (such as sugar-sweetened beverage consumption). For some indicators, including the use of alcohol, we see the reverse pattern. Those from more affluent families are more likely to be 'current drinkers' and have been drunk twice or more in their lifetime. More affluent adolescents are also more likely to report a medically-attended injury.

3   Quality Health Services for Adolescents

Adolescence presents unique health challenges especially in terms of sexual and reproductive health, mental health and engagement in substance use. These issues can be compounded by what is often an uncomfortable relationship with mainstream health services. Young people report relatively low satisfaction with such services compared to older adults, citing concerns about confidentiality, stigma, discrimination and poor alignment to their specific needs.

WHO urges countries to honour their commitments made in the United Nations Convention on the Rights of the Child (United Nations 1989) and provide all adolescents with access to the health care they need. This age group requires accessible, acceptable and appropriate services. WHO supports the implementation of adolescent-friendly health services based around core principles of protection, confidentiality, non-discrimination, non-judgement and respect.

Providing a holistic approach to health and wellbeing (i.e., not being merely clinical services) can enhance young people's attendance at, and perception of these services (Whitehead et al. 2018). Making use of 'soft' entry points such as being based around leisure activities or peer-led discussion groups may also be helpful. These services have a significant role in the promotion of young people's health and wellbeing. Appropriately designed, they can both provide diagnosis and management of health problems and enable signposting to other health and social service providers, as appropriate.

Adolescent friendly health services provide an accessible and de-stigmatised mechanism for service delivery and health promotion. Their quality, and utility also stands to benefit substantially from including youth in the design, delivery and evaluation of services.

Such services are particularly important in the context of sexual and reproductive health. In most settings, health care providers are not specifically trained in dealing with adolescents and in some countries, doctors incorrectly tell adolescents that contraception is harmful. Based on their undertaking made in the UNCRC, to which all European countries have signed, adolescents must be able to access health services based on their maturity. To assess this, all health providers need to be trained to assess the maturity of the adolescent, as it is for example taught in the EUTeach training materials (EUTeach 2020). A sufficiently trained workforce is a prerequisite for the provision of quality health services to adolescents in health services and also in schools.

4   The WHO Pocket Book of Primary Health Care for Children and Adolescents

In 2018, a regional review of the implementation of the UNICEF/WHO strategy on the Integrated Management of Childhood Illnesses (IMCI) was conducted (Carai et al. 2018) in order to assess what services are provided to children and adolescents in the context of universal health coverage. This review highlighted that children and adolescents currently do not always receive the care they need, particularly at the primary health care level. This is precipitating preventable mortality, morbidity and disability as well as impeding the achievement of the full potential of children and adolescents resulting in personal tragedies, waste of resources for health systems, as well as society at large.

A Pocket Book of Primary Health Care for Children and Adolescents is currently being developed to guide medical practitioners working with children and adolescents at primary health care level. These guidelines will form the basis for standards of care in universal health coverage and benefits packages for health insurance, thus being tightly incorporated into the health system at large. The Pocket Book will include chapters on health promotion and prevention from birth through adolescence, newborn health, the child or adolescent presenting with a specific complaint or a specific disease or condition, adolescent health, and emergencies and traumas.

5   The Example of Sexual and Reproductive Health in the Region

The 2017/2018 HBSC survey showed that at age 15, 1 in 4 boys (24 %) and 1 in 7 girls (14 %) report having had sexual intercourse (Inchley et al. 2020a), with particularly high prevalence amongst girls in Nordic countries, and boys in eastern Europe. The survey also indicated that 1 in 4 adolescents who have sex are having unprotected sex, with particularly low levels of condom or pill use in Malta, the Republic of Moldova and Wales. At the same time, the ease with which adolescents can access contraceptives is inconsistent across the European Region. In many countries adolescents cannot access contraceptives (except condoms) without parental consent before they are 18 years old. Only 1 in 4 countries allow adolescents to access contraceptives (excluding condoms) based on their maturity (see Fig. 1). Compounding this issue, the countries where this is not permitted also tend to not provide comprehensive sexuality education in schools. In stark contrast to contraceptive accessibility, the age of criminal responsibility of adolescents across Europe is in many countries lower than the age of being able to consent to one's medical treatment (Fig. 1).

Adolescent birth rates vary considerably across the region from 1/1000 adolescent girls to 54/1000 adolescent girls (Fig. 2) and are significantly higher in countries with higher ages for legal access to contraception. Rates are generally higher in Eastern European countries and Central Asia and lower in Western Europe.

6   WHO Tools and Frameworks for Progress

When *Investing in Children: the European Child and Adolescent Health Strategy* 2015–2020 (WHO 2014) was adopted, supporting evidence was needed to monitor the strategy's implementation. Progress since then has been tracked using a number of publicly available tools to increase transparency around monitoring. These include: (1) implementation tools for national work; (2) online country profiles; (3) two questionnaire-based surveys to Ministers of Health (2017 and 2020), (4) country feedback forms; and (5) two reports that analyzed survey findings and put them in context for the region (2018 and 2020).

The WHO Regional Office has developed guidance for countries on how to develop national strategies for child and adolescent health. This covers planning and implementing strategic plans, programmes and interventions, and

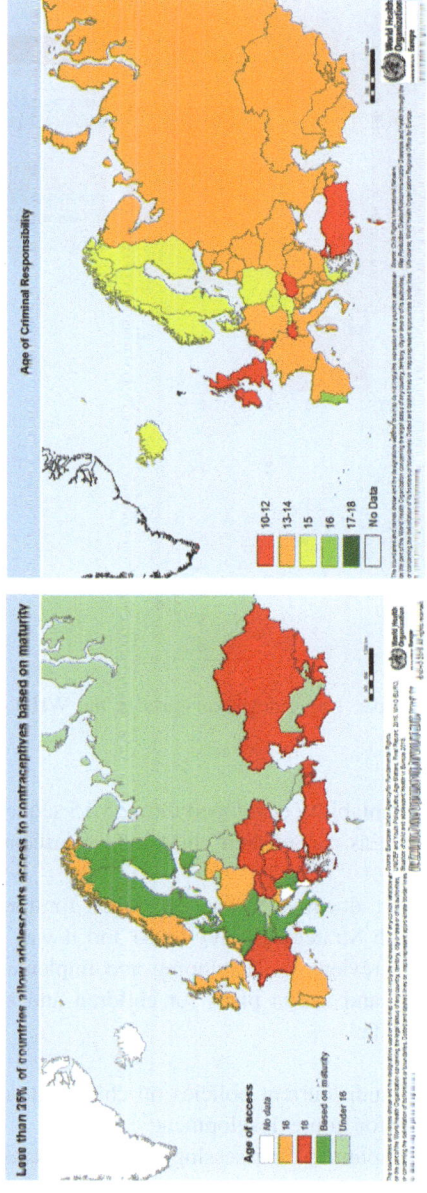

Fig. 1 Adolescent access to contraceptives based on maturity (left) and age of criminal responsibility (right) in the WHO European Region (by country). (Source: Created by Author)

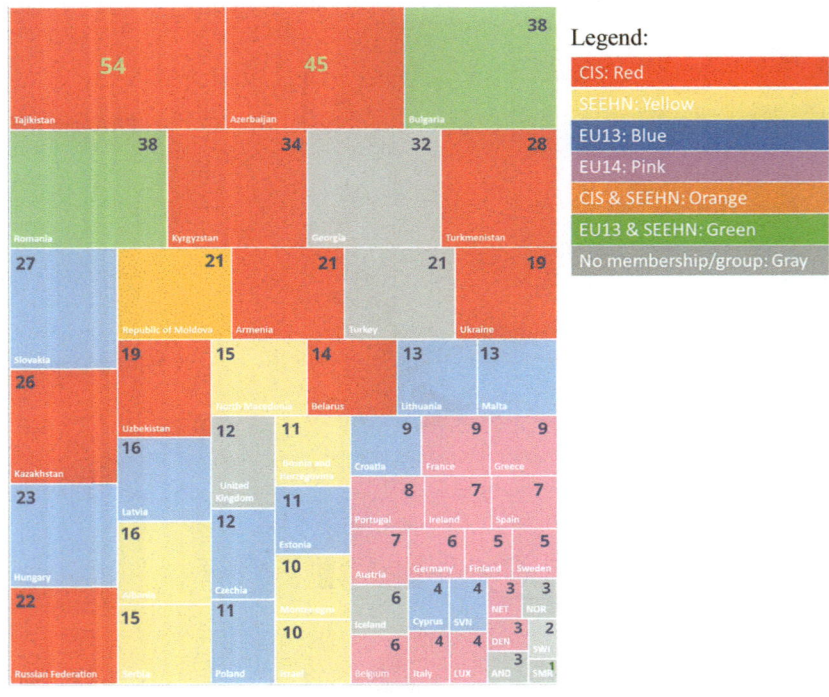

Fig. 2 Adolescent birth rates per 1000 adolescent girls in the WHO European region. (Source: Created by Author)

strengthening national accountability developed through 15 sequential steps. This has been piloted in Romania as part of their child and adolescent health strategy development process.

A toolkit containing four documents was developed for the first European Child and Adolescent Health Strategy (WHO 2005) and it was revised in 2015 to assist Member States in reviewing, developing and implementing their own national policies, strategies and action plans for children and adolescents. The individual components include:

- an assessment tool—to audit current policies on child and adolescent health and identify possibilities for future development;
- an action tool—to assist countries in assessing existing policies and strategies;

- an information tool—to identify necessary data and information to aid policy and strategy development; and.
- a gender tool—that enables countries to incorporate gender analysis into their child and adolescent health programmes and identify effective interventions that have a gender perspective.

A set of country profiles were developed for all 53 Member States of the WHO European Region (WHO European Health Information Gateway 2019). Profile indicators were selected on the basis of how accurately and holistically they represented child and adolescent health, assessed through expert consultation and collaboration with other WHO programme areas. These brought together the best available data on child and adolescent health, including an overview of population and health systems for each country, information on childhood infectious diseases. sexual and maternal health, risk behaviours, nutrition, and mental health and well-being. They also highlight inequities such as gender differences in six of the indicators. These profiles were the foundation of an initial dataset that would inform the development of regional surveys to monitor the strategy. Shared with Member States, these profiles form the basis of the development of national strategies and are accessible through the European Health Information Gateway.

While these profiles provided an overview of existing data, some key bits of information on child and adolescent health for each country were missing, hampering efforts to evaluate the strategy's progress. To address this gap, two monitoring surveys were sent out to the Ministries of Health in the member states of the WHO European region. These have been central tools to capture the state of, and apparent investment in, child and adolescent health and related policies and have been used to track changes over the course of the strategy implementation period.

The first of these surveys was sent to countries in 2017 (WHO European Health Information Gateway 2018) and a midterm report was submitted to the WHO WHO Regional Committee for Europe in 2018 (WHO 2018). A policy paper (Alemán-Díaz et al. 2018) was additionally produced to accompany the report and inform stakeholders in the wider child and adolescent health community.

The second survey, completed in 2020, concluded monitoring of the 2015–2020 strategy and laid ground for strategic development beyond 2020. The 2017 survey consisted of 82 questions, while the 2020 survey consisted of 66 questions. Experts at the Regional Office (e.g. programme managers on violence and injury prevention, nutrition, tobacco, alcohol and maternal health, among others) and WHO collaborating centres in the European Region provided their input and made suggestions for new items in both processes. Data from both surveys are available via the WHO European Health Gateway.

The final report on the 2015–2020 strategy was presented to the representatives of member states at the 70th session of the WHO Regional Committee for Europe (WHO 2020c). The Regional Office is committed to collaboration with countries to improve child and adolescent health and provide transparency on the data collected. As part of this process, country feedback forms were produced to highlight findings from the country profiles and survey exercise and have been used to initiate dialogue with Ministers of Health about areas where further investment could be useful.

7   Support for Countries

In 2019 the WHO Regional Office published "Adolescent health in the European Region: can we do better?" to encourage action and investment to improve the physical, mental and social well-being of young people in the region (Scott et al. 2019). This document provides an adaptation of global AA-HA! guidance with a focus on the European region, urging investment in adolescent health to enable countries to meet the goals of the 2015–2020 European Child and Adolescent Health Strategy and achieve the United Nations Sustainable Development Goals by 2030. Divided into three sections, the first focuses on making the case for investing in adolescent health. The second provides an analysis of the current state of adolescent health in the Region, including highlighting disparities within and between countries. The final section presents a four-phase guide for countries on planning, developing, implementing and monitoring action taken on adolescent health.

The regional office has also developed tools to support countries develop their own child and adolescent health strategies. Several Member States have recently worked with WHO in the development of their national child and adolescent health strategies, including the Republic of Moldova, Romania, Tajikistan, Turkmenistan, Uzbekistan and the United Kingdom of Great Britain and Northern Ireland (Scotland).

WHO collaborating centres for child and adolescent health in Germany, Ireland, Italy, Norway, the Russian Federation, Switzerland and the United Kingdom have contributed significantly to the implementation of the current European Child and Adolescent Health Strategy. Collaborating centres form part of an institutional collaborative network set up by WHO to support its technical work. Collaborating centres are designated (typically for a period of four years) following an extensive review of the centre's scientific and technical competencies, its stability and ability to link with, and influence national and international institutions.

8 Health Promoting Schools and the Schools for Health in Europe (SHE) Network

Children spend a substantial proportion of their time, over a long period of their life in schools. We know that schools have the potential to be protective environments and that children can learn what they need to know about health, and practice it (health literacy and life skills). Schools are also a setting where children can receive the healthcare they need. WHO is therefore supporting the health promoting schools programme. In terms of school health promotion, the objective is "to make every school a health promoting school". This was endorsed by a high level meeting of Ministries of Health and Education in Europe in Paris 2016 (WHO 2017b).

8.1 Components of Health Promoting Schools

Key components of health promoting schools as identified in the WHO framework for health promoting schools are outlined in Fig. 3 (WHO 2017b).

The features of health promoting schools go far beyond merely what happens in classrooms. For instance, where schools have invested in infrastructure such as sports and play facilities, there should be efforts made to make these available outside school hours to encourage sports and leisure activities. Additionally, cities need to plan for journeys to and from school through active transport, for example by being cycle-friendly, or having safe footpaths. Thought needs to be given to ways in which city planning can help reduce pollution and young people's exposure to it on their journey to and from school.

Health promoting schools are based on the Ottawa Charter, adopted at the First International Conference on Health Promotion, held in November 1986. It stated that health promotion is "the process of enabling people to increase control over, and to improve, their health". Strategies to promote health include:

- Strengthening community action
- Developing personal skills

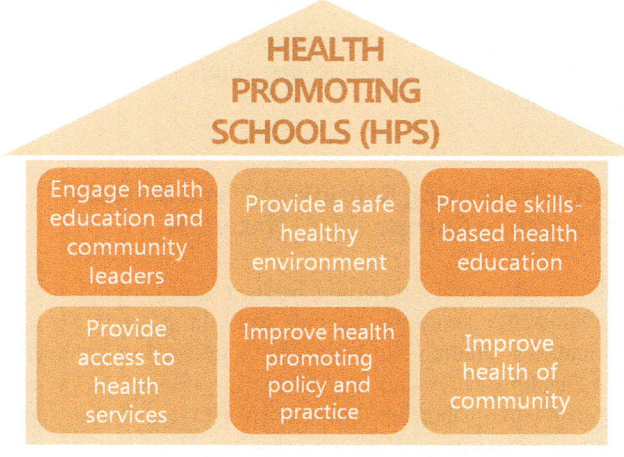

Key features of HPS

Fig. 3 The six components of health promoting schools. (Source: Created by Author)

- Creating supportive environments
- Enabling, mediating, advocating
- And reorienting health services

8.2   Schools for Health in Europe (SHE) Network Foundation

Over the past 30 years, across the region the health promoting schools approach has been adopted to improve the health of school children effectively. A network to establish the approach has gradually developed and consolidated as the School for Health in Europe (SHE) network foundation. SHE aims to improve the health of children and young people in Europe, including reducing health inequalities, through a specific focus on the school setting. There are SHE national coordinators in over 30 countries across the WHO region.

The network is coordinated by the University of Southern Denmark. For the countries of the former Soviet Union, which often have Russian as a second language of communication, a WHO collaborating centre, the Scientific Institute of Pediatrics in Moscow, is taking a coordinating role in translating the materials and process into Russian and supporting country orientation and pilot processes. Several countries in Central Asia and the Caucasus have become members of the network.

The SHE network provides a wealth of materials for achieving the objectives of school health promotion. In 2019, SHE published the 'SHE School Manual 2.0', to encourage national/regional SHE coordinators, school principals, school management, teachers, other school staff, pupils and community partners to be involved in the development of health promoting schools. These materials and details of national coordinators are available from the SHE website (www. schoolsforhealth.org). The network organises regular meetings which share the experiences and approaches which countries have found useful. A yearly summer school is also run by the network to train staff across Europe, with a focus on research methodology (Fig. 4).

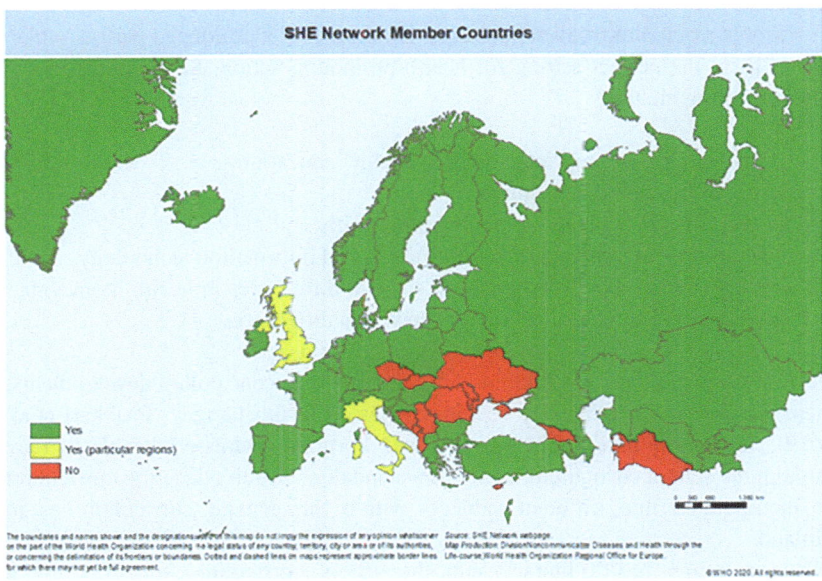

Fig. 4 Members of the SHE Network. (Source: Created by Author)

8.3   School Support for Health Literacy

Health literacy consists of „the personal, cognitive and social skills which determine the motivation and ability of individuals to gain access to, understand and use information in ways which promote and maintain good health" (Nutbeam 2000).

A key component of health promoting schools is the acquisition of health literacy, as this falls into the core teaching competencies of the schools. The education system as a whole and schools, in particular, are important settings for the development of health literacy among children. Health literacy skills benefit the health, growth and development of children, as well as their health in later life and the health of the broader society.

Researchers using data from the Health Behaviour in School-aged Children (HBSC) survey in Finland have recently found that health literacy is one of the main factors contributing to health differences and is associated with educational outcomes such as academic achievement and post-school aspirations (Paakkari et al. 2019).

Schools reach almost all school-aged children over a prolonged period, which makes them the perfect setting for health-promoting action. Key benefits of the schools setting include:

- Access to age-appropriate school health education via a whole-school approach and school curriculum.
- Opportunities to develop lifelong learning skills.
- Access to free exchange health information and information technology
- Well-resourced schools can equalize societal differences in health literacy, but wide variations in school resources can widen differences.

Despite health literacy in children being a focus of recent policy developments, there are only a few education sector policies on health literacy (Paakkari et al. 2019). Education policies in Finland and Portugal addressed health literacy through the school curriculum, either as a standalone health education curriculum or incorporated into different subjects within the general curriculum, as in Finland.

Incorporating health literacy into the school curriculum, supported by a whole-school approach, is the most promising strategy to ensure that all children can gain the necessary knowledge and skills to support their health and well-

being across the life-course. To achieve this, the health and education sectors
need to work together.

9   Using the Health Behaviour in School-Aged Children (HBSC) Study to Support Countries

The 2015–2020 European CAH Strategy sought to make children's lives visible
in the region. Reliable data on child and adolescent health provide an essential
foundation to achieve this and provides a critical underpinning for evidence-
informed policy making and effective child health programming.

Data from the Health Behaviour in School-aged Children (HBSC) study
has been an essential component of monitoring the healthy development of
young people in participating countries since 1983. Every four years, children
and young people (aged approximately 11–15 years) in participating countries
take part in the survey, providing valuable trend data and intra- and international comparisons. The most recent survey was conducted in 2018, with
two international reports published in 2020; one summarising findings across
all participating countries and (Inchley et al. 2020a), another with more
comprehensive detail on collected data (Inchley et al. 2020b).

There has been an increasing interest in the study as evidenced by the
inclusion of new participating countries in every survey cycle to date, the
publication of an external survey protocol in 2013[1] and public terms of
reference in 2014 (CAHRU 2014). An increasingly public face for the study, has
complemented these efforts. The 2013–2014 and 2017–2018 waves of HBSC data
are included in the WHO European Health Information Gateway, HBSC trend
data is included in the European Child and Adolescent Health Country Profiles
and the Situation of Child and Adolescent Health in Europe report (WHO 2018),
both key elements of the monitoring process on the implementation of the CAH
strategy.

Since the adoption of the 2015–2020 Child and Adolescent Health
Strategy, seven new countries (Azerbaijan, Cyprus, Georgia, Kazakhstan,
Kyrgyzstan, Serbia and Uzbekistan) have joined the study, leading to a total of
46 participating countries in the Region (Fig. 5). Most states in the region now

---

[1] Protocol available upon request at www.hbsc.org (N.B. 2009–2010 was the first external
protocol officially produced).

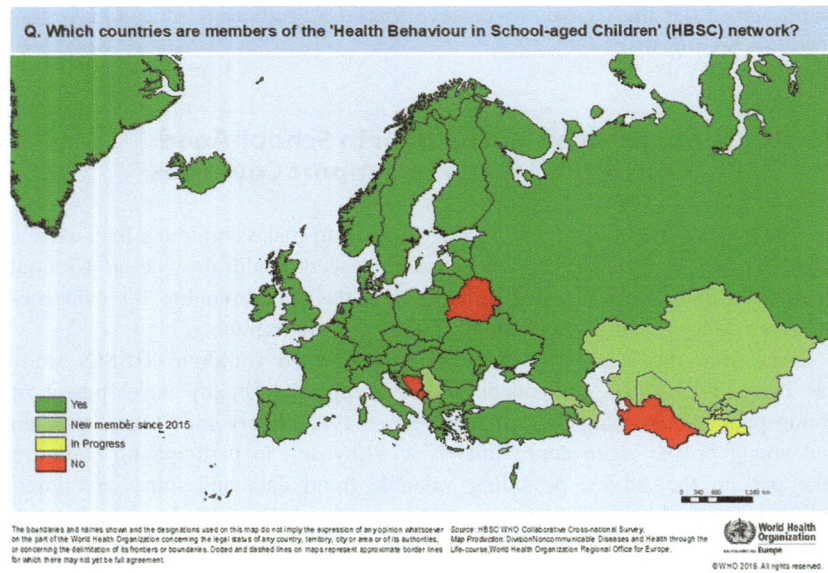

Fig. 5 Map of HBSC Network member countries in the WHO European region. (Source: Created by Author)

participate in the study increasing it's value across the region and as a tool for monitoring of child and adolescent health by WHO.

9.1   WHO Support for Membership of HBSC

New study members are currently limited to countries within the WHO Euro Region. Interested member states have expressed interest to the WHO Regional Office or the HBSC International Coordinating Centre (ICC) who, with support of HBSC members from Armenia, Croatia, Kazakhstan, Latvia, Republic of Macedonia and Russia, have organized introductory sessions to the HBSC survey. These sessions have led to countries conducting pilot HBSC surveys in preparation for a formal application to participate in the HBSC study.

9.2   HBSC SHE Collaboration

HBSC provides a wealth of data on the situation of children in schools, and several aspects of their well-being can best be addressed through school-based interventions. In many countries, both networks are coordinated by the same group of people, facilitating deep collaboration and knowledge exchange. To learn more about this process, WHO has recently formalized the cooperation in a number of countries, building on the experience in Wales and Scotland, where HBSC data are obtained in schools and used for the design and monitoring of interventions. In this process, investigators from both networks jointly analyse data and provide feedback to schools, teachers, parents and pupils. Findings are discussed in multi-disciplinary teams and interventions are optimised, taking into account objective feedback. The focus of this process is to ensure that schools can make best use of HBSC data information to measure health and well-being related to the school context. Ways on how this information can be used and indicators for successful implementation of the health promoting school concept are continuously being explored. There is a substantial focus on involvement of children and young people. Pupils generally engage well with the topics and are interested and motivated to give their opinions. The data sets are also often used by older adolescents who can benefit from getting a better understanding of research methodology and formal data analysis.

10   Moving Forward—Remaining Adolescent Health Challenges and a New Strategic Direction

As good progress has been made in the region to reduce child and adolescent mortality, reduced death rates have led to the general misconception that the health and wellbeing of children and adolescents no longer constitute a priority in Europe. This has resulted in a lack of focus and less attention to adolescent health issues.

Significant health issues remain for Europe's adolescents, addressing these will have an impact now, throughout their life and also the next generation. Challenges which the countries of Europe need to address as a priority to make progress include children's rights, health promotion, disease prevention and specific availability of services for adolescents. A recent survey of key stake-holders identified the problems outlined in Table 1. Factsheets and support

Table 1 Health related problems of adolescents in Europe. (Source: Created by Author)

Problems faced by adolescents in the WHO European Region
Obesity is on the rise: 1 in 3 11-year-olds is overweight or obese. Levels of overweight and obesity have risen since 2014, and now affect 1 in 5 young people, with higher levels among boys and younger adolescents; 1 in 4 adolescents perceive themselves as too fat, especially girls. Marketing is poorly regulated: unhealthy food is aggressively promoted.
Adolescent mental and behavioral health problems are increasing and a major cause of mortality. Suicide is the 1st leading cause of death among adolescents in low- and middle-income countries, and 2nd leading cause in high-income countries in the WHO European Region. Rates of anxiety and depressive symptoms are increasing over time: mental health and wellbeing represents the largest contributor to years of healthy life loss during adolescence. School health services focus on screening: Mental health services and counselling are not available.
Children are killed or seriously injured on roads in the WHO European Region. More than 3000 children under the age of 15 are killed on roads in the WHO European Region each year. Road traffic accidents are the most common cause of death among 15-19 year olds in the European region. Violence against children is a major public health problem, affecting at least 55 million children in Europe.
Adolescents do not receive the care they need: Most primary care providers have not been trained in adolescent care. Adolescents cannot universally access health services by themselves: the age of consent for health services is often higher than the age of criminal responsibility. Less than 25% of countries allow adolescents access to health services based on maturity without parental consent. Adolescents do not receive the care they need: Most primary care providers have not been trained in adolescent care. Out-of-pocket payments for health care of children and adolescents are too high: Care and treatment is often too expensive for parents or adolescents to afford. Entitlements are not clear: adolescents (and their parents) are not aware what services they are entitled to. Adolescents face barriers in accessing particularly sexual reproductive health services.
Schools are not a healthy environment: Food is not healthy, drinking water not provided, hand washing often not possible and physical activity is not a priority. Schools do not teach life skills: Children and adolescents do not learn the health competencies they need for their future. School health services focus on screening: Mental health services and counselling are not available.

(continued)

Table 1 (continued)

Children and adolescents in Europe exceed the recommended daily screen time. Electronic media use represents a new challenge for adolescents' physical and mental health.
Lifetime trajectories of non-communicable diseases, such as diabetes, **are established during adolescence** and are linked to diet and physical activity.
Prevention, detection and treatment of tuberculosis has been neglected amongst adolescents. Adolescents are neglected in the regional response to tuberculosis. Less than 5% of children with multidrug-resistant Tuberculosis are diagnosed and treated.
Too many adolescents are not fully protected from vaccine-preventable diseases. The WHO European Region has the 2nd highest number of measles cases globally.
Tobacco use among adolescents in the WHO European Region is the second highest globally; 8.9% (2.7 million) children aged 13-15 smoke cigarettes in the WHO European Region. The availability, pricing and marketing of tobacco products facilitates uptake amongst young people.
Migration can be a risk factor for children's health. Over 9 million children in the WHO European Region are refugees or migrants in 2019.
Tooth decay is the most common noncommunicable disease; 18-98% of 6-year-olds have dental caries in their primary teeth. There is room for improvement in toothbrushing behaviour: whilst rates of twice-daily brushing have increased over time, they remain strongly patterned by socio-demographic factors including sex and socioeconomic status.
Data are not made public: countries do not report key aspects of child epidemiology. Adolescents at risk are invisible: Countries do not collect data required to improve the situation, and the adolescent age group is often invisible in official statistics.

materials are available for each of the specific problems that children and adolescents face in the WHO European Region (WHO 2020a).

The problems highlighted are major areas for action and will be foci of WHO Europe's upcoming Child and Adolescent Health Strategy, which will guide policy development in the region up until 2030.

In the 2020 monitoring survey, European Member states of WHO were asked whether these problem areas were of concern in their respective countries.

Table 2 Selected answers to problems statements of adolescent health by Member States in a survey by the WHO secretariat. (Source: Created by Author)

Country grouping		Adolescent access to health services		Substantial out-of-pocket payments for health care of children and adolescents		Adolescent mental health problems		Increasing number of children who are overweight or obese		Schools are not a health promoting environment		Children are not taught in schools what they need to know about their health, present and future		High rates of road and other injuries		Increasing gambling and gaming among adolescents	
		Yes	No	Yes	No	Yes	No	Yes	No	Yes	No	Yes	No	Yes	No	Yes	No
% Overall	Yes, No	60	40	18	82	84	16	89	11	44	56	36	64	47	53	47	53
% EU14	Yes, No	57	43	14	86	79	21	86	14	43	57	36	64	43	57	36	64
% EU13	Yes, No	46	54	38	62	77	23	77	23	38	62	38	62	54	46	38	62
% CIS	Yes, No	70	30	0	100	80	20	80	20	50	50	30	70	40	60	60	40
% SEEHN	Yes, No	67	33	17	83	67	33	67	33	50	50	50	50	50	50	17	83

A summary of responses by some selected country groupings is presented in Table 2. The majority of countries agreed that mental health of adolescents is a major issue, as is increasing rates of obesity. Fewer countries were concerned about out of pocket payments or access to services for children and adolescents.

11 The Next WHO Child and Adolescent Health Strategy for Europe

The current WHO Child and adolescent health strategy for Europe runs until 2020. The Regional Office began the development of the next strategy for child and adolescent health in 2019. This new strategy will cover the period up to 2030 in line with the Sustainable Development Goals and the Global Strategy for Women's, Children's and Adolescents' Health (WHO 2016). It will also draw on WHO's Thirteenth General Programme of Work, 2019–2023, and the European Programme of Work, 2020–2025 "United Action for Better Health in Europe." (WHO 2020b). This whole-of-region strategy aims to consolidate all European regional programmes around children and adolescents, thus seeking to eliminate duplication and fragmentation in matters relating to children and young people. Early work around the strategy has focused around four key priority areas:

1) early childhood development (ECD)
2) school-aged children
3) quality of care for children and adolescents
4) social and environmental determinants of health.

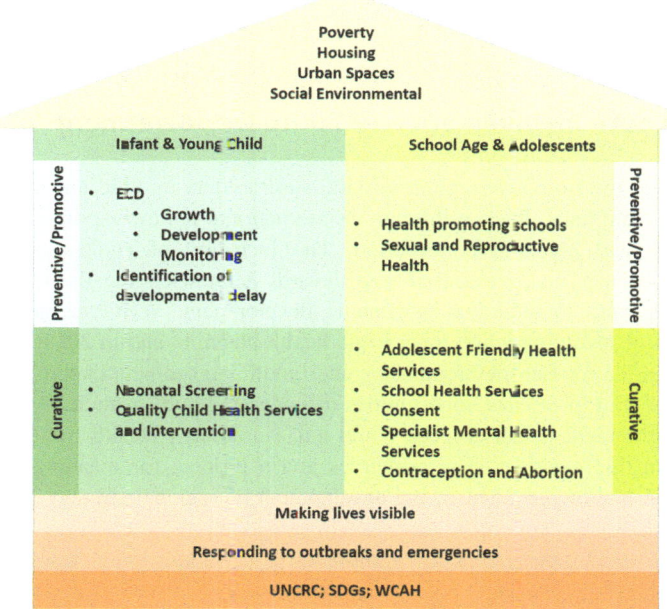

Fig. 6 Conceptual diagram of strategy for CAH after 2020.[2] (Source: Created by Author)

The new strategy development and its actions will stem from broad consultation to build momentum towards additional national investments. The priority areas envisioned in Fig. 6 arise from monitoring implementation of the previous strategies and consultation work with stakeholders, including children and adolescents. The strategy focuses on both health promotion activity and actions to address specific acute issues, each framed by social determinants of health and international commitments. Stakeholder views are critical elements of a holistic effort to support ministries of health, other ministries and stakeholders in the Region can also help identify whole system actions to improve the health of its children and young people. In 2020 the regional office is actively organizing

---

[2] ECD—Early Childhood Development; UNCRC—United Nations Convention on the Rights of the Child; SDGs—Sustainable Development Goals; GWCAH—Global Strategy for Women's, Children's and Adolescents' Health.

consultations with relevant stakeholders on initial drafts of the forthcoming strategy to gather further input and support on these early conceptualizations.

12   Youth Involvement and Youth Empowerment

The youth of the European region are vital stakeholders in child and adolescent health, yet from local practice through to international policy, we often overlook their views and potential contribution. The inclusion of adolescents in the 2030 Agenda marked an essential step towards acknowledging the importance of young people to attaining sustainable development. WHO recognizes the importance of involving youth in strategic health planning and in 2019 the WHO Regional Office for Europe brought together youth engagement experts from the European region to discuss opportunities to integrate youth from across the area in the development of a European Child and Adolescent Health Strategy post-2020. From this meeting basic principles and a process for meaningful youth consultation and engagement in the development of regional strategy post-2020 emerged.

Moving forward there was a commitment to including youth from the start of the strategy development process and transparency about what will happen with their input. In 2019, youth engagement experts from across the European Region—from Armenia, Denmark, Ireland, the Republic of Moldova, Poland, Portugal and the United Kingdom (Scotland) —consulted with around 350 children and young people aged between 9 and 23 years on their priorities for child and adolescent health.

The central theme emerging from their responses was the need for a sharper focus on mental health and well-being. Family relationships and leisure time were also of high importance. Many young people highlighted the pressing need for a more sustainable lifestyle and national action aimed at tackling climate change, reducing air pollution and promoting a cleaner environment.

As part of the iterative process of youth engagement in the strategy development, an online consultation survey focused on the key areas for action included in the draft strategy has been completed by 11–19 year olds across the region. The survey also asks for young people's views about how WHO could help children and young people in regard to the COVID-19 outbreak. The survey went live in June 2020 to gather the views of children and adolescents across the region. The insights from this survey will be included in the next iteration of the regional strategy and will inform areas and recommendations for action.

Provisional findings indicate that it is essential to our young people that they participate in decisions that affect their health. They firmly believe that schools should actively promote health behaviours among students but fewer report that this happens. Support for mental health and wellbeing, how to deal with violence and bullying, access to youth-friendly health services with skilled staff are priorities. Reducing poverty, providing housing and taking care of the environment are viewed as essential actions that governments can take to promote young people's health and wellbeing.

The goal of these initiatives was to establish a mechanism to provide for the ongoing engagement and consultation of young people across the Region. Ultimately they have proven the potential for participation of children and young people from across the region in international strategic development.

13   The impact of the COVID-19 virus

As this chapter was being written, the COVID-19 pandemic emerged with significant consequences for health and its socio-ecological determinants across the region. Whilst children and adolescents are less likely to suffer the direct health consequences of COVID19, the crisis and its consequent control measures are expected to have a significant impact on their health, wellbeing and development.

> 'All children, of all ages, and in all countries, are being affected, in particular by
> the socio-economic impacts and, in some cases, by mitigation measures that may
> inadvertently do more harm than good. This is a universal crisis and, for some
> children, the impact will be lifelong' (United Nations 2020)

Adolescents across the region have experienced disruption to routine health services, closure of education facilities, lack of access to safe outside space and opportunities to play and interact in social relationships. Societal lockdown poses a particular challenge for young people experiencing abuse or for those exposed to interpersonal violence, with the double burden of increased exposure to violence alongside disruption or withdrawal of support services.

These impacts will not be experienced equally. They will exacerbate the existing inequalities we see for adolescents living in the poorest circumstances and with the greatest existing disadvantages in the region. Addressing these issues will be a critical focus for the WHO Child and Adolescent health programme and European child and adolescent health strategy in the years to come.

14 Conclusion

Adolescence is a key developmental period, often neglected in national health promotion programmes and clinical health services. This age group is therefore at the centre of WHO's child and adolescent strategy. Countries must invest into this life stage, and get a better understanding of the situation of adolescents, through surveys such as HBSC. A particular challenge to adolescent health is the unequal distribution of positive outcomes and health-protecting assets (which are key given that some degree of experimentation and risk are normal parts of adolescent development). It is vital, therefore, that collected data are able to be disaggregated by key socio-demographic characteristics, particularly on the basis of socioeconomic status, in order to identify where inequalities in health outcomes exist. This evidence then must be used to shape effective policies, which are in line with the commitments of the UNCRC. Such efforts must take into account that consequences of income inequalities on adolescents' health arise both through the impact on individual socioeconomic factors, as well as systemic underinvestment in health services, and social and financial support at national levels.

Investments into adolescents and their future health yields long term returns in health, development, well-being and future of a country. The COVID-19 pandemic has made this long-term vision all the more important, with significant implications for adolescents' living conditions, mental health, education, and job prospects. Ongoing measures to control the spread of transmission must be carefully planned in order to minimisethe social and economic impacts, with particular attention paid to the implications for adolescents' development and education. Adolescents at greater risk of deprivation because of the pandemic must also be prioritised and receive tailored support, for example those at risk of malnutrition as a result of missing meals provided at school, and those for whom remote learning is difficult or impossible due to circumstantial or material factors. This is even more important to emphasise as incomes are shrinking and debt incurred will need to be paid off by the current adolescent generation.

To move this agenda forward, WHO Europe's forthcoming Child and Adolescent Health strategy will support countries in the region achieve these goals, as well as address the issues identified. It is vital that youth play a role in shaping it.

References

Alemán-Díaz AY, Backhaus S, Siebers LL... and Weber MW. 2018. Child and adolescent health in Europe: monitoring implementation of policies and provision of services. The Lancet Child and Adolescent Health.https://www.thelancet.com/journals/lanchi/article/PIIS2352-4642(18)30286-4/fulltext

Carai, S., Kuttumuratova, A. & Weber, M. (2018). Review of Integrated Management of Childhood Illnesses (ICMI) in Europe. Copenhagen: WHO Regional Office for Europe. https://www.euro.who.int/__data/assets/pdf_file/0006/369883/imci-review-euro-eng.pdf

Child and Adolescent Health Research Unit (CAHRU) 2014. Health Behaviour in School-aged Children (HBSC) Study: Terms of Reference. http://www.hbsc.org/about/HBSC%20ToR.pdf

Clark, H., Coll-Seck, A. M., Banerjee, A., ... & Costello, A. (2020). A future for the world's children? A WHO–UNICEF–Lancet Commission. https://www.thelancet.com/commissions/future-child

EUTeach (2020). Lausanne: Division interdisciplinaire de santé des adolescents.https://www.unil.ch/euteach/en/home/menuinst/about-euteach/key-concepts.html

Inchley J, Currie D, Budisavljevic S, Torsheim T, Jåstad A, Cosma A et al., (Eds.) Spotlight on adolescent health and well-being. Findings from the 2017/2018 Health Behaviour in School-aged Children (HBSC) survey in Europe and Canada. International report. Volume 1. Key findings. Copenhagen: WHO Regional Office for Europe; 2020a. http://www.hbsc.org/publications/international/

Inchley J, Currie D, Budisavljevic S, Torsheim T, Jåstad A, Cosma A et al., (Eds.) Spotlight on adolescent health and well-being. Findings from the 2017/2018 Health Behaviour in School-aged Children (HBSC) survey in Europe and Canada. International report. Volume 2. Key data. Copenhagen: WHO Regional Office for Europe; 2020b. http://www.hbsc.org/publications/international/

Institute for Health Metrics and Evaluation (IHME) 2020: Global Burden of Disease Results Tool. http //ghdx.healthdata.org/gbd-results-tool

Nutbeam, D. (2000). Health literacy as a public health goal: a challenge for contemporary health education and communication strategies into the 21st century, Health Promotion International, 15,3. https://academic.oup.com/heapro/article/_5/3/259/551108

Paakkari, L., Torppa, M., Paakkari, O., Välimaa, R., Ojala, K. & Tynjälä, J. (2019). Does health literacy explain the link between structural stratifiers and adolescent health? European Journal of Public Health, 29, 5. https://academic.oup.com/eurpub/article-abstract/29/5/919/5308386?redirectedFrom=fulltext

Schools for Health in Europe (SHE) https://www.schoolsforhealth.org/

Scott, E., Whitehead, R., Aleman-Diaz, A. & Weber, M. (2019). Adolescent Health and Development in the WHO European Region: Can we do better? Copenhagen: WHO Regional Office for Europe. https://www.euro who.int/__data/assets/pdf_file/0005/407219/AA-HA-adaptation-V7_maket_10.07.19_e_book_2.pdf

United Nations (1989). UN Convention on the Rights of the Child (UNCRC) https://downloads.unicef.org.uk/wp-content/uploads/2010/05/UNCRC_united_nations_convention_on_the_rights_of_the_child.pdf?_ga=2.130404615.901361749.1592223119-1387548312.1592223119

United Nations (2015). Sustainable Development Goals Knowledge Platform https://
    sustainabledevelopment.un.org/
United Nations (2020). Policy Brief: The Impact of COVID-19 on children. https://unsdg.
    un.org/resources/policy-brief-impact-covid-19-children
Whitehead, R., Arnot, J., Armour, G., Scott, E. & Reid, G. (2018). Youth health services:
    Reviewing the benefits of a holistic approach. NHS Health Scotland. http://www.
    healthscotland.scot/media/2121/youth-health-services-reviewing-the-benefits-of-a-
    holistic-approach.pdf
WHO (1986). The Ottowa Charter for Health Promotion. https://www.who.int/health-
    promotion/conferences/previous/ottawa/en/
WHO (2005). Assessment Tool: European strategy for child and adolescent health and
    development. https://www.euro.who.int/__data/assets/pdf_file/0009/82368/Assesment_
    tool.pdf
WHO (2014). Investing in children: the European child and adolescent health strategy
    2015–2020. Copenhagen: WHO Regional Office for Europe; 2014 (document EUR/
    RC64/12; http://www.euro.who.int/__data/assets/pdf_file/0010/253729/64wd12e_Invest
    CAHstrategy_140440.pdf?ua=1
WHO (2016). The Global Strategy For Women's, Children's, and Adolescent's Health
    (2016–2030). Geneva: World Health Organization https://www.who.int/life-course/
    partners/global-strategy/global-strategy-2016-2030/en/
WHO (2017a). Global Accelerated Action for the Health of Adolescents (AA-HA!):
    guidance to support country implementation. Geneva: World Health Organization;
    2017. Licence: CC BY-NC-SA 3.0 IGO https://apps.who.int/iris/bitstream/han
    dle/10665/255415/9789241512343-eng.pdf?sequence=1
WHO (2017b). Health Promoting School: an effective approach for early action on NCD risk
    factors. https://www.who.int/healthpromotion/publications/health-promotion-school/en/
WHO (2018). Situation of child and adolescent health in Europe. Copenhagen:
    WHO Regional Office for Europe. http://www.euro.who.int/__data/assets/pdf_
    file/0007/381139/situation-child-adolescent-health-eng.pdf?ua=1
WHO (2020a). WHO support materials for RC69 technical briefing on child and
    adolescents' health in the WHO European Region. http://www.euro.who.int/en/health-
    topics/Life-stages/child-and-adolescent-health/publications/who-support-materials-for-
    rc69-technical-briefing-on-child-and-adolescents-health-in-the-who-european-region
WHO. (2020b). United action for better health in Europe Draft European Programme of
    Work, 2020–2025. Copenhagen: WHO Regional Office for Europe. https://www.euro.
    who.int/__data/assets/pdf_file/0005/445712/27s4e25_EPW_200412.pdf
WHO (2020c). Final reports on Investing in Children: the European Child and Adolescent
    Health Strategy 2015–2020 and the European Child Maltreatment Prevention Action
    Plan 2015–2020. https://www.euro.who.int/en/about-us/governance/regional-committee-
    for-europe/70th-session/documentation/working-documents/eurrc7081-final-reports-on-
    investing-in-children-the-european-child-and-adolescent-health-strategy-20152020-and-
    the-european-child-maltreatment-prevention-action-plan-20152020
WHO European Health Information Gateway (2019). Child and adolescent health profiles.
    https://gateway.euro.who.int/en/datasets/cah/.

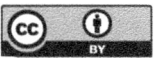

Printed and bound by CPI Group (UK) Ltd, Croydon, CR0 4YY
28/04/2026
02098501-0003